MCQs in Obstetrics & Gynecology
for MD & DM Entrance Exam

MCQs in Obstetrics & Gynecology
for MD & DM Entrance Exam

Editor-in-Chief

Ruchika Garg
MD Fellow - Indian College of Obstetricians and Gynecologists
Member – National Academy Medical Sciences
FIAOG FICMCH FMAS
Associate Editor
Journal of Midlife Health and
Journal of SAFOG
Professor
Department of Obstetrics and Gynecology
SN Medical College
Agra, Uttar Pradesh, India

Editors

Rajshree Dayanand Katke
MBBS MD (Obs & Gyne) FMAS FICOG
Professor and Unit Chief
Department of Obstetrics and Gynecology
Grant Government Medical College
Mumbai, Maharashtra, India

Jai Bhagwan Sharma
MD DNB FRCOG (London) PhD MFFP FAMS FICOG FIMSA
Professor
Department of Obstetrics and Gynecology
All India Institute of Medical Sciences
New Delhi, India

Forewords

Arup Kumar Majhi
Jaydeep Tank

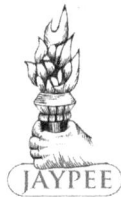

JAYPEE BROTHERS MEDICAL PUBLISHERS
The Health Sciences Publisher
New Delhi | London

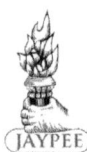 **Jaypee Brothers Medical Publishers (P) Ltd.**

Headquarters
Jaypee Brothers Medical Publishers (P) Ltd
EMCA House, 23/23-B
Ansari Road, Daryaganj
New Delhi 110 002, India
Landline: +91-11-23272143, +91-11-23272703
+91-11-23282021, +91-11-23245672
Email: jaypee@jaypeebrothers.com

Overseas Office
JP Medical Ltd.
83, Victoria Street, London
SW1H 0HW (UK)
Phone: +44 20 3170 8910
Email: info@jpmedpub.com

Corporate Office
Jaypee Brothers Medical Publishers (P) Ltd
4838/24, Ansari Road, Daryaganj
New Delhi 110 002, India
Phone: +91-11-43574357
Fax: +91-11-43574314
Email: jaypee@jaypeebrothers.com

EU GPSR Authorised Representative
Logos Europe, 9 rue Nicolas Poussin
17000, La Rochelle, France
Phone: +33 (0) 6 67 93 73 78
E-mail: Contact@logoseurope.eu

Website: www.jaypeebrothers.com
Website: www.jaypeedigital.com

© 2024, Jaypee Brothers Medical Publishers

The views and opinions expressed in this book are solely those of the original contributor(s)/author(s) and do not necessarily represent those of editor(s) or publisher of the book.

All rights reserved. No part of this publication may be reproduced, stored or transmitted in any form or by any means, electronic, mechanical, photo copying, recording or otherwise, without the prior permission in writing of the publishers.

All brand names and product names used in this book are trade names, service marks, trademarks or registered trademarks of their respective owners. The publisher is not associated with any product or vendor mentioned in this book.

Medical knowledge and practice change constantly. This book is designed to provide accurate, authoritative information about the subject matter in question. However, readers are advised to check the most current information available on procedures included and check information from the manufacturer of each product to be administered, to verify the recommended dose, formula, method and duration of administration, adverse effects and contra indications. It is the responsibility of the practitioner to take all appropriate safety precautions. Neither the publisher nor the author(s)/editor(s) assume any liability for any injury and/or damage to persons or property arising from or related to use of material in this book.

This book is sold on the understanding that the publisher is not engaged in providing professional medical services. If such advice or services are required, the services of a competent medical professional should be sought.

Every effort has been made where necessary to contact holders of copyright to obtain permission to reproduce copyright material. If any have been inadvertently overlooked, the publisher will be pleased to make the necessary arrangements at the first opportunity.

Inquiries for bulk sales may be solicited at: jaypee@jaypeebrothers.com

MCQs in Obstetrics & Gynecology for MD & DM Entrance Exam

First Edition: **2024**
ISBN: 978-93-5696-886-8

Dedicated to

The tireless pursuit of knowledge in the field of gynecology, and to the postgraduate students who embark on the challenging journey of mastering its intricacies. May this book serve as a guiding light on your path to excellence, and may your passion for advancing women's health shine brightly in your future endeavors.

Contributors

Ananya Girish MBBS MS (Obs & Gyne)
Junior Resident
Department of Obstetrics and Gynecology
Vinayaka Missions Kirupananda Variyar Medical College
and Hospital
Salem, Tamil Nadu, India

Ankita Aghav
Junior Resident
Department of Obstetrics and Gynecology
Grant Government Medical College
Mumbai, Maharashtra, India

Anuja Bhalerao
Professor and Head
Department of Obstetrics and Gynecology
NKPSALVE Institute of Medical Sciences
Nagpur, Maharashtra, India

Archana Kumari MBBS MS
Assistant Professor
Department of Obstetrics and Gynecology
All India Institute of Medical Sciences
New Delhi, India

Arnav Pai MBBS MS (Obs & Gyne)
Private Practice
Department of Obstetrics and Gynecology
Mumbai, Maharashtra, India

Arun Kumar Dora MD (Obs & Gyne)
Professor
Department of Obstetrics and Gynecology
All India Institute of Medical Sciences
Bhopal, Madhya Pradesh, India

Aruna M Biradar MBBS MS
Professor
Department of Obstetrics and Gynecology
BLDE(DU) Shri BM Patil Medical College Hospital and Research Center
Vijayapura, Karnataka, India

Aruna Verma
MD (Obs & Gyne) FICOG FMAS
Professor
Department of Obstetrics and Gynecology
LLRM Medical College
Meerut, Uttar Pradesh, India

Ashwini Bhalerao-Gandhi
MD DGO DFP FCPS DNB FICOG
Consultant
Department of Gynecology
PD Hinduja Hospital and Medical Research Center
Mumbai, Maharashtra, India

Astha Lalwani MBBS DNB FICOG
Professor
Department of Obstetrics and Gynecology
TMMC and RC
Moradabad, Uttar Pradesh, India

Athulya Shajan MBBS MS (Obs & Gyne) FIRM FAGE
Consultant
Reproductive Medicine and Surgery
CIMAR, The Women's Hospital
Thrissur, Kerala, India

Beena Kumari MD (Obs & Gyne)
ACHD and Head
Department of Obstetrician and Gynecologist
Dr Babasaheb Ambedkar Central Railway Hospital
Mumbai, Maharashtra, India

Bhumika Kotecha Mundhe
DGO DNB (Obs & Gyne) MNAMs (India) FICOG
Consultant
Department of Obstetrician and Gynecologist
Saifee Hospital
Masina Hospital
Wockhardt Hospital
St Elizabeth Hospital
Narayana Healthcare- SRCC Hospital
Mumbai, Maharashtra, India

Charmila Ayyavoo
MD DGO DFP FICOG PGDCR
Director
Department of Obstetrics and Gynecology
Aditi Hospital and Parvathy Ayyavoo Fertility Center
Trichy, Tamil Nadu, India

Deep Kamal MD DNB
Classified Specialist
Department of Medicine
Indian Navy
Naval Hospital
Mumbai, Maharashtra, India

Deepa Chaudhary
MBBS MS FMAS FARM Dip in Urogynecology
Professor
Department of Obstetrics and Gynecology
SMS Medical College
Jaipur, Rajasthan, India

Deepa Kala
MBBS MD (Obs & Gyne) FICOG MA YOGASUTRA
Professor and HOD
Department of Obstetrics and Gynecology
Terna Medical College and TSHRC
Mumbai, Maharashtra, India

Deepa Singh MBBS
Resident
Department of Obstetrics and Gynecology
King George's Medical University
Lucknow, Uttar Pradesh, India

Deepali Kapote
MBBS MS DGO FCPS DFP FICOG FMAS
PGD in Reproductive Medicine (Infertility), Gynecological Endoscopy (Kiel, Germany) and Professional Diploma in Aesthetic Gynecology
Additional Professor
Department of Obstetrics and Gynecology
LTMMC and LTMGH Sion
Mumbai, Maharashtra, India

Dhara Singh
MS (Gold Medalist), DNB (Obs & Gyne)
Assistant Professor
Department of Obstetrics and Gynecology
MGM Medical College and MTH Hospital
Indore, Madhya Pradesh, India

Divya Pandey MS MNAMS FICOG FICMCH
Professor
Department of Obstetrics and Gynecology
Vardhan Mahavir Medical College and Safdarjung Hospital
New Delhi, India

Divya Suman MD (Obs & Gyne) FIMAS
Consultant
Department of Obstetrics and Gynecology
Vaidyam Super Specialty Hospital
Patna, Bihar, India

Ganesh Dangal MBBS MD FICS FRCOG
Professor
Department of Obstetrics and Gynecology
Kathmandu Model Hospital, Under National Academy of Medical Sciences (NAMS)
Guide/Preceptor/Supervisor-PG/MD/Fellowship in Urogynecology of NAMS and FCPS (Obs & Gyne)
Senior Consultant, Kathmandu Model Hospital
Academic Director, phect-NEPAL/KMHIHS
Kathmandu Model Hospital Institute of Health Sciences (KMHIHS)

Garima Gupta
MS (Obs & Gyne) DNB DMAS FMAS FART CIMP
Associate Professor
Department of Obstetrics and Gynecology
GSVM Medical College
Kanpur, Uttar Pradesh, India

Gayathri AK MBBS
Junior Resident
Department of Obstetrics and Gynecology
Grant Government Medical College
Mumbai, Maharashtra, India

Geetha Balsarkar MD DGO DNB FCPS
Professor and Unit Chief
Department of Obstetrics and Gynecology
Nowrosjee Wadia Maternity Hospital
Seth GS Medical College
Mumbai, Maharashtra, India

Harshada Thakur MS (Obs & Gyne)
Additional Associate Professor
Department of Obstetrics and Gynecology
Seth GS Medical College and KEM Hospital
Mumbai, Maharashtra, India

Hemant Damle MD (Obs & Gyne)
Professor
Department of Obstetrics and Gynecology
SKN Medical College
Pune, Maharashtra, India

Honey M Gemavat
MBBS MS DNB MRCOG (Obs & Gyne)
Assistant Professor
Department of Obstetrics and Gynecology
Lokmanya Tilak Municipal Medical College and General Hospital
Mumbai, Maharashtra, India

Jai Bhagwan Sharma
MD DNB FRCOG (London) PhD MFFP FAMS FICOG FIMSA
Professor
Department of Obstetrics and Gynecology
All India Institute of Medical Sciences
New Delhi, India

Jayashree V Kanavi
MBBS MS (Obs & Gyne)
Consultant
Department of Obstetrics and Gynecology
Manipal Hospitals
Bengaluru, Karnataka, India

Jyothi GS MBBS MD (Obs & Gyne) PGDMLE FICOG FICMCH
Professor and Unit Chief
Department of Obstetrics and Gynecology
Ramaiah Medical College and Hospitals
Bengaluru, Karnataka, India

Kalpana Basany MD DNB MRCOG
Professor and Head
Department of Obstetrics and Gynecology
MediCiti Institute of Medical Sciences
Secunderabad, Telangana, India

Kalpana Kumari MBBS MD (Obs & Gyne)
Professor and Head
Department of Obstetrics and Gynecology
UPUMS
Saifai, Uttar Pradesh, India

Kalyani Sai Dhandapani
DGO DNB (Obs & Gyne) MNAMS (Obs & Gyne)
Medical Director and HOD
Department of Obstetrics and Gynecology
Chief Gynecologist
S Railway HQ Hospital
Chennai, Tamil Nadu, India

Kanchan Dwidmuthe
MBBS DGO DNB (Obs & Gyne)
Assistant Professor
Department of Obstetrics and Gynecology
Nkpsims and RC and LMH
Nagpur, Maharashtra, India

Kanchan Rani
MS (Obs & Gyne) FICOG FRM
Professor
Department of Obstetrics and Gynecology
TMMC and RC
Moradabad, Uttar Pradesh, India

Kavita Mandrelle Bhatti
MD FICOG FMAS Fellowship in Reproductive Medicine ACME CIMP
Professor and Head
Department of Obstetrics and Gynecology
Christian Medical College and Hospital
Ludhiana, Punjab, India

Kavita Tilwani
MBBS DNB (Obs & Gyne) DGO FMAS
Associate Professor
Department of Surgery
Grant Government Medical College
Mumbai, Maharashtra, India

Kinjal Shah
MBBS DNB Diploma in Laparoscopy (Germany)
Consultant
Department of Obstetrics and
Gynecology
Bhatia Hospital
Ruxmani Hospital
Wockhardt Hospital
SRCC Children Hospital
Mumbai, Maharashtra, India

Kiranmai Devineni MD FICOG
Professor
Department of Obstetrics and
Gynecology
GMC, Wanaparthy, Kaloji University of
Health Sciences
Warangal, Telangana, India

Komal N Chavan
MD DNB MNAMS FCPS DGO FICOG Diploma in
Reproductive Medicine (UKSH Germany)
Senior Consultant, Unit Chief, and
DNB Teacher
Department of Obstetrics and
Gynecology
VN Desai Hospital
Mumbai, Maharashtra, India
Vice President Elect FOGSI 2025

Kunjal Bathija MD DGO FCPS DFP
Assistant Professor
Department of Obstetrics and
Gynecology
Bombay Hospital and Medical Research
Center
Mumbai, Maharashtra, India

Madhura Mandlik MBBS MS
Senior Resident
Department of Obstetrics and
Gynecology
LTMMC and LTMGH
Mumbai, Maharashtra, India

Mandakini Megh
MD DGO FICOG FICMCH FICMU
Medical Director
Department of Obstetrics and
Gynecology
Dr Megh' Gynaeo Care Clinics
Mumbai, Maharashtra, India
National President AMWI, International
Vice President (Central Asia), MWIA

Meenal S Sarmalkar
MS DNB DGO DFP (Obs & Gyne)
Associate Professor
Department of Obstetrics and
Gynecology
Lokmanya Tilak Municipal Medical
College and General Hospital
Mumbai, Maharashtra, India

Meera Jayaprakash
MS (Obstetrics and Gynecology) FCPS
Fellowship in Fetal Medicine (MUHS)
Consultant
Siddhivinayak Hospital
Lakhani, Maharashtra, India

Meher Narain MD (Obs & Gyne)
Senior Resident
Department of Obstetrics and
Gynecology
King George's Medical University
Lucknow, Uttar Pradesh, India

Mona Asnani
MD (Obs & Gyne) FIAMS MNAMS FICOG
Additional Professor
Department of Obstetrics and
Gynecology
King George's Medical University
Lucknow, Uttar Pradesh, India

Monica Agrawal
MS DGO DNB MNAMS (Obs & Gyne) FICOG
Additional Professor
Department of Obstetrics and
Gynecology
King George's Medical University
Lucknow, Uttar Pradesh, India

Mugdha L Jungari
MBBS MS DNB FMAS
Consultant
Department of Obstetrics and
Gynecology
Nagpur, Maharashtra, India

Naisargi Patel MBBS DGO DNB DCG
Consultant
Department of Obstetrics and
Gynecology
Gayatri Maternity and Nursing Home
Patan, Gujarat, India

Nandita Palshetkar
MD FCPS FICOG FRCOG (UK)
Professor Emeritus in Obstetrics
and Gynecology
DY Patil School of Medicine
Navi Mumbai, Maharashtra, India
Infertility Specialist
Lilavati Hospital IVF Center
Mumbai
Scientific Director and
Co-Founder, Bloom IVF
Scientific Director and
Co-Founder, BAUFICI Genetics
President
Indian Society of Assisted Reproduction
(2022–2024)
President
Association of Maharashtra
Obstetric and Gynecological
Societies (2020–2022)
Past President
FOGSI, IAGE, MOGS and MSR

Neelima Mantri
MS (Obs & Gyne) FMAS FACS
Associate Professor
Department of Obstetrics and
Gynecology
Bombay Hospital and
Medical Research Center
Mumbai, Maharashtra, India

Neha Khairnar MBBS MS (Obs & Gyne)
Senior Resident
Department of Obstetrics and
Gynecology
Lokmanya Tilak Municipal Medical
College and General Hospital
Mumbai, Maharashtra, India

Neha Sharma MBBS MS DNB
Senior Resident
Department of Obstetrics
and Gynecology
LHMC
New Delhi, India

Neharika Malhotra MBBS MS
Consultant
Department of Gynecology
Malhotra Nursing Home
Agra, Uttar Pradesh, India

Contributors

Nidhi Sharma Chauhan
MBBS MS (Obs & Gyne) MRCOG (UK) Dip Pelvic Endoscopy (Kiel School, Germany)
D. ART (Artificial Reproductive Technology, Kiel School, Germany)
Clinical Accreditation in IVF (NUH, Crest, Singapore) FMas & D.Mas (Dams, New Delhi)
Consultant
Department of Obstetrician and Gynecologist
Ex Assistant Professor
Sir Ji Group of Hospitals, DY Patil Hospital and Medical College
Saifee Hospital, Bhatia Hospital, SRCC Hospital, and Haji Ali
Mumbai, Maharashtra, India

Nishita Shah MBBS DGO MD
Consultant
Department of Obstetrics and Gynecology
St Elizabeth and Saifee Hospitals
Mumbai, Maharashtra, India

Nishma Bajracharya MBBS FCPS
Registrar
Department of Obstetrics and Gynecology
Alka Hospital Pvt Ltd
Kathmandu, Nepal

Pavika Lal
MBBS MD (AIIMS, New Delhi) DNB FICOG CIMP
Associate Professor
Department of Obstetrics and Gynecology
GSVM Medical College
Kanpur, Uttar Pradesh, India

Pinky Mishra
DGO DNB (Obs & Gyne) Fellow AGOI (Gyne Oncology)
Assistant Professor
Department of Obstetrics and Gynecology
Government Institute of Medical Sciences
Greater Noida, Uttar Pradesh, India

Poonam Yadav MBBS MS
Professor
Department of Obstetrics and Gynecology
SN Medical College
Agra, Uttar Pradesh, India

Prabhat Agrawal
MBBS MD FRCP (Edinburgh, Glasgow)
Professor
Department of Medicine
SN Medical College
Agra, Uttar Pradesh, India

Prachi Yadav MBBS
Junior Resident
Department of Obstetrics and Gynecology
Grant Government Medical College
Mumbai, Maharashtra, India

Pradnya Changede
MS (Obs & Gyne) FICOG FCPS DGO MBBS IBCLC
Associate Professor
Department of Obstetrics and Gynecology
Lokmanya Tilak Municipal Medical College and General Hospital
Mumbai, Maharashtra, India

Preeti Nitsure Deshpande
MS MRCOG FICOG
Consultant
Department of Obstetrics and Gynecology
Sambhav Clinic, Raheja-Fortis Hospital, and Guru Nanak Hospital
Mumbai, Maharashtra, India

Prema Kania MD (Obs & Gyne)
Assistant Professor and Consultant
Department of Obstetrics and Gynecology
Bombay Hospital Institute of Medical Sciences
Mumbai, Maharashtra, India

Priya Vora DNB FICOG FCPS DFP
Consultant Obstetrician and Gynecologist
Dr Vora's Hospital, Haji-Ali
St Elizabeth Hospital
Ruxmani Hospital
Bhatia Hospital
Mumbai, Maharashtra, India

Priyanka Rai MS (Obs & Gyne)
Associate Professor
Department of Obstetrics and Gynecology
All India Institute of Medical Sciences
Deoghar, Jharkhand, India

Priyankur Roy
MBBS MS (Obs & Gyne) FIRM FAGE
Associate Professor
Department of Gynae-Endoscopy and Reproductive Medicine
Roy's Clinic and Multispecialty Hospital
Siliguri, West Bengal, India

Punit S Bhojani
MS DNB FICOG FCPS DGO DFP
Consultant
Department of Obstetrics and Gynecology
Bhojani Clinic, Matunga
Attached to Surya, SRCC, Masina and KJ Somaiya Hospitals
Mumbai, Maharashtra, India

Purnima Satoskar MD DNB FRCOG
Professor
Department of Obstetrics and Gynecology
Seth GS Medical College and Nowrosjee Wadia Maternity Hospital
Mumbai, Maharashtra, India

Pushpa Lata Sankhwar
MS (Obs & Gyne) FICS MNAMS FICOG
Professor
Department of Obstetrics and Gynecology
King George's Medical University
Lucknow, Uttar Pradesh, India

Radhika Chetan
MBBS MS (Obs & Gyne)
Associate professor
Department of Obstetrics and Gynecology
Bangalore Medical College and Research Institute
Bengaluru, Karnataka, India

Rajat Agrawal MS (Obs & Gyne)
Senior Resident
Department of Obstetrics and Gynecology
Lokmanya Tilak Municipal Medical College and General Hospital
Mumbai, Maharashtra, India

Contributors xi

Rajeshwari Laxman Khyade
MBBS DGO DNB FMAS FICOG
Senior Consultant and DNB Teacher
Department of Obstetrics and Gynecology
KBBH Bhabha Bandra, Breach Candy Hospital, and HN Reliance Hospital
Mumbai, Maharashtra, India

Rajshree Dayanand Katke
MBBS MD (Obs & Gyne) FMAS FICOG
Professor and Unit Chief
Department of Obstetrics and Gynecology
Grant Government Medical College
Mumbai, Maharashtra, India

Rani Daruwale
MBBS DNB (Obs & Gyne) FMAS FART
Assistant Professor
Department of Obstetrics and Gynecology
Seth GS Medical College and KEM Hospital
Mumbai, Maharashtra, India

Rao Preethi Venkatachala MBBS DNB
Assistant Professor
Department of Obstetrics and Gynecology
St John's Medical College Hospital
Bengaluru, Karnataka, India

Rashmi Bala DNB (Obs & Gyne)
Senior Resident
Department of Obstetrics and Gynecology
All India Institute of Medical Sciences
Deoghar, Jharkhand, India

Rekha Rani MBBS MS
Professor
Department of Gynecology
SN Medical College
Agra, Uttar Pradesh, India

Renu Gupta MBBS MD DNB FICOG MNAMS
Professor and Unit Head
Department of Obstetrics and Gynecology
GSVM Medical College
Kanpur, Uttar Pradesh, India

Richa Singh MBBS MS
Professor and Head
MS Department Obstetrics and Gynecology
SN Medical College
Agra, Uttar Pradesh, India

Rishma Dhillon Pai
MD DNB DGO FCPS FICOG
Honorary Consultant Gynecology
Jaslok and Lilavati Hospitals
Director, Everywoman Cliniqs and Pearl Center Hospital
Mumbai, Maharashtra, India

Ritika Pathak
MBBS MD (Obs & Gyne) DNB (Obs & Gyne)
Fellowship in Fetal Medicine Fellowship in IVF PGDUS PGMO
PGMO
Department of Obstetrics and Gynecology
VN Desai Hospital
Mumbai, Maharashtra, India

Ritu Santwani MBBS MD FICOG FIAOG
AMRCOG ART-Singapore
Founder and CEO
Department of Obstetrics and Gynecology
360 Degree Healthcare Studio
Pune, Maharashtra, India

Ritu Sharma
MD (Obs & Gyne) FICMCH ACME Fellow DCR
Professor and Head
Department of Obstetrics and Gynecology
Government Institute of Medical Sciences
Greater Noida, Uttar Pradesh, India

Rohan Palshetkar
MS (Obs & Gyne) FRM ADRME BDRME
Professor
DY Patil School of Medicine
Navi Mumbai, Maharashtra, India
Head of Unit, Bloom IVF, Nerul
Consultant, Sir HN Reliance Foundation Hospital, Surya Hospital
Breach Candy, Palshetkar Patil Nursing Home
Chairperson, FOGSI Young Talent Promotion Committee (2024–2027)
Treasurer, AMOGS; Joint Treasurer, MAGE; Managing Committee Member, MSR & MOGS

Ruchika Garg
MD Fellow - Indian College of Obstetricians and Gynecologists Member - National Academy Medical Sciences FIAOG FICMCH FMAS
Associate Editor Journal of Midlife Health and Journal of SAFOG
Professor, Department of Obstetrics and Gynecology
SN Medical College
Agra, Uttar Pradesh, India

Rutuja Bodake
Resident
Department of Obstetrics and Gynecology
Bombay Hospital Institute of Medical Sciences and Research Center
Mumbai, Maharashtra, India

S Karthikeyan DCH DNB AASC
Assistant Professor
Department of Pediatrics
KAPV Government Medical College
Trichy, Tamil Nadu, India

Sahana Girish MBBS MS DNB
Obstetrician and Gynecologist (Fetal Medicine)
Bangalore Fetal Medicine Center
Bengaluru, Karnataka, India

Sangamesh S Mathapati MBBS MS
Associate Professor
Department of Obstetrics and Gynecology
BLDE(DU) Shri BM Patil Medical College Hospital and Research Center
Vijayapura, Karnataka, India

Sarita Bhalerao MD DNB FRCOG
Consultant
Department of Obstetrics and Gynecology
Bhatia, Saifee, Reliance HNH, and Breach Candy Hospital
Mumbai, Maharashtra, India

Savita Somalwar MBBS DGO DNB
Associate Professor
Department of Obstetrics and Gynecology
NKP Salve Institute of Medical Sciences and Research Center
Nagpur, Maharashtra, India

Sebanti Goswami
MBBS MD (Obs & Gyne)
Consultant Gynecologist
Department of Obstetrics and Gynecology
Amri Hospital Mukundapur
Kolkata, West Bengal, India

Seema Mehrotra
MBBS MD (Obs & Gyne)
Professor
Department of Obstetrics and Gynecology
King George Medical University
Lucknow, Uttar Pradesh, India

Shaifali Singh MBBS
Resident
Department of Obstetrics and Gynecology
SN Medical College
Agra, Uttar Pradesh, India

Shakun Tyagi
Professor
Department of Obstetrics and Gynecology
Maulana Azad Medical College and LNJP Hospital
Govt of NCT, New Delhi, India

Shashi Lata Maheshwari (Kabra)
MD FICOG FMAS Dip MAS AMASI
Senior Specialist
Department of Obstetrics and Gynecology
Deen Dayal Upadhyay Hospital
Govt of NCT, New Delhi, India

Shashi R Goyal MD (Obs & Gyne)
Associate Professor
Department of Obstetrics and Gynecology
Bombay Hospital Institute of Medical Sciences
Mumbai, Maharashtra, India

Sheela Jain MBBS DGO CIMP
Senior Resident
Department of Obstetrics and Gynecology
NKP Salve Institute of Medical Sciences and Research Center
Nagpur, Maharashtra, India

Shefali Singh MS (Obs & Gyne)
Junior Resident
SN Medical College
Agra, Uttar Pradesh, India

Shelly Agarwal MS (Obs & Gyne) FICOG
Professor
Department of Obstetrics and Gynecology
School of Medical Sciences and Research
Sharda University
Greater Noida, Uttar Pradesh, India

Shikha Seth MD FICS FICOG
Professor
Department of Obstetrics and Gynecology
All India Institute of Medical Sciences
Gorakhpur, Uttar Pradesh, India

Shilpi Srivastava MBBS MS (Obs & Gyne)
Assistant Professor
Department of Obstetrics and Gynecology
UPUMS
Saifai, Uttar Pradesh, India

Shivam Yadav MBBS
PG Resident
Department of Obstetrics and Gynecology
VMMC and Safdarjung Hospital
New Delhi, India

Shobana Mahadevan
MD DipNB (Obs & Gyne) FRCOG (UK)
Consultant
Department of Obstetrics and Gynecology
Seethapathy Clinic and Hospital
Chennai, Tamil Nadu, India

Shreedevi Tanksale
DNB DGO FMAS Fellowship in Reproductive Medicine
Director
OB GYN Infertility Specialist
Little Miracles Fertility clinic
Mumbai, Maharashtra, India

Shrutika Thakkar MS DNB FICOG
Director
Department of Obstetrics and Gynecology
Medansh Multispecialty Hospital
Mumbai, Maharashtra, India

Shubhangi Nawarange
MBBS MS (Obs & Gyne)
Assistant professor
Department of Obstetrics and Gynecology
GGMC and JJ Hospital
Mumbai, Maharashtra, India

Shubhra Agarwal MBBS MS DNB
Professor
Department of Obstetrics and Gynecology
TMMC and RC
Moradabad, Uttar Pradesh, India

Sippy Agrawal MS
Professor
Department of Obstetrics and Gynecology
MLB Medical College
Jhansi, Uttar Pradesh, India

Somya Suman
MBBS DNB, Fellowship in Minimal Invasive Surgery
Senior Resident
Department of Obstetrics and Gynecology
Saifee Hospital
Mumbai, Maharashtra, India

Soniya Dhiman MBBS MD
Assistant Professor
Department of Obstetrics and Gynecology
All India Institute of Medical Sciences
New Delhi, India

Sreelatha S MBBS MD
Professor
Department of Obstetrics and Gynecology
ESICMC and PGIMSR
Bengaluru, Karnataka, India

Suchi Jain
MBBS MS (Obs & Gyne) FICS PhD (Obs & Gyne) MCH IMS BHU
Associate Professor
Department of Obstetrics and Gynecology
Varanasi, Uttar Pradesh, India

Sukriti Atram MD (Anesthesiology)
Associate Professor
Department of Anesthesiology
Grant Government Medical College
Mumbai, Maharashtra, India

Suman Chaudhary MBBS MS FMAS
Professor
Department of Obstetrics and Gynecology
SMS Medical College
Jaipur, Rajasthan, India

Sunil Tambvekar
MBBS DNB MNAMS DFP FMAS PGDMLS
Assistant Professor
Department of Obstetrics and Gynecology
Nowrosjee Wadia Maternity Hospital
Seth GS Medical College
Mumbai, Maharashtra, India

Sunita Samal
MBBS MD (Obs & Gyne) FICOG FMAS ACME
Professor and Senior Consultant
Department of Obstetrics and Gynecology
Apollo Women's Hospital
Chennai, Tamil Nadu, India

Surekha Tayade
MBBS DNB MNAMS FICOG PGDHHM FIME MPH FAIMER Fellow MEd (HPE) PhD
Professor
Department of Obstetrics and Gynecology
Jawaharlal Nehru Medical College
Wardha, Maharashtra, India

Suvarna Khadilkar
MD DGO FICOG CIMP PG Diploma in Endocrinology (South Wales UK)
Professor and Head
Department of Obstetrics and Gynecology
Consultant, Endocrinologist and Gynecologist
Bombay Hospital Institute of Medical Sciences and Research Centre
Mumbai, Maharashtra, India

Swapnil Bala MS (Obs & Gyne)
Senior Resident
Department of Obstetrics and Gynecology
All India Institute of Medical Sciences
Deoghar, Jharkhand, India

Tejal Poddar MS (Obs & Gyne) Fellowship Reproductive Medicine
Director - Little Miracles Fertility Clinic
Department of Obstetrics and Gynecology
Little Miracles Fertility Clinic
Mumbai, Maharashtra, India

Urvashi Verma MBBS MS FICOG FICMCH
Professor
Department of Obstetrics and Gynecology
SN Medical College
Agra, Uttar Pradesh, India

Vaidehi Thakur
MD (Obs & Gyne) DGO CTGO
Specialist (Obs & Gyne)
Department of Obstetrics and Gynecology
Indian Navy
Naval Hospital
Mumbai, Maharashtra, India

Vandana Bansal
MD DGO DNB FICOG FRCOG FNB (High Risk Pregnancy and Perinatology)
Additional Professor
Department of Obstetrics and Gynecology and Fetal Medicine
Nowrosjee Wadia Maternity Hospital and Seth GS medical College
Mumbai, Maharashtra, India

Vandana Solanki
MS (Obs & Gyne) FICOG
Additional Professor
Department of Obstetrics and Gynecology
King George's Medical University
Lucknow, Uttar Pradesh, India

Veena M Vernekar
MBBS MS (Obs & Gyne) DNB (Obs & Gyne)
Senior Resident
Department of Obstetrics and Gynecology
ESIC MC and PGIMSR
Bengaluru, Karnataka, India

Vejainty Chauhan MBBS MD FMAS
Consultant, Private Practitioner
Department of Obstetrics and Gynecology
Haridwar, Uttarakhand, India

Vertika Singh MBBS
Resident
Department of Obstetrics and Gynecology
King George's Medical University
Lucknow, Uttar Pradesh, India

Vidya Thobbi
Professor and Head
Department of Obstetrics and Gynecology
Alameen Medical College
Vijayapur, Karnataka, India

Vineeta MS (Obs & Gyne)
Associate Professor
Department of Obstetrics and Gynecology
All India Institute of Medical Sciences
Deoghar, Jharkhand, India

Vivek Tilwani
MBBS MS (General Surgery) FMAS FIAGES LLB PGDMLS
Professor
Department of Surgery
Grant Government Medical College
Mumbai, Maharashtra, India

Foreword

In the modern education system, Multiple Choice Questions are an indispensable resource for medical students, residents, and healthcare professionals seeking a comprehensive review of the fundamental concepts in this specialized field. The editors in this book of "Multiple Choice Questions in Obstetrics and Gynecology" compiled by experts in obstetrics and gynecology, have fulfilled all the all the qualities to serve as a valuable tool for both learning and exam preparation.

The book's structure follows a systematic approach, covering a wide spectrum of topics within obstetrics and gynecology. From reproductive anatomy to high-risk pregnancies and gynecological malignancies, the multiple-choice questions (MCQs) encompass essential information that reflects the latest developments in the field. Each chapter is strategically organized, providing readers with a logical progression of concepts that aids in building a solid foundation.

One of the standout features of this book is its extensive question bank. With more than thousand carefully crafted MCQs, readers are exposed to a variety of clinical scenarios, encouraging critical thinking and problem-solving skills. Additionally, the questions are designed to mimic the format of many standardized medical exams, ensuring that readers are well-prepared for their assessments.

Each question is accompanied by a detailed explanation that not only provides the correct answer but also offers insightful discussions on the reasoning behind each choice. This feature enhances the learning experience by allowing readers to grasp the underlying principles and nuances of each topic. The explanations encompass alternative perspectives or clinical scenarios.

All the contributors are experts and doyens in the subject with immense experience and updated knowledge. Editors must be congratulated for this herculean task. All the contributors are experts in the subject, and they have penned down their extensive experience.

In conclusion, "Multiple Choice Questions in Obstetrics and Gynecology" is a commendable resource for anyone looking to solidify their knowledge in this specialized medical field. Its thorough coverage of key topics, extensive question bank, and detailed explanations make it a valuable tool for exam preparation and self-assessment. The book remains an excellent companion for medical professionals seeking to excel in obstetrics and gynecology.

Arup Kumar Majhi MD DNB FICOG
Professor
Department of Obstetrics and Gynecology
Santiniketan Medical College, Bolpur
Kolkata, West Bengal, India
Former Professor and Head
Department of Obstetrics and Gynecology
RG Kar Medical College
Kolkata, West Bengal, India
President, Indian Society of Obstetrics and Gynaecology (ISOPARB)

Foreword

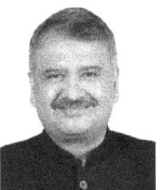

The Book *"Multiple Choice Questions in Obstetrics and Gynecology"* is an invaluable resource for medical students, residents, and practitioners seeking to test and reinforce their knowledge in the field of women's health. Authored by experts in obstetrics and gynecology, this book serves as an excellent companion for exam preparation, self-assessment, and continuous learning.

The book's structure is well-organized, presenting a wide range of multiple-choice questions that cover the entire spectrum of obstetrics and gynecology. Divided into various sections, each corresponding to a different aspect of the field, readers can easily navigate to specific areas they want to focus on. This segmentation makes it an ideal tool for targeted studying and quick reference.

One of the book's strengths lies in its comprehensive coverage of both common and complex topics. The questions are thoughtfully curated to encompass core concepts, emerging trends, and evidence-based practices, reflecting the dynamic nature of obstetrics and gynecology. This approach not only supports exam preparation but also facilitates a deeper understanding of the subject matter.

Furthermore, the explanations provided for each question are clear, concise, and well-referenced. This is particularly beneficial for learners seeking to consolidate their understanding of the material. The book also offers rationales for incorrect answers, which helps in addressing common misconceptions and refining critical thinking skills.

The inclusion of clinical scenarios and images enhances the book's practicality, bridging the gap between theoretical knowledge and real-world application. This feature makes it an ideal resource for medical students transitioning to clinical rotations and for junior doctors aiming to enhance their diagnostic and decision-making abilities. The book provides breadth, depth and expansive research from many medical experts in the field of reproductive and sexual health. The book honors fact-based information and provides cutting edge interpretation of various Obstetrics and gynecology in its both sections. The book provides up to date resources and extensive question bank in Obstetrics and Gynecology.

Jaydeep Tank
President FOGSI 2024-25
Mumbai, Maharashtra, India

From the Desk of Editor

The book *"Multiple Choice Questions in Obstetrics and Gynecology"* is a valuable resource that fills a much-needed gap in the field of medical education. This book offers a comprehensive collection of multiple-choice questions (MCQs) tailored specifically to the realm of obstetrics and gynecology.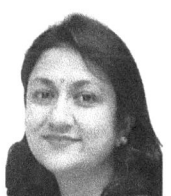

The book is organized into sections that cover a wide range of topics within obstetrics and gynecology, including pregnancy, labor, gynecological disorders, reproductive health, and more. Each section is well-structured and presents MCQs that challenge the reader's knowledge and critical thinking skills. The questions vary in difficulty, providing a balanced approach suitable for both medical students preparing for exams and practicing professionals seeking to refresh their knowledge.

One of the notable strengths of this book is the detailed explanations provided for each question. After attempting a question, readers can refer to the comprehensive explanations that accompany the answers. These explanations not only clarify the correct answer but also delve into the reasoning behind the other choices, helping readers understand the nuances of each topic.

Furthermore, the book incorporates up-to-date information and follows the latest guidelines in the field. Medical knowledge is constantly evolving, and this book ensures that readers are equipped with the most current information, enhancing its relevance and utility.

Concise explanations could enhance the overall readability and make it easier for readers to grasp key concepts quickly. Multiple choice, could add diversity to the learning experience.

In conclusion, "Multiple Choice Questions in Obstetrics and Gynecology" is a commendable resource that addresses the need for a comprehensive collection of MCQs in this specialized medical field. Its detailed explanations, wide coverage of topics, and adherence to current medical standards make it an excellent aid for both medical students and professionals seeking to bolster their understanding. Our all authors are experts with extensive experience. We thank them with utmost gratitude for bringing out this up-to-date guide for medical undergraduates, postgraduates, and DNB students, those preparing for DM and fellowship exams and those who want to test their knowledge. This book has the potential to become an indispensable tool in the study and practice of obstetrics and gynecology.

Ruchika Garg
Rajshree Dayanand Katke
Jai Bhagwan Sharma

Preface

Welcome to the world of learning and assessment in Obstetrics and Gynecology! This book, dedicated to postgraduate students seeking a comprehensive understanding of the field, aims to be a valuable resource in your educational journey. The multiple-choice questions included are carefully crafted to not only test your knowledge but also to deepen your insights into the intricate realm of women's health.

Structured to cover a wide spectrum of topics, this collection serves as a tool for self-assessment, helping you reinforce concepts, identify areas for further study, and prepare for examinations. The questions are designed to challenge your critical thinking and clinical reasoning skills, reflecting the dynamic nature of obstetrics and gynecology.

As you navigate through these pages, envision this book as a companion on your path to mastery. Whether you are a dedicated student, a resident, or a practitioner refreshing your knowledge, may this resource contribute to your growth and proficiency in providing optimal care to women at every stage of life.

Your commitment to advancing healthcare in obstetrics and gynecology is commendable, and I hope this book enhances your journey of continuous learning and professional development.

Best wishes for success in your academic and clinical pursuits.

Ruchika Garg

Acknowledgments

We wish to thank all our authors who responded to our requests with promptness and have contributed immensely and added vital, contemporaneous information with their vast experience.

We wish to appreciate the efforts of Jaypee Brothers Medical Publishers for bringing out this book in its final shape with their talent of skillfully and expediently coordinating and overseeing composition. We thank Shri Jitendar P Vij (Group Chairman), Mr Ankit Vij (Managing Director), Ms Chetna Malhotra (Senior Director—Professional Publishing, Marketing, and Business Development), Asmi Bharati (Development Editor), and Ashish Kumar (Commissioning Editor) as their thoughtful, creative efforts for our book were like pearls. Their attention to details and accurate renderings added important academic support to our words.

We express my utmost gratitude to Dr Prabhat Agrawal, loving kids Pratham, Palakshi, parents Mahesh Chandra Agrawal, Dr Anuradha and Dr JK Garg, as this herculean task would not have seen the light of day without them. We bow with respect to Prof Gangadhar Sahoo Sir , Dr Narendra Malhotra Sir, and Dr Jaideep Malhotra Madam for being our mentor. We express gratitude to the learned faculty of Department of Obstetrics and Gynecology, Sarojini Naidu Medical College (SNMC), Agra, Uttar Pradesh, India with Prof Richa Singh, Prof Nidhi Gupta, and Prof Shikha Singh, for their support and cooperation. Our special appreciation and thanks to all our colleagues and friends who supported our idea of bringing out this series and gave us the confidence to finish this book.

Contents

SECTION 1: Obstetrics

1. **Anatomy of Female Reproductive Organs** 3
   Aruna Verma, Neha Sharma

2. **Safe Motherhood: Epidemiology in Obstetrics** 8
   Punit S Bhojani

3. **Placenta and Fetal Membranes** 15
   Bhumika Kotecha Mundhe

4. **Physiological Changes during Pregnancy** 22
   Kalpana Kumari, Shilpi Srivastava

5. **Diagnosis of Pregnancy** 26
   Komal N Chavan, Ritika Pathak

6. **Fetus in Utero** 31
   Rajshree Dayanand Katke

7. **Fetal Skull and Maternal Pelvis** 35
   Rajshree Dayanand Katke, Ankita Aghav

8. **Antenatal Care, Preconceptional Counseling, and Care** 39
   Preeti Nitsure Deshpande

9. **Antenatal Assessment of Fetal Well-being** 49
   Seema Mehrotra, Neharika Malhotra

10. **Fetal Monitoring during Labor** 53
    Kinjal Shah

11. **Prenatal Genetic Counseling, Screening, and Diagnosis** 60
    Purnima Satoskar

12. **Normal Labor** 65
    Prema Kania

13. **Postpartum Hemorrhage** 67
    Rajshree Dayanand Katke

14. **Normal Puerperium** 71
    Neelima Mantri

15. **Abnormalities of the Puerperium: Part 1** 75
    Deepa Kala

16. **Abnormalities of Puerperium: Part 2** 79
    Deepali Kapote, Madhura Mandlik

17. **Bleeding in Early Pregnancy** 84
    Kunjal Bathija

18. **Vomiting in Early Pregnancy** 89
    Kunjal Bathija

19. **Gestational Trophoblastic Neoplasia** 92
    Jayashree V Kanavi

20. **Recurrent Abortions** 95
    Jyothi GS, Sahana Girish

21. **Spontaneous Abortion, Ultrasound Findings, and Septic Abortion** 102
    Radhika Chetan, Ananya Girish

22. **Ectopic Pregnancy** 108
    Priyanka Rai, Swapnil Bala

23. **Multifetal Gestation** 115
    Pavika Lal, Garima Gupta

24. **Oligohydramnios and Polyhydramnios** 122
    Pradnya Changede, Neha Khairnar, Rajat Agrawal

25. **Abnormalities of the Placenta and Umbilical Cord** 127
    Rajshree Dayanand Katke

26. **Hypertensive Disorders in Pregnancy** 130
    Shubhangi Nawarange, Rajshree Dayanand Katke

27. **Anemia in Pregnancy** 136
    Somya Suman, Sarita Bhalerao

28. **Rh Isoimmunization** 143
    Soniya Dhiman

29. **Liver Dysfunction in Pregnancy** 154
    Shashi Lata Maheshwari (Kabra), Shakun Tyagi

30. **Renal Disorders in Pregnancy** 163
    Kavita Mandrelle Bhatti

31. **Thrombocytopenia in Pregnancy** 166
    Harshada Thakur, Rani Daruwale

32. **Viral Infections in Pregnancy** 171
    Sreelatha S, Veena M Vernekar

33. **Malaria and Dengue in Pregnancy** 175
    Sunita Samal

34. **Antepartum Hemorrhage** 180
    Sebanti Goswami

35. **Gynecological Problems in Pregnancy** 183
    Hemant Damle

36. Preterm Labor	**186**
Shikha Seth	
37. Preterm Premature Rupture of Membranes	**191**
Geetha Balsarkar, Sunil Tambvekar	
38. Postmaturity	**196**
Arnav Pai, Rishma Dhillon Pai	
39. Intrauterine Fetal Demise	**199**
Vaidehi Thakur, Mandakini Megh, Deep Kamal	
40. Malpresentation, Malposition, and Cephalopelvic Disproportion	**204**
Surekha Tayade	
41. Abnormal Uterine Action Section Malpresentations	**211**
Mugdha L Jungari	
42. Breech	**217**
Shrutika Thakkar	
43. Quiz on Occipitoposterior Position	**222**
Shashi R Goyal	
44. Transverse Lie, Brow, and Face	**225**
Rajshree Dayanand Katke, Gayathri AK	
45. Medicolegal Aspects in Gynecology and Obstetrics	**230**
Kavita Tilwani, Vivek Tilwani	
46. Cord Prolapse	**235**
Priya Vora, Nishita Shah	
47. Prolonged Labor, Obstructed Labor, and Dystocia	**240**
Suvarna Khadilkar, Rutuja Bodake	
48. Placenta Accreta Spectrum	**246**
Poonam Yadav	
49. Gestational Diabetes Mellitus	**249**
Kiranmai Devineni, Kalpana Basany	
50. Genital Tract Injuries	**257**
Rajeshwari Laxman Khyade	
51. Term Newborn Infant	**261**
Charmila Ayyavoo, S Karthikeyan	
52. Induction of Labor	**269**
Rajshree Dayanand Katke, Prachi Yadav	
53. Operative Obstetrics	**275**
Nandita Palshetkar, Rohan Palshetkar	
54. Intrauterine Growth Restriction	**282**
Priyankur Roy	
55. Imaging in Obstetrics	**289**
Vandana Bansal, Meera Jayaprakash	

56. **Anesthesia and Analgesia in Obstetrics** 295
   Sukriti Atram, Ruchika Garg

57. **HIV in Pregnancy** 307
   Arun Kumar Dora, Prabhat Agrawal

58. **Principles of Drugs in Pregnancy and Categories of Drugs (Category B)**..317
   Jayashree V Kanavi

59. **Neurological Disorders in Pregnancy** 321
   Aruna M Biradar, Sangamesh S Mathapati

60. **Disseminated Intravascular Coagulation in Pregnancy** 328
   Meenal S Sarmalkar, Honey M Gemavat

61. **Blood Transfusion**...337
   Kalyani Sai Dhandapani, Ruchika Garg

62. **Fetal Growth Restriction** 340
   Shobana Mahadevan, Ruchika Garg

63. **Physiology of Pregnancy**...346
   Kalpana Kumari, Shilpi Srivastava

SECTION 2: Gynecology

64. **Ultrasound in Infertility** 353
   Astha Lalwani, Shubhra Agarwal

65. **Ovarian Reserve**..358
   Astha Lalwani, Shubhra Agarwal

66. **Laparoscopy in Infertility**..364
   Astha Lalwani, Shubhra Agarwal

67. **Hysteroscopy in Infertility** 369
   Shubhra Agarwal, Astha Lalwani

68. **Amenorrhea** 373
   Vejainty Chauhan, Shefali Singh

69. **Polycystic Ovary Syndrome** 386
   Mona Asnani, Meher Narain

70. **Endometriosis**..397
   Ganesh Dangal, Nishma Bajracharya

71. **Ovulation Induction** 405
   Anuja Bhalerao

72. **Tubal Factor Infertility**...408
   Archana Kumari, Ruchika Garg

73. **Female Genital Tuberculosis** 411
   Sippy Agarwal, Prabhat Agrawal

74. **Male Infertility** 415
   Divya Pandey, Shivam Yadav

75. Intrauterine Insemination 421
Kanchan Rani, Divya Suman

76. In vitro Fertilization 427
Shreedevi Tanksale, Tejal Poddar

77. Preimplantation Genetic Diagnosis 434
Athulya Shajan

78. Mullerian Anomalies 438
Shelly Agarwal

79. Fibroid 446
Deepa Chaudhary

80. Endocrinology of Reproduction 454
Nidhi Sharma Chauhan, Rajshree Dayanand Katke

81. Menstruation 459
Urvashi Verma, Rekha Rani

82. Abnormal Uterine Bleeding 462
Renu Gupta, Pavika Lal

83. Premenstrual Syndrome 469
Vandana Solanki, Deepa Singh

84. Postmenopausal Bleeding 474
Pushpa Lata Sankhwar

85. Vaginal Infection and Pelvic Inflammatory Diseases 479
Suman Chaudhary, Ruchika Garg

86. Hyperprolactinemia 489
Shubhra Agarwal

87. Prolapse Uterus: Part 1 493
Beena Kumari, Rajshree Dayanand Katke

88. Prolapse Uterus: Part II 496
Ruchika Garg

Etiology, Supports of Uterus, Classification, Risk Factors, Symptoms, Examination, and Differential Diagnosis 496
Savita Somalwar, Kanchan Dwidmuthe

Management 499
Anuja Bhalerao, Sheela Jain

89. Urogynecology 502
Vineeta, Rashmi Bala, Priyanka Rai

90. Contraception 508
Suchi Jain, Ruchika Garg

91. Vulvodynia 513
Richa Singh, Shaifali Singh

92. Contraception Miscellaneous 516
Vidya Thobbi

93. Premature Ovarian Insufficiency 518
Ritu Sharma, Pinky Mishra

94. Myomectomy 527
Kanchan Rani, Divya Suman

95. Ovarian Hyperstimulation Syndrome: Part 1 531
Kanchan Rani, Divya Suman

96. Ovarian Hyperstimulation Syndrome: Part 2 536
Athulya Shajan

97. Thyroid in Pregnancy 541
Savita Somalwar, Anuja Bhalerao, Sheela Jain, Prabhat Agrawal

98. Cervical Cancer 544
Monica Agrawal

99. Human Papillomavirus and Vaccination 555
Ritu Santwani, Naisargi Patel

100. Carcinoma of Ovary 562
Rajshree Dayanand Katke

101. Germ Cell Tumors 566
Vandana Solanki, Vertika Singh

102. Menopause General: Part 1..572
Rao Preethi Venkatachala, Ruchika Garg

103. Menopause General: Part 2 575
Ashwini Bhalerao-Gandhi

104. Vaginal Discharge 579
Dhara Singh, Ruchika Garg

Section 1

Obstetrics

Chapter Outline

1. Anatomy of Female Reproductive Organs
2. Safe Motherhood: Epidemiology in Obstetrics
3. Placenta and Fetal Membranes
4. Physiological Changes during Pregnancy
5. Diagnosis of Pregnancy
6. Fetus in Utero
7. Fetal Skull and Maternal Pelvis
8. Antenatal Care, Preconceptional Counseling, and Care
9. Antenatal Assessment of Fetal Well-being
10. Fetal Monitoring during Labor
11. Prenatal Genetic Counseling, Screening, and Diagnosis
12. Normal Labor
13. Postpartum Hemorrhage
14. Normal Puerperium
15. Abnormalities of the Puerperium: Part 1
16. Abnormalities of Puerperium: Part 2
17. Bleeding in Early Pregnancy
18. Vomiting in Early Pregnancy
19. Gestational Trophoblastic Neoplasia
20. Recurrent Abortions
21. Spontaneous Abortion, Ultrasound Findings, and Septic Abortion
22. Ectopic Pregnancy
23. Multifetal Gestation
24. Oligohydramnios and Polyhydramnios
25. Abnormalities of the Placenta and Umbilical Cord
26. Hypertensive Disorders in Pregnancy
27. Anemia in Pregnancy
28. Rh Isoimmunization
29. Liver Dysfunction in Pregnancy
30. Renal Disorders in Pregnancy
31. Thrombocytopenia in Pregnancy
32. Viral Infections in Pregnancy
33. Malaria and Dengue in Pregnancy
34. Antepartum Hemorrhage
35. Gynecological Problems in Pregnancy
36. Preterm Labor
37. Preterm Premature Rupture of Membranes
38. Postmaturity
39. Intrauterine Fetal Demise
40. Malpresentation, Malposition, and Cephalopelvic Disproportion
41. Abnormal Uterine Action Section Malpresentations
42. Breech
43. Quiz on Occipitoposterior Position
44. Transverse Lie, Brow, and Face
45. Medicolegal Aspects in Gynecology and Obstetrics
46. Cord Prolapse
47. Prolonged Labor, Obstructed Labor, and Dystocia
48. Placenta Accreta Spectrum
49. Gestational Diabetes Mellitus
50. Genital Tract Injuries
51. Term Newborn Infant
52. Induction of Labor
53. Operative Obstetrics
54. Intrauterine Growth Restriction
55. Imaging in Obstetrics
56. Anesthesia and Analgesia in Obstetrics
57. HIV in Pregnancy
58. Principles of Drugs in Pregnancy and Categories of Drugs (Category B)
59. Neurological Disorders in Pregnancy
60. Disseminated Intravascular Coagulation in Pregnancy
61. Blood Transfusion
62. Fetal Growth Restriction
63. Physiology of Pregnancy

Chapter 1: Anatomy of Female Reproductive Organs

Aruna Verma, Neha Sharma

QUESTIONS

1. **The "Pudenda" word is used for:**
    a. Pudendal nerve
    b. Pudendal artery
    c. Vulva
    d. Mons pubis

2. **All statements regarding labia majora are true, *except*:**
    a. Labia majora are homologous to the male scrotum embryologically
    b. These are continuous with the mons veneris superiorly
    c. Round ligaments terminate at their upper border
    d. Posteriorly, they taper and merge into the skin overlying the anus

3. **Which one of the venous plexus engorges commonly during pregnancy to develop vulval varicosities?**
    a. Labia majora
    b. Labia minora
    c. Skin and subcutaneous tissue over the perineum
    d. Skin and subcutaneous tissue covering the mons pubis

4. **The demarcating line or area on the inner surface of labia minora from where keratinized stratified squamous epithelium changes to nonkeratinized squamous epithelium.**
    a. Hart line
    b. Arcuate line
    c. White line
    d. Perineal membrane

5. **True facts regarding vestibule are all, *except*:**
    a. It is derived from the embryonic urogenital membrane
    b. It is almond-shaped
    c. It is enclosed by white line laterally
    d. The posterior portion between the fourchette and vaginal opening is called the fossa navicularis

6. **Following trauma or infection, which of the following duct may swell and obstruct to form a cyst or abscess:**
    a. Skene gland duct
    b. Bartholin gland duct
    c. Minor vestibular gland duct
    d. Cowper gland duct

7. **Anteriorly, the vagina is separated from the bladder and urethra by connective tissue called:**
    a. The urogenital septum
    b. The vesicovaginal septum
    c. The vesicourethral septum
    d. The rectovaginal septum

8. **All are true regarding vagina, *except*:**
    a. Makes an angle of 45° with the horizontal in an erect posture
    b. Appears as letter "H" on the cross-section
    c. Its long axis is parallel to the plane of pelvic inlet and at a right angle to that of the uterus
    d. Lined by keratinized stratified squamous epithelium

9. **True about ischioanal fossa are all, *except*:**
    a. Single fat-filled wedge-shaped space and constitutes the little part of anal triangle
    b. Injuries to vessels in anal triangle can lead to hematoma formation in the fossa
    c. Double fat-filled space on either side of the anal canal
    d. The fat in the fossa provides support to the surrounding organs and allows vaginal stretching during delivery

10. **Anatomical changes during pregnancy are all, *except*:**
    a. Remarkable uterine growth due to muscle fiber hypertrophy

b. Flattened convexity of uterine fundus changes into dome-shaped convexity
c. Round ligament appears to insert at the junction of middle and lower third of the uterus
d. Fallopian tubes elongate but both ovaries are grossly unchanged

11. **Concerning the endometrium, the true statement is:**
    a. The basal artery comes directly from the arcuate artery
    b. Spiral arteries extend directly from radial arteries
    c. The spiral arteries extend directly from the arcuate artery
    d. Functionalis layer contains spiral arteries and radial arteries

12. **Isthmus of the uterus is:**
    a. Bounded by histological internal ors above and anatomical internal ors below
    b. Bounded by anatomical internal ors above and histological internal ors below
    c. Bounded by uterus above and anatomical internal ors below
    d. Bounded by histological internal ors above and external ors below

13. **In uncontrollable PPH, all of the following arteries can be ligated,** *except:*
    a. Uterine artery
    b. Anterior division of the internal iliac artery
    c. Posterior division of the internal iliac artery
    d. Ovarian artery

14. **Regarding cervical changes in early pregnancy, the correct statement is/are:**
    a. Increased vascularity within the cervical stroma beneath the epithelium creates blueness in ectocervix termed as "Chadwick sign"
    b. Cervical edema leads to softening—"Godell sign"
    c. Isthmic softening, termed as "Hegar sign"
    d. All of the above

15. **Not considered as true support of the uterus:**
    a. Uterosacral ligament b. Broad ligament
    c. Sacrospinous ligament d. Both b and c

16. **Pick up the incorrect pair (depicting embryological origin):**
    a. *Clitoris:* Genital tubercle
    b. *Skene gland:* Urogenital sinus
    c. *Labia minora:* Genital swelling
    d. *Ovary:* Genital ridge

17. **Which of the following is not true?**
    a. Ovarian arteries arise from the abdominal aorta
    b. Both ovarian veins drain into the inferior vena cava
    c. Uterine artery arises from anterior division of the internal iliac artery
    d. Cornual area of the uterus drains into the superficial inguinal lymph node

18. **During LSCS, Pfannenstiel incision is preferred as:**
    a. Better field of vision
    b. Time of surgery reduces
    c. Repeat LSCS, if required becomes easier
    d. In the lower abdominal wall, Langer's lines are arranged transversely and Pfannenstiel incision follows them and gives superior cosmetic results

19. **Pick up the incorrect statement with respect to the internal iliac artery:**
    a. Posterior division branches extend to the buttock and thigh and are superior gluteal, iliolumbar, and lateral sacral
    b. Anterior division supplies pelvic organs and perineum, which are inferior gluteal, internal pudendal, middle rectal, vaginal, uterine, obturator, and superior vesical artery
    c. During PPH management, internal iliac ligation is advocated distal to posterior division
    d. None of the above

20. **True statements regarding pelvic diaphragm are all,** *except:*
    a. Found deep to the anterior and posterior triangles
    b. Composed of the levator ani and the coccygeus muscle
    c. Vaginal birth causes damage to the only coccygeus muscle and its innervation
    d. The injury to the pelvic diaphragm may predispose to pelvic organ prolapse and stress urinary incontinence

21. **After ligation of the uterine or internal iliac artery to control the PPH, which arterial supply prevents uterine ischemia?**
    a. Vaginal artery
    b. Ovarian artery
    c. Descending cervical artery
    d. Lateral sacral artery

22. A 30-year-old female presented to gynecological outpatient department (OPD) with vaginal discomfort and dyspareunia for the last 2 weeks. She also felt a mass on the external aspect of her vagina. On physical examination, there is a 2-cm unilateral erythematous swelling on the right side of the posterolateral labia minora. Diagnosis is:
    a. Bartholin cyst/abscess   b. Labial cyst/abscess
    c. Gartner's cyst/abscess   d. Vulval cyst/abscess

23. Regarding the fallopian tube, which one of the following is true?
    a. Sympathetic innervation of the tubes is extensive in contrast to their parasympathetic innervation
    b. The nerve supply derives solely from the ovarian plexus
    c. The nerve supply derives solely from the utero-vaginal plexus
    d. Sensory afferent fibers ascend to L1 spinal cord level

24. The uterine musculature during pregnancy is arranged in which of the following layers:
    a. *Inner:* Longitudinal
    b. *Intermediate:* Interlacing
    c. *Outer:* Circular
    d. *All layers:* Interlacing

25. Which statement is false regarding blood supply of external genitalia?
    a. Superficial external pudendal artery supplies the skin of pubic region
    b. Deep external pudendal artery supplies the labia majora
    c. Internal pudendal artery supplies perineal and vulval structures
    d. Superior epigastric artery supplies the mons pubis

26. Which of the following gland secretes fluid into the vagina?
    a. Mammary gland   b. Sebaceous gland
    c. Bartholin gland   d. Gartner gland

27. Mark the incorrect statement with respect to fallopian tubes.
    a. Fallopian tubes, also known as oviducts, extend laterally 8–14 cm from uterine cornua
    b. All four portions (interstitial, isthmus, ampulla, and infundibulum) are covered by mesosalpinx
    c. Tubal mucosa is lined by columnar epithelium with a direction of flow toward the uterine cavity
    d. Ampulla of tubes is the most common site for tubal ectopic pregnancy

28. With regard to the nerve supply of the pelvis, all are correct, *except:*
    a. The sensory component of the pudendal nerve supplies the skin of vulva, clitoris, perineum, and lower vagina
    b. Motor component of the pudendal nerve supplies all muscles of the pelvic floor
    c. Anterior half of vulva is supplied by the ilioinguinal and genitofemoral nerve
    d. Posterior half of vulva is supplied by the ilioinguinal nerve

29. Which pair is false in regard to pain perception during pregnancy?
    a. Early labor → T10-L1
    b. Late labor → S2-S4
    c. Cesarean section → blockage from T4 segment
    d. Painless labor → blockage to be given from T12

30. Following are various statements with regard to pelvic joint mobility:
    1. Upward gliding of sacroiliac joint is maximum in dorsal lithotomy
    2. Sacroiliac joint mobility aids Mac Robert's maneuver in shoulder dystocia management
    3. Squatting position increases interspinous diameter and pelvic outlet
    4. Pelvic joint mobility/relaxation remains same in early gestation and at term

    Which of the above statements are correct?
    a. 1, 2, and 3   b. 1 and 2
    c. 2 and 3   d. 1, 2, 3, and 4

ANSWERS

1. **c.** The pudenda—commonly designated the vulva—includes all structures visible externally from the symphysis pubis to the perineal body. This includes the mons pubis, labia majora and minora, clitoris, hymen, vestibule, urethral opening, greater vestibular or Bartholin glands, minor vestibular glands, and paraurethral glands.
(Reference: Williams Obstetrics, 25th edition, page 16)

2. **d.** Embryologically, the labia majora are homologous with the male scrotum. Labia vary somewhat in appearance, principally according to the amount of fat they contain. They are 7–8 cm in length, 2–3 cm in

depth, and 1–1.5 cm in thickness. They are continuous directly with the mons pubis superiorly, and the round ligaments terminate at their upper borders. Posteriorly, the labia majora taper and merge into the area overlying the perineal body to form the posterior commissure.
(Reference: Williams Obstetrics, 25th edition, page 16)

3. **a.** During pregnancy, this vasculature commonly develops varicosities, especially in parous women, from increased venous pressure created by the enlarging uterus. They appear as engorged tortuous veins or as small grapelike clusters, but they are typically asymptomatic.
(Reference: Williams Obstetrics, 25th edition, page 16)

4. **a.** Thinly keratinized stratified squamous epithelium covers the outer surface of each labium. On their inner surface, the lateral portion is covered by this same epithelium up to a demarcating line—Hart line. Medial to this line, each labium is covered by squamous epithelium that is nonkeratinized.
(Reference: Williams Obstetrics, 25th edition, page 17)

5. **c.** This is the functionally mature female structure derived from the embryonic urogenital membrane. In adult women, it is an almond-shaped area that is enclosed by the Hart line laterally, the external surface of the hymen medially, the clitoral frenulum anteriorly, and the fourchette posteriorly. The vestibule usually is perforated by six openings: The urethra, the vagina, two Bartholin gland ducts, and at times, two ducts of the largest paraurethral glands—the Skene glands. The posterior portion of the vestibule between the fourchette and the vaginal opening is called the fossa navicularis.
(Reference: Williams Obstetrics, 25th edition, page 17)

6. **b.** The bilateral Bartholin glands, also termed greater vestibular glands, are major glands that measure 0.5–1 cm in diameter. On their respective side, each lies inferior to the vascular vestibular bulb and deep to the inferior end of the bulbocavernosus muscle. The duct from each measures 1.5–2 cm long and opens distal to the hymeneal ring—one at 5 and the other at 7 o'clock on the vestibule. Following trauma or infection, either duct may swell and obstruct to form a cyst or, if infected, an abscess.
(Reference: Williams Obstetrics, 25th edition, page 17)

7. **b.** Anteriorly, the vagina is separated from the bladder and urethra by connective tissue—the vesicovaginal septum.
(Reference: Williams Obstetrics, 25th edition, page 18)

8. **d.** The vaginal lining is composed of nonkeratinized stratified squamous epithelium and underlying lamina propria.
(Reference: Williams Obstetrics, 25th edition, page 18)

9. **a.** Also known as ischiorectal fossae, these two fat-filled wedge-shaped spaces are found on either side of the anal canal and comprise the bulk of the posterior triangle. The fat found within each fossa provides support to surrounding organs yet allows rectal distention during defecation and vaginal stretching during delivery. Clinically, injury to vessels in the posterior triangle can lead to hematoma formation in the ischioanal fossa, and the potential for large accumulation in these easily distensible spaces.
(Reference: Williams Obstetrics, 25th edition, page 21)

10. **c.** Pregnancy stimulates remarkable uterine growth due to muscle fiber hypertrophy. The uterine fundus, a previously flattened convexity between tubal insertions, now becomes dome-shaped. Moreover, the round ligaments appear to insert at the junction of the middle and upper thirds of the organ. The fallopian tubes elongate, but the ovaries grossly appear unchanged.
(Reference: Williams Obstetrics, 25th edition, page 21)

11. **b.** The main artery provides a branch of considerable size to the upper cervix and then numerous other medial branches serially penetrate the body of the uterus to form the arcuate arteries. As indicated by the name, each branch arches across the organ by coursing within the myometrium just beneath the serosal surface. Arcuate vessels from each side anastomose at the uterine midline. Radial artery branches originate at right angles from the arcuate arteries and travel inward through the myometrium, enter the endometrium/decidua, and branch there to become either basal arteries or coiled spiral arteries. The spiral arteries supply the functionalis layer. Also called the straight arteries, the basal arteries extend only into the basalis layer.
(Reference: Williams Obstetrics, 25th edition, page 26)

12. **b.** *(Reference: Williams Obstetrics, 25th edition, page 23)*

13. **c.** *(Williams Obstetrics 25th edition page 27)*

14. **d.** In early pregnancy, increased vascularity within the cervix stroma beneath the epithelium creates an ectocervical blue tint that is characteristic of

CHAPTER 1: Anatomy of Female Reproductive Organs 7

Chadwick sign. Cervical edema leads to softening—Goodell sign, whereas isthmic softening is Hegar sign.
(Reference: Williams Obstetrics, 25th edition, page 24)

15. **d.** The round and broad ligaments provide no substantial uterine support, which contrasts with the cardinal and uterosacral ligaments.
(Reference: Williams Obstetrics, 25th edition, page 24)

16. **c.** *(Reference: Williams Obstetrics, 25th edition, page 38)*

17. **b.** Left ovarian vein drains into left renal vein and right ovarian vein directly drains into the inferior vena cava.
(Reference: Williams Obstetrics, 25th edition, page 26)

18. **d.** Langer lines describe the orientation of dermal fibers within the skin. In the anterior abdominal wall, they are arranged transversely. As a result, vertical skin incisions sustain greater lateral tension and thus, in general, develop wider scars. In contrast, low transverse incisions, such as the Pfannenstiel, follow Langer lines and lead to superior cosmetic results.
(Reference: Williams Obstetrics, 25th edition, page 14)

19. **d.** The anterior division provides blood supply to the pelvic organs and perineum and includes the inferior gluteal, internal pudendal, middle rectal, vaginal, uterine, and obturator arteries, as well as the umbilical artery and its continuation as the superior vesical artery. The posterior division branches extend to the buttock and thigh and include the superior gluteal, lateral sacral, and iliolumbar arteries. For this reason, during internal iliac artery ligation, many advocate ligation distal to the posterior division to avoid compromised blood flow to the areas supplied by this division.
(Reference: Williams Obstetrics, 25th edition, page 27)

20. **c.** Found deep to the anterior and posterior triangles, this broad muscular sling provides substantial support to the pelvic viscera. The pelvic diaphragm is composed of the levator ani and the coccygeus muscles. The levator ani, in turn, contains the pubococcygeus, puborectalis, and iliococcygeus muscles. The pubococcygeus muscle is also termed the pubovisceral muscle and is subdivided based on points of insertion and function. These include the pubovaginalis, puboperinealis, and puboanalis muscles, which insert into the vagina, perineal body, and anus, respectively. Vaginal birth conveys significant risk for damage to the levator ani or to its innervation.
(Reference: Williams Obstetrics, 25th edition, page 21)

21. **b.** In addition to the uterine artery, the uterus receives blood supply from the ovarian artery. This artery is a direct branch of the aorta and enters the broad ligament through the infundibulopelvic ligament. At the ovarian hilum, it divides into smaller branches that enter the ovary. As the ovarian artery runs along the hilum, it also sends several branches through the mesosalpinx to supply the fallopian tubes. Its main stem, however, traverses the entire length of the broad ligament toward the uterine cornu. Here, it forms an anastomosis with the ovarian branch of the uterine artery. This dual uterine blood supply creates a vascular reserve to prevent uterine ischemia if ligation of the uterine or internal iliac artery is performed to control postpartum hemorrhage.
(Reference: Williams Obstetrics, 25th edition, page 26)

22. **a.** *(Reference: Williams Obstetrics, 25th edition, page 17)*

23. **a.** The tubes are supplied richly with elastic tissue, blood vessels, and lymphatics. Their sympathetic innervation is extensive, in contrast to their parasympathetic innervation. This nerve supply derives partly from the ovarian plexus and partly from the uterovaginal plexus. Sensory afferent fibers ascend to T10 spinal cord levels.
(Reference: Williams Obstetrics, 25th edition, page 28)

24. **b.** The muscles are arranged as inner circular, outer longitudinal, and intermediate interlacing.
(Reference: Williams Obstetrics, 25th edition, page 24)

25. **d.** Inferior epigastric artery, a branch of the external iliac artery, supplies the mons pubis.

26. **c.** Bartholin gland
(Reference: Williams Obstetrics, 25th edition, page 17)

27. **b.** Interstitial part of tube not covered by mesosalpinx
(Reference: Williams Obstetrics, 25th edition, page 28)

28. **d.** Posterior half by posterior cutaneous nerve of thigh.
(Reference: DC Dutta's textbook of Gynecology 8th edition, page 3)

29. **d.** Complete analgesia of pain for labor and delivery necessitate a block from T10 to the S5 dermatome.
(Reference: Williams Obstetrics, 25th edition, pages 28 and 493)

30. **a.** Pelvic joint mobility increases at term.
(Reference: Williams Obstetrics, 25th edition, page 29)

Chapter 2

Safe Motherhood: Epidemiology in Obstetrics

Punit S Bhojani

QUESTIONS

1. Safe motherhood initiative aims to improve women's health through all the following interventions, *except:*
   a. Community
   b. Political
   c. Economic
   d. Social

2. Which among the following is false?
   a. Maternal mortality cannot be reduced with limited policy interventions
   b. Maternal mortality is a social disadvantage
   c. Safe motherhood is considered a basic human right
   d. Maternal mortality is not merely health disadvantage

3. Lifetime risk is defined as the probability of dying of a woman in her reproductive age (15–49 years) due to causes in pregnancy, childbirth, or within 6 weeks of childbirth. In India, presently it is?
   a. 0.3%
   b. 1%
   c. 1.5%
   d. 2.5%

4. To improve the maternal mortality situation in India, all the states have been categorized into groups: (A) Empowered Action Group (EAG), (B) Southern states, (C) Other states. Which among the following is not included in EAG?
   a. Uttar Pradesh
   b. Himachal Pradesh
   c. Chhattisgarh
   d. Madhya Pradesh

5. Which among the following is not an aim of Reproductive and Child Health (RCH)?
   a. Safe motherhood
   b. Anemia prevention
   c. Reducing risk of sexually transmitted infections (STIs)
   d. Family planning

6. Three cleans of intrapartum care include all the following, *except:*
   a. Clean hands
   b. Clean cord tie
   c. Clean perineal area
   d. Clean birth canal

7. Maternal mortality ratio (MMR) in India currently is:
   a. 126/100,000
   b. 103/100,000
   c. 97/100,000
   d. 97/10,000

8. Life-saving drugs in the context of obstetrics care include all the following, *except:*
   a. Misoprostol
   b. Injection $MgSO_4$
   c. Injection metronidazole
   d. Injection amikacin

9. "Maternal mortality" is defined as death of a woman while pregnant or within___days of the termination of pregnancy irrespective of the duration and the site of pregnancy, from any cause related to or aggravated by the pregnancy or its management but not from accidental or incidental causes.
   a. 28 days
   b. 42 days
   c. 60 days
   d. 180 days

10. All the following factors are mainly recognized as the factors responsible for high maternal and perinatal deaths in the developing countries, *except:*
    a. Instrumental delivery
    b. Unsafe abortion
    c. Inadequate antenatal care
    d. Lack of trained birth attendants

11. Among the following, which contributes the least to MMR?
    a. Eclampsia
    b. Obstructed labor
    c. Sepsis
    d. Embolism

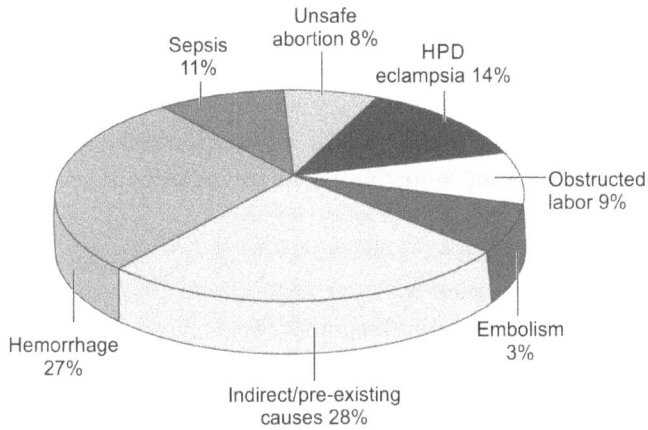

12. Which among the following is an indirect cause of "maternal mortality"?
    a. Preeclampsia
    b. Postpartum hemorrhage
    c. Anemia
    d. Ectopic gestation

13. Which among the following is not a proven intervention to prevent hemorrhagic conditions in obstetric care?
    a. Use of tocolytics in time
    b. Blood transfusion, if severe hemorrhage
    c. Skilled attendant at birth
    d. Treating anemia in pregnancy

14. Which among the following is not a proven strategy to prevent maternal mortality due to anemia?
    a. Routine iron supplementation during gestation
    b. Deworming
    c. Treating malaria, HIV
    d. Admit if Hb <9

15. In partograms recommended by the "WHO", the distance between the alert and action lines is:
    a. 1 hour   b. 2 hours
    c. 4 hours   d. 5 hours

16. "Maternal Near Miss" is defined as follows:
    a. "A woman who nearly died but survived a complication that occurred during pregnancy, childbirth, or within 42 days of termination of pregnancy"
    b. "A woman who required admission but survived a complication that occurred during pregnancy, childbirth, or within 42 days of termination of pregnancy"
    c. "A woman who nearly died but had a debilitating complication that occurred during pregnancy, childbirth, or within 42 days of termination of pregnancy"
    d. "A woman who nearly died but required ICU admission for >2 weeks due to a complication that occurred during pregnancy, childbirth, or within 42 days of termination of pregnancy"

17. Basic emergency obstetric services include all, *except:*
    a. Parenteral oxytocics
    b. Antibiotics and anticonvulsants
    c. Manual extraction of the placenta
    d. Blood transfusions

18. Perinatal mortality is defined as:
    a. Deaths of fetuses weighing 700 g or more at birth who die before or during delivery or within the first 10 days of delivery
    b. Deaths of fetuses weighing 1,000 g or more at birth who die before or during delivery or within the first 14 days of delivery
    c. Deaths of fetuses weighing 500 g or more at birth (28 weeks' gestation) who die before or during delivery or within the first 7 days of delivery
    d. Deaths among fetuses weighing 1,000 g or more at birth (28 weeks' gestation) and who die before or during delivery or within the first 7 days of delivery

19. Which among the following is not an epidemiological determinant of perinatal mortality?
    a. Age over 30 years and teenagers
    b. Parity above 5
    c. Low socioeconomic condition
    d. Poor maternal nutritional status

20. All are done in active management of third stage of labor, *except:*
    a. Early cord clamping
    b. Injection oxytocin at delivery of anterior shoulder
    c. Fundal massage
    d. Controlled cord traction

21. Weight of the fetus around 22nd week of gestation is around?
    a. 500 g   b. 750 g
    c. 625 g   d. 900 g

22. FIGO recommended dose of misoprostol for PPH prevention is:
    a. 600 µg orally   b. 600 µg sublingual
    c. 800 µg orally   d. 800 µg rectally

23. Stillbirth is defined as:
a. A stillbirth is the birth of a newborn after 22nd completed week (weighing 1,000 g or more) when the baby does not breathe or show any sign of life after delivery
b. A stillbirth is the birth of a newborn after 28th completed week (weighing 1,000 g or more) when the baby does not breathe or show any sign of life after delivery
c. A stillbirth is the birth of a newborn after 28th completed week (weighing 500 g or more) when the baby does not breathe or show any sign of life after delivery
d. A stillbirth is the birth of a newborn after 24th completed week (weighing 500 g or more) when the baby does not breathe or show any sign of life after delivery

24. Neonatal death is defined as:
a. Neonatal death is the death of the infant within 14 days after birth. Neonatal mortality rate is the number of such deaths per 1,000 live births
b. Neonatal death is the death of the infant within 28 days after birth. Neonatal mortality rate is the number of such deaths per 100 live births
c. Neonatal death is the death of the infant within 28 days after birth. Neonatal mortality rate is the number of such deaths per 1,000 live births
d. Neonatal death is the death of the infant within 48 days after birth. Neonatal mortality rate is the number of such deaths per 1,000 live births

25. Sustainable Development Goal (SDG) target is to achieve MMR of __ by 2030.
a. 60
b. 80
c. 70
d. 90

26. The key five strategies toward ending preventable maternal mortality by 2030 are all, *except*:
a. To address inequities in access to quality of sexual, maternal, reproductive, and newborn healthcare facilities
b. To ensure universal and comprehensive healthcare for sexual, maternal, reproductive, and newborn health
c. To strengthen health system for the needs and priorities of women and girls
d. To ensure efficient and robust data is available for obstetrics and maternal healthcare

27. Half-life of IV oxytocin is:
a. 3 minutes
b. 30 minutes
c. 3 hours
d. 45–60 minutes

28. 41 weeks, primigravida, presents with features of obstructed labor. Management includes all, *except*:
a. IV fluids
b. Oxytocin
c. Antibiotics
d. Lower (uterine) segment cesarean section (LSCS)

29. A 28-year-old primigravida with 33 weeks of pregnancy suddenly complains of headache, oliguria, and blurred vision. Her BP is 180/110 mm Hg and urine albumin is +3. The line of further management is:
a. Wait and watch
b. Labetelol and LSCS
c. $MgSO_4$, labetelol, and induction of labor
d. $MgSO_4$, labetelol, and deliver at 37 weeks

30. A 35-year-old female comes with obstructed labor and is febrile and dehydrated with intrauterine fetal demise (IUFD) and cephalic presentation. Which is the best way to manage?
a. Craniotomy
b. Decapitation
c. Cesarean section
d. Forceps extraction

ANSWERS

1. **b.** Safe motherhood initiative (SMI) is a global effort, and it is designed to operate through partners: (a) Government agencies, (b) Nongovernment agencies, and (c) Other groups and individuals. Safe motherhood initiative aims to improve women's health through social, community, and economic interventions.

2. **a.** Experts from WHO, UNFPA, UNICEF, IPPFF, the World Bank, the population council, and other national and international agencies concerned with safe motherhood concluded that it is possible to reduce maternal mortality significantly with limited investment and effective policy interventions. According to national and international human rights treaties (1948), safe motherhood is considered as a human rights issue. Therefore, it is considered that maternal death is the reflexion of "social disadvantage" not merely a "health disadvantage".

3. **a.** Lifetime risk is defined as the probability of dying of a woman in her reproductive age (15–49 years) due to causes in pregnancy, childbirth, or within 6 weeks of childbirth. In India, presently it is 0.3%.

4. **b.** To improve the maternal mortality situation in India, all the states have been categorized into groups: (A) Empowered Action Group (EAG). The states in this group are Bihar, Jharkhand, Madhya Pradesh, Chhattisgarh, Orissa, Rajasthan, Uttar Pradesh, Uttarakhand, and Assam. (B) Southern states: Andhra Pradesh, Karnataka, Kerala, Tamil Nadu, and (C) Other states.

5. **b.** *The aims of RCH care are:* (i) Safe motherhood, (ii) Child survival, (iii) Adolescent health, (iv) Family planning, and (v) Prevention and management of infections [STI/reproductive tract infection (RTI)]. New initiatives have been taken by the Government of India [The National Rural Health Mission (NRHM), 2005] to improve RCH care. Partnership for maternal, newborn, and child health (PMNCH) was initiated to reach the Millennium Development Goals 4 and 5.

   The new initiatives include: (a) To provide basic and comprehensive emergency obstetric care (EmOc) and essential newborn care, (b) To strengthen and to make all primary healthcare centers (PHCs), the community health centers (CHCs), and first referral units (FRUs) operational as 24 hours delivery centers in a phased manner.

6. **d.** Clean birth and postnatal care practices according to the World Health Organization's (WHO) "six cleans" are:
   1. Handwashing of birth attendant
   2. Clean birth surface
   3. Clean perineum
   4. Cutting of the umbilical cord using a clean instrument
   5. Clean cord tie, and
   6. Clean cloth for drying

7. **c.** India has improved its maternal mortality ratio (MMR)—number of deaths per 100,000 live births—to 97 deaths per lakh in 2018–2020 from 103 deaths per lakh in 2017–2019.

8. **d.** Life-saving drugs are misoprostol [prevention of postpartum hemorrhage (PPH)], injection oxytocin, (Management of PPH), injection $MgSO_4$ (eclampsia), ampicillin, metronidazole (infection), and the life-saving interventions are: Digital removal of products of conception (incomplete abortion with bleeding), active management of third stage of labor, maintaining a partograph.

9. **b.** Death of a woman while pregnant or within 42 days of the termination of pregnancy irrespective of the duration and the site of pregnancy, from any cause related to or aggravated by the pregnancy or its management but not from accidental or incidental causes.

10. **a.** Unregulated fertility, unsafe abortion, inadequate antenatal care, and lack of trained birth attendants are mainly recognized as the factors responsible for high maternal and perinatal deaths in the developing countries.

11. **d**

12. **c.** Anemia is the most common indirect cause of maternal mortality.
    Hemorrhage is the most common direct cause.

13. **a.** Hemorrhage (mostly due to PPH) is the most common cause of maternal mortality.
    Proven interventions include:
    - Skilled attendant at birth
    - Treating anemia in pregnancy
    - Use of oxytocics in time
    - Blood transfusion, if severe hemorrhage
    - Replace fluid loss

14. **d.** Anemia is the most common indirect cause of maternal mortality.
    Effective interventions include: Routine iron and folic acid supplementation during gestation, deworming (for hookworm), treating malaria, human immuno-deficiency virus (HIV) and admit if Hb <7 g/dL.

15. **c.** 4 hours
    Partogram is a composite graphical record of key data (maternal and fetal) entered against time on a single sheet of paper, during labor.
    It provides an accurate record of the progress of labor, and any delay or deviation from normal may be detected quickly and treated accordingly. It was first devised by Freidman in 1954.

    Components:
    - *Patient's identification:* Name, gravida, and parity
    - *Time:* Recorded at an interval of 1 hour. Zero time for spontaneous labor is the time of admission in

the labor ward, and for induced labor it is the time of induction.
- *Fetal heart rate:* Recorded every 30 minutes.
- *Membranes and color of liquor:* "I" designates intact membranes, "C" designates clear, and "M" designates meconium-stained liquor.
- Cervical dilatation and descent of head
- *Uterine contractions:* Squares in vertical columns are shaded according to intensity and duration.
- Drugs and fluids given to patient in labor
- Blood pressure
- Pulse rate
- *Oxytocin:* If it is used, then concentration (U/L) is noted down in the upper box, whereas dose (drops/minute) is noted in the lower box.
- Urine analysis
- Temperature record

The concept of "alert line" and "action line" was introduced by Philpott and Castle in 1972.

The action line can be placed at 2–4 hours gap to the right and parallel to alert line.

In partograms recommended by the "WHO", the distance between the alert and action lines is 4 hours.

(Reference: DC Dutta's Textbook of Gynecology, 7th Edition, page 531).

16. **a.** *Maternal Near Miss (MNM):* Women who experienced and survived a severe health condition during pregnancy, childbirth, or postpartum are considered as maternal near miss or severe acute maternal morbidity (SAMM) cases. Maternal near miss is defined as: "A woman who nearly died but survived a complication that occurred during pregnancy, childbirth, or within 42 days of termination of pregnancy" (WHO). MNM incidence ratio (MNMIR) refers to the number of maternal near miss cases per 1,000 live births (MNM IR = MNM/1,000 LB).

17. **d.** Blood transfusions

Basic emergency obstetric services include:
- Parenteral oxytocics
- Antibiotics and anticonvulsants
- Assisted deliveries
- Manual extraction of the placenta
- Removal of retained products

Comprehensive emergency obstetric services include:
- Basic services
- Cesarean sections
- Blood transfusions

(Reference: WHO Bulletin)

18. **d.** Perinatal mortality is defined as deaths among fetuses weighing 1,000 g or more at birth (28 weeks' gestation) who die before or during delivery or within the first 7 days of delivery.

19. **a.** *Epidemiological determinants of perinatal mortality are:* Age over 35 years, teenagers, parity above 5, low socioeconomic condition, and poor maternal nutritional status.

20. **a.** Early cord clamping

Active management of the third stage of labor (AMTSL): Current evidence indicates AMTSL (administration of uterotonic drugs, controlled cord traction, and fundal massage after delivery of the placenta) can reduce the incidence of PPH by up to 60%.

WHO recommends that "Clamp and cut the cord following strict hygienic techniques after cord pulsations have ceased or approximately 2–3 minutes after birth of the baby, whichever comes first".

Delay in clamping for 2–3 minutes or till cessation of the cord pulsation facilitates transfer of 80–100 mL of blood from the compressed placenta to a baby, when placed below the level of uterus. But, early clamping should be done in cases of Rh incompatibility (to prevent transfer of antibodies from the mother to the baby) or babies born asphyxiated.

21. **a.** Weight of the fetus around 22 weeks is about 500 g, 1 kg at 28 weeks, and 2.5 kg at 37 weeks.

22. **a.** 600 µg orally

Students to read the question carefully as dose and route for prevention and treatment of PPH are different.

WHO and FIGO independently conducted extensive expert reviews of the scientific data and concluded that misoprostol is a safe and effective therapy for the prevention of PPH when oxytocin is not available or cannot be used.

In 2012, FIGO finalized guidelines on the prevention and treatment of PPH with misoprostol. The guidelines include evidence-based recommendations.

For PPH, prophylaxis recommended dose is 600 µg orally, single dose.

For PPH, treatment recommended dose is 800 µg sublingual, single dose.

(Reference: FIGO Guidelines.)

23. **b.** A stillbirth is the birth of a newborn after 28th completed week (weighing 1000 g or more) when the baby does not breathe or show any sign of life after delivery. It includes macerated and fresh stillbirths.
24. **c.** Neonatal death is the death of the infant within 28 days after birth. Neonatal mortality rate is the number of such deaths per 1,000 live births.

    About two-thirds of neonatal deaths are related to prematurity.
25. c
26. **d.**

    The key five strategies toward ending preventable maternal mortality by 2030 are all:
    1. To address inequities in access to quality of sexual, maternal, reproductive, and newborn healthcare facilities
    2. To ensure universal and comprehensive healthcare for sexual, maternal, reproductive, and newborn health
    3. To strengthen health system for the needs and priorities of women and girls
    4. To address all causes of maternal mortality, morbidities, and related disabilities
    5. To ensure accountability to improve quality care and equity
27. **a.** 3 minutes

    As per the WHO and the ACOG guidelines, oxytocin is the first-line DOC for atonic PPH.

    Rapid and continuous infusion of dilute IV oxytocin (40–80 U) in 1 L NS should be started.
    - An IV bolus of 10 units of oxytocin causes a transient but marked fall in arterial BP that is followed by an abrupt increase in cardiac output.

    Hence, it should not be given intravenously as a large bolus, but rather as a much more dilute solution by continuous IV infusion or as an intramuscular injection.
    - The half-life of intravenously infused oxytocin is approximately 3 minutes. Prolonged oxytocin administration can cause water intoxication because of its antidiuretic action.

    (Reference: Williams Obstetrics, 24th Edition, page 785).
28. **b.** Oxytocin use

    Two main principles in management of obstructed labor are:
    1. Never wait and watch and
    2. Never use oxytocin.

    In patients of obstructed labor, the uterine contractions (power) are always adequate or even more.

    By increasing the power (by giving oxytocin), there is risk of rupture uterus.

    Uterus is already contracting, and so there is no point in increasing the contractions further in a case of obstructed labor.

    The patient should be given IV fluids to correct the dehydration and ketoacidosis. Patient should be given antibiotics to prevent infection, and then steps should be taken to immediately relieve the obstruction either by instrumental deliver or by LSCS.

    (Reference: Williams Obstetrics, 22nd Edition, pages 608, 613, and 826)
29. **c.** $MgSO_4$, labetelol, and induction of labor

    The patient is a case of severe preeclampsia with impending eclampsia.

    The dangerous symptoms that indicate impending eclampsia in case of preeclampsia are:
    - Headache
    - Oliguria
    - Epigastric pain
    - Nausea and vomiting
    - Blurring of vision

    Whenever the above symptoms develop in a case of severe preeclampsia the patient is at a risk of eclampsia; the patient should first be given anticonvulsant ($MgSO_4$) and antihypertensive medication, and the pregnancy should then be terminated by induction of labor irrespective of the weeks of gestation (delivery is the definitive treatment).
    - Magnesium sulfate is the drug of choice for eclampsia and also for impending eclampsia.
    - Prophylactic magnesium sulfate decreases the risk of convulsion, abruption, and maternal mortality in this scenario.
    - Labetalol is the DOC for hypertensive crisis followed by hydralazine.
    - Never wait and watch in case of impending eclampsia and never directly proceed for LSCS as it can be fatal for the mother.

    Vaginal delivery is safest for mother, and hence labor should be induced after stabilization of mother (after $MgSO_4$ and antihypertensive medications).

If after induction of labor there is fetal distress or failure of induction, then LSCS can be done. The indications for termination of pregnancy (irrespective of the weeks of gestation) in a case of preeclampsia are:
- Severe preeclampsia with impending eclampsia
- Eclampsia (give $MgSO_4$ first, followed by induction of labor)
- Hemolysis, elevated liver enzymes, low platelet count (HELLP) syndrome

(Reference: Williams Obstetrics, 24th Edition, pages 750, 764-65.)

30. c. Cesarean section

Two main principles in the management of obstructed labor are:
1. Never wait and watch
2. Never use oxytocin

In patients of obstructed labor, the uterine contractions (power) are always adequate.

The patient should be given IV fluids to correct the dehydration and ketoacidosis, which usually develop due to prolonged labor. Patient should be given antibiotics to prevent infection and then steps should be taken to immediately relieve the obstruction by LSCS.
- LSCS may have to be done (even if the baby is dead) if vaginal delivery is not possible, or else, rupture uterus will occur.
- In modern-day obstetrics, destructive operations (decapitation, craniotomy, evisceration, etc.) are never to be performed as they are more dangerous and can lead to complications like rupture uterus and bladder injury.
- LSCS is much safer than destructive operations.

Chapter 3: Placenta and Fetal Membranes

Bhumika Kotecha Mundhe

QUESTIONS

1. **Placenta has following functions, *except*:**
   a. Physiological
   b. Immunological
   c. Metabolic
   d. Endocrinal

2. **Based on the histology, human placenta is:**
   a. Endotheliochorial
   b. Hemochorial
   c. Epitheliochorial
   d. None of the above

3. **Human placenta is derived from:**
   a. Allantois
   b. Chorion
   c. Amnion
   d. Chorion and allantois

4. **Human chorionic gonadotropin (hCG) was secreted by:**
   a. Syncytiotrophoblast
   b. Cytotrophoblast
   c. Extraembryonic mesoderm
   d. None of the above

5. **Primary villi formed from:**
   a. Syncytiotrophoblast
   b. Cytotrophoblast
   c. Extraembryonic mesoderm
   d. Allantois

6. **hCG produced by the syncytiotrophoblast is detected in maternal blood and urine by as early as _____ day pregnancy**
   a. 5th day
   b. 4th day
   c. 10th day
   d. 3rd day

7. **Extra-embryonic mesoderm is between all of the following, *except*:**
   a. Cytotrophoblast
   b. Syncytiotrophoblast
   c. Amnion
   d. Yolk sac

8. **The yolk sac is covered by the following:**
   a. Extraembryonic somatic mesoderm
   b. Extraembryonic visceral mesoderm
   c. Amnion
   d. Cytotrophoblast

9. **The connecting stalk which is the primordium of the umbilical cord is formed by _____**
   a. Amnion
   b. Syncytiotrophoblast
   c. Extraembryonic visceral mesoderm
   d. Extraembryonic somatic mesoderm

10. **Fetal circulation flows from the fetus to maternal end is via:**
    a. Two umbilical arteries (deoxygenated) and single umbilical vein (oxygenated)
    b. One umbilical artery (oxygenated) and one umbilical vein (deoxygenated)
    c. Two umbilical arteries (oxygenated) and single umbilical vein (deoxygenated)
    d. One umbilical artery (deoxygenated) and one umbilical vein (oxygenated)

11. **The types of cord insertion are:**
    a. *Four types:* Central, eccentric, marginal, and velamentous
    b. *Three types:* Central, marginal, and velamentous
    c. *Four types:* Central, marginal, velamentous, and lateral
    d. *Three types:* Central, eccentric, and velamentous

12. **Eccentric location of cord insertion which is usually not of grave concern is:**
    a. >2 cm from the placental margin
    b. <2 cm from the placental margin
    c. >3 cm from the placental margin
    d. <3 cm from the placental margin

13. **The most hazardous type of cord insertion:**
    a. Marginal cord insertion/Battledore placenta
    b. Velamentous cord insertion
    c. Eccentric cord insertion
    d. Central cord insertion

14. The three shunts of the fetomaternal circulation are all, *except*:
    a. Ductus arteriosus
    b. Foramen magnum
    c. Ductus venosus
    d. Foramen ovale

15. The following are the possible types of twin pregnancy, *except*:
    a. Dichorionic diamniotic pregnancy
    b. Monochorionic diamniotic pregnancy
    c. Monochorionic monoamniotic pregnancy
    d. Dichorionic monoamniotic pregnancy

16. Which one of the following decidua fuses to obliterate the uterine cavity?
    a. Decidua basalis and decidua parietalis
    b. Decidua parietalis and decidua capsularis
    c. Decidua capsularis and decidua basalis
    d. Decidua parietalis and decidua myometria

17. The amnion has the following functions:
    a. It protects the fetus physically
    b. It provides room for fetal movements
    c. It helps to regulate fetal body temperature
    d. All of the above

18. Which of the following statements about the amniotic fluid are true?
    a. Produced by dialysis of fetal and maternal blood
    b. Later-fetal urination contributes to the volume of amniotic fluid
    c. Fetal swallowing decreases the volume of amniotic fluid
    d. All of the above

19. Choriocarcinoma is a malignant tumor arising from the following:
    a. Normal pregnancy
    b. Blighted ovum
    c. Hydatiform mole
    d. All of the above

20. Which of the following cross fetoplacental barrier, *except*?
    a. Steroidal hormones
    b. Bacteria and viruses
    c. Free fatty acids
    d. Vitamins

21. Which of the following abnormality is associated with oligohydramnios?
    a. Potter syndrome
    b. Microcephaly
    c. Annular pancreas
    d. Esophageal atresia

22. The spectrum of morbidly adherent placenta includes all, *except*:
    a. Placenta accreta
    b. Placenta previa
    c. Placenta increta
    d. Placenta percreta

23. The types of placenta previa are:
    a. Marginal placenta, complete placenta previa, and partial placenta previa
    b. Low-lying placenta previa, complete placenta previa, and partial placenta previa
    c. Marginal placenta, complete placenta previa, partial placenta previa, low-lying placenta previa
    d. Complete placenta previa, partial placenta previa, and low-lying placenta previa

24. Association of vasa previa with:
    a. Velamentous cord insertion
    b. Vessels crossing between lobes in succenturiate or bilobate placentas
    c. Both of the above
    d. None of the above

25. The structural abnormalities of placenta include:
    a. Bilobed/Multilobed placenta
    b. Circumvallate placenta
    c. Placenta membranacea
    d. Succenturiate placenta
    e. All of the above

26. This placental anomaly may be mistaken for partial hydatiform mole:
    a. Circumvallate placenta
    b. Placental chorioangioma
    c. Placental mesenchymal dysplasia
    d. None of the above

27. Placental infection can be due to which of the following infective agents?
    a. *Cytomegalovirus*
    b. Toxoplasmosis
    c. *Listeria monocytogenes*
    d. All of the above

28. Morphologically placenta is:
    a. 20–22 cm in diameter, 2–2.5 cm thick and weighs about one-sixth of fetal birthweight
    b. 20–22 cm in diameter, 4–5 cm thick and weighs about one-sixth of fetal birthweight
    c. 30–40 cm in diameter, 2–2.5 cm thick and weighs about one-sixth of fetal birthweight
    d. 20–22 cm in diameter, 2–2.5 cm thick and weighs about one-tenth of fetal birthweight

29. The placental abnormalities can be:
    a. Structural abnormalities
    b. Infectious abnormalities
    c. Abnormal implantation abnormalities
    d. All of the above

30. **Which of the following are acellular?**
    a. Syncytiotrophoblast   b. Cytotrophoblast
    c. Both   d. None of the above

ANSWERS

1. **c.** Metabolic
   It helps in physiological exchange of gases and nutrients between the maternal and fetal tissues. It avoids fetal allograft rejection on immunological basis. It secretes various hormones important for the maintenance of pregnancy.[1]

2. **b.** Hemochorial
   Epitheliochorial type: Superficial one, no significant invasion of uterine lining, trophoblasts loosely attached to the epithelium of the uterine lining.
   Endotheliochorial type: Fetal trophoblasts come in contact with the maternal endometrium.
   Hemochorial type: Most invasive type, all maternal tissue layers disappear with implantation and maternal blood in contact with fetal trophoblasts.[2]

3. **b.** Chorion
   Human placenta is derived from chorion. However, amniotic sac is formed by chorion and amnion.[1]

4. **a.** Syncytiotrophoblast
   The syncytiotrophoblast produces hCG whereas the cytotrophoblast produces hormones that allow penetration of cytotrophoblasts.[3]

5. **b.** Cytotrophoblast
   Placenta consists of the syncytiotrophoblast, cytotrophoblast, and extraembryonic mesoderm. The cytotrophoblast extends into the syncytiotrophoblast as finger-like projections which are called the primary chorionic villi. The extraembryonic mesoderm divides into somatic and splanchnic mesoderm, of which the somatic mesoderm grows into the primary villi creating the secondary villi. The mesenchyme gives rise to blood cells and vessels, which is tertiary villi.[4]

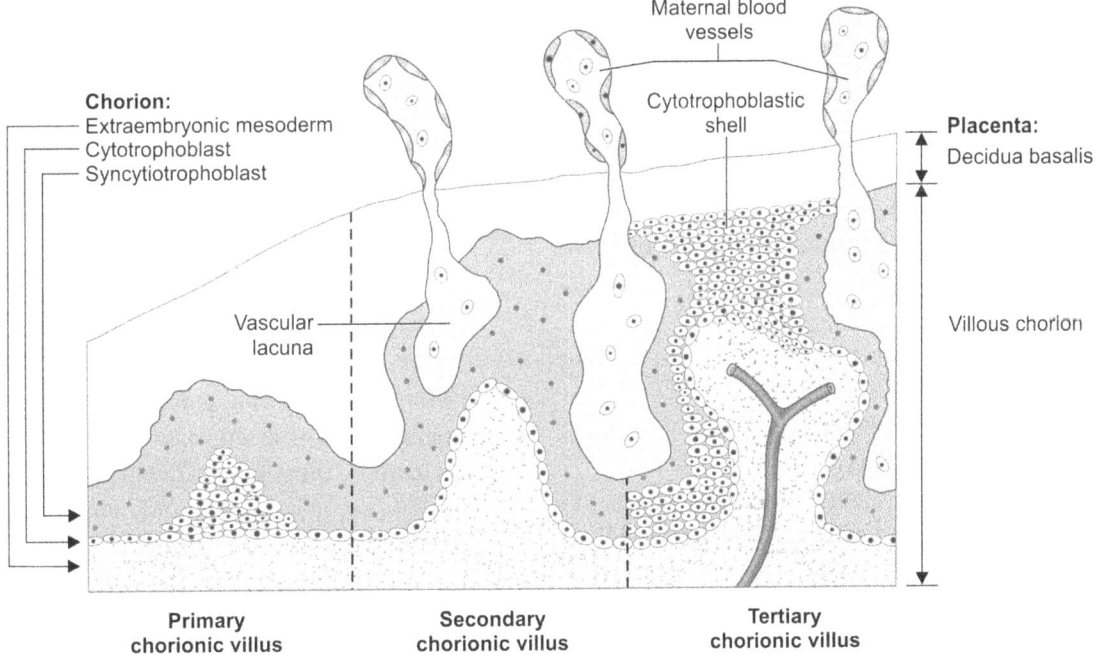

6. **c.** 10th day
   hCG in maternal blood and urine which is the basis of pregnancy tests can be detected as early as 10th day of pregnancy.[5]

7. **b.** Syncytiotrophoblast

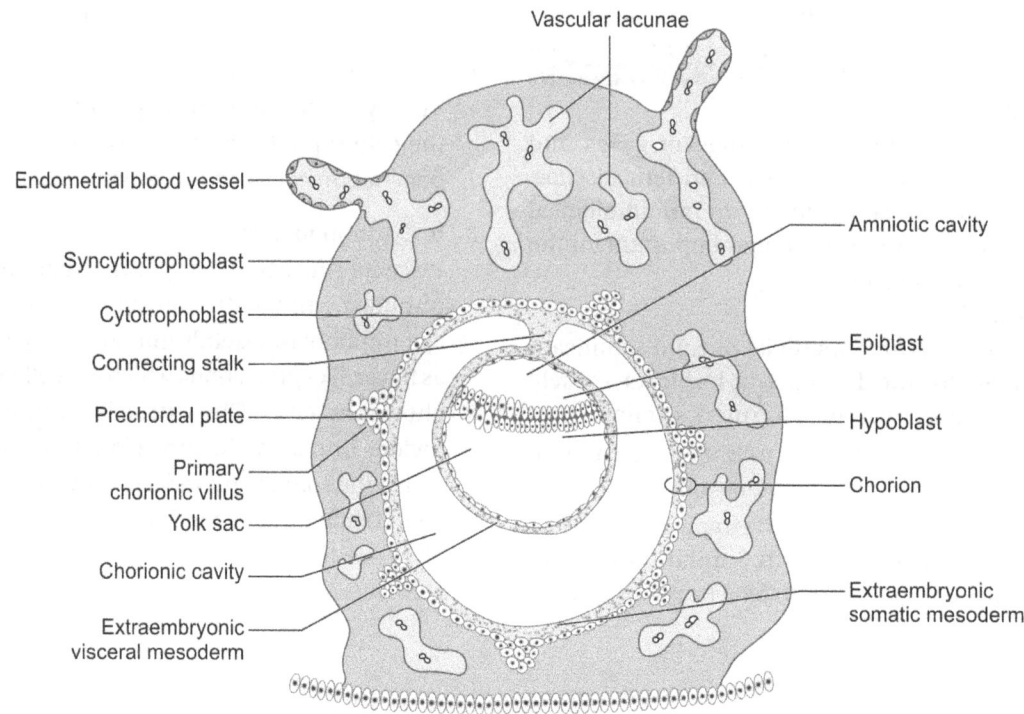

Diagram: Day 14 blastocyst showing structure of the placenta.
Extraembryonic mesoderm is between cytotrophoblast, amnion, and yolk sac.[5]

8. **b.** Extraembryonic visceral mesoderm
Extraembryonic visceral mesoderm covers the yolk sac.[5]

9. **d.** Extraembryonic somatic mesoderm
Extraembryonic somatic mesoderm forms the umbilical cord.[5]

10. **a.** Two umbilical arteries (deoxygenated) and single umbilical vein (oxygenated)
Fetal circulation starts with blood flow from the fetus via two umbilical arteries (deoxygenated) to chorionic arteries in the cotyledons. With exchange of gases, with the maternal blood occurring at the level of capillary bed. A single umbilical vein (oxygenated) carries blood back to the fetus.[4]

11. **a.** *Four types:* Central, eccentric, marginal, and velamentous
There are four main types of cord insertion. They are central, marginal, velamentous, and eccentric types of cord insertion.[6]

12. **a.** >2 cm from the placental margin
Eccentric cord insertion is the type where the cord is inserted >2 cm from the placental margin and is usually of no much harm to the mother or fetus.[6]

13. **b.** Velamentous cord insertion
In velamentous cord insertion, the umbilical cord inserts into the amniotic sac. It occurs in 5.4% of pregnancies. It is most dangerous due to its connection with vasa previa. In case of velamentous cord insertion not being diagnosed antenatally and patient being delivered vaginally may land into vasa previa where the vessels of the umbilical cord into the amniotic sac may rupture and patient may land into bleeding from both maternal and fetal side.[7]

14. **b.** Foramen magnum
The ductus venosus helps which allows blood from the placenta to bypass the liver, and the ductus arteriosus and foramen ovale, which together allow blood to bypass the developing lungs.[4]

15. **d.** Dichorionic monoamniotic pregnancy
Determination of zygosity, chorionicity, and amniosity

Zygosity: It estimates the genetic origin of the twin. It is of two types: Dizygotic and monozygotic.

Dizygotic twins: Each of the twin has originated from a separate oocyte and a separate spermatocyte. It is always in a dichorionic diamniotic pregnancy.

Monozygotic twins: A single zygote will undergo cleavage and form two embryos. Depending on the timing of cleavage, its chorionicity and amniosity are determined.[8]

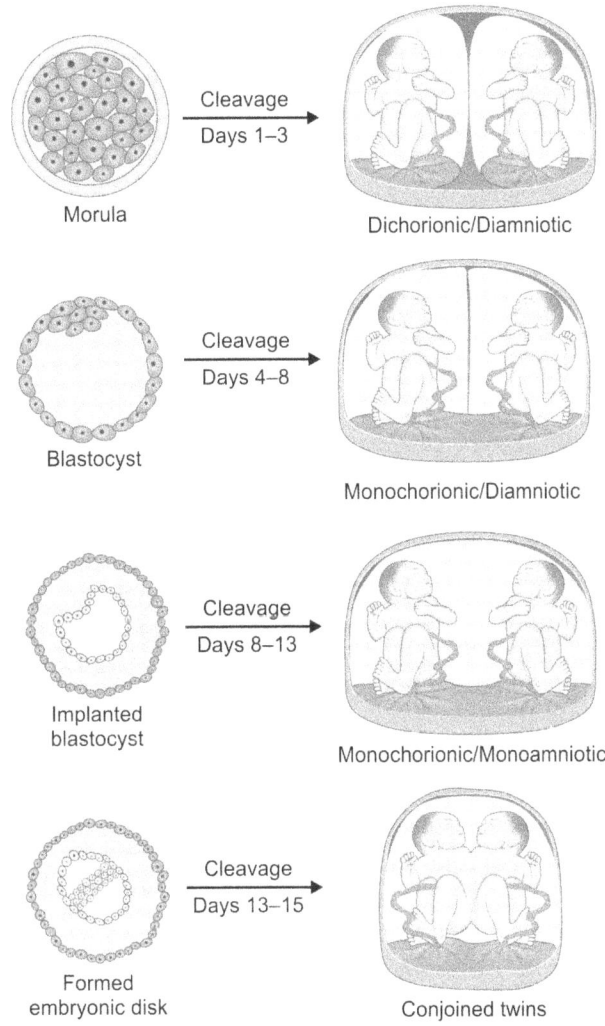

Diagram representing chorionicity and amniosity of a twin gestation.[8]

16. **b.** Decidua parietalis and decidua capsularis

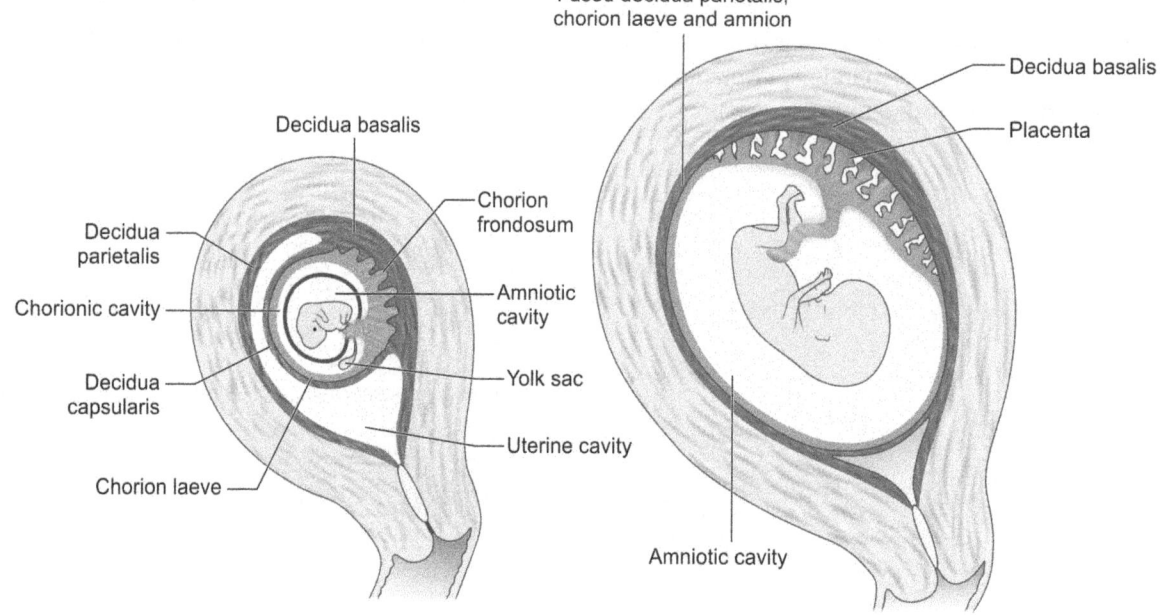

As the fetus enlarges the decidua capsularis fuses with the decidua parietalis and obliterates the uterine cavity.[4]

17. **d.** All of the above
The amnion helps by physical protection to the fetus, room for fetal movements, and fetal temperature regulation.[4]

18. **d.** All of the above
The amniotic fluid is produced by dialysis of fetal and maternal blood. As the fetal developmental process progresses, the fetal urination contributes to the volume of amniotic fluid. The fetus swallows the amniotic fluid and may contribute to its reduction.

19. **d.** All of the above
Choriocarcinoma is a malignant tumor which may arise from normal pregnancy, blighted ovum, and hydatiform mole.

20. **d.** Vitamins
Substances that cross fetoplacental barrier.[4]

Beneficial	
Gases	Oxygen and carbon dioxide
Nutrients	Glucose, amino acids, free fatty acids, and vitamins
Metabolites	Carbon dioxide, urea, uric acid, bilirubin, creatine, and creatinine

Contd...

Electrolytes	Na^+, K^+, Cl^-, Ca^{2+}, PO_4^{2-}
Erythrocytes	Fetal and maternal both (a few)
Maternal serum proteins	Serum albumin, some protein hormones (thyroxin and insulin)
Steroid hormones	Cortisol and estrogen (unconjugated only)
Immunoglobins	IgG (confers fetal passive immunity)
Harmful	
Poisonous gases	Carbon monoxide
Infectious agents	Viruses (HIV, *Cytomegalovirus*, rubella, coxsackie, variola, varicella, measles, and poliomyelitis), bacteria (tuberculosis and treponema), and protozoa (Toxoplasma)
Drugs	Cocaine, alcohol, caffeine, nicotine, warfarin, trimetadione, phenytoin, tetracycline, cancer chemotherapeutic agents, anesthetics, sedatives, and analgesics
Immunoglobins	Anti-Rh antibodies

21. **a.** Potter syndrome
Potter syndrome is a congenital anomaly associated with renal agenesis. This condition is incompatible with life as these fetuses have pulmonary hypoplasia. Potter sequence and Otter syndrome are interchangeably used terminologies with similar consequences.[9]

22. **b.** Placenta previa
    Morbidly adherent placenta or abnormally invasive placenta includes three types as follows:
    1. *Placenta accreta:* Placenta villi attach to myometrium.
    2. *Placenta increta:* Placenta villi penetrate the myometrium.
    3. *Placenta percreta:* Placental villi extend up to uterine serosa and/or adjacent organs.

    However, placenta previa is a condition where the placenta is overlying the internal cervical os.[10]

23. **c.** Marginal placenta, complete placenta previa, partial placenta previa, and low-lying placenta previa
    - *Marginal placenta previa:* Placenta edge close to the edge of the cervical os.
    - *Complete placenta previa:* Placenta covering the internal os of the cervix.
    - *Partial placenta previa:* Placenta partially covering the internal os of the cervix.
    - *Low-lying placenta previa:* Placental edge is within 2 cm from the edge of the cervical os.[10]

24. **c.** Both of the above
    A few recent reports have concluded a strong association between velamentous cord insertion and vessels crossing between lobes in succenturiate or bilobate placentas.[10]

25. **e.** All of the above
    Bilobed/Multilobed placenta: Placenta separated into two or more lobes with membranes in between
    Circumvallate placenta: Annular placenta with raised edges
    Placenta membranacea: Thin structure occupying the entire chorion periphery
    Succenturiate placenta: A small accessory placenta develops in the membranes.[10]

26. **c.** Placental mesenchymal dysplasia
    Placental mesenchymal dysplasia: Rare vascular anomaly with hyperplasia of mesenchymal stem villous.
    Placental chorioangioma: Benign vascular tumor, malformation of primitive tissue of placenta perfused with fetal circulation.[10]

27. **d.** All of the above
    Placental infections can be because of following infections: Malaria, *Cytomegalovirus,* herpes simplex virus, *Listeria monocytogenes,* streptococcal infection, syphilis, toxoplasmosis, and *Chlamydia psittaci*.[10]

28. **a.** 20–22 cm in diameter, 2–2.5 cm thick and weighs about one-sixth of fetal birthweight
    The human placenta is a round- or oval-shaped organ and is roughly 22 cm in diameter. It is about 2–2.5 cm thick and weighs about one-sixth of the fetal birthweight.[10]

29. **d.** All of the above
    The placental abnormalities can be structural, vascular, infectious, functional and abnormal implantation.[10]

30. **a.** Syncytiotrophoblast
    Syncytiotrophoblast is acellular and does not expand mitotically.
    Cytotrophoblast is cellular and expands mitotically into the syncytiotrophoblast to form primary chorionic villi.[5]

REFERENCES

1. Ahokas R, McKinney ET. Development and Physiology of the Placenta and Membranes. Glob Libr Women Med. 2008.
2. Herrick EJ, Bordoni B. Embryology, Placenta. Treasure Island (FL): StatPearls Publishing; 2023.
3. Cole LA. Biological functions of hCG and hCG-related molecules. Reprod Biol Endocrinol. 2010;8:102.
4. University of Michigan Medical School. (2000). Placenta and extraembryonic membranes. [online] Available from: https://www.med.umich.edu/lrc/coursepages/m1/embryology/embryo/06placenta.htm [Last accessed December, 2023].
5. University of Michigan Medical School. (2000). Second week (Days 8-14). [online] Available from: https://www.med.umich.edu/lrc/coursepages/m1/embryology/embryo/04secondweek.htm. [Last accessed December, 2023].
6. Radiopedia.org. (2021). Variation in cord insertion. [online] Available from https://radiopaedia.org/articles/variation-in-cord-insertion [Last accessed December, 2023].
7. Birth Injury Help Center. (2023). Velamentous cord insertion. [online] Available from: https://www.birthinjuryhelpcenter.org/abnormal-cord-insertion.html [Last accessed December, 2023].
8. OBG Project for Physicians, by Physicians™. (2019). Twin pregnancy: Ultrasound Evaluation and Monitoring. [online] Available from: https://www.obgproject.com/2019/06/12/uncomplicated-twin-pregnancy-ultrasound-evaluation-and-monitoring/ [Last accessed December, 2023].
9. Bhandari J, Thada PK, Sergent SR. Potter's Syndrome. Treasure Island (FL): StatPearls Publishing; 2023.
10. Drăgușin RC, Șorop-Florea M, Pătru CL, Zorilă L, Marinaș C, Șorop BV, et al. (2018). Abnormalities of placenta. [online] Available from: https://www.researchgate.net/publication/324914739_Abnormalities_of_the_Placenta. [Last accessed December, 2023].

Chapter 4

Physiological Changes during Pregnancy

Kalpana Kumari, Shilpi Srivastava

QUESTIONS

1. Which one of the following hormonal changes occurs during pregnancy?
   a. Decreased levels of human chorionic gonadotropin (hCG)
   b. Increased levels of estrogen and progesterone
   c. Decreased levels of prolactin
   d. Increased levels of thyroid-stimulating hormone (TSH)

2. Which one of the following endocrine glands enlarges during pregnancy?
   a. Adrenal glands
   b. Pituitary gland
   c. Thyroid gland
   d. Pancreas

3. What is the primary hormone responsible for maintaining the uterine lining during pregnancy?
   a. Human chorionic gonadotropin (hCG)
   b. Progesterone
   c. Follicle-stimulating hormone (FSH)
   d. Estrogen

4. What gastrointestinal symptom is commonly experienced during pregnancy?
   a. Increased appetite
   b. Constipation
   c. Decreased sense of taste
   d. Decreased saliva production

5. Which one of the following changes occurs in the immune system during pregnancy?
   a. Increased susceptibility to infections
   b. Decreased cellular immunity
   c. Decreased inflammatory response
   d. Increased autoimmune activity

6. Which one of the following changes occurs in the endocrine system during pregnancy?
   a. Decreased insulin production
   b. Increased cortisol levels
   c. Suppressed thyroid function
   d. Elevated parathyroid hormone levels

7. What is the term used to describe the increased pigmentation of the skin during pregnancy?
   a. Melanosis   b. Chloasma
   c. Erythema   d. Xerosis

8. Which one of the following changes occurs in the urinary system during pregnancy?
   a. Decreased kidney size
   b. Decreased glomerular filtration rate (GFR)
   c. Increased bladder capacity
   d. Decreased urine production

9. What is the hormone responsible for stimulating milk production after childbirth?
   a. Progesterone
   b. Estrogen
   c. Prolactin
   d. Oxytocin

10. Which one of the following changes occurs in the musculoskeletal system to accommodate the growing fetus?
    a. Increased joint stability
    b. Decreased muscle mass
    c. Increased spinal curvature
    d. Widening of the ribcage

11. Which one of the following changes occurs in the respiratory system during pregnancy?
    a. Decreased oxygen consumption
    b. Decreased residual volume
    c. Decreased respiratory rate
    d. Increased airway resistance

12. **Which one of the following changes occurs in the skin during pregnancy?**
    a. Increased oil production leading to dry skin
    b. Decreased melanin production leading to lighter complexion
    c. Increased pigmentation, especially in areas such as the abdomen and nipples
    d. Decreased blood flow to the skin resulting in paleness

13. **Which one of the following changes occurs in the urinary system during pregnancy?**
    a. Increased bladder capacity
    b. Increased renal blood flow
    c. Increased urine production
    d. Decreased sensitivity to antidiuretic hormone (ADH)

14. **Which one of the following changes occurs in the cardiovascular system during pregnancy?**
    a. Decreased blood volume
    b. Decreased cardiac output
    c. Decreased blood pressure
    d. Increased blood volume

15. **What is the hormone responsible for stimulating uterine contractions and milk ejection during breastfeeding?**
    a. Estrogen   b. Progesterone
    c. Oxytocin   d. Prolactin

16. **Which one of the following changes occurs in the gastrointestinal system during pregnancy?**
    a. Increased gastric acid secretion
    b. Decreased gastric motility
    c. Decreased appetite
    d. Decreased nutrient absorption

17. **Which one of the following changes occurs in the renal system during pregnancy?**
    a. Decreased glomerular filtration rate (GFR)
    b. Decreased urine production
    c. Decreased renal blood flow
    d. Increased sensitivity to antidiuretic hormone (ADH)

18. **Which one of the following changes occurs in the endocrine system during pregnancy?**
    a. Decreased thyroid hormone production
    b. Decreased insulin resistance
    c. Decreased adrenal gland activity
    d. Increased production of human placental lactogen (hPL)

19. **Which one of the following changes occurs in the hematological system during pregnancy?**
    a. Decreased blood volume
    b. Decreased red blood cell production
    c. Increased clotting factors
    d. Decreased white blood cell count

20. **Which one of the following changes occurs in the cardiovascular system during pregnancy?**
    a. Decreased cardiac output
    b. Increased blood pressure
    c. Decreased blood volume
    d. Increased heart rate

21. **Which one of the following changes occurs in the urinary system during pregnancy?**
    a. Decreased bladder capacity
    b. Decreased urine production
    c. Increased glomerular filtration rate (GFR)
    d. Decreased sensitivity to antidiuretic hormone (ADH)

22. **Which one of the following changes occurs in the hematological system during pregnancy?**
    a. Decreased blood clotting factors
    b. Increased red blood cell count
    c. Decreased platelet count
    d. Increased blood viscosity

23. **In pregnancy which parameter related to respiratory system among the following have no change?**
    a. Tidal volume
    b. Inspiratory reserve volume
    c. Vital capacity
    d. Total lung capacity

24. **What is the direction of shift of apex beat during pregnancy?**
    a. Up and Out   b. Up and In
    c. Down and Out   d. Down and In

25. **When is cardiac output maximum?**
    a. 32 weeks
    b. During second stage of labor
    c. Immediate postpartum
    d. After 1 hour post delivery

26. **When does cardiac output return to prelabor values?**
    a. 1 hour postpartum
    b. 6 hours postpartum
    c. 2 weeks postpartum
    d. 4 weeks postpartum

27. Which one of these findings in heartbeat is abnormal during pregnancy?
    a. Ejection systolic murmur
    b. Diastolic murmur
    c. S_3
    d. S_4

28. Values of which of the following coagulation factors do not change during pregnancy?
    a. Factor 11   b. Factor 10
    c. Factor 5   d. Factor 7

29. Which of the following factor has maximum rise in values during pregnancy?
    a. Factor 1   b. Factor 7
    c. Factor 10   d. Factor 8

ANSWERS

1. **b.** Both estrogen and progesterone increase significantly during pregnancy. Estradiol increases from nonpregnant values of 0.1–0.6 to 15–20 during pregnancy and progesterone increases from values of nonpregnant state, i.e., 0.1–40 to 250–600 during pregnancy.
   (Reference: Williams Obstetrics, 25th Edition, Chapter 5, page 98)

2. **c.** During pregnancy thyroid gland boosts production of thyroid hormones by 40–100% to meet maternal and fetal needs. To accomplish this, the thyroid gland undergoes moderate enlargement during pregnancy caused by glandular hyperplasia and greater vascularity.
   (Reference: Williams Obstetrics, 25th Edition, Chapter 4, page 69)

3. **b.** *(Reference: Williams Obstetrics, 25th Edition, Chapter 5, page 66)*

4. **b.** Due to lower peristalsis wave and increased gastric emptying time one may experience constipation during pregnancy and it may be so severe that it may lead to hemorrhoids.
   (Reference: Williams Obstetrics, 25th Edition, Chapter 4, page 68)

5. **b.** During pregnancy Th-1-mediated immunity shift to Th-2-mediated immunity. This suppressed Th-1 response is requisite for human pregnancy.
   (Reference: Williams Obstetrics, 25th Edition, Chapter 4, page 59)

6. **b.** The serum concentration of circulating cortisol rises during pregnancy but much of it is in bound by transcortin.
   (Reference: Williams Obstetrics, 25th Edition, Chapter 4, page 71)

7. **b.** During pregnancy there are irregular brownish patch of varying size on face and neck giving rise to chloasma or melasma gravidarum-the mask of pregnancy.
   (Reference: Williams Obstetrics, 25th Edition, Chapter 4, page 53)

8. **c.** Hyperplasia of bladder muscle and connective tissue elevate the trigone and thicken its intraureteric margin. Continuation of this process to term produces marked deepening and widening of trigone.
   (Reference: Williams Obstetrics, 25th Edition, Chapter 4, page 68)

9. **c.** With delivery, maternal serum levels of progesterone and estrogen decline abruptly and this drop removes the inhibitory influence of progesterone and this progesterone withdrawal allows prolactin to unopposed action in its stimulation of alpha lactoglobulin and milk production.
   (Reference: Williams Obstetrics, 25th Edition, Chapter 4, page 656)

10. **d.** During pregnancy subcostal angle widens from 68.5° to 103.5° at 37 weeks which results in increase in transverse diameter by 2 cm and increase in thoracic circumference by 6 cm.
    (Reference: Williams Obstetrics, 25th Edition, Chapter 4, page 64)

11. **b.** During pregnancy residual volume decreases by 20–25% or 200–400 mL.
    (Reference: Williams Obstetrics, 25th Edition, Chapter 4, page 656)

12. **c.** Hyperpigmentation develops in 90% of women and usually more in dark-skinned people. The specific sites are pigmented skin line in the midline of anterior abdominal wall called linea nigra. Pigmentation around nipples also increases.
    (Reference: Williams Obstetrics, 25th Edition, Chapter 4, page 53)

13. **b.** Renal plasma flow increases by approximately 80% before the end of first trimester.
    (Reference: Williams Obstetrics, 25th Edition, Chapter 4, page 65)

CHAPTER 4: Physiological Changes during Pregnancy

14. **d.** Hypervolemia associates with normal pregnancy average up to 40-45% above the nonpregnant after 32-34 weeks.
    (Reference: Williams Obstetrics, 25th Edition, Chapter 4, page 57)

15. **c.** Milk ejection, or letting down, is a reflex initiated especially by suckling, which stimulates the posterior pituitary to liberate oxytocin.
    (Reference: Williams Obstetrics, 25th Edition, Chapter 36, page 657)

16. **b.** During labor, however, and especially after administration of analgesics, gastric emptying time may be appreciably prolonged.
    (Reference: Williams Obstetrics, 25th Edition, Chapter 4, page 68)

17. **d.** Osmotic thresholds for AVP release and thirst decrease thus sensitivity increase.
    (Reference: Williams Obstetrics, 25th Edition, Chapter 4, page 66)

18. **d.** HPL production is proportional to placental mass and near term is 1 g/dL—it is by far the maximum hormone production.
    (Reference: Williams Obstetrics, 25th Edition, Chapter 5, page 101)

19. **c.** During normal pregnancy, both coagulation and fibrinolysis are augmented but remain balances to maintain hemostasis. Evidence of activation includes increased concentrations of all clotting factors except factors XI and XIII.
    (Reference: Williams Obstetrics, 25th Edition, Chapter 4, page 59)

20. **d.** The heart rate rises on an average of 10 bpm during pregnancy but physiological increase always remains <100 bpm.
    (Reference: Williams Obstetrics, 25th Edition, Chapter 4, page 60)

21. **c.** The GFR increases as much as 25% by 2nd week of pregnancy to 50% by 2nd trimester of pregnancy.
    (Reference: Williams Obstetrics, 25th Edition, Chapter 4, page 65)

22. **b.** There is 20-30% in RBC count during pregnancy.
    (Reference: Williams Obstetrics, 25th Edition, Chapter 4, page 62)

23. **c.** During pregnancy vital capacity has no change because it is sum of TV + ERV + IRV. The ERV decreases during pregnancy and IRV increases during pregnancy. So, both these effects nullify each other's effect and tidal volume remaining unchanged is major determinant in determining the vital capacity.
    (Reference: Williams Obstetrics, 25th Edition, Chapter 4, page 656.)

24. **a.** Apex beat is shifted upward and outward during pregnancy. It shifts from 5th intercostal space to 4th intercostal space 2.5 cm away from mid-clavicular line.
    (Reference: Williams Obstetrics, 25th Edition, Chapter 4, page 60)

25. **c.** Cardiac output is maximum during immediate postpartum up to 60-80% increase from prepregnancy values. It is also because compression on IVC is relieved postdelivery and sudden contraction of uterus results in approximately 500 mL of more blood in circulation.
    (Reference: Williams Obstetrics, 25th Edition, Chapter 4, page 60)

26. **a.** Cardiac output returns to prelabor values after 1 hour of delivery.
    (Reference: Williams Obstetrics, 25th Edition, Chapter 4, page 60)

27. **b.** During pregnancy, diastolic murmurs are abnormal.
    Normal findings in heartbeat during pregnancy are: S_3, S_4, ejection systolic murmur, S_1 split, bounding/collapsing pulse, relative sinus tachycardia, and few ectopic beats.
    (Reference: Williams Obstetrics, 25th Edition, Chapter 4, page 60)

28. **c.** Pregnancy being hypercoagulable state all factors increase during pregnancy except factors 11 and 13 which decrease and factors 2, 5, and 12 which remain unchanged during pregnancy.

29. **a.** Factor 1 also known as fibrinogen has maximum rise during pregnancy which is increased by 50%.

Chapter 5: Diagnosis of Pregnancy

Komal N Chavan, Ritika Pathak

QUESTIONS

1. **Chadwick's sign is:**
   a. Bluish discoloration of the vaginal mucosa
   b. Softening of lower part of uterus felt on bimanual examination
   c. Tenderness and enlargement of the breasts
   d. Weak uterine contractions felt on bimanual examination

2. **Goodel's sign is:**
   a. Bluish discoloration of the vaginal mucosa
   b. Softening of lower part of uterus felt on bimanual examination
   c. Tenderness and enlargement of the breasts
   d. Softening of cervix

3. **Palmer's sign is:**
   a. Bluish discoloration of the vaginal mucosa
   b. Weak uterine contractions felt on bimanual examination
   c. Tenderness and enlargement of the breasts
   d. Softening of lower part of uterus felt on bimanual examination

4. **Hegar's sign is:**
   a. Bluish discoloration of the vaginal mucosa
   b. Tenderness and enlargement of the breasts
   c. Softening of lower part of uterus felt on bimanual examination
   d. Weak uterine contractions felt on bimanual examination

5. **On examination of a 22-year-old primigravida whose last menses began 7 weeks ago, you notice that the vaginal mucosa has bluish color. This sign suggestive of pregnancy is called:**
   a. Hegar's sign   b. Palmer's sign
   c. Goodel's sign   d. Jacquemier's sign

6. **The uterus starts to be felt abdominally at:**
   a. 12 weeks   b. 14 weeks
   c. 20 weeks   d. 24 weeks

7. **In a singleton pregnancy, the uterus is normally felt at the level of xiphisternum at about:**
   a. 12 weeks   b. 24 weeks
   c. 32 weeks   d. 36 weeks

8. **Regarding the diagnosis of pregnancy, all of the following is true, *except*:**
   a. Frequency of micturition starts early in pregnancy
   b. Breast changes are reversible by the end of pregnancy
   c. Beta-human chorionic gonadotropin (hCG) can be detected in the blood 1 week before the missed period
   d. Beta-hCG can be detected in urine few days after the missed period

9. **Regarding the diagnosis of pregnancy, which of the following is true?**
   a. Abdominal ultrasound is preferable than vaginal ultrasound in early pregnancy
   b. Hegar's sign is positive throughout pregnancy
   c. Hormone withdrawal bleeding is a modern method for diagnosis of pregnancy
   d. Fetal heart sound is the most reliable sign

10. **The average date of quickening in the primigravida is around:**
    a. 12 weeks   b. 16 weeks
    c. 20 weeks   d. 24 weeks

11. **Counting from the first day of last menstrual period, all healthy gestational sacs should be visualized using TVS by:**
    a. 20–25 days   b. 25–30 days
    c. 30–35 days   d. 40–45 days

12. A gestational sac can be visualized during sonography by:
    a. 5–6 weeks
    b. 7–8 weeks
    c. 9–10 weeks
    d. 11–12 weeks

13. A pregnant woman who is 7 weeks from her last menstrual period (LMP) comes to the OPD for her first antenatal visit. Her previous pregnancy ended in a missed abortion in the first trimester. The patient is very anxious about the well-being of this pregnancy.

    Which of the following modalities will allow you to best document fetal heart sound?
    a. Doppler
    b. Regular stethoscope
    c. Transvaginal ultrasound (TVS)
    d. Transabdominal sonography (TAS)

14. A patient comes to your OPD with LMP 4 weeks ago. She denies any symptoms such as nausea, vomiting, and frequency. She thinks that she may be pregnant because her menses are delayed and is very anxious to find out because she has a history of previous ectopic pregnancy and wants to be sure to get early antenatal care.

    Which of the following evaluation methods is most sensitive in diagnosing pregnancy?
    a. No evaluation to determine pregnancy is needed because the patient is asymptomatic
    b. Abdominal USG
    c. Beta-hCG
    d. Detection of fetal heart sound by Doppler

15. On examination of a primigravida whose last menses began 7 weeks ago, you notice that the vaginal mucosa has a bluish color. This sign suggestive of pregnancy is called:
    a. Hegar's sign
    b. Palmer's sign
    c. Goodel's sign
    d. Jacquemier's sign

16. A 25-year-old patient presents to your clinic with a missed period and frequency of micturition, proper management would include all of the following, *except:*
    a. Pelvic sonography
    b. General and local examination
    c. Pregnancy test
    d. Medroxyprogesterone for 5 days

17. Softening and cyanosis of the cervix occurring in early pregnancy are due to:
    a. Increased vascularity
    b. Decreased stromal edema
    c. Action of melanocyte stimulating hormone
    d. Atrophy of cervical glands

18. Pigmentation of the skin of cheeks and a part of the nose during pregnancy is called:
    a. Striae gravidarum
    b. Linea nigra
    c. Melasma
    d. Chloasma

19. Dilated sebaceous glands visible on the breast areola in pregnancy are called:
    a. Goodel's sign
    b. Hegar's sign
    c. Montgomery's tubercles
    d. Bartholin's glands

20. The rule used for the calculation of the estimated due date (EDD) by adding 9 months and 7 days to the 1st day of LMP is known as:
    a. Naegele
    b. Pinard
    c. Montgomery
    d. Braxton-Hick

21. Your pregnant patient had her LMP on August 2nd, 2022. Her EDD should be on:
    a. 9.5.2023
    b. 2.5.2023
    c. 30.4.2023
    d. 16.5.2023

22. A 22-year-old woman who is 6 weeks by dates has come to OPD with vaginal spotting. USG shows a fetal pole with a crown-rump length (CRL) of 4 mm. There is no fetal heart action noted. The ovaries and adnexa appear normal. What is the most likely diagnosis?
    a. Heterotopic pregnancy
    b. Viable intrauterine pregnancy
    c. Could be a viable pregnancy
    d. Nonviable pregnancy

23. External ballottement can be elicited from:
    a. 12–16 weeks
    b. 16–18 weeks
    c. 20–26 weeks
    d. 32–36 weeks

24. Earliest diagnosis of pregnancy can be established safely by:
    a. USG for fetal cardiac activity
    b. Fetal cardiac Doppler study
    c. Human chorionic gonadotropin levels
    d. MRI pelvis

25. **Double bleb sign in USG is depictive of:**
    a. Intrauterine two gestational sac
    b. Amniotic sac and yolk sac
    c. Ectopic pregnancy
    d. Heterotopic pregnancy
    e. Twin pregnancy

26. **Which is the most reliable and conclusive sign for the diagnosis of pregnancy?**
    a. Fetal heart sound
    b. Amenorrhea
    c. Nausea and vomiting with amenorrhea
    d. Enlargement of abdomen

27. **Fundal height reaches the level of umbilicus at about:**
    a. 16–18 weeks
    b. 22–24 weeks
    c. 24–26 weeks
    d. 30–32 weeks

28. **Crown-rump length (CRL) cut-off for diagnosing pregnancy failure in absence of cardiac activity:**
    a. 4 mm
    b. 7 mm
    c. 9 mm
    d. 12 mm

29. **Sonographic findings suspicious for failed intrauterine pregnancy:**
    a. Empty amnion
    b. Enlarged yolk sac
    c. Empty gestational sac with mean sac diameter (MSD) between 16 and 24 mm
    d. All of the above

30. **Which of the following parameter is used in calculation of estimated fetal weight using Hadlock formula?**
    A. Head circumference (HC)
    b. Mean sac diameter (MSD)
    c. Crown-rump length (CRL)
    d. Foot length

31. **What is Piskacek's sign?**
    a. One-half of uterus is more firm than other half
    b. Bleeding per vaginum
    c. Breast engorgement
    d. False pregnancy

32. **Regarding pseudocyesis, all are true, *except*:**
    a. Quickening
    b. Enlargement of uterus
    c. Amenorrhea
    d. False labor

33. **Chadwick' sign is seen in:**
    a. Pregnancy
    b. Adenomyosis
    c. Endometriosis
    d. All of the above

34. **A 38-year-old diabetic female comes to your OPD with complaint of heavier, more intense period with more intense cramping about a week later than usual. Examination findings are unremarkable but pregnancy test comes to be positive. No sac or adnexal mass is seen on sonography. What could be the cause?**
    a. Ectopic pregnancy
    b. Pelvic inflammatory disease
    c. Endometriosis
    d. Chemical pregnancy

35. **Softening of uterine isthmus is called:**
    a. Hegar's sign
    b. Ladin's sign
    c. Palmer's sign
    d. Goodell's sign

36. **A 42-year-old pregnant in vitro fertilization (IVF)-conceived patient has come to OPD with scan report showing two gestational sacs corresponding to 7.9 weeks of gestation, each containing an embryo with heartbeat.**

    This patient comes for follow-up scan after 4 weeks. Scan report shows one normal fetus with cardiac activity, and a second, much smaller fetus without cardiac activity. Subsequent scans showed no evidence of demised twin or its gestational sac.

    This is a case of:
    a. Missed abortion
    b. Chemical pregnancy
    c. Vanishing twin
    d. Heterotopic pregnancy

37. **A 36-year-old morbidly obese female comes to OPD with sonography report showing an intrauterine embryo of 9 mm length without cardiac activity. What advice you will give to patient?**
    a. Repeat scan after 7 days
    b. Repeat scan after 14 days
    c. Termination of pregnancy
    d. Hormonal support

38. **A 42-year-old IVF-conceived female has come to OPD with sonography report showing single gestational sac of 5 weeks' gestation. Follow-up scan was done after 1 week showing two embryos with heart beats located within a single gestational sac. What is your probable diagnosis?**
    a. Heterotopic pregnancy
    b. Monochorionic twins
    c. Dichorionic twins
    d. None of the above

ANSWERS

1. **a.** Chadwick's sign is a nonspecific, early sign of pregnancy that is typically characterized by a bluish discoloration of the cervix, vagina, and vulva. It can typically be observed as early as 6–8 weeks after conception, and commonly disappears shortly after birth. It does not commonly present with any other specific signs and symptoms such as pain.

2. **d.** Goodell's sign is significant softening of the vaginal portion of the cervix from increased vascularization. This vascularization is a result of hypertrophy and engorgement of the vessels below the growing uterus. This sign occurs at approximately 6 weeks' gestation. Goodell's sign is named after William Goodell (1829–1874).

3. **b.** Uterine contractions are palpable between 4 and 8 weeks on bimanual examination (Palmer's sign).

4. **c.** The abdominal and vaginal fingers can be apposed below the body of uterus due to softness of isthmus (Hegar's sign)-8–12 weeks. Hegar's sign is more difficult to recognize in multiparous women. It is named after Ernst Ludwig Alfred Hegar, German gynecologist, in 1895.

5. **d.** The Jacquemier's or Chadwick's sign is a nonspecific, early sign of pregnancy that is typically characterized by a bluish discoloration of the cervix, vagina, and vulva.

6. **a.** The uterus starts to be felt abdominally at 12 weeks.

7. **d.** Uterus is felt at the level of xiphisternum at about 36 weeks of singleton pregnancy.

8. **b.** Breast changes continues throughout pregnancy and even after delivery. After delivery, breast becomes more active for lactation.

9. **d.** Fetal heart sound is the most reliable and conclusive sign for the diagnosis of pregnancy.

10. **c.** Quickening appears around 18–20 weeks in primigravida. Multiparous women appreciate it 2 weeks earlier due to their past experience.

11. **c.** Timing of appearance of ultrasound findings in early pregnancy on TVS:

Gestational sac	4.5 weeks
Yolk sac	5 weeks
Fetal node	5.5 weeks
Fetal heart	6 weeks

12. **a.** Gestational sac can be seen during sonography by 5–6 weeks.

13. **c.** Early pregnancy findings are best documented on transvaginal sonography.

14. **c.** hCG is the earliest and most sensitive indicator in diagnosis of early pregnancy. Measurement of β-hCG every 48 hours helps in determining viability of early intrauterine pregnancies.

15. **d.** Bluish discoloration of cervix and vagina is called Jacquemier's sign or Chadwick's sign.

16. **d.** Hormone withdrawal bleeding is contraindicated in suspected case of pregnancy.

17. **a.** Softening and cyanosis of cervix and vagina, occurring in early pregnancy is due to increased vascularity of genital organs in pregnancy leading to congestion of blood vessels. It is detected between the 4th and 8th weeks, increases in intensity to peak at 16th week, and persists throughout pregnancy.

18. **d.** During pregnancy, there is increased pigmentation of face (chloasma) and abdomen (linea nigra).

19. **c.** Montgomery tubercles are dilated sebaceous glands visible on areola of the breast during pregnancy.

20. **a.** *Naegele's rule:* For calculation of estimated due date (EDD), add 7 days to the first day of last menstrual period and count forward by 9 months.

21. **a.** Naegele's rule to be applied as described above.

22. **c.** Crown-rump length (CRL) of 7 mm is the cut-off for diagnosing pregnancy failure in the absence of cardiac activity.

23. **c.** External ballottement can be elicited from 20th to 26th week of gestation when the fetus is small as compared with the amount of liquor.

24. **c.** Human chorionic gonadotropin (hCG) levels can be used for the earliest diagnosis of pregnancy.

25. **b.** Double bleb sign is a sonographic feature where there is visualization of a gestational sac containing a yolk sac and amniotic sac giving an appearance of two small bubbles. The embryonic disk is located between the two bubbles. It is an important feature of an intrauterine pregnancy and thus distinguishes a pregnancy from a pseudogestational sac or decidual cast cyst. It should not be confused with the double decidual sac sign.

26. **a.** Fetal heart sound is the most reliable and conclusive sign for the diagnosis of pregnancy.
27. **b.** Fundal height reaches the level of umbilicus at about 22–24 weeks of gestation.
28. **b.** Crown-rump length (CRL) of 7 mm is the cut-off for diagnosing pregnancy failure in the absence of cardiac activity.
29. **d.** Sonographic findings suspicious (but not definitive) for failed intrauterine pregnancy.

Category	Findings suspicious for pregnancy failure
Embryo with no cardiac activity	CRL < 7 mm
Gestational sac containing no embryo with heartbeat	MSD 16–24 mm
Empty amnion	Amnion seen adjacent to yolk sac, with no visible embryo
Expanded amnion	Embryo with no cardiac activity, with amnion visible around it
Enlarged yolk sac	>7 mm

30. **a.** Hadlock formula uses the following parameters for calculation of estimated fetal weight—Head circumference, abdominal circumference, femur length, and biparietal diameter.
31. **a.** In lateral implantation, there is asymmetrical enlargement of the uterus. One-half of the uterus where the implantation occurred is firm while the other half is soft. This is known as "Piskacek's sign". The sign is named after Ludwig Piskaçek.
32. **b.** Pseudocyesis is a condition in which the patient has all signs and symptoms of pregnancy except for the confirmation of the presence of a fetus. In the case of pseudocyesis, i.e., phantom pregnancy, there is abdominal distention, enlargement of the breasts, enhanced pigmentation, cessation of menses, morning sickness and vomiting, typical lordotic posture on walking, inverted umbilicus, increased appetite, and weight gain. There is no enlargement of uterus in pseudocyesis.
33. **d.** Chadwick's sign is a nonspecific, early sign of pregnancy that is typically characterized by a bluish discoloration of the cervix, vagina, and vulva. While the Chadwick's sign is commonly associated with pregnancy, some conditions that may mimic signs of pregnancy and have a positive Chadwick's sign, include cervical endometriosis, adenomyosis, and pseudocyesis.
34. **d.** Chemical pregnancy is a very early miscarriage that usually happens before 5 weeks' gestation. It can only be detected through a pregnancy test, which shows elevated hormone levels. Such pregnancy cannot be verified through an ultrasound or fetal heartbeat. Risk factors for chemical pregnancy are: aged 35 years or older, atypically shaped uterus, hormonal imbalance, sexually transmitted infections (STI), polycystic ovarian syndrome (PCOS), and diabetes. Signs of chemical pregnancy: Experiencing a heavier, more intense period with more intense cramping about a week later than usual.
35. **b.** Ladin's sign is a clinical sign of pregnancy in which there is softening in the midline of the uterus anteriorly at the junction of the uterus and cervix. It is detectable with bimanual examination at about 6 weeks gestation.
36. **c.** Vanishing twin syndrome is a condition in which one of a set of twins or multiple embryos dies in utero, disappears, or gets resorbed partially or entirely with an outcome of a spontaneous reduction of a multi-fetus pregnancy to a singleton pregnancy, portraying the image of a vanishing twin.
37. **c.** Crown-rump length (CRL) of 7 mm is the cut-off for diagnosing pregnancy failure in the absence of cardiac activity. Thus, termination of pregnancy should be advised.
38. **b.** This is a case of "Appearing" twin. Since both fetuses are located within a single gestational sac, it indicates that they are monochorionic twins.

Chapter 6

Fetus in Utero

Rajshree Dayanand Katke

QUESTIONS

1. Which one of the following complications is associated with short cord?
    a. Failure of external version
    b. It prevents descent of the presenting part especially during labor
    c. It causes separation of normally situated placenta
    d. All of the above

2. Which of the following complication is associated with long cord?
    a. Cord prolapse
    b. Entanglement of cord around the neck or the body of fetus
    c. It prevents external version
    d. (a) + (b)

3. What is percentage incidence of single umbilical artery?
    a. 1–2%
    b. 4–5%
    c. 3–4%
    d. 8–10%

4. Single umbilical artery is associated in which of the following congenital anomalies?
    a. Renal anomalies
    b. Genital anomalies
    c. Trisomy 18
    d. All of the above

5. Which of the following condition is associated with placenta marginata?
    a. Antepartum hemorrhage
    b. Hepatitis
    c. Retained placenta or membranes
    d. (a) + (c)

6. At what gestation placental and fetal weights are nearly equal?
    a. 12 weeks
    b. 17 weeks
    c. 20 weeks
    d. 28 weeks

7. After what weeks gestation end diastolic flow appears during Doppler study to assess fetal well-being?
    a. 10 weeks
    b. 15 weeks
    c. 20 weeks
    d. 28 weeks

8. What is most accurate measure to assess gestational age during 1st trimester on USG?
    a. Crown-rump length
    b. Biparietal diameter
    c. Head circumference
    d. Femur length

9. Which vessel traverses the liver to enter the inferior vena cava directly?
    a. Umbilical vein
    b. Ductus venosus
    c. Ductus arteriosus
    d. Umbilical artery

10. Which of the following statement is/are true?
    a. After birth umbilical vessels, ductus arteriosus, foramen ovale, and ductus venosus normally constrict or collapse
    b. Intra-abdominal remnant of the umbilical vein forms the ligamentum teres
    c. Ductus venosus after birth ultimately forms the ligamentum venosum
    d. All of the above

11. What is sequence of production of hemoglobin in fetus over period of gestation?
    a. Liver > Yolk sac > Bone marrow
    b. Yolk sac > Bone marrow > Liver
    c. Yolk sac > Liver > Bone marrow
    d. Bone marrow > Yolk sac > Liver

12. Which of the following is/are composition of surfactant in utero?
    a. Dipalmitoyl phosphatidylcholine
    b. Phosphatidylglycerol
    c. Phosphatidylinositol
    d. All of the above

SECTION 1: Obstetrics

13. At what gestation surfactant production starts in utero?
    a. 20 weeks b. 16 weeks
    c. 24 weeks d. 28 weeks

14. What is the length of umbilical cord to say it is short?
    a. <30 cm b. <40 cm
    c. <45 cm d. <50 cm

15. What is the weight of normal placenta at term?
    a. 250 g b. 350 g
    c. 500 g d. 550 g

16. What is the % incidence of true knots?
    a. 1% b. 2%
    c. 3% d. 4%

17. Ultrasonographically "Hanging noose" sign is seen in which of the following condition?
    a. True knots b. Cord stricture
    c. Cord loops d. Nuchal cord

18. What is the presenting part in funic presentation?
    a. Feet b. Buttock
    c. Umbilical cord d. None of the above

19. What is the incidence of neural tube defect inheritance in females without periconceptional folic acid supplementation?
    a. 1–2% b. 3–5%
    c. 8–10% d. 5–7%

20. Which of the following complications are associated with post-term pregnancy?
    A. Stillbirth b. Neonatal convulsions
    c. Postmaturity syndrome d. All of the above

21. Which of the following pathway is/are involved in amniotic fluid volume regulation?
    a. Fetal urination
    b. Fetal lung fluid secretion
    c. Fetal swallowing
    d. All of the above

22. Which of the following is not seen in tetralogy of Fallot?
    a. Anterior displacement of the conotruncal septum
    b. Pulmonary stenosis
    c. Hypertrophy of the right ventricle
    d. Hypertrophy of the left ventricle

23. Which of the following structure is derived from intermediate mesoderm?
    a. Heart b. Kidney
    c. Blood vessels d. Muscle

24. Which of the following structure arises from ectoderm?
    a. Brain b. Bone
    c. Gonads d. Stomach

25. Umbilical cord is derived from which of the following?
    a. Chorion b. Connecting stalk
    c. Primary villi d. Secondary villi

26. What is amniotic fluid index in severe polyhydramnios?
    a. >35 cm b. >25 cm
    c. >30 cm d. >40 cm

27. Which of the following fetal anomalies are associated with hydramnios?
    a. Anencephaly
    b. Cleft lip/palate
    c. Ureteropelvic junction obstruction
    d. All of the following

28. At what gestational age, fetal kidneys are the main contributor to amnionic fluid volume?
    a. 12 weeks b. 14 weeks
    c. 18 weeks d. 22 weeks

29. Which of the following abnormalities are amenable to fetal surgical treatment?
    a. Congenital cystic adenomatoid malformation (CCAM)
    b. Myelomeningocele
    c. Sacrococcygeal teratoma
    d. All of the following

30. Which of the following statement is/are true about intrauterine fetus?
    a. Heart development is completed by 6 weeks of gestation
    b. Liver development starts by 8 weeks
    c. Brain development completes by 16 weeks
    d. Reproductive system development starts at 8 weeks

ANSWERS

1. **d.** Short cord may cause following:
   - Failure of external version
   - Prevent descent of the presenting part during labor
   - It can cause separation of normally situated placenta.
   - Malpresentation
   - It can cause fetal distress in labor.

2. **d.** In long cord, there are increased chance of:
   - Cord prolapse
   - Cord entanglement around the neck or the body of the fetus
   - Long cord may be associated with true knot, but is rare.

3. **a.** Single umbilical artery is present in about 1–2% of cases. It is due to failure of development of one artery or due to its atrophy in later months.

4. **d.** Single umbilical artery is associated with congenital malformation of the fetus (20–25%).

   It is associated with following congenital malformations of the fetus:
   - Renal anomalies
   - Genital anomalies
   - Trisomy 18

5. **d.** Condition is associated with placenta marginata are as follows:
   - Antepartum hemorrhage
   - Preterm delivery
   - Retained placenta or membranes
   - Abortion
   - Hydrorrhea gravidarum (excessive watery vaginal discharge)
   - Growth retardation of the baby

6. **b.** At 17 weeks' gestation placental and fetal weights are nearly equal.

7. **a.** After 10 weeks of gestation end-diastolic flow appears during Doppler study to assess fetal well-being.

8. **a.** Crown-rump length is the most accurate measure to assess gestational age during 1st trimester on USG. Clinically, crown-rump length is not measured beyond 13 weeks, which corresponds to approximately 8.4 cm. Instead, biparietal diameter, head circumference, abdominal circumference, and femur length are measured. Fetal weight in the 2nd and 3rd trimesters is assessed from a combination of these measurement.

9. **a.** Oxygen and nutrients required for fetal growth and maturation from the placenta are supplied through single umbilical vein, single umbilical vein divides into the ductus venosus and the portal sinus. The ductus venosus is the major branch of the umbilical vein. Ductus venosus traverses the liver to enter the inferior vena cava directly.

10. **d.** After birth, umbilical vessels, ductus arteriosus, foramen ovale, and ductus venosus normally constrict or collapse.

    Intra-abdominal remnants of the umbilical vein form the ligamentum teres.

    The ductus venosus constricts after birth and is anatomically closed around 2–3 weeks and ultimately forms the ligamentum venosum.

11. **d.** Fetal blood is first produced in the yolk sac, where hemoglobins Gower 1, Gower 2, and Portland are formed. Erythropoiesis then occurs in liver, where fetal hemoglobin F is produced. Hemopoiesis finally moves to the bone marrow, where adult-type hemoglobin A1 appears in fetal red blood cells.

12. **d.** The principal active component that constitutes half of surfactant is a lecithin, which is dipalmitoyl phosphatidylcholine (DPPC or PC). Phosphatidylglycerol (PG) is almost 8–15%. The other major constituent is phosphatidylinositol (PI).

13. **c.** By 24 weeks' gestation, surfactant production initiated by secretory type II pneumocytes.

14. **a.** Most umbilical cords at delivery measure about 40–70 cm in length. Short cord measures <30 cm, may lead to fetal distress, abruptio placentae, and prolonged labor.

15. **c.** Weight of typical placenta at term is 450 g.

16. **a.** % incidence of true knots is 1%.

17. **a.** Knots are found incidentally during antepartum sonography, and sign is called "hanging noose" sign.

18. **c.** In a funic presentation, the umbilical cord is the presenting part. These are uncommon and most often are associated with fetal malpresentations.

    Once identified at term, cesarean delivery is typically recommended in cases of funic presentation.

19. **b.** Risk of neural-tube defect inheritance without periconceptional folic acid supplementation is 3–5%.

20. **d.** Following complications are associated with post-term pregnancy:
    - Stillbirth
    - Neonatal convulsions
    - Postmaturity syndrome
    - Infections
    - Meconium aspiration syndrome

21. **d.** Following pathways are involved in amniotic fluid volume regulation:
    a. Fetal urination
    b. Fetal lung fluid secretion
    c. Fetal swallowing
    d. Intramembranous fluid transfer across and into fetal vessels on the placental surface
    e. Transmembranous fluid across amniotic membrane

22. **d.** In tetralogy of Fallot (TOF), there is an anterior displacement of the conotruncal septum.

    It is characterized by pulmonary stenosis, a ventricular septal defect (VSD), an overriding aorta, and hypertrophy of the right ventricle.

    The pulmonary stenosis forces the deoxygenated blood to travel through the VSD from the right side to the left side, leading to right ventricular hypertrophy.

    Because of the deoxygenated blood crossing over into systemic circulation, the baby presents with early cyanosis in cases of tetralogy of Fallot.

23. **b.** Structures derived from mesoderm: Muscle, bone, connective tissue, notochord, kidney, gonads, and circulatory system

    Structures derived from intermediate mesoderm: Kidneys, adrenal gland, and urogenital system

    Structures derived from lateral plate mesoderm: Heart, blood vessel, organ muscle, and body wall.

24. **a.** Structures derived from ectoderm: Epidermis (outer layer of skin), hair, nails, brain, spinal cord, and peripheral nervous system

    Structures derived from mesoderm: Muscle, bone, connective tissue, notochord, kidney, gonads, and circulatory system

    Structures derived from endoderm: Epithelial lining of the digestive tract: Stomach, colon, liver, pancreas, bladder, and lung.

25. **b.** Umbilical cord is derived from connecting stalk.

26. **a.**
    - Polyhydramnios is categorized as: Mild if the amniotic fluid index (AFI) is 25–29.9 cm; moderate, if the AFI is 30–34.9 cm; and severe, if ≥35 cm.
    - Using a single deepest pocket of amnionic fluid, mild polyhydramnios is defined as 8–9.9 cm, moderate as 10–11.9 cm, and severe hydramnios as ≥12 cm.

27. **d.** Fetal anomalies associated with hydramnios are as follows:
    a. Anencephaly
    b. Cleft lip/palate
    c. Ureteropelvic junction obstruction
    d. Diaphragmatic hernia
    e. Cardiomyopathy

28. **c.** By 18 weeks of gestation, the fetal kidneys mainly contribute to amnionic fluid volume.

29. **d.** Abnormalities amenable to fetal surgical treatment are as follows:
    a. Congenital cystic adematoid malformation (CCAM)
    b. Myelomeningocele
    c. Sacrococcygeal teratoma
    d. Pulmonary sequestration
    e. Twin-twin transfusion syndrome

30. **a.**

	Start weeks	Complete develop weeks
a. Heart development	3 weeks	6 weeks
b. Liver development	3–4 weeks	12 weeks
c. Brain development	3 weeks	28 weeks
d. Reproductive system	5 weeks	7 weeks

REFERENCES

1. Cunningham FG, Leveno KJ, Dashe JS, Hoffman BL, Spong CY (Eds). Williams Obstetrics, 26th edition. New York: McGraw Hill/Medical; 2022.
2. Konar H. DC Dutta's Textbook of Obstetrics, 10th edition. New Delhi: Jaypee Brothers Medical Publishers (P) Ltd.; 2022.

Chapter 7: Fetal Skull and Maternal Pelvis

Rajshree Dayanand Katke, Ankita Aghav

QUESTIONS

1. **Which of the following are the boundaries of lambdoid suture?**
   a. It lies between two parietal bones
   b. It lies between two frontal bones
   c. It runs between parietal and frontal bones on either side
   d. It separates the occipital bone and two parietal bones

2. **What are the clinical importance of sutures?**
   a. It permits gliding movement of one bone over the other during molding of the head
   b. It gives an idea of manner of engagement of the head
   c. It gives an idea of degree of internal rotation of the head and degree of molding of the head
   d. All of the above

3. **Which among the following is true about anterior fontanel?**
   a. It is also known as Bregma
   b. Sinciput lies posterior to the anterior fontanel
   c. It ossifies after 18 months of birth
   d. It facilitates molding of head
   e. All of the above

4. **Which among the following is the longest AP diameter of the fetal skull?**
   a. Occipitofrontal   b. Mentovertical
   c. Submento-vertical   d. Suboccipito-frontal

5. **What is the length of "Bimastoid Diameter"?**
   a. 8 cm   b. 8.5 cm
   c. 7.5 cm   d. 9 cm

6. **Which will be the engaging diameter of fetus in occipito-posterior position?**
   a. Biparietal   b. Bimastoid
   c. Subparietal   d. Bitemporal

7. **Define area of brow presentation.**
   a. Part of skull between anterior fontanel and root of nose
   b. Part of skull lying between anterior fontanel and posterior fontanel
   c. Part of skull between root of nose and chin
   d. Area of face

8. **Fetus skull is formed by how many bones?**
   a. Six   b. Five
   c. Four   d. Seven

9. **Which of the following is true regarding grades of molding of head?**
   a. *Grade 1:* The bones touching but not overlapping
   b. *Grade 2:* Bones overlapping but easily separated
   c. *Grade 3:* Fixed overlapping
   d. All of the above

10. **What among the following is true about "Caput Succedaneum"?**
    a. Caput gives idea about long-standing fetal head at perineum
    b. It is as same as cephalohematoma
    c. It occurs because of overlapping of sutures
    d. It gives idea about engagement of head

11. **On per vaginal examination with two fingers, you noticed that your finger reaches the sacral promontory with difficulty. What does it indicate?**
    a. Inadequate anteroposterior diameter
    b. Inadequate transverse diameter
    c. Inadequate oblique diameter
    d. None of the above

12. **If on per vaginal examination, you noticed that the sagittal sutures are irreducible and overlapping. What is the grade of molding in this case?**
    a. Grade 1   b. Grade 2
    c. Grade 3   d. Grade 4

13. Pelvic inlet is formed by:
    a. Pubic symphysis
    b. Pectineal line and iliopubic eminence
    c. Sacral promontory
    d. All of the above

14. How much is the anatomical conjugate?
    a. 10 cm   b. 12 cm
    c. 11 cm   d. 13 cm

15. What is the longest diameter of pelvic inlet?
    a. Transverse diameter
    b. Oblique diameter
    c. Anatomical conjugate
    d. Anteroposterior diameter

16. Define anatomical conjugate?
    a. It is measured between the upper edge of symphysis and midpoint of sacral promontory
    b. It is the distance between lower border of symphysis pubis to the midpoint of sacral promontory
    c. It is measured between the midpoint of sacral promontory to prominent bony projection in the midline on the inner surface of symphysis pubis
    d. None of the above

17. How much is the transverse diameter of pelvic outlet?
    a. 12 cm   b. 13 cm
    c. 10.5 cm   d. 12.5 cm

18. What is the smallest diameter of mid cavity of pelvis?
    a. Anteroposterior diameter
    b. Oblique diameter
    c. Interspinous diameter
    d. Transverse diameter

19. What is the importance of ischial spine?
    a. Internal rotation of fetal head
    b. Pudendal block during surgery
    c. To assess the station
    d. All of the above

20. What are the boundaries of the outlet of maternal pelvis?
    a. Sacrotuberous ligament   b. Sacral promontory
    c. Coccyx   d. Ischial bones
    e. All of the above

21. How much is the posterior sagittal diameter?
    a. 11 cm   b. 8.5 cm
    c. 9 cm   d. 9.5 cm

22. You notice in a patient that the pubic arch is very narrow. What does it signify?
    a. Subpubic angle <70°   b. Subpubic angle <85°
    c. Subpubic angle >85°   d. None of the above

23. Which of the following diameters can be seen in vertex presentation?
    a. Suboccipito bregmatic   b. Suboccipito frontal
    c. Occipital frontal   d. All of the above

24. What are the types of pelvis?
    a. Android pelvis   b. Anthropoids' pelvis
    c. Platypelloid pelvis   d. Gynecoid pelvis
    e. All of the above

25. Which of the following is not a type of deformed pelvis?
    a. Robert's pelvis   b. Rachitic pelvis
    c. Platypelloid pelvis   d. Kyphotic pelvis

26. What are the joints of pelvis?
    a. Sacroiliac joints   b. Sacrococcygeal joint
    c. Symphysis pubis   d. All of the above

27. Sacroiliac joint is a what type of joint?
    a. Synovial joint   b. Ball and socket joint
    c. Saddle joint   d. Hinge joint

28. How much is the "Subpubic Angle"?
    a. 100°   b. 90°
    c. 85°   d. 80°

29. On examining the pelvic outlet, you noticed that your four-knuckle fist is not going inside. What does it signify clinically?
    a. Transverse diameter of outlet is adequate
    b. Transverse diameter of outlet is not adequate
    c. Oblique diameter is adequate
    d. Anteroposterior diameter is adequate

30. On per vaginal examination, if the bispinous diameter is inadequate, what will be the difficulty you can expect during labor?
    a. Fixing of head
    b. Difficulty in internal rotation
    c. Difficulty in extension
    d. Difficulty in engagement of the head

31. On clinical examination per vaginally, you can feel that ala of the sacrum is absent, then what is the type of pelvis in this patient?
    a. Rachitic pelvis   b. Robert's pelvis
    c. Gynecoid pelvis   d. Osteomyelitic pelvis

ANSWERS

1. **d.**
   Sutures are of four types:
   1. Sagittal suture lies between two parietal bones.
   2. Coronal sutures run between parietal and frontal bones on either side.
   3. The frontal suture lies between two frontal bones.
   4. Lambdoid suture separates the occipital bone and two parietal bone.

2. **d.**
   Clinical importance of sutures:
   - It permits gliding movement of one bone over the other during molding of the head.
   - It gives an idea of the manner of engagement if the head (asynclitism or synclitism)
   - Degree of internal rotation of the head and degree of molding of head

3. **e.** Anterior fontanel is formed by joining the four sutures in the midplane:
   1. It is diamond-shaped.
   2. It is also known as bregma.
   3. It facilitates molding of head.
   4. It ossifies at 18 months after birth.

4. **b.** Longest AP diameter of the skull is mentovertical diameter—14 cm.
   Occipitofrontal: 11.5 cm
   Submento-vertical: 11.5 cm
   Suboccipito-frontal: 10 cm

5. **c.** Bimastoid diameter: 7.5 cm

6. **a.** Engaging diameter of fetal head in occipito-posterior position: Biparietal diameter

7. **a.** Brow presentation is defined as part of skull between anterior fontanel and root of nose.

8. **a.** Fetal skull is formed by *six* bones.
   1. Frontal bone
   2. Occipital bone
   3. Two parietal bones
   4. Two temporal bones

9. **d.** All of the above
   There are three gradings for molding of the head.
   1. *Grade 1:* The bones touching but not overlapping.
   2. *Grade 2:* Overlapping but easily separated
   3. *Grade 3:* Fixed overlapping

10. **a.**
    - Caput succedaneum is the formation of swelling due to stagnation of fluid in the layers of the scalp beneath the girdle of contact.
    - Caput gives idea about long-standing of fetal head at perineum.

11. **a.** Anteroposterior (AP) diameter extends from the inferior border of the symphysis pubis to the tip of the sacrum.
    If on per vaginal (P/V) examination finger reaches the sacral promontory with difficulty, it indicates that AP diameter is inadequate.

12. **c.** There are three gradings for molding of the head.
    1. *Grade 1:* The bones touching but not overlapping.
    2. *Grade 2:* Overlapping but easily separated
    3. *Grade 3:* Fixed overlapping

13. **d.**
    Pelvic inlet is formed by all of the below:
    - Pubic symphysis
    - Pectineal line and iliopubic eminence
    - Sacral promontory
    - Anterior border of the ala of sacrum
    - Pubic tubercle

14. **c.**
    - Anatomical or *true* conjugate measures 11 cm.
    - Obstetric conjugate: 10 cm
    - Diagonal conjugate: 12 cm

15. **a.**
    - Longest diameter of pelvis is transverse diameter.
    - Transverse diameter: 13 cm
    - Oblique diameter: 12 cm
    - Anatomical conjugate: 11 cm
    - Anteroposterior diameter: 11 cm

16. **a.** *Anatomical conjugate* is measured between the upper edge of symphysis and midpoint of sacral promontory.

17. **b.** Transverse diameter of the pelvic outlet is 13 cm.

18. **c.** Smallest transverse diameter of midcavity of pelvis is interspinous 10.5 cm

19. **d.** All of the above
    Importance of ischial spines is as follows:
    - Internal rotation of fetal head occurs here.
    - Pudendal block during surgery can be given at this level.
    - To assess the station of fetal head.

20. **d.** Ischial bones
21. **b.** *Posterior sagittal diameter* is 8.5 cm.
    It is the anteroposterior distance between the sacrococcygeal joint and the midpoint of the transverse diameter of the outlet.
22. **b.** In case of narrow pubic arch, the subpubic angle <85°.
23. **d.** All of the above
24. **e.** All of the above
    There are four types of pelvis:
    1. Android pelvis
    2. Anthropoids' pelvis
    3. Platypelloid pelvis
    4. Gynecoid pelvis
25. **c.** Platypelloid pelvis is a type of normal pelvis. Other three are a type of deformed pelvis.
    1. *Robert's pelvis:* Both sacral alae are absent.
    2. *Rachitic pelvis:* Flat pelvis due to softening of bones
    3. *Kyphotic pelvis:* Characterized by increase in the conjugate diameter at pelvic from and decrease of the transverse diameter at the outlet.
26. **d.** All of the above
    - Sacroiliac Joints
    - Sacrococcygeal joint
    - Symphysis pubis
27. **a.** *Sacroiliac joint* is a type of synovial joint. It is a freely movable joint.
28. **c.** Subpubic angle measures 85 cm.
29. **a.** Transverse diameter of the outlet (TDO) is the distance between inner border of ischial tuberosities. If the four-knuckle fist is not going inside on P/V examination, then it signifies that the TDO is adequate.
30. **b.** Bispinous diameter is the distance between the tip of two ischial spines, measuring 10.5 cm.
    If it is inadequate, there will be difficulty in internal rotation of the fetal head.
31. **b.** In Robert's pelvis, ala of the sacrum is absent.

Chapter 8

Antenatal Care, Preconceptional Counseling, and Care

Preeti Nitsure Deshpande

QUESTIONS

1. **What is the hemoglobin level to define anemia of pregnancy?**
   a. <11 g in first trimester, <10.5 g in the second and third trimester
   b. <10 g in first trimester, <9.5 g in the second and third trimester
   c. <12 g in first trimester, <11 g in the second and third trimester
   d. <9.5 g in first trimester, <9 g in the second and third trimester

2. **What is the best diagnostic test for iron deficiency in pregnancy?**
   a. Serum ferritin level
   b. Serum iron level
   c. Transferrin saturation
   d. Total iron-binding capacity

3. **What is the daily requirement of calcium in pregnancy?**
   a. 1,200 mg/day
   b. 1,000 mg/day
   c. 500 mg/day
   d. 750 mg/day

4. **Total iron requirement in the entire pregnancy is:**
   a. 1,200 mg
   b. 1,000 mg
   c. 500 mg
   d. 750 mg

5. **What is the sequence/chronology of changes before iron-deficiency anemia develops?**
   a. Fall in serum ferritin, decrease in transferrin saturation, and alteration in red blood cell (RBC) indices
   b. Decrease in transferrin saturation, fall in serum ferritin, and alteration in RBC indices
   c. Alteration in RBC indices, decrease in transferrin saturation, fall in serum ferritin
   d. Fall in serum ferritin, fall in hemoglobin, fall in RBC indices

6. **After Rubella vaccination, pregnancy needs to be avoided for:**
   a. 4 weeks
   b. 8 weeks
   c. 12 weeks
   d. 16 weeks

7. **At what gestation, pertussis vaccine is recommended?**
   a. 20-24 weeks
   b. 24-28 weeks
   c. 28-38 weeks
   d. 16-20 weeks

8. **When is flu vaccine recommended?**
   a. After 12 weeks
   b. After 28 weeks
   c. 20-28 weeks
   d. All stages of pregnancy

9. **What is the current recommendation for vaccination for tetanus in pregnancy, if the patient has previously received diphtheria, tetanus, and pertussis (DPT) vaccines?**
   a. Two doses tetanus toxoid (TT)/diphtheria and tetanus (dT)
   b. One dose TT/dT
   c. Three doses TT/dT
   d. No need to vaccinate against TT

10. **When is the blood volume the maximum in pregnancy?**
    a. 32nd week
    b. 36th week
    c. 24th week
    d. 12th week

11. **When is routine antenatal anti-D prophylaxis (RAADP) recommended for a patient with Rh-negative blood group?**
    a. 150 μg at 28 and 34 weeks
    b. 300 μg at 28 and 34 weeks
    c. 300 μg at 28 weeks
    d. 300 μg at 34 weeks

12. In a Rh-negative patient who has an episode of bleeding per vagina after 20 weeks of pregnancy, what is the recommended dose of anti-D immunoglobulin?
    a. 50 μg
    b. 100 μg
    c. 150 μg
    d. 300 μg

13. Which is a high-risk factor for preeclampsia indicating the need to start aspirin among these?
    a. Diabetes mellitus type 1/type 2
    b. Age ≥40 years
    c. Body mass index (BMI) ≥35
    d. Nulliparity

14. Which one is a moderate risk factor for development of preeclampsia?
    a. Chronic hypertension
    b. Autoimmune disease
    c. Renal disease
    d. Multiple pregnancy

15. By what gestational age must aspirin be started to reduce the risk of fetal growth retardation?
    a. 12 weeks
    b. 16 weeks
    c. 20 weeks
    d. 24 weeks

16. Gestational diabetes testing is offered for women at risk, with 75 g 2 hours oral glucose tolerance test (OGTT) at 24–28 weeks. What is the indication for early OGTT after booking?
    a. Body mass index (BMI) >30 kg/m^2
    b. Previous macrosomic baby weighing 4.5 kg or more
    c. Previous history of gestational diabetes
    d. Family history of diabetes (in a first-degree relative)

17. Gestational diabetes testing is offered for women at risk, with 75 g 2 hours oral glucose tolerance test (OGTT) at 24–28 weeks. What is one of the indications for early OGTT after booking?
    a. BMI > 35 kg/m^2
    b. History of preeclampsia and stillbirth
    c. Maternal age > 45 years
    d. Family history of diabetes (in a first-degree relative)

18. In a known case of diabetes, below what value should the HbA1c be preconception, so that the pregnancy can be safely planned?
    a. Less than 48 mmol/mol (6.5%)
    b. Less than 86 mmol/mol (10%)
    c. Less than 39 mmol/mol (5.7%)
    d. More than 39 mmol/mol (5.7%)

19. What is the risk of nausea-vomiting in pregnancy?
    a. 80%
    b. 50%
    c. 60%
    d. 20%

20. What is the maximum number of days for which metoclopramide can be safely prescribed?
    a. 7 days
    b. 5 days
    c. 3 days
    d. 1 day

21. What is the recommended dose of folic acid in pregnancy?
    a. 400 μg
    b. 500 μg
    c. 1 mg
    d. 5 mg

22. All cross the placenta, *except:*
    a. Phenytoin
    b. Diazepam
    c. Heparin
    d. Coumarin

23. Which drug is contraindicated in pregnancy?
    a. Nifedipine
    b. Atenolol
    c. Diazoxide
    d. Enalapril

24. At what size of gestational sac should the fetal pole be visible on a transvaginal scan (TVS)?
    a. 20 mm
    b. 10 mm
    c. 22 mm
    d. 25 mm

25. If the fetal pole is not visible on transvaginal scan (TVS) in a gestational sac of 25 mm, what will be your next step?
    a. Repeat the TVS after 3 days
    b. Repeat the TVS after 5 days
    c. Repeat the TVS after 7 days
    d. Repeat the TVS after 10 days

26. At what size of crown-rump length (CRL) should the cardiac activity be visible?
    a. 5 mm
    b. 6 mm
    c. 7 mm
    d. 8 mm

27. At a false positive of 5% which test has the best detection rate for Down syndrome?
    a. Nuchal translucency
    b. Double marker
    c. Quadruple marker
    d. Combined screening

28. What does combined screening include?
    a. Age, nuchal thickness, and double marker
    b. Nuchal thickness, ductus venosus, and nasal bone
    c. Age, nuchal thickness, and nasal bone
    d. Double marker, nuchal thickness, and quadruple marker

29. At what gestational age is combined screening done?
   a. 11-13^{+6} weeks
   b. 11-12 weeks
   c. 11-13 weeks
   d. 11^{+2}-14^{+1} weeks

30. At what gestational age is quadruple screen recommended?
   a. 11^{+2}-14^{+1} weeks
   b. 14^{+2}-20 weeks
   c. 15^{+1}-18^{+2} weeks
   d. 15^{+1}-20 weeks

ANSWERS

1. **a.** Parvord et al. recommended that a diagnosis of anemia is made for women with a hemoglobin of <110 g/L in the first trimester and <105 g/L in the second and third trimester and <100 g/L during the postpartum period.
(Reference: Percy L, Mansour D. Iron Deficiency and iron-deficiency anaemia in women's health. Obstet Gynaecol. 2017)

2. **a.** Serum ferritin is the most reliable indicator of iron deficiency in the absence of inflammation or chronic disease. Serum ferritin levels below 15 ng/mL are consistent with a diagnosis of iron deficiency. Sensitivity is improved from 25 to 92% using cut-off of 30 ng/mL and specificity remains high at 98%. When acute or chronic inflammation, hepatocellular damage, and some malignancies are present, transferrin saturation may be a more useful investigation for assessing iron deficiency. Transferrin saturation of <16% is indicative of insufficient iron supply for erythropoiesis.

   During pregnancy anemia is best assessed using serum ferritin. Ferritin rises initially and then gradually declines as pregnancy continues so that by 32-week levels are 50% less than prepregnancy. Treatment should be instigated when levels fall below 30 μg/L.
(Reference: Percy L, Mansour D. Iron Deficiency and iron-deficiency anaemia in women's health. Obstet Gynaecol. 2017)

3. **b.** The required intake of calcium in pregnancy is 1,000 mg/day, however, it is suggested that only 6% of pregnant women reach this daily quantity. Maternal risks of calcium deficiency in pregnancy include osteopenia, osteoporosis, tremor, paresthesia, muscle cramps and tetany. Calcium also has a role in fetal bone mineralization and in the prevention of fetal growth restriction.

   Serum calcium levels have been found to be reduced in patients with coexisting preeclampsia and calcium deficiency has also been linked to other pregnancy morbidities such as preterm labor.
(Reference: Mone F, Mc Auliffe FM. Low dose aspirin and calcium supplementation for the prevention of pre-eclampsia. Obstet Gynaecol. 2014;16:246-50)

4. **a.** Pregnancy results in an increased iron requirement of 1,200 mg for the entirety of pregnancy and this must be met through nutritional changes and supplementation, where necessary.

   First-line management of iron deficiency and iron-deficiency anemia is oral iron supplementation containing ferrous ions which is inexpensive and effective. Ferric compounds have been researched but they tend to be less soluble and have poor bioavailability.

   Following commencement of oral iron therapy, a further full blood count and serum ferritin level should be undertaken 3-4 weeks later (2 weeks later in pregnancy). Hemoglobin should rise by 20 g/L every 3-4 weeks or 1.2 g/L/day.

   Once hemoglobin and serum ferritin levels are normal treatment should be continued for 3 months **(Table 1)**.

TABLE 1: Iron content in different oral iron preparations.

Iron salt	Amount	Ferrous iron content
Ferrous fumarate	200 mg	65 mg
Ferrous gluconate	300 mg	35 mg
Ferrous sulfate	300 mg	60 mg
Ferrous sulfate (dried)	200 mg	65 mg

(Reference: Percy L, Mansour D. Iron Deficiency and iron-deficiency anaemia in women's health. Obstet Gynaecol. 2017)

5. **a.** Before iron deficiency develops many parameters of iron deficiency become abnormal and the chronology of these changes is as per this table **(Table 2)**.

TABLE 2: Chronology of changes to laboratory investigations in iron deficiency.

	Laboratory test	Laboratory finding
Early changes	• Serum ferritin • Serum iron • Transferrin saturation • Total iron-binding capacity • Red cell count • Red cell distribution width • Mean corpuscular volume	• <40 µg/L • <50 µg/dL • <15% • >450 µg/dL • <4 × 10^6/mm^3 • >14.5% • <80 fl
Late changes	Hemoglobin	<130 g/L, men <120 g/L, menstruating women

(Reference: Percy L, Mansour D. Iron Deficiency and iron-deficiency anaemia in women's health. Obstet Gynaecol. 2017)

6. **a.** Vaccines contraindicated in pregnancy are the Bacillus Calmette–Guérin (BCG) vaccine, measles, mumps, rubella, varicella, and human papillomavirus (HPV) vaccine.

   Where a woman is known to be rubella-susceptible, the vaccine should be given in the postpartum period. A single dose of measles, mumps, and rubella (MMR) vaccine will suffice. Women are advised to avoid conception for 28 days after administration.

   The children of pregnant women can be vaccinated without risk to the mother and fetus since the infection is not transmitted from the recently immunized individuals.
   (Reference: Arunakumari PS, Kalburgi S, Sahare A. Vaccination in pregnancy. Obstet Gynaecol. 2015;17: 257-63)

7. **c.** The purpose of the program is to passively protect the infant in the first few months of life before they reach the age of routine infant vaccination at about 8 weeks. This is achieved by vaccinating pregnant women between 28 and 38 weeks of gestation in order to maximize the transplacental transfer of pertussis antibody.
   (Reference: Arunakumari PS, Kalburgi S, Sahare A. Vaccination in pregnancy. Obstet Gynaecol. 2015;17: 257-63)

8. **d.** Influenza is associated with greater morbidity in pregnant women. Women in the second and third trimester are at an increased risk of hospitalization from influenza. Vaccination reduces the risk of serious maternal medical complication and provides passive protection to the neonate. It is recommended that all pregnant women have influenza vaccine whatever stage of pregnancy they are at.
   (Reference: Arunakumari PS, Kalburgi S, Sahare A. Vaccination in pregnancy. Obstet Gynaecol. 2015;17: 257-63)

9. **b.** Diphtheria and tetanus (dT) vaccination is WHO prequalified since 1995. As per WHO/UNICEF joint communication recommends dT to replace tetanus toxoid (TT).

   If four doses of diphtheria-tetanus-pertussis (DTP) were taken in childhood, one dose of TT is sufficient in the first and subsequent pregnancies at intervals of 1 year. If only three doses of DTP were taken in infancy—two doses of TT/dT in the first pregnancy and then one dose in subsequent pregnancies suffices.

   The last dose of TT should be at least 2 weeks prior to delivery.
   [Reference: WHO. (2007). Standards for Maternal and Neonatal Care. Maternal immunization against Tetanus. Integrated management of pregnancy and child birth (IMPAC). (online) Available from: http://www.who.int/publications-detail-redirect/standards-for-maternal-and-neonatal-care (Last accessed December, 2023)]

10. **a.** As early as 6 weeks of gestation, an increase in plasma volume and reduction in peripheral vascular resistance occurs because of activation of renin-angiotensin system and a mild decrease in plasma atrial natriuretic peptide levels. The increase in blood volume continues until it plateaus at a level of 140–150% at around 32 weeks of gestation compared to nonpregnant state. Cardiac output increases steadily until 25 weeks of gestation, initially secondary to increase in stroke volume and later because of an increase in maternal heart rate.

During labor and delivery, further hemodynamic changes occur. The heart rate and blood pressure increase significantly as a result of pain, anxiety, and uterine contraction. The increase in heart rate is similar to that observed during moderate to heavy physical exercise.

Cardiac output increases by 50% with each contraction. About 300–400 mL of blood is transferred from the uterus into the circulation with each contraction. In the active phase of the second stage of labor, the Valsalva maneuver results in larger variations in the central venous pressure.

(Reference: Wuntakal R, Shetty N, Ioannou E, Sharma S, Kurian J. Myocardial infarction and pregnancy. Obstet Gynaecol. 2013;15:247-55)

11. **c.** All D negative pregnant women who have not been previously sensitized should be offered routine antenatal prophylaxis with anti-D immunoglobulin (RAADP) either with a single dose regimen at around 28 weeks or two-dose regimen given at 28 and 34 weeks.

It is important that the 28 weeks sample for blood group and antibody screen is taken prior to the first routine prophylactic anti-D immunoglobulin injection being given. This forms the second screen required in pregnancy as stated in the British Committee for Standards in Haematology (BCSH) guidelines for blood grouping and red cell antibody testing during pregnancy.

Routine antenatal anti-D immunoglobulin prophylaxis (RAADP) should be regarded as a separate entity and administered regardless of, and in addition to, any anti-D immunoglobulin that may have been given for a potentially sensitizing event.

If using the two-dose regimen, a minimum dose of anti-D immunoglobulin 500 IU is recommended at 28 and 34 weeks.

Alternatively, a single dose of anti-D immunoglobulin, 1,500 IU should be administered between 28 and 30 weeks. The single dose regimen may be more cost effective, potentially enabling better compliance and providing logistic benefits.

500 IU = 100 μg
1,500 IU = 300 μg

(Reference: Qureshi H, Massey E, Kirwan D, Davies T, Robson S, White J, et al. British Committee for Standards in Haematology Guideline for the use of anti-D immunoglobulin for prevention of haemolytic disease of the fetus and newborn. Clin J Br Blood Trans Soc. 2014;24:8-20)

12. **b.** For potentially sensitizing events between 12 and 20 weeks' gestation, a minimum dose of 250 IU should be administered within 72 hours of the event. A test for fetomaternal hemorrhage is not required.

For potential sensitizing events after 20 weeks gestation, a minimum dose of anti-D immunoglobulin dose of 500 IU should be administered within 72 hours of the event. A test for fetomaternal hemorrhage is required.

250 IU = 50 μg
500 IU = 100 μg

(Reference: Qureshi H, Massey E, Kirwan D, Davies T, Robson S, White J, et al. British Committee for Standards in Haematology Guideline for the use of anti-D immunoglobulin for prevention of haemolytic disease of the fetus and newborn. Clin J Br Blood Trans Soc. 2014;24:8-20)

13. **a.** Advise pregnant women at high risk of preeclampsia to take 75–150 mg of aspirin daily from 12 weeks until the birth of the baby.

Women at high risk are those with any of the following:
- Hypertensive disease during a previous pregnancy
- Chronic kidney disease
- Autoimmune diseases such as systemic lupus erythematosus or antiphospholipid syndrome
- Type 1 or type 2 diabetes
- Chronic hypertension

[Reference: NICE. (2019). Hypertension in pregnancy: diagnosis and management (NG133). (online) Available from: https://www.nice.org.uk/guidance/ng133 (Last accessed December, 2023)]

14. **d.** Advise pregnant women at high risk of preeclampsia to take 75–150 mg of aspirin daily from 12 weeks until the birth of the baby.

Women at high risk are those with any of the following:
- Hypertensive disease during a previous pregnancy
- Chronic kidney disease
- Autoimmune diseases such as systemic lupus erythematosus or antiphospholipid syndrome
- Type 1 or type 2 diabetes
- Chronic hypertension

Advise pregnant women with more than 1 moderate risk factor for preeclampsia to take 75–150

mg of aspirin daily from 12 weeks until the birth of the baby. Factors indicating moderate risk are:
- First pregnancy
- Age 40 years or older
- Pregnancy after a gap of >10 years
- Body mass index (BMI) of 35 kg/m² or more at first visit
- Family history of preeclampsia
- Multi-fetal pregnancy

[Reference: NICE. (2019). Hypertension in pregnancy: diagnosis and management (NG133). (online) Available from: https://www.nice.org.uk/guidance/ng133 (Last accessed December, 2023)]

15. b. A recent systematic review and meta-analysis of five trials, with 414 women, has suggested that with respect to women at risk of preeclampsia, the timing of commencement of aspirin is important. Where aspirin was started at 16 weeks of gestation or less the relative risk of a small for gestational age SGA infant was 0.47 (95% CI: 0.3–0.74) and the number needed to treat was 9 (95% CI: 5.0–17.0). No reduction in risk of an SGA was found when aspirin was started after 16 weeks of gestation (RR: 0.92, 95% CI: 0.78–1.10).

A systematic review of nine trials of aspirin, in 1,317 women with abnormal uterine artery Doppler, concluded that aspirin started before 16 weeks of pregnancy reduced the incidence of preeclampsia as well as SGA birth (RR: 0.51, 95% CI: 0.28–0.92), number needed to treat = 10 (95% CI: 5–50). Aspirin started after 20 weeks was not effective in reducing the risk of the SGA infant. It is not possible to determine to what extent the effect of aspirin is due to the reduction of preeclampsia in these women.

[Reference: Royal College of Obstetricians and Gynecologists. (2016). The Investigation and Management of the small-for-gestational-age fetus (Green Top Guideline no 31). (online) Available from: www.rcog.org.uk/globalassets/documents/guidelines/gtg_31.pdf. (Last accessed December, 2023)]

16. c. Assess risk of gestational diabetes using risk factors in a healthy population. At the booking appointment, determine the following risk factors for gestational diabetes—body mass index >30 kg/m², baby weight 4.5 kg or more, previous history of gestational diabetes, family history of diabetes mellitus (first-degree relative with diabetes), minority ethnic family origin with a high prevalence of diabetes.

[Reference: NICE (2015). Diabetes in pregnancy: Management from preconception to postnatal period (NG3). (online) Available from: https://www.nice.org.uk/guidance/ng3. (Last accessed December, 2023)]

17. c. Medical literature uses the term "very advanced maternal age (VAMA)" to refer to women who are aged 45 years or more the time of delivery.

Women of very advanced maternal age are nine times more likely to require insulin to treat gestational diabetes mellitus than younger women. We recommend offering screening at 16–18 weeks of gestation in addition to screening at 26–28 weeks of gestation.

(Reference: Howell A, Blott M. Very Advanced Maternal Age. Obstet Gynaecol. 2021)

18. a. Advise women with diabetes who are planning to become pregnant to aim to keep their HbA1c level below 48 mmol/mol (6.5%) if this is achievable without causing problematic hypoglycemia.

[Reference: NICE (2015). Diabetes in pregnancy: Management from preconception to postnatal period (NG3). (online) Available from: https://www.nice.org.uk/guidance/ng3. (Last accessed December, 2023)]

19. a. Nausea vomiting affects up to 80% of pregnant women and is one of the most common indications for hospital admission among pregnant women with typical stays of 3 and 4 days.

Hyperemesis gravidarum is a severe form of nausea vomiting in pregnancy which affects about 0.3–3.6% of pregnant women.

[Reference: RCOG. (2016). The Management of nausea and vomiting of pregnancy and hyperemesis gravidarum. Green Top Guideline No 69. (online) Available from: https://www.rcog.org.uk/guidance/browse-all-guidance/green-top-guidelines/the-management-of-nausea-and-vomiting-of-pregnancy-and-hyperemesis-gravidarum-green-top-guideline-no-69/ (Last accessed December, 2023)]

20. b. Due to the risk of extrapyramidal effects with metoclopramide it should be used as second-line therapy. A review of metoclopramide conducted by European Medical Agency's committee for medicinal products for human use has confirmed the risks of short-term extrapyramidal disorders and tardive dyskinesia particularly in young people.

The review recommends metoclopramide should only be prescribed for short-term use (maximum dose of 30 mg in 24 hours or 0.5 mg/kg body weight in 24 hours (whichever is lowest) and maximum duration of 5 days and intravenous doses should be administered by slow bolus injection over at least 3 minutes to help to minimize these risks. Dystonic reactions have been shown to be significantly less common in non-pregnant patients receiving a slow infusion as opposed to a bolus injection of 10 mg of metoclopromide.

[Reference: RCOG. (2016). The Management of nausea and vomiting of pregnancy and hyperemesis gravidarum. Green Top Guideline No 69. (online) Available from: https://www.rcog.org.uk/guidance/browse-all-guidance/green-top-guidelines/the-management-of-nausea-and-vomiting-of-pregnancy-and-hyperemesis-gravidarum-green-top-guideline-no-69/ (Last accessed December, 2023)]

21. a. Women intending to become pregnant should be informed that delivery supplementation with folic acid before conception and up to 12 weeks gestation reduces the risk of having a baby with neural tube defects. The recommended dose is 0.4 mg/day. For women who have previously had an infant with a neural tube defect or who are receiving antiepileptic medication or who have diabetes, a higher dose of 5 mg/day is recommended.

[Reference: NICE. (2017). Fertility problems: assessment and treatment (CG 156). (online) Available from: https://www.nice.org.uk/guidance/cg156/resources/fertility-problems-assessment-and-treatment-35109634660549 (Last accessed December, 2023)]

Women with BMI 30 kg/m² or greater wishing to become pregnant should be advised to take 5 mg folic acid supplementation daily, starting at least 1 month before conception and continuing during the first trimester of pregnancy.

[Reference: Denison FC, Aedla NR, Keag O, Hor K, Reynolds RM, Milne A, et al.; Royal College of Obstetricians and Gynaecologists. Care of women with Obesity in Pregnancy. Green Top Guideline No. 72. BJOG. 2019;126(3):e62-e106]

Folic acid (5 mg) should be given once daily both preconceptually and through pregnancy.

[Reference: Royal College of Obstetricians and Gynaecologists. Management of Sickle Cell Disease in Pregnancy. Green Top Guideline No. 61. (online) Available from: https://www.mkuh.nhs.uk/wp-content/uploads/2022/10/Sickle-Cell-Disease-in-Pregnancy.pdf (Last accessed December, 2023)]

Folic acid (5 mg) is recommended preconceptually to all women to prevent neural tube defects.

Women with thalassemia have a much higher demand for folic acid so high-dose supplementation is needed. Folic acid 5 mg daily should be commenced 3 months prior to conception.

(Reference: Royal College of Obstetricians and Gynaecologists. Management of Beta Thalassaemia in Pregnancy. Green Top Guideline No. 66. London: RCOG; 2014)

22. c. Heparin is a large, highly ionized molecule, therefore not absorbed orally. It also does not cross the blood-brain barrier or placenta (it is the anticoagulant of choice during pregnancy)

[Reference: Tripathi KD. Essentials of Medical Pharmacology. New Delhi: Jaypee Brothers Medical Publishers (P) Ltd.; 2018]

There is evidence that low-molecular weight heparins do not cross the placenta.

(Reference: Kyei-Mensah, Legit C. Green Top Guideline: Thromboembolic disease in pregnancy and puerperium: Acute management. Green Top Guideline No. 37b. 2015)

23. d. Offer women with chronic hypertension referral to a specialist in hypertensive disorders of pregnancy to discuss risks and benefits of treatment.

Advise women who take angiotensin-converting enzyme inhibitors (ACEi) or angiotensin II receptor blockers (ARBs):

- That there is an increased risk of congenital abnormalities if these drugs are taken during pregnancy.
- To discuss alternative antihypertensive treatment with the healthcare provider responsible for managing their hypertension, if they are planning for pregnancy.
- To discuss alternative treatment with the healthcare provider responsible for managing their condition, if the ACEi or ARBs are being taken for other conditions such as renal disease

- Stop antihypertensive treatment in women taking ACEi or ARBs, if they become pregnant (preferably in 2 working days of notification of pregnancy) and offer alternatives.

Advise women who take thiazide or thiazide-like diuretics:
- That there may be an increased risk of congenital abnormality and neonatal complication if these drugs are taken during pregnancy.
- To discuss alternative antihypertensive treatment with the healthcare provider responsible for managing their hypertension, if they are planning of pregnancy.
- Advise women who take antihypertensive treatment other than ACEi, ARBs, thiazide, thiazide-like diuretics that the limited evidence available has not shown an increased risk of congenital malformations with such treatment.

Consider labetalol to control treatment of chronic hypertension in pregnant women, consider nifedipine for women in whom labetalol is not suitable, or methyldopa if both labetalol and nifedipine are not suitable.

[Reference: NICE. (2019). Hypertension in pregnancy: diagnosis and management (NG133). (online) Available from: https://www.nice.org.uk/guidance/ng133 (Last accessed December, 2023)]

24. **d.** If the mean gestational sac diameter is <25.0 mm with a transvaginal ultrasound scan and there is no visible fetal pole, perform a second scan a minimum of 7 days after the first before making a diagnosis. Further scans may be needed before a diagnosis can be made.

If the mean gestational sac diameter 25.0 mm or more using a transvaginal ultrasound scan and there is no visible fetal pole:
- Seek a second opinion on the viability of the pregnancy and/or
- Perform a second scan a minimum of 7 days after the first before making a diagnosis.

[Reference: Ectopic pregnancy and miscarriage: diagnosis and initial management (NG126). London: National Institute for Health and Care Excellence (NICE); 2023]

25. **c.** If the mean gestational sac diameter is <25.0 mm with a transvaginal ultrasound scan and there is no visible fetal pole, perform a second scan a minimum of 7 days after the first before making a diagnosis. Further scans may be needed before a diagnosis can be made.

If the mean gestational sac diameter is 25.0 mm or more using a transvaginal ultrasound scan and there is no visible fetal pole:
- Seek a second opinion on the viability of the pregnancy and/or
- Perform a second scan a minimum of 7 days after the first before making a diagnosis

[Reference: Ectopic pregnancy and miscarriage: diagnosis and initial management (NG126). London: National Institute for Health and Care Excellence (NICE); 2023]

26. **c.** If the crown-rump length (CRL) is <7.0 mm with a transvaginal ultrasound scan and there is no visible heartbeat, perform a second scan a minimum of 7 days after the first before making a diagnosis. Further scans may be needed before a diagnosis can be made.

If the CRL is 7.0 mm or more with a transvaginal ultrasound scan and there is no visible heartbeat:
- Seek a second opinion on the viability of the pregnancy and/or
- Perform a second scan a minimum of 7 days after the first before making a diagnosis

[Reference: Ectopic pregnancy and miscarriage: diagnosis and initial management (NG126). London: National Institute for Health and Care Excellence (NICE); 2023]

27. **d.** (Table 3)

TABLE 3: Comparison of different methods of screening for fetal trisomy-21.

Method of screening	Detection rate (%)	False positive rate (%)
Maternal age	30%	5%
• Second trimester serum biochemistry		
• Double test (AFP and β-hCG)	60–65%	5%
• Triple test (AFP, β-hCG, and u E3)	65–70%	5%
• Quadruple test (AFP, β-hCG, u E3, and inhibin)	70–75%	5%
First trimester combined screen	90%	5%
Cell-free DNA test	99%	5%

(AFP: α-fetoprotein, β-hCG: beta-human chorionic gonadotropin; u E3: unconjugated estriol)

At a false-positive rate of 5%, the detection rate increased from 30% using maternal age alone to 60–65% using double test (a combination of maternal age and serum α-fetoprotein and free β-hCG), to 65–70% using triple test (double test with addition of unconjugated estriol), and 70–75% using the quadruple test (triple test with the addition of inhibin A).

In 1990s, it was discovered that in fetuses with trisomy-21 there was an increase in the accumulation of subcutaneous fluid behind the fetal neck (nuchal translucency) that can be assessed by ultrasonography at 11–13 weeks of gestation. It was subsequently found that in trisomy-21 pregnancies at 11–13 weeks, the maternal serum concentration of free β-hCG is about twice as high and pregnancy-associated plasma protein A (PAPP-A) is reduced to half compared with euploid pregnancies. Maternal age was combined with fetal nuchal translucency and serum biochemistry to develop a screening test with a detection rate of about 90% at an FPR of 5%.

(Reference: Al Mahri GA, Nicolaides KH. Evolution in screening for Down Syndrome. Obstet Gynaecol. 2019)

28. **a.** In 1990s, it was discovered that in fetuses with trisomy-21 there was an increase in the accumulation of subcutaneous fluid behind the fetal neck (nuchal translucency) that can be assessed by ultrasonography at 11–13 weeks of gestation. It was subsequently found that in trisomy-21 pregnancies at 11–13 weeks, the maternal serum concentration of free β-hCG is about twice as high and pregnancy-associated plasma protein A (PAPP-A) is reduced to half compared with euploid pregnancies. Maternal age was combined with fetal nuchal translucency and serum biochemistry to develop a screening test with a detection rate of about 90% at an FPR of 5%.
   (Reference: Al Mahri GA, Nicolaides KH. Evolution in screening for Down Syndrome. Obstet Gynaecol. 2019)

29. **d.** Offer pregnant women an ultrasound scan to take place between 11^{+2} and 14^{+1} weeks to:
   - Determine gestational age
   - Detect multiple pregnancy
   - And, if opted for, screen for Down syndrome, Edward syndrome, and Patau syndrome

   [Reference: National Institute for Health and Care Excellence Antenatal Care (NG201). Developed by the National Guideline Alliance, which is part of the Royal College of Obstetricians and Gynaecologists. 2021]

THE COMBINED TEST

The combined test assesses the chance of the baby having trisomy-21 (T-21), trisomy-18 (T-18), or trisomy-13 (T-13) by using:
- Maternal age
- Biochemical markers—free β-human chorionic gonadotrophin (β-hCG) and pregnancy-associated plasma protein-A (PAPP-A)
- Ultrasound measurements—nuchal translucency (NT) and crown rump length (CRL)

The NT measurement must be used in combination with a maternal blood sample for calculating the chance result. It must not be used alone.

The eligibility criteria for the combined test is when the CRL is between 45.0 and 84.0 mm.

If the CRL is <45.0 mm, the woman is recalled for a further ultrasound scan to measure the NT and remeasure the CRL.

If the CRL is >84.0 mm, the gestational age is calculated using the head circumference (HC). The quadruple test is offered if the criteria is met.

The CRL and NT measurements must be taken on the same day.

The combined test gives the woman more time to consider screening options.

In practice, there are two ways the combined test can be performed and this determines how the woman receives the chance result. The maternal blood sample can be:
- Taken at the time of ultrasound scan
- Taken before the ultrasound scan (from 10 weeks onward)

(Reference: https://www.gov.uk/government/publications/fetal-anomaly-screening-programme-handbook/screening-for-downs-syndrome-edwards-syndrome-and-pataus-syndrome--3#the-combined-test)

30. **b.** Quadruple test screens for T-21 only.
   The quadruple test is offered when the:
   - Nuchal translucency (NT) measure cannot be obtained.
   - Crown-rump length (CRL) measurement is >84.0 mm and the HC is between 101.0 and 172.0 mm.

The quadruple test uses the maternal age and the four following biochemical markers measured from 14^{+2} to 20^{+0} weeks.

i. Alpha-fetoprotein
ii. Human chorionic gonadotropin (hCG) or free β-hCG
iii. Inhibin-a
iv. Unconjugated estriol uE-3

The combination of markers has a lower detection rate (DR) and a higher screen positive rate (SPR) than the combined test. For a woman present in second trimester, an ultrasound scan is required to measure the HC to date the pregnancy and complete the quadruple test.

If the HC is >172.0 mm, the quadruple test must not be offered. The woman is offered the 20-week screening scan.

(Reference: https://www.gov.uk/government/publications/fetal-anomaly-screening-programme-handbook/screening-for-downs-syndrome-edwards-syndrome-and-pataus-syndrome--3#the-quadruple-test)

Chapter 9: Antenatal Assessment of Fetal Well-being

Seema Mehrotra, Neharika Malhotra

QUESTIONS

1. **Middle cerebral artery Doppler evaluation is useful in the following conditions, *except*:**
   a. Rh isoimmunization
   b. Monochorionic twin gestation
   c. Fetal growth restriction
   d. Fetal cardiac anomaly

2. **All of the following statements are true regarding uterine artery Doppler waveform, *except*?**
   a. Increased resistance to flow and development of diastolic notch is associated with development of gestational hypertension, preeclampsia, and fetal growth restriction
   b. Positive predictive value of first trimester uterine artery Doppler for early onset of preeclampsia is very high
   c. Normal uterine artery waveform is characterized by high diastolic flow velocities and by highly turbulent flow
   d. Recent studies support its role to predict preeclampsia between 11 and 14 weeks and to start aspirin if pulsatility index (PI) comes to be raised

3. **Modified biophysical profile includes:**
   a. Nonstress test (NST) and fetal movement
   b. NST and fetal tone
   c. NST and amniotic fluid index (AFI)
   d. NST and fetal breathing movement

4. **The variables to be affected first and the last in biophysical profile respectively are:**
   a. Nonstress test (NST) and the fetal one
   b. Fetal breathing movement and fetal tone
   c. NST and fetal tone
   d. Gross fetal movement and fetal breathing movement

5. **Which of the following statement is not true about umbilical artery (UA) Doppler?**
   a. Umbilical artery (UA) pulsatility index (PI) depends on the angle of insonation
   b. The best place to assess UA-PI is in the middle of the free loop
   c. Higher resistance is seen at the fetal end of the cord
   d. Lower resistance is seen at the placental end of the cord

6. **Which of the following is not true about early deceleration in cardiotocography (CTG)?**
   a. Early deceleration is indicative of fetal hypoxia
   b. Occurs due to head compression
   c. The nadir of deceleration corresponds to peak of contractions
   d. They usually occur in the late first stage or in the second stage

7. **Which of the following is true about variable deceleration? They occur because of:**
   a. Head compression
   b. Poor oxygen reserve in placental pool
   c. Cord compression
   d. Fetomaternal hemorrhage

8. **Nonreassuring features in a cardiotocography (CTG) includes all, *except*:**
   a. Baseline fetal heart rate (FHR) between 100 and 109 beats/min
   b. Beat-to-beat variability of <5 for ≥40 minutes but <90 minutes
   c. Early deceleration
   d. Late deceleration

9. **Component of abnormal cardiotocography (CTG) is:**
   a. Baseline fetal heart rate (FHR) between 100 and 109 beats/min

b. Beat-to-beat variability of <5 for ≥40 minutes but <90 minutes
c. Sinusoidal pattern
d. Early deceleration

10. Maternal medications which affect the fetal heart rate pattern include:
a. Beta-blocker
b. Betamethsone
c. Opiates
d. All of the above

11. Which of the following maternal causes can lead to fetal tachycardia, *except*?
a. Pyrexia
b. Dehydration
c. Hypothyroidism
d. Hypovolemia

12. Which of the following is not true about shouldering seen in fetal CTG?
a. It is a brief period of increase in baseline before deceleration
b. Occurs due to cord compression
c. Feature of variable deceleration
d. Indicates severe fetal hypoxia

13. A suspicious cardiotocography (CTG) is one which
a. All features fall into nonreassuring category
b. All features fall into abnormal category
c. Two features fall into reassuring category
d. Features fall into one of the nonreassuring categories and the remainder of the features are reassuring

14. Which of the following is the thresholds for reassurance of fetal well-being?
a. Perception of at least 10 fetal movements (FMs) over up to 2 hours when the mother is at rest and focused on counting
b. Perception of at least 10 FMs during 12 hours of normal maternal activity
c. Perception of at least 4 FMs in 1 hour when the mother is at rest and focused on counting
d. All of the above

15. Before 32 weeks of gestation a reactive nonstress test (NST) is defined as:
a. As two accelerations that rise at least 10 beats/min above baseline and have a duration of at least 10 seconds
b. As two or more accelerations reaching a peak of at least 15 beats per minute (bpm) above the baseline rate and lasting at least 15 seconds
c. As two accelerations that rise at least 20 bpm above baseline and have a duration of at least 20 seconds
d. As two accelerations that rise at least 30 bpm above baseline and have a duration of at least 30 seconds

16. _____ is a reassuring sign reflective of adequate fetal oxygenation and normal brain function.
a. Absent fetal heart rate (FHR) variability
b. Decreased FHR variability
c. Moderate FHR variability
d. Marked FHR variability

17. How are variable fetal heart rate (FHR) decelerations frequently addressed?
a. Vagolytic drugs (e.g., atropine)
b. Changes in maternal positioning
c. Cesarean delivery
d. Intravenous (IV) fluid

18. Following are the cardiotocography (CTG) trace readings:
Baseline fetal heart rate (FHR): 110 beats/min; baseline variability: <5 beats/min for 90 minutes; acceleration: Nil; Deceleration: Variable deceleration with biphasic pattern.
The impression is:
a. Normal CTG
b. Suspicious CTG
c. Pathological CTG
d. None of the above

19. Which of the BPP parameter reflects the chronic fetal status?
a. Fetal tone
b. Fetal heart rate (FHR)
c. Gross fetal movement
d. Amniotic fluid volume (AFV)

20. The sequence of affection of BPP parameter in response to hypoxemia is:
a. Loss of fetal heart rate (FHR) acceleration, fetal breathing movement, decrease fetal movement (FM), and loss of fetal tone
b. Loss of fetal tone, decrease fetal movement, loss of FHR acceleration, and loss of fetal breathing movement
c. Decrease in fetal movement, loss of fetal tone, loss of FHR acceleration, and loss of fetal breathing movement
d. Loss of fetal breathing movement, decrease in fetal movement, loss of fetal tone, and loss of FHR acceleration

21. **Which of the following is not true about BPP?**
    a. Administration of antenatal corticosteroids affect BPP
    b. Intra-amniotic infusion in a patient with prelabor rupture of membrane may be associated with low BPP
    c. Preterm labor may be associated with absence of fetal breathing movement
    d. Maternal anemia affects fetal biophysical activities

22. **Which of the following is not true about assessment of fetal movement?**
    a. Fetal movement peaks about 32 weeks
    b. The fetus is most active between 9:00 PM and 1:00 AM
    c. The perception of 10 distinct movements in 2 hours is commonly regarded as reassuring
    d. Placental location can affect maternal perception of movement

23. **Sinusoidal pattern in nonstress test (NST) is associated with:**
    a. Maternal anemia   b. Fetal anemia
    c. Maternal infection   d. Fetal infection

24. **Biphasic waveform is the feature of:**
    a. Middle cerebral artery (MCA) Doppler
    b. Umbilical artery (UA) Doppler
    c. Uterine artery Doppler
    d. Ductus venosus Doppler

25. **Reversed diastolic flow in the umbilical arterial circulation represents placental arterial obliteration of:**
    a. 20–30%   b. 35–45%
    c. 50–60%   d. >70%

26. **For accurate MCA-PSV measurement, angle of insonation should be:**
    a. 30°   b. 20°
    c. 10°   d. 0°

27. **The predictive value of uterine artery Doppler for development of preeclampsia:**
    a. 98%   b. 78%
    c. 58%   d. 48%

28. **Bilateral uterine artery notching at 11–13 weeks 6 days is seen in ....% of normal first trimester pregnancy.**
    a. 20%   b. 30%
    c. 40%   d. 50%

29. **A 28-year-old female gravida 2 para 1^{+0}, 33 weeks gestation comes with USG report showing estimated fetal weight (EFW) <3rd centile and cerebroplacental ratio (CPR) <5th centile, AFI: 5 cm. NST: normal. Next course of action should be:**
    a. Immediate cesarean delivery
    b. Steroid coverage and delivery by induction of labor (IOL)
    c. Steroid coverage, weekly monitoring and delivery at 37 weeks
    d. Delivery at 40 weeks

30. **Which of the following statement is correct about fetal Doppler?**
    a. Pulsatility index (PI) gives a better estimate of the characteristics of the waveform than does resistive index (RI) or S/D ratio
    b. PI shows a linear correlation with vascular resistance, as opposed to both S/D ratio and RI, which show a parabolic relationship with increasing vascular resistance
    c. Additionally, PI does not approach infinity when there are absent or reversed diastolic values
    d. All of the above are correct

ANSWERS

1. **d.** Rh isoimmunization is associated with increase in middle cerebral artery-peak systolic velocity (MCAPSV). Centralization of the flow or the brain sparing effect in fetal MCA is seen in placental insufficiency in singleton/twin pregnancy.

2. **b.** First-trimester Doppler examination of the uterine arteries can predict 47.8% of cases of early PE (7.9% false-positive rate).

3. **b.** The modified biophysical combines the nonstress test with amniotic fluid index as an indicate of long-term function of the placenta.

4. **a.** First one to be affected is the nonstress test (NST) followed by fetal breathing movement and then gross fetal movements. Fetal tone is last to be affected.

5. **a.** Umbilical artery (UA), pulsatility index (PI), resistive index (RI), and S/D ratio are independent of angle of insonation.

6. **a.**

7. **c.** Variable decelerations are the most common type of deceleration seen during labor usually due to cord

compression. They are variable in shape, size, and timing in reference to uterine contractions depending upon the severity of cord compression.

8. **d.** Late deceleration feature of abnormal cardiotocography (CTG).

9. **c.** a, b, and d are features of nonreassuring cardiotocography (CTG).

10. **d.**
    Opiates: Prolong NREM sleep pattern
    Beta blockers: Decrease baseline FHR and decrease frequency of accelerations.
    Betamethasone: Decreases baseline variability.

11. **c.** Maternal hyperthyroidism can lead to fetal tachycardia.

12. **d.** Shouldering reflects fetal compensatory mechanism which is intact in a so far well-oxygenated fetus.

13. **d.**

14. **d.**

15. **a.**

16. **c.**

17. **b.** Variable decelerations, which are the most common periodic FHR pattern, are often corrected by changing the maternal position to relieve pressure on the umbilical cord.

18. **c.** Beat-to-beta <5 for >90 minutes and variable deceleration with biphasic pattern indicating atypical variation—two findings in abnormal category—Pathological CTG.

19. **d.** AFV. Amniotic fluid volume is not an acute parameter since decrease in AFV in response to chronic uteroplacental insufficiency generally occurs gradually. Fetal breathing movement, FHR acceleration, gross FM reflects acute fetal status.

20. **a.** As a result of different sensitivities to hypoxemia, fetal biophysical profile activities respond to hypoxemia in a predictable physiologically based cascade.

21. **d.**

22. **a.** Fetal movement peaks at 38 weeks.

23. **b.**

24. **d.**

25. **d.**

26. **d.**

27. **d.** A recent meta-analysis (*Ultrasound Obstet Gynecol.* 2014;43:500-7.) reported that first-trimester Doppler examination of the uterine arteries can predict 47.8% of cases of early PE (7.9% false-positive rate), 26.4% of cases of PE at any stage (6.6% false-positive rate), when using as a cut-off the 90th centile of PI or RI. However, combined screening [including maternal factors, maternal mean arterial blood pressure, uterine artery Doppler and placental growth factor (PlGF) measurement] has superior predictive performance (as detailed later) and, if available, should be preferred over Doppler-based screening.

28. **d.**

29. **c.**

30. **d.**

Chapter 10: Fetal Monitoring during Labor

Kinjal Shah

QUESTIONS

1. **The gold standard test for antenatal surveillance of the pregnancy at-risk for an adverse pregnancy outcome with the lowest false negative rate is:**
    a. Biophysical profile
    b. Cardiotocography (CTG) only
    c. CTG and an estimation of the amniotic fluid volume
    d. Contractions stress test

2. **How does the fetus usually respond to a lack of oxygen during labor?**
    a. There is an increase in fetal movements
    b. There is a decrease in the fetal heart rate
    c. There is an increase in the fetal heart rate
    d. There is a decrease in fetal movements

3. **The fetal heart rate pattern should be monitored:**
    a. During a contraction
    b. Before a contraction
    c. After a contraction
    d. Before, during, and after a contraction

4. **Despite the presence of other fetal heart rate (FHR) patterns, _____ is a reassuring sign reflective of adequate fetal oxygenation and normal brain function.**
    a. Decreased FHR variability
    b. Moderate FHR variability
    c. Marked FHR variability
    d. Absent FHR variability

5. **Which of the following is the preferred method for stimulating the fetus in the case of an external fetal monitoring tracing indicating decreased or absent variability without spontaneous accelerations?**
    a. Vibroacoustic stimulation
    b. Allis clamp scalp stimulation
    c. Fetal scalp sampling
    d. None of the above

6. **When is vaginal delivery appropriate in the presence of a persistently nonreassuring FHR pattern?**
    a. If there is evidence of fetal acidosis
    b. If there is evidence that delivery is imminent
    c. If there is evidence of progressive fetal hypoxia
    d. If there is meconium stain liquor

7. **Early decelerations:**
    a. Start at the beginning of a contraction and return to the baseline at the end of a contraction
    b. Start at the beginning of a contraction and end 30 seconds or more after the contraction
    c. Do not have any relation to contractions
    d. Occur during the period of uterine relaxation

8. **What are late decelerations?**
    a. Decelerations that occur after 38 weeks gestation
    b. Decelerations that are only present at the end of the first stage of labor
    c. Decelerations that start 30 seconds or more after the beginning of the contraction
    d. Decelerations that return to the baseline 30 seconds or more after the end of the contraction

9. **A baseline tachycardia:**
    a. Indicates that the fetus is in good condition
    b. Is common when the mother is given pethidine
    c. May be caused by infection of the placenta and membranes
    d. Indicates that the fetus is dying from lack of oxygen

10. **A baseline bradycardia:**
    a. Is a safe pattern
    b. Is a pattern which indicates an increased risk of fetal distress
    c. Indicates severe fetal distress
    d. Is usually caused by infection of the placenta and membranes

11. **Which form of meconium in the liquor is most likely to indicate the presence of fetal distress?**
    a. Fresh meconium indicates definite fetal distress and is an indication for an emergency cesarean section
    b. Old meconium indicates that there was a problem but that there is no need to be concerned
    c. Yellow meconium is of no clinical importance
    d. The management is the same as it does not matter what the consistency or color of the meconium is

12. **What is the most common cause of a reduced supply of oxygen to the fetus during labor?**
    a. Uterine contractions
    b. Partial placental separation
    c. Placental insufficiency
    d. Infection of the membranes

13. **Which of the following is least likely to be a cause of fetal bradycardia?**
    a. Fetal arrhythmia
    b. Prolapsed umbilical cord
    c. Worsening fetal acidosis
    d. Beta-agonists (e.g., terbutaline) given to the woman

14. **Which of the following statement is true?**
    a. Recurrent late fetal heart rate decelerations are probably due to compression of the umbilical cord
    b. Late fetal heart rate decelerations are a sign of a healthy fetus
    c. An abnormal nonstress test is an indication for an emergency cesarean delivery
    d. Giving the woman oxygen may help correct an abnormal fetal heart rate pattern

15. **Which is the first to disappear in biophysical profile (BPP)?**
    a. Fetal breathing
    b. Fetal tone
    c. Nonstress test (NST)
    d. Fetal movements

16. **Which of the following is most likely an indication of fetal intolerance to labor?**
    a. Increased variability
    b. Fetal heart rate accelerations
    c. Absent variability
    d. Early fetal heart rate decelerations

17. **In which of the following pregnancies would biophysical profile testing be recommended for fetal assessment?**
    a. Fetus in breech presentation
    b. Woman with gestational hypertension
    c. Woman with four previous deliveries
    d. Woman with group B beta-hemolytic *Streptococcus* cervical colonization

18. **Which of the following statements describes a reactive nonstress test?**
    a. No increase in fetal heart rate with fetal activity
    b. No more than one fetal heart rate acceleration of 15 beats per minute with fetal activity during a 20-minute period
    c. At least two fetal heart rate accelerations of at least 15 beats per minute and lasting at least 15 seconds during a 20-minute period
    d. Variable decelerations of at least 15 beats per minute and lasting at least 15 seconds occurring with fetal activity during a 20-minute period

19. **All the following statements about biophysical profile testing are accurate, *except*:**
    a. It is indicated only if an abnormal contraction stress test is obtained
    b. It includes nonstress testing
    c. A score of 4 or lower usually requires immediate delivery
    d. It includes ultrasound evaluation of amniotic fluid volume

20. **Which of the following is false?**
    a. Fetal heart rate response to auditory stimulation may be used as an indication of fetal well-being
    b. A normal nonstress test result occurs when there are no fetal heart rate accelerations with fetal activity
    c. An abnormal nonstress test result should be followed by a contraction stress test or biophysical profile
    d. Early fetal heart rate decelerations are usually not associated with fetal compromise

21. **Fetal tachycardia, without accompanying decelerations, may be caused by:**
    a. Maternal fever
    b. Fetal hypothyroidism
    c. Post-term fetus
    d. Narcotics given to the laboring woman

22. A 25-year-old primigravida at 40 weeks of gestation presented with labor pains. On examination, uterus showing three contractions lasting for 25 seconds in 10 minutes. On pervaginal examination cervix is 2 cm dilated, well effaced, membranes present, station-2.

What is the next management?

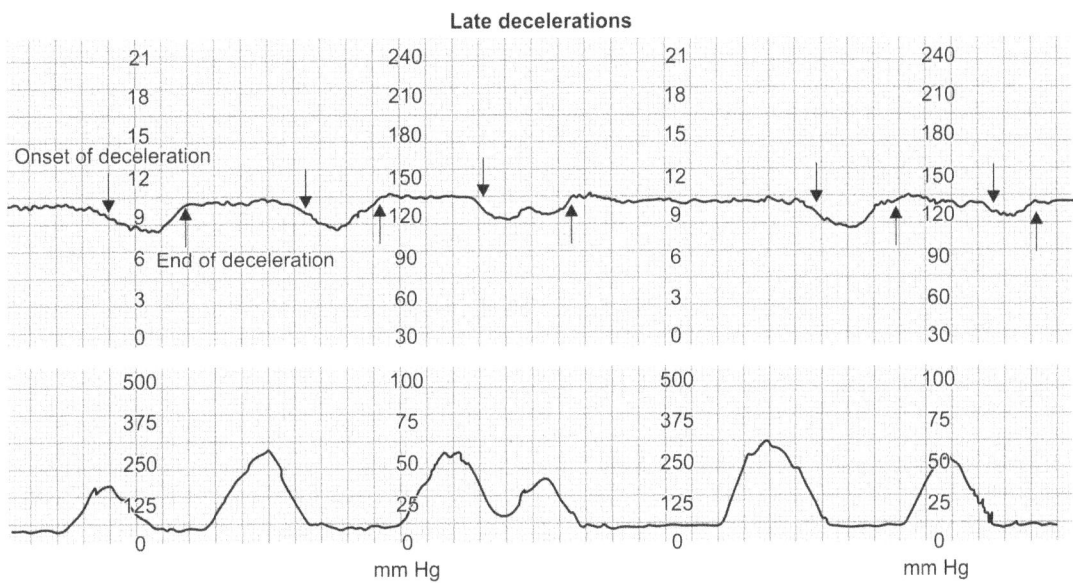

a. Wait and watch
b. ARM (artificial rupture of membranes)
c. Forceps delivery
d. Lower segment cesarean section (LSCS)

23. Interpret the CTG.

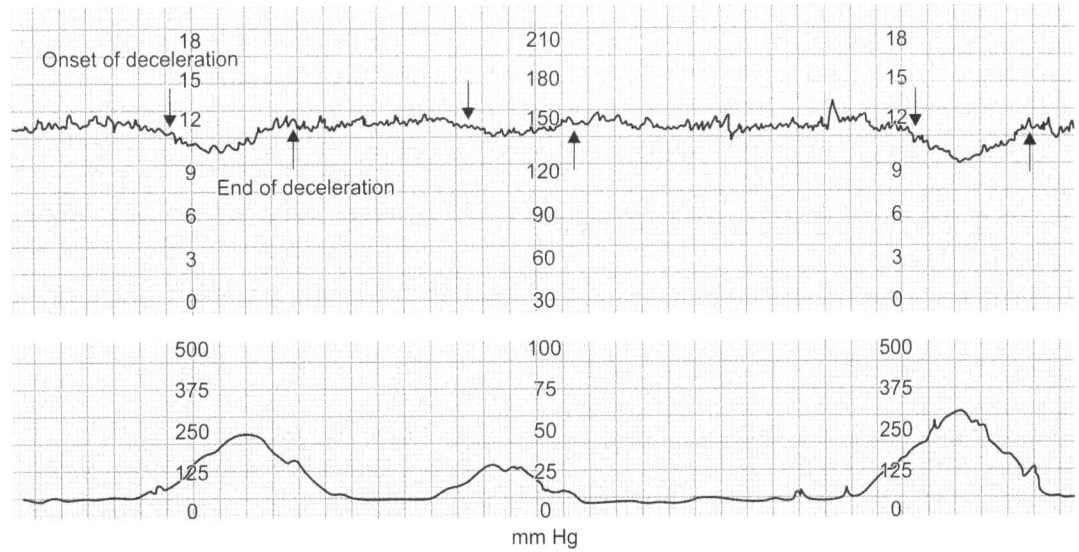

a. Reassuring
b. Cord compression
c. Head compression
d. Fetal distress

24. **Primi with 40 weeks GA underwent NST for fetal wellbeing.**

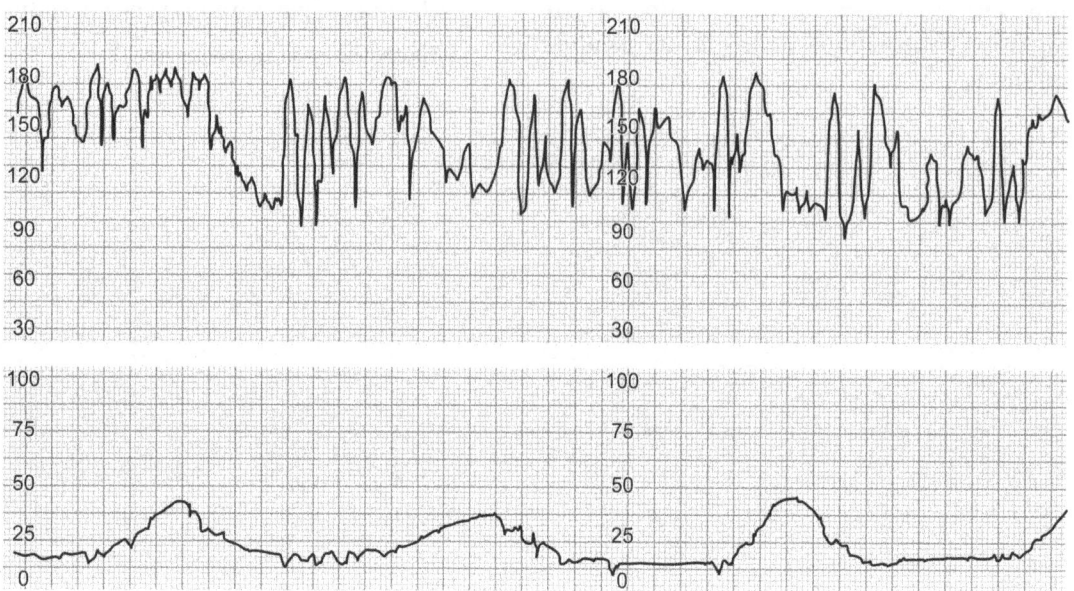

 NST as above
 She is advised:
 a. Repeat NST after 6 hours
 b. To get admitted for induction of labor
 c. Follow-up in OPD after 1 week and report earlier if any complaints
 d. To get admitted for cesarean

25. **The following statement is true about umbilical artery Doppler:**
    a. Increased impedance correlates with neonatal mortality
    b. Accurate CTG interpretation irrespective of umbilical artery Doppler findings has been shown to improve neonatal mortality
    c. Impedance values are higher at the fetal end of the cord and lower at the placental end
    d. The timing of umbilical artery Doppler changes is similar in early or late onset FGR

26. **The following is true regarding middle cerebral artery (MCA) Doppler:**
    a. The cerebroplacental ratio (CPR) is strongly predictive for perinatal morbidity in late-onset FGR
    b. A reduced MCA to umbilical Doppler impedance ratio is associated with the risk of cesarean section in labor in the presence of normal umbilical artery Doppler
    c. MCA Doppler interpretation is important in advising timing of delivery in early onset FGR
    d. The CPR is a better marker for timing of delivery than MCA Doppler alone

27. **The following statement correctly describes the role of uterine artery Doppler:**
    a. The uterine artery Doppler is a better predictor of FGR when recorded in the first, compared to the second, trimester
    b. The uterine artery Doppler recorded in the third trimester has no additive value in identifying the fetuses at risk at term
    c. The uterine artery Doppler is significantly associated with the risk of stillbirth
    d. The uterine artery Doppler is significantly associated with the risk of stillbirth, even after adjusting for estimated fetal weight and CPR

28. **Which Doppler parameters are virtually always normal in late-onset fetal growth restriction?**
    a. Umbilical artery only
    b. Ductus venosus only
    c. Middle cerebral artery only
    d. Umbilical artery and ductus venosus

29. **The following features in a CTG can be interpreted as follows:**
    a. A normal stable baseline FHT of 110–160 bpm with periods of accelerations with fetal movement

indicates that the fetus shows no evidence of diminished oxygen availability

b. A fetus who exhibits a baseline FHT of 170 bpm with absent decelerations suggests the presence of hypoxia

c. A fetus with a normal baseline FHT with moderate and frequent variable decelerations that return promptly to the previous baseline rate requires no intervention or further evaluation

d. A fetus with a previously normal baseline FHT and moderate variability and variable decelerations that return promptly to the previous baseline rate suddenly reveals a stable baseline tachycardia to 170 with absent variability and diminished amplitude of decelerations requires no intervention or further evaluation

30. **With regards to the CTG in the severely preterm fetus (i.e., less than 32 weeks):**
    a. Accelerations may be seen in a proportion of fetuses
    b. The baseline is typically lower than that in the term fetus
    c. The tracing is uninterpretable in over 20% of cases
    d. V-shaped decelerations lasting for 15 seconds are a sign of fetal compromise

ANSWERS

1. **d.** The biophysical profile (BPP) has a false negative rate of 0.6/1000. CTG only has a false negative rate of 1.9-5/100. CTG and estimation of the amniotic fluid volume have a false negative rate of 0.8/1,000. The contraction stress test has a false negative rate of 0.4/1,000.

2. **b.** Decreased fetal heart rate is directly related to fetal hypoxia and fetal distress.

3. **d.** Cardiotocography is done during labor to assess the fetal well-being. Therefore, a continuous graph of 20 minute is taken to rule out any decelerations.

   Decelerations are temporary drops in the fetal heart rate. There are three basic types of decelerations: early decelerations, late decelerations, and variable decelerations. Early decelerations are generally normal and not concerning. Late and variable decelerations can sometimes be a sign the baby is not doing well.

4. **b.** Moderate FHR variability is a reassuring sign reflecting adequate fetal oxygenation and normal brain function, regardless of what other FRH patterns exist.

5. **a.** Of all the techniques available to stimulate the fetus, vibroacoustic and digital scalp stimulation are the least invasive and thus preferred methods.

6. **c.** Cesarean delivery is warranted with evidence of progressive fetal hypoxia and acidosis, but vaginal delivery is appropriate if delivery is deemed imminent.

7. **a.** Early deceleration is defined as a symmetrical decrease and return of fetal heart rate (FHR) that is associated with a uterine contraction.

   Early decelerations in FHR are caused by compression of the fetus's head during a uterine contraction. As the uterine muscles get tighter and shorter, the size of the uterus decreases, thereby limiting the available space for the fetus.

8. **d.** Late deceleration is defined as a visually apparent, gradual decrease in the fetal heart rate typically following the uterine contraction. The gradual decrease is defined as—from onset to nadir taking 30 seconds or more. Typically, late decelerations are shallow, with slow onset and gradual return to normal baseline. The usual cause of the late deceleration is uteroplacental insufficiency.

9. **c.** Fetal tachycardia causes:
   - Excessive thyroid hormone secretion by the mother (maternal hyperthyroidism)
   - Fetal anemia (reduced oxygen in the blood)
   - Fetal distress
   - Fetal infection
   - Fever in the mother
   - Infection in the mother's uterus
   - Stimulants (drugs that speed up activities in the body)

10. **c.** Fetal bradycardia
    Causes include:
    - Fetal distress
    - Maternal autoimmune diseases such as lupus erythematous or Sjögren's syndrome
    - Maternal medications

11. **d.** Meconium stain liquor is an indicator of fetal distress. The management is to deliver the baby

immediately either by vaginal route if the patient is fully dilated or by an emergency cesarean section to prevent meconium aspiration and prevent neonatal morbidity and mortality.

12. **a.** Cause of acute fetal bradycardia is acute fetal hypoxia due to hyperstimulation of the uterus (with oxytocin or prostaglandin) in nearly all cases.

13. **d.** Beta agonist causes maternal and fetal tachycardia.

14. **d.** In cases of fetal distress, we give the mother left lateral tilt along with nasal oxygen with prongs which improves the fetal hypoxia.

15. **c.** Fetal tone
Fetal tone appears at 7.5–8.5 weeks
Fetal movements appears at 9 weeks
Fetal breathing appears at 20–21 weeks
NST at 28 weeks
Fetal tone is the first to appear and last to disappear

16. **c.** Absent variability and severe decelerations (either late or variable type) imply poor fetal condition and a more rapid delivery is mandated.

17. **b.** The indications for a biophysical profile are most commonly a nonreactive nonstress test or the presenting complaint of decreased fetal movement. However, many high-risk obstetric and fetal conditions require this study to help guide management.

18. **c.** A NST is considered reassuring if the fetal heart rate increases at least 15 beats per minute over the baseline (between 120 and 160 beats per minute), lasting at least 15 seconds, within a 20-minute timeframe. This is called a "reactive NST."

19. **a.** The indications for a biophysical profile are most commonly a nonreactive nonstress test or the presenting complaint of decreased fetal movement.

    However, many high-risk obstetric and fetal conditions require this study to help guide management.

    During the biophysical profile, your provider is looking at five main areas to check your baby's health: body movements, muscle tone, breathing movements, amniotic fluid, and heartbeat. Each of these five areas is given a score of either 0 (abnormal) or 2 (normal).

20. **b.** An NST is considered reassuring if the fetal heart rate increases at least 15 beats per minute over the baseline (between 120 and 160 beats per minute), lasting at least 15 seconds, within a 20-minute timeframe. This is called a "reactive NST."

    There have to be accelerations with fetal movements.

21. **a.** Maternal fever causes tachycardia in the mother, leading to tachycardia in the fetus. Therefore, when NST is done for fetal well-being, there is evidence of tachycardia (fetal heart rate above 140) without decelerations.

22. **b.** The NST shows late decelerations which is ideally seen in cases of fetal distress. Artificial rupture of membranes will tell if the amniotic fluid is clear or meconium stained which will help in decision making for delivering the baby immediately by cesarean section as the mother is only 2 cm dilated with late decelerations.

23. **c.** The baseline heart rate is 140 bpm with early decelerations suggestive of head compression.

24. **c.** The NST is reactive with good variability; therefore, according to American College of Obstetricians and Gynecologist (ACOG) guidelines, we can wait for spontaneous labor till 40+6 weeks.

25. **c.** Although there is evidence that the use of umbilical artery Doppler findings can reduce the mortality by 29% in high-risk pregnancies, high resistance to umbilical arterial flow can only help define growth restriction rather than predict adverse perinatal outcomes. Umbilical artery reverse flow has been shown to predict neonatal mortality. CTG interpretation in conjunction with umbilical artery Doppler velocimetry findings has been shown to reduce not only neonatal mortality but also to reduce hospital stay. Most reference charts report the umbilical artery Doppler in a free loop of cord. Impedance values are higher at the fetal end of the cord and lower at the placental end. The etiopathogenesis of early and late onset FGR is different; hence, the pattern of deterioration of umbilical artery Doppler velocimetry is often not similar. In early onset fetal growth restriction (FGR), there is a reduction of villi, unlike in late onset where there is mainly impaired maturation. Therefore, the deterioration of umbilical artery Doppler waveform may not occur until very late in late onset FGR.

26. **b.** While several studies have shown that the cerebroplacental ratio is associated with adverse perinatal outcomes in late third trimester FGR, none have shown that it is strongly predictive. The middle cerebral artery (MCA)–umbilical artery Doppler ratio is associated with emergency cesarean

section even in the presence of normal umbilical artery Doppler velocimetry. The MCA Doppler is a useful tool to evaluate cerebral vasodilatation and multicenter studies have shown that it is associated with poor perinatal outcome; however, it does not inform the timing of delivery. CPR < 1 is associated with fetal hypoxia and is present in a quarter of cases of late onset FGR prior to delivery. Although one study has shown that CPR correlates with adverse perinatal outcomes, there is still uncertainty about the interpretation of findings in association with timing of delivery.

27. **c.** The uterine artery Doppler, whether recorded in the first, second, or third trimester, is significantly associated with the risk of stillbirth. It is true that in longitudinal studies, the uterine artery Doppler recorded in the third trimester is likely to be a better predictor of the fetuses at risk at term, when compared to the second trimester uterine artery Doppler. The uterine artery Doppler is a better predictor of FGR when recorded in the second, compared to the first, trimester. The uterine artery Doppler recorded in the third trimester has an additive value in identifying the fetuses at risk at term. The uterine artery Doppler is significantly associated with the risk of stillbirth, but not after adjusting for estimated fetal weight and CPR.

28. **d.** The etiopathogenesis of early and late onset FGR is different; hence, the pattern of deterioration of umbilical artery Doppler velocimetry is often not similar. In early onset FGR, there is a reduction of villi, unlike in late onset where there is mainly impaired maturation. Therefore, the deterioration of umbilical artery Doppler waveform may not occur until very late in late onset FGR.

29. **a.** CTG patterns permit more comprehensive assessment of the fetus than simply the presence or absence of hypoxia/acidemia. The features described including: a normal stable baseline FHT of 110–160 bpm with periods of accelerations with fetal movement and absent decelerations with contractions indicate rest/activity or sleep/wake cycles in the fetus and represent a high order of neurological integration. A baseline heart rate of 170 bpm with absent variability is not reflective of fetal hypoxia. Tachycardia reflects hypoxia only in association with decelerations. With absent decelerations, the more likely diagnosis is maternal fever, medication, fetal "anxiety" response (where the tachycardia will be limited in duration), or possibly neurological injury. This emphasizes the role of decelerations in the detection of head compression or other mechanical problems of labor.

30. **a.** After 30 weeks, an increasing number of fetuses have a mature pattern of heart rate acceleration that is equivalent to that seen at term. The baseline of the preterm fetus is higher than the term fetus. Given an understanding of the immature heart rate accelerative pattern in fetuses < 30 weeks, a reactive pattern can be identified in normal fetuses. V-shaped decelerations lasting approximately 15 seconds are common changes seen on the baseline and are benign.

Chapter 11: Prenatal Genetic Counseling, Screening, and Diagnosis

Purnima Satoskar

QUESTIONS

1. At what level of beta human chorionic gonadotropin (BHCG) should a gestational sac be visible on transvaginal ultrasound?
   a. 600 mIU/mL
   b. 3,000 mIU/mL
   c. 600 mIU/L
   d. 1,500 mIU/L

2. At what period of gestation is the combined test done for screening for Down syndrome?
   a. Between 6 and 10^{+6} weeks
   b. Between 11 and 13^{+6} weeks
   c. Between 14 and 16 weeks
   d. Between 16 and 20 weeks

3. What should be the crown-rump length for nuchal translucency measurement?
   a. 39–45 mm
   b. 45–95 mm
   c. 45–84 mm
   d. None of the above

4. Which of the following statements is *wrong* with respect to first-trimester screening?
   a. Pregnancy-associated plasma protein A (PAPP-A) < 0.5 MoM correlates with adverse perinatal outcome
   b. Low PAPP-A is found in Down syndrome
   c. Low beta-human chorionic gonadotropin (hCG) is suggestive of Down syndrome
   d. Both PAPP-A and HCG are low in Trisomy 18

5. The detection rate of noninvasive prenatal screening for Down syndrome is:
   a. 88%
   b. 95%
   c. 96%
   d. 99%

6. At how many weeks, can noninvasive prenatal screening be done?
   a. As soon as pregnancy is detected
   b. After 9 weeks
   c. From 11 to 14 weeks only
   d. Before 20 weeks

7. Which test is recommended for early diagnosis of Down syndrome if one of the parents is carrying a 14/21 translocation?
   a. Chorionic villus sampling (CVS) at 9 weeks with fluorescence in situ hybridization (FISH)
   b. CVS at 9 weeks with karyotyping
   c. CVS at 11 weeks with karyotyping
   d. CVS at 11 weeks with FISH

8. Which of the following diagnostic techniques is of no value for the diagnosis of neural tube defects?
   a. Amniocentesis
   b. Chorion villus sampling (CVS)
   c. Maternal serum screening
   d. Ultrasonography

9. The most common approach for intrauterine transfusion is:
   a. Umbilical artery at fetal insertion of cord
   b. Umbilical vein at placental insertion of cord
   c. Umbilical artery at placental insertion of cord
   d. Umbilical vein at fetal insertion of cord

10. The recommendation for genetic testing for structurally anomalous fetus at 17 weeks on amniotic fluid is:
    a. FISH and karyotype
    b. Chromosomal microarray
    c. Karyotype is sufficient
    d. Store DNA

11. Which of the following is the least likely complication of amniocentesis?
    a. Leaking PV
    b. Bloody tap
    c. Fetal bradycardia
    d. Chorioamnionitis

12. A patient undergoes chorionic villous sampling for a positive combined screening for Down syndrome. The report shows 46**/Trisomy 21 mosaicism. What advice will you give?
    a. Repeat chorionic villous sampling immediately
    b. Final decision after anomaly scan
    c. Amniocentesis and karyotype at 17 weeks
    d. Terminate the pregnancy in view of Trisomy 21

13. A G2P1 Rh negative with 30 weeks with previous lower segment cesarean section (LSCS) has an Rh antibody titer of 1:128. Middle cerebral artery peak systolic velocity (MCA-PSV) is 2 MoM. How will you proceed?
    a. Repeat MCA-PSV in 2 weeks
    b. Repeat MCA-PSV in 1 week
    c. Amniocentesis for spectrophotometry
    d. Cordocentesis and transfusion

14. First trimester combined test in a primi is high risk for trisomy 21 in a pair of diamniotic dichorionic twins at 13 weeks. Placenta is fused and posterior reaching os. After counseling, patient says she wants a definite answer with a single test. How will you proceed?
    a. Repeat the test to rule out erroneous report
    b. Proceed with chorionic villous sampling by combined transabdominal and transvaginal approach
    c. Advise amniocentesis from each sac after anomaly scan
    d. Advise noninvasive prenatal testing

15. A patient with previous beta thalassemia major child presents at 23 weeks. Ultrasonography shows anterior placenta. What test will you advise?
    a. Placental biopsy
    b. Cordocentesis
    c. Amniocentesis
    d. Too late for testing

16. Noninvasive prenatal testing (NIPT) done in a primigravida shows high risk for Turner syndrome. What will you advise?
    a. Explain features of Turner and offer termination
    b. Explain features of Turner and advise continuation if anomaly scan rules out coarctation of aorta
    c. Confirm with amniocentesis and karyotyping
    d. Can proceed with termination due to very high sensitivity of the test

17. Both husband and wife are carriers for CFTR gene responsible for cystic fibrosis. Which of the following is true?
    a. The risk of having an affected child is 100%
    b. The risk of having an unaffected child is 75%
    c. The risk of having an affected child is 50%
    d. The risk of having a child which is also carrier is 25%

18. What are the chances of having an affected offspring if one parent is affected with an autosomal dominant disorder?
    a. 100%
    b. 75%
    c. 50%
    d. 25%

19. Which of the following is an example of abnormality of chromosomal number?
    a. Trisomy
    b. Monosomy
    c. Polyploidy
    d. All of the above

20. Which of the following is not true about Fragile X syndrome?
    a. Most common inherited form of intellectual disability
    b. Males are more severely affected than females
    c. Caused by expansion of CGG repeats at X chromosome
    d. The risk of full mutation in offspring is less if CGG repeats are more than 200

21. Which technique is used for preimplantation genetic screening/preimplantation genetic diagnosis?
    a. Polar body analysis
    b. Blastomere biopsy
    c. Trophectoderm biopsy
    d. All of the above

22. A couple have a third-degree marriage. There is a strong history of neonatal deaths in the family due to an unexplained cause. No genetic tests were ever performed on the neonate. What is the next best step in evaluation of the couple?
    a. Karyotype of the couple
    b. Whole exome sequencing of the couple
    c. No tests can be offered as genetic cause of neonatal deaths not established
    d. They can plan pregnancy without any evaluation as risk of recurrence is only 25%

23. A primigravida at 32 weeks was diagnosed on ultrasonography (USG), to have a severely growth restricted fetus with presence of intrahepatic calcification and echogenic bowel. A TORCH profile was done on maternal serum. Which of the following result will show evidence of a recent cytomegalovirus (CMV) infection?
    a. CMV IgM positive and IgG negative
    b. CMV IgM negative and IgG positive
    c. CMV IgG positive with low avidity
    d. CMV IgG positive with high avidity

24. Which investigation will you suggest for a couple facing recurrent pregnancy loss?
    a. Karyotype
    b. Whole exome sequencing
    c. Chromosomal microarray
    d. Sanger's sequencing

25. Which of the following is *not* true about trisomy 18 (Edward's syndrome)?
    a. It has high intrauterine mortality
    b. It is associated with low levels on free β-hCG and PAPP-A on dual marker test
    c. Risk of recurrence in 50%
    d. It is associated with major cardiovascular and central nervous system (CNS) anomalies

26. Which of the following is *not* a cause of nonimmune hydrops?
    a. Hemoglobinopathies   b. Infections
    c. Rh alloimmunization   d. Structural anomalies

27. What is true about inheritance of mitochondrial diseases?
    a. Mitochondria are inherited from both set of parents
    b. Mitochondria are inherited majorly from mother and in lesser amount from father
    c. Mitochondria are inherited exclusively from mother
    d. Mitochondria are inherited exclusively from father

28. What is *not* true about Robertsonian translocation?
    a. Involve only acrocentric chromosomes -13, -14, -15, -21, -22
    b. Incidence of abnormal offspring is more if translocation is carried by mother
    c. Karyotype helps in picking up the translocation
    d. They are a major cause of miscarriage

29. Which of the following is *not* a cause of polyhydramnios?
    a. Rh alloimmunized pregnancy
    b. Suspected tracheoesophageal fistula in fetus
    c. Gestational diabetes in mother
    d. Lower urinary tract obstruction (LUTO)

30. DiGeorge syndrome is an autosomal dominant disorder, due to microdeletion in *22q11* gene. Which statement best is *not* true regarding the disorder?
    a. It is a rare microdeletion
    b. Features include thymic dysplasia, cardiovascular abnormalities, and developmental delay
    c. Also known as velocardiofacial syndrome
    d. More than 90% cases occur from de novo mutations

ANSWERS

1. **b.** An intrauterine gestational sac is visible on transvaginal ultrasonography (TVS) at a serum beta-hCG level of 3,000 mIU/mL due to the high resolution of TVS probe, while the threshold is much higher using the transabdominal approach (approximately 6,000 mIU/mL).

2. **b.** Combined test includes serum dual marker test as well as nuchal scan which is done from 11 to 13^{+6} weeks.

3. **c.** 45–84 mm as per Fetal Medicine Foundation (FMF) guidelines

4. **c.** High beta-hCG is suggestive of Down syndrome.

5. **d.** The detection rate of noninvasive prenatal screening for Down syndrome is 99% but it is less for other aneuploidies.

6. **b.** Noninvasive prenatal testing (NIPT) can be done from 9 weeks onward as the fetal fraction may be low before this period. Fetal fraction of at least 4% is necessary or it is reported as a *No call*.

7. **c.** Chorion villus sampling (CVS) at 11 weeks with karyotyping as CVS should not be performed before 9 weeks due to risk of limb defects. FISH will not pick up translocations.

8. **b.** Chorion villus sampling (CVS). Maternal serum alpha-fetoprotein has been used as a screening method. Elevated alpha-fetoprotein levels in amniotic fluid have been used in the past for further

work up. The best way to pick up a neural tube defect is on ultrasonography. A neural tube defect will be missed very rarely with high-resolution ultrasound by an experienced operator.

9. **b.** The most common approach for intrauterine transfusion is the umbilical vein as the blood is directed toward the fetal heart. An arterial entry may lead to spasm with bradycardia or spurting and cord hematoma. The placental insertion of cord is relatively immobile, hence preferred.

10. **b.** Chromosomal microarray (CMA) is now the recommended test for structural anomalies as it gives a 5% additional yield of microdeletion/duplication.

11. **c.** Complications of amniocentesis include bloody tap, leaking PV, chorioamnionitis, and Rh isoimmunization. Fetal bradycardia is highly unlikely if procedure is carried out under ultrasonography guidance, avoiding the umbilical cord.

12. **c.** Amniocentesis and karyotype at 17 weeks will give the definite answer. Most likely the fetus is normal and the report is due to sampling of confined placental mosaicism.

13. **d.** Cordocentesis and transfusion should be done immediately as MCA-PSV of 2 MoM correlates with severe fetal anemia and the fetus is premature.

14. **c.** Advise amniocentesis from each sac after anomaly scan. Never repeat a positive screen. CVS is difficult without mixing the samples and a second test may be needed if the report shows mosaicism. Anomaly scan will identify any additional markers and make it easy to map the fetuses.

15. **b.** Cordocentesis will give a definite result before 24 weeks.

16. **c.** Noninvasive prenatal screening (NIPS) is a screening test and termination should never be offered without diagnostic testing.

17. **b.** Cystic fibrosis is an autosomal recessive disease. As both husband and wife are carriers, the chance of an affected child is 25% and unaffected child is 75%. 50% of the offsprings will be carrier.

18. **c.** Carriers have a 50% chance of passing the affected gene with each conception.

19. **d.** Trisomy and monosomy refer to an extra chromosome or loss of one chromosome respectively. Polyploidy refers to an abnormal number of haploid chromosomal sets, such as triploidy.

20. **d.** Fragile X is the most common inherited form of intellectual disability. It is caused by expansion of a repeated trinucleotide DNA (CGG) at X chromosome. Although transmission is X linked, the factors determining the degree of impairment are the sex of the individual and the number of CGG repeats. Intellectual disability is generally more severe in males. Women with Fragile X permutation, i.e., >55 CGG repeats are at a very high risk of having a full mutation in the offspring.

21. **d.**
    - Polar body analysis is used to diagnose whether a developing oocyte is affected by a maternally inherited genetic disorder. The first and second polar bodies are normally extruded from the developing oocyte following meiosis I and II, and their sampling should not affect fetal development.
    - Blastomere biopsy is done at the 6- to 8-cell stage and allows both maternal and paternal genomes to be evaluated. A limitation of this technique is that because of mitotic nondisjunction, mosaicism of the blastomeres may not reflect the chromosomal complement of the developing embryo. Also, the implantation rate of normal embryos is slightly lower following this technique.
    - Trophectoderm biopsy involves removal of 5-7 cells from a 5- to 6-day blastocyst. An advantage is that the trophectoderm cells give rise to the trophoblast the placenta—no cells are removed from the developing embryo. Disadvantage is—because the procedure is performed later in development, if genetic analysis cannot be performed rapidly, then cryopreservation and embryo transfer during a later IVF cycle may be required.

22. **b.** For preconceptional counseling of a consanguineous couple with strong family history of any illness, it is necessary to offer a test that encompasses the largest number of genes possible.

23. **c.** IgG avidity is defined as the strength with which IgG binds to antigenic epitopes. Low avidity is an accurate indicator of primary infection within the preceding 3-4 months, whereas high avidity excludes primary infection within the preceding 3 months.

24. **a.** Chromosomal abnormalities are observed in majority of spontaneous pregnancy losses as well as recurrent pregnancy losses. Parental karyotyping and genetic testing of products of conception may aid in defining the underlying etiology and in counseling patients.
25. **c.** Risk of recurrence is around 1%, as for all autosomal trisomies.
26. **c.** Rh alloimmunization is a cause of immune hydrops.
27. **c.** Oocytes contain about 100,000 mitochondria. Sperms hold only about 100 mitochondria, which are destroyed after fertilization. Hence, mitochondria are inherited exclusively from mother.
28. **d.** The incidence of abnormal offspring approximates 15% if a Robertsonian translocation is carried by the mother and 2% if carried by the father. Robertsonian translocations are not a major cause of miscarriage and are found in fewer than 5% of couples with recurrent pregnancy loss.
29. **d.** Lower urinary tract obstruction (LUTO) causes oligohydramnios.
30. **a.** It is the most common microdeletion with prevalence of 1 in 3,000–6,000 births.

Chapter 12

Normal Labor

Prema Kania

QUESTIONS

1. **Cardinal movements of labor are:**
   a. Engagement → descent → flexion → internal rotation → extension → restitution → external rotation → expulsion
   b. Engagement → extension → descent → internal rotation → flexion → expulsion
   c. Engagement → flexion → descent → internal rotation → expulsion → external rotation
   d. Engagement → extension → external rotation → internal rotation → expulsion

2. **During active labor, cervical dilatation per hour in primigravida is:**
   a. 1.2 cm   b. 1.6 cm
   c. 1.8 cm   d. 2.1 cm

3. **Living ligature of the uterus is:**
   a. Inner layer of myometrium
   b. Middle layer of myometrium
   c. Perimetrium
   d. All of the above

4. **The most common cause of nonengagement at term, in primigravida is:**
   a. Cephalopelvic disproportion (CPD)
   b. Polyhydramnios
   c. Face presentation
   d. Breech presentation

5. **True labor pain includes all, *except*:**
   a. Painful, progressive uterine contraction
   b. Shortening of vagina
   c. Cervical dilatation and effacement
   d. Progressive descent of presenting part of fetus

6. **Factors which help in descent of the presenting part during labor are all, *except*:**
   a. Progressive uterine contraction and retraction
   b. Straightening of the fetal ovoid
   c. Bearing down efforts by mother
   d. Resistance from the pelvic floor muscles

7. **The prerequisites for internal rotation of the head are all, *except*:**
   a. Well-flexed fetal head
   b. Uterine contraction and retraction
   c. Shape of maternal pelvis
   d. Tone of abdominal muscles

8. **Which is included in active management of 3rd stage in labor to prevent PPH?**
   a. Direct oxytocin injection after delivery of shoulder
   b. Prophylactic misoprost
   c. Controlled and sustained cord traction
   d. All of the above

9. **Pain in early labor is limited to dermatomes:**
   a. T10–L1   b. L1–L3
   c. L4–L5   d. S1–S2

10. **Assessment of progress of labor is best done by:**
    a. Station of head
    b. Cervical dilation only
    c. Cardiotocography (CTG)
    d. Partogram

ANSWERS

1. **a.** Engagement → descent → flexion → internal rotation → extension → restitution → external rotation → expulsion *(Reference: Dutta Obstetrics, 7th edition, page 128)*

2. **a.** 1.2 cm *(Reference: Williams Obstetrics, 22nd edition, pages 422, 423; 23rd edition, page 388)*
   Labor is said to active when:
   - Cervix is dilated to at least 3–4 cm
   - Regular uterine contractions are present
   - Rate of dilatation is at least 1.2 cm/h for nulliparous and 1.5 cm/h for parous women.

3. **b.** Middle layer of myometrium *(Reference: Dutta Obstetrics, 7th edition, page 46)*
   Muscle fibers in uterus are arranged in three layers:
   1. Outer longitudinal
   2. Inner circular
   3. Intermediate—is the strongest and thickest layer arranged in crisscross fashion.
      - Through this layer blood vessels run.
      - Apposition of two double curve muscle fiber gives the figure of 8 form.
      - When the muscles contract, they occlude the blood vessels running through the fibers and hence called living ligature

4. **a.** CPD *(Reference: Dutta Obstetrics, 7th edition, pages 81, 82, 352)*
   Engagement is said to occur when the greatest transverse diameter of the presenting part has passed through the pelvic inlet. In all cephalic presentations, the greatest transverse diameter is always the biparietal.
   Engagement occurs in multipara with commencement of labor in the late Ist stage after rupture of membranes and in nullipara during the last few weeks of pregnancy, i.e., ≈ 38 weeks.
   In primi's, the most common cause of non-engagement at term is deflexed head or occipitoposterior position followed by cephalopelvic disproportion (CPD). Since deflexed head or occipitoposterior is not given in option, we will go for CPD as the answer.

5. **b.** Short vagina *(Reference: Dutta Obstetrics, 7th edition, page 117)* Cervical changes (dilatation and effacement) present only in true labor.

6. **d.** Resistance from the pelvic floor *(Reference: Dutta Obstetrics, 7th edition, page 124)*
   Descent: Descent is a continuous process provided there is no undue bony or soft tissue obstruction. It is slow or insignificant in first stage but pronounced in second stage. It is completed with the expulsion of the fetus. In primigravidae, with prior engagement of the head, there is practically no descent in first stage; while in multiparae, descent starts with engagement.
   Head is expected to reach the pelvic floor by the time the cervix is fully dilated.
   Factors facilitating descent are—(1) uterine contraction and retraction, (2) bearing down efforts, and (3) straightening of the fetal ovoid especially after rupture of the membranes.

Note: Resistance offered by the pelvic floor promotes flexion of head and not descent.

7. **d.** Tone of abdominal muscles *(Reference: Dutta Obstetrics, 7th edition, page 125)*

8. **d.** All of the above
   (Reference: Dutta Obstetrics, 7th edition, pages 141, 142)

   Active management of the third stage of labor includes:
   - Administration of a uterotonic soon after birth (best is oxytocin followed by misoprost
   - Delayed cord damping
   - Delivery of placenta by controlled cord traction
   - Uterine massage

   Now, this leaves us with no doubt that "early cord clamping" should not be included in active management of labor.
   Reason: Why early cord clamping is being discouraged is because if cord is clamped immediately the cord blood present in it (80–100 mL) will go waste whereas, if delayed cord clamping is done, the cord blood goes to the newborn and there are less chances of anemia, intraventricular hemorrhage, and late onset sepsis especially in preterm infants.
   In order to facilitate the cord blood to reach the newborn, the tray with the baby should be placed at a lower level than the mother's abdomen after delivery and before cord is cut.
   The only drawback of active management of 3rd stage of labor is—since uterotonic agent is given at the delivery of shoulder before the delivery of placenta, it can lead to increased chances of retained placenta.

9. **a.** i.e., T10–L1 *(Reference: Dutta Obstetrics, 7th edition, page 117)*
   In the early stages of labor, pain is mainly uterine in origin because of painful uterine contraction
   "The pain of uterine contractions is distributed along the cutaneous nerve distribution of T10 to L1" *(Reference: Dutta Obstetrics, 6th edition, page 118)*
   In later stages, pain is due to dilatation of the cervix.
   "The pain of cervical dilatation and stretching is referred to the back through sacral plexus." *(Reference: Dutta Obstetrics, 6th edition, page 118)*

10. **d.** Partogram *(Reference: Dutta Obstetrics, 7th edition, page 530; Williams Obstetrics, 23rd edition, page 406)*
    Partogram is the best method to assess progress of labor.

Chapter 13: Postpartum Hemorrhage

Rajshree Dayanand Katke

QUESTIONS

1. How much is the blood loss to say as postpartum hemorrhage in vaginal delivery?
   a. 500 mL
   b. 400 mL
   c. 1,500 mL
   d. 250 mL

2. What are the types of postpartum hemorrhage?
   a. Primary
   b. Tertiary
   c. Secondary
   d. Both a and c

3. What are the various causes of PPH?
   a. Tone
   b. Tissue
   c. Trauma
   d. Thrombin
   e. All of the above

4. What are the conditions in which postpartum hemorrhage is common?
   a. Grand multipara
   b. Overdistension
   c. Antepartum hemorrhage
   d. Malnutrition
   e. All of the above

5. How much is the quantity of blood loss following cesarean section to say as postpartum hemorrhage?
   a. 700 mL
   b. 500 mL
   c. 1,000 mL
   d. 800 mL

6. What are placental causes of postpartum hemorrhage?
   a. Placenta accreta
   b. Placenta percreta
   c. Retained placenta
   d. All of the above

7. After vaginal delivery if patient is bleeding profusely, on per abdominal examination it is flabby, what is your diagnosis?
   a. Atonic uterus
   b. DIC
   c. Traumatic PPH
   d. All of the above

8. In traumatic postpartum hemorrhage, what are the various conditions?
   a. Lacerations of cervix
   b. Episiotomy wound hematoma
   c. Rupture uterus
   d. All of the above

9. Disseminated intravascular coagulation (DIC) as cause of PPH is developed in which of the following conditions?
   a. Abruptio placenta
   b. Jaundice in pregnancy
   c. HELLP syndrome
   d. Severe preeclampsia thrombocytopenic puerperia
   e. All of the above

10. Patient came in the emergency ward with profuse bleeding per vaginum after forceps delivery on per abdomen examination, the uterus was contracted. What could be the cause of bleeding?
    a. Atonic PPH
    b. Traumatic PPH
    c. All of the above
    d. Traumatic + atonic PPH

11. What preventive measures and precautions we should take to prevent postpartum hemorrhage antenatally?
    a. Diagnosis and corrections of anemia and nutritional care
    b. Early diagnosis of pregnancy-induced hypertension and treatment
    c. Diagnosis of high-risk cases and treatment timely
    d. All of the above

12. The patient has delivered per vaginally spontaneously but after delivery of baby even after 30 minutes placenta has not been delivered, what could be the cause of it?
    a. Impartially separated placenta
    b. Morbid adherent placenta
    c. a and b
    d. None of the above

13. What are the various oxytocic drugs used to control postpartum hemorrhage?
    a. Oxytocin
    b. Methergine
    c. Misoprostol
    d. All of the above

14. What is the contraindication of using injection methergine in cases of postpartum hemorrhage?
    a. Severe hypertension
    b. Severe diabetes
    c. None of above
    d. AIDS

15. What are the types of sutures taken to control the bleeding of postpartum hemorrhage?
    a. B-Lynch suture
    b. Cerclage operation
    c. Vertical mattress sutures
    d. None of the above

16. In atonic postpartum hemorrhage, what are the steps to be taken to do management?
    a. Uterine bimanual massage
    b. Use of oxytocics and misoprostol to contract uterus
    c. Compression suture
    d. All of the above

17. Patient is in hemorrhagic shock due to postpartum hemorrhage. Intraoperatively what are the various measures should be taken to control the bleeding?
    a. Bilateral uterine ligation
    b. B-lynch
    c. Bilateral internal iliac artery ligation
    d. All of the above

18. Which is the drug as rectal suppositories to keep in cases of atonic postpartum hemorrhage?
    a. Oxytocics
    b. Methergine
    c. Misoprostol 800 mg
    d. Cerviprime gel

19. What is the effect of bilateral anterior division of internal iliac ligation?
    a. Reduction of blood flow by 85% and pulse pressure by 46%
    b. Reduction of blood flow by 50% and pulse pressure by 50%
    c. Reduction of blood flow by 75% and pulse pressure by 40%
    d. Reduction of blood flow by 68% and pulse pressure by 20%

20. Which is the branch ligated in internal iliac ligation to control bleeding in postpartum hemorrhage?
    a. Posterior branch of internal iliac artery
    b. Anterior branch of internal iliac artery
    c. Internal pudendal branch of iliac artery
    d. Superior vesical branch

21. At what level, the anterior branch of internal iliac artery ligated to control the bleeding in PPH?
    a. 3.5–4 cm after the division of posterior division of internal iliac artery
    b. 2 cm below the division of anterior division of internal iliac artery
    c. 8 cm above iliac artery
    d. 6 cm above iliac artery

22. Misoprostol dose for the PPH for rectal administration:
    a. 600 µg
    b. 400 µg
    c. 1,000 µg
    d. 800 µg

23. In which patients, misoprostol should not be used in PPH?
    a. Hypertension
    b. Diabetes mellitus
    c. Bronchial asthma
    d. Rh-negative pregnancy

24. What are the complications of B-lynch sutures?
    a. Ischemic necrosis of uterus
    b. Ischemic necrosis of ovaries
    c. Infection of uterus
    d. All of the above

25. What are the complications of internal iliac artery ligation?
    a. Injury to ureter
    b. Injury to external iliac vein
    c. Injury to internal iliac vein
    d. All of the above

26. How much % is the PPH contributing in maternal mortality?
    a. 25%
    b. 10%
    c. 20%
    d. 50%

27. What is the role of Non-Pneumatic Anti-shock Garment (NASG)?
    a. It reverses shock by decreasing blood flow to the abdomen and lower body
    b. It keeps patient with postpartum hemorrhage alive for 48 hours
    c. It reverses shock by returning blood to the vital organs heart, lungs, and brain
    d. All of the above

28. How to assess blood loss in postpartum hemorrhage?
    a. Weighing soaked gauze
    b. Blood in the suction machine
    c. Hypovolemic shock
    d. All of the above

29. **For embolization of internal iliac artery to control the bleeding in postpartum hemorrhage, what catheters and material are used?**
    a. Gelfoam polyvinyl alcohol particles (size 300–500 μm) or coils
    b. Plastic catheter
    c. Steel catheter
    d. None of the above

30. **What are the major complications of embolization of internal iliac artery in cases of postpartum hemorrhage?**
    a. Necrosis of uterus
    b. Blockage of popliteal artery
    c. Groin hematoma
    d. All of the above

ANSWERS

1. **a.** Postpartum hemorrhage is defined as blood loss of >500 mL after normal vaginal delivery and 1000 mL during cesarean section.

2. **d.** *There are two types of postpartum hemorrhage (PPH):* Primary PPH is when it occurs within 24 hours of delivery and it is divided into mild when blood loss is (500–1,000 mL), moderate when blood loss is (1,000–2,000 mL), and severe when blood loss is >2000 mL.
   Secondary PPH is hemorrhage occurring after 24 hours of delivery until 6 weeks postpartum period.

3. **e.** *Various causes of postpartum hemorrhage:*
   - Tone (uterine atony): 70%
   - Trauma (laceration/rupture): 20%
   - Tissue (retained placenta): 10%
   - Thrombin (coagulopathy): 1%

4. **e.** All of the above
   The conditions in which atonic postpartum hemorrhage is common are:
   - Grand multipara
   - Overdistended uterus
   - Antepartum hemorrhage
   - Malnutrition

5. **c.** Postpartum hemorrhage has been defined as estimated blood loss of 1,000 mL after cesarean delivery.

6. **d.** *Placental causes of postpartum hemorrhage are:*
   - Placenta accreta
   - Placenta increta
   - Placenta percreta
   - Retained placenta

7. **a.** If after VgD if patient is bleeding and uterus is flabby then it is known as atonic PPH.

8. **d.** All of the above
   Various conditions in traumatic postpartum hemorrhage are:
   - Cervical laceration
   - Episiotomy wound hematoma
   - Uterine rupture

9. **e.** *Disseminated intravascular coagulation (DIC) as cause of PPH is developed in following conditions:*
   - Abruptio placenta
   - Jaundice in pregnancy
   - HELLP syndrome
   - Severe preeclampsia thrombocytopenic puerperia

10. **b.** Patient came to emergency ward with profuse vaginal bleeding following forceps delivery and uterus was well contracted then the cause of bleeding is traumatic PPH caused due to forceps application.

11. **d.** Following preventive measures and precautions should be taken to prevent postpartum hemorrhage antenatally:
    - Early diagnosis and corrections of anemia and nutritional care
    - Early diagnosis of pregnancy-induced hypertension and treatment
    - Diagnosis of high-risk cases and timely treatment

12. **c.** *After vaginal delivery of baby if even after 30 minutes placenta has not been delivered, following are causes:*
    - Impartially separated placenta
    - Morbidly adherent placenta

13. **d.** *Oxytocic/uterotonic drugs used to control postpartum hemorrhage:*
    - *First-line drugs:* Oxytocin and Carbetocin
    - *Second-line drugs:* Misoprostol
    - Methylergometrine
    - Carboprost

14. **a.** Methergin is contraindicated in patients with severe hypertension.

15. **a.** *B-Lynch sutures:* In this pair, vertical brace sutures are secured around uterus with number 2 chromic catgut.
    This suture works by compressing anterior and posterior wall placental bed, thus reducing uterine blood loss.

16. **d.** *In atonic postpartum hemorrhage management, following steps are needed:*
    - *Compression techniques:* Uterine bimanual compression, uterine tamponade
    - Use of oxytocics and misoprostol to contract uterus
    - *Compression suture:* B-Lynch sutures, hymen (modified B-Lynch) suture, Cho stitches
17. **d.** *When patient is in hemorrhagic shock due to postpartum hemorrhage, intraoperatively following measures should be taken to control the bleeding:*
    - Bilateral uterine artery ligation
    - B-lynch suture, hymen (modified B-Lynch)suture, Cho stitches
    - Bilateral internal iliac artery ligation
18. **c.** Tablet misoprostol 800 µg is kept per rectally as a rectal suppository in case of atonic PPH.
19. **a.** Effect of bilateral anterior division of internal iliac ligation is reduction of blood flow by 85% and pulse pressure by 46%.
20. **b.** Anterior branch of internal iliac artery is ligated 4–5 cm away from its origin to control bleeding in postpartum hemorrhage.

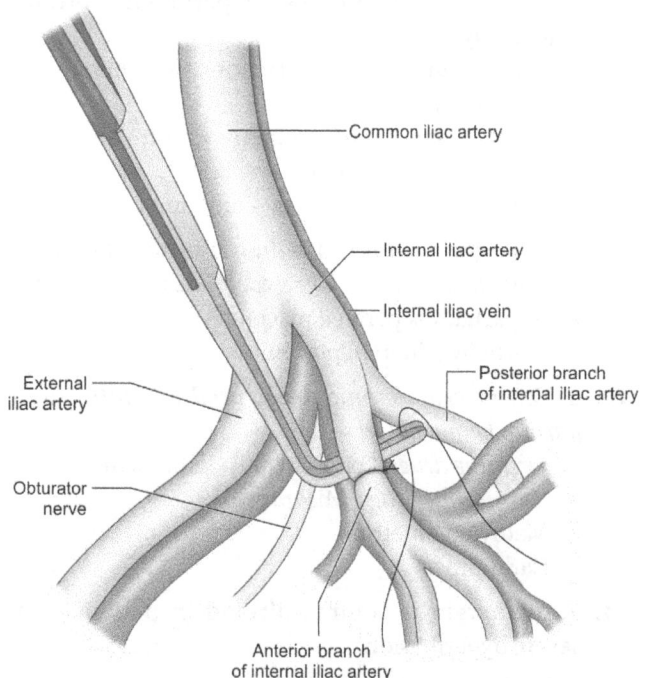

21. **a.** Anterior branch of internal iliac artery ligated 3.5–4 cm after the division of posterior division of internal iliac artery to control the bleeding in PPH.
22. **d.** 800 µg misoprostol is used for rectal administration in PPH.
23. **c.** Misoprostol is contraindicated in PPH in patients with allergic reactions like bronchial asthma.
24. **d.** *Complications of B-Lynch sutures are as follows:*
    - Ischemic necrosis of uterus
    - Ischemic necrosis of ovaries
    - Infection of uterus
25. **d.**
    Complications of internal iliac artery ligation are as follows:
    - Injury to ureter
    - Injury to external iliac vein
    - Injury to internal iliac vein
26. **a.** Postpartum hemorrhage contributes 25% in maternal mortality.
27. **d.** *Roles of nonpneumatic antishock garment (NASG) are as follows:*
    - It reverses shock by decreasing blood flow to the abdomen and lower body
    - It reverses shock by returning blood to the vital organs heart, lungs, and brain
    - It keeps patient with postpartum hemorrhage alive for 48 hours
28. **d.** *Blood loss in postpartum hemorrhage is assessed by following ways:*
    - Weighing soaked gauze
    - Blood in the suction machine
    - Hypovolemic shock
29. **a.** Gelfoam polyvinyl alcohol particles (size 300–500 µm) or coils are used for embolization of internal iliac artery to control the bleeding in postpartum hemorrhage.
30. **d.** *Major complications of embolization of internal iliac artery in cases of postpartum hemorrhage are as follows:*
    - Necrosis of the uterus
    - Blockage of popliteal arteries
    - Groin hematoma formation

REFERENCES

1. Cunningham. Williams Textbook, 26th edition. New York: McGraw Hill/Medical; 2022.
2. Garg R. Labour and delivery: an updated guide. Singapore: Springer Nature Singapore Pte Ltd;2023.
3. Katke RD. Ovarian necrosis of both ovaries with uterine ischemic changes following B-Lynch sutures: A rare complication and review of literature. J Int Med Res Health Sci. 2021;1(1):1-6.

Chapter 14: Normal Puerperium

Neelima Mantri

QUESTIONS

1. **Postpartum decidual secretions present are referred to as:**
   a. Lochia
   b. Show
   c. Vasa-previa
   d. Decidua parietalis

2. **Lochia in correct order: during puerperium:**
   a. Rubra, serosa, alba
   b. Serosa, mucosa, alba
   c. Alba, serosa, mucosa
   d. Alba, rubra, serosa

3. **Approximate size of uterus at 8 weeks postpartum is:**
   a. 100 g
   b. 500 g
   c. 300 g
   d. 600 g

4. **In comparison to breast milk, colostrum has higher content of:**
   a. Protein
   b. Fat
   c. Sodium
   d. Calcium

5. **Which of the following is more correct about breast infection during lactation?**
   a. Due to microbes from infant's saliva
   b. Mastitis does not affect the child
   c. Streptococcus is the only organism
   d. Can lead to abscess and I and D may be required

6. **Contraceptive method of choice in lactating mothers is:**
   a. Barrier method
   b. Progesterone only pill
   c. Lactational amenorrhea
   d. None of the above

7. **Common route of spread of puerperal sepsis:**
   a. Lymphatic
   b. Direct invasion
   c. Skip lesion
   d. Hematogenous

8. **The cause of "postpartum blues" is:**
   a. Decreased estrogen
   b. Decreased dopamine, increased prolactin
   c. Decreased progesterone
   d. Decreased estrogen and progesterone

9. **All are complication of formula fed baby over human milk fed baby, *except*:**
   a. Necrotizing enterocolitis
   b. Otitis media
   c. Hypocalcemia
   d. Vitamin K deficiency

10. **Most common immunoglobulin secreted by mother in milk and colostrum is:**
    a. IgA
    b. IgG
    c. IgM
    d. IgD

11. **The uterus becomes pelvic organ after delivery in:**
    a. 10-12 days
    b. 12-14 days
    c. 15-17 days
    d. 18-20 days

12. **Without breastfeeding, the first menstrual flow usually begins __ weeks after delivery:**
    a. 2-4 weeks
    b. 6-8 weeks
    c. 10-12 weeks
    d. 12-14 weeks

13. **Which of the following sets of condition is attributed to normal physiology of puerperium?**
    a. Tachycardia and weight gain
    b. Increased frequency of micturition, constipation, and weight gain
    c. Constipation, tachycardia, and urinary urgency
    d. Retention of urine and constipation

14. **Initiation of lactation is affected by:**
    a. Oxytocin
    b. Prolactin
    c. HPL
    d. All of the above

15. **Decrease lactation seen in:**
    a. Maternal anxiety
    b. Cracked nipple
    c. Breast abscess
    d. All of the above

16. **A 24-year-old P^{2+0} woman presents to the emergency department complaining of pain in her right breast. The patient is postpartum day 10 from an uncomplicated spontaneous vaginal delivery at 42 weeks. She reports no difficulty breastfeeding for the first several days postpartum, but states that for the past week her daughter has had difficulty latching on. 3 days ago, her right nipple became dry and cracked, and since yesterday, it has become increasingly swollen and painful. Her temperature is 38.3°C (101°F). Her right nipple and areola are warm, swollen, red, and tender. There is no fluctuance or induration, and no pus can be expressed from the nipple.**
    a. Continue breastfeeding from both the breasts
    b. Breastfeed from unaffected breast only
    c. Immediately start antibiotics and breastfeed only when antibiotics are discontinued
    d. Stop breastfeeding immediately

17. **M/C nerve injured during normal vaginal delivery is:**
    a. Obturator N
    b. Lateral femoral cutaneous N
    c. Genitofemoral nerve N
    d. Pudendal N

18. **Which of the following steps helps in decreasing puerperal infection following cesarean section:**
    a. Closure of peritoneum
    b. Double layer uterine closure
    c. Administration of single dose of ampicillin or 1st-generation cephalosporin at the time of cesarean delivery
    d. Skin closure with staples than with suture

19. **A 23-year-old primi patient who had delivered a 2.7 kg baby boy 2 days back comes to the casualty. She had a normal vaginal delivery and placenta delivered spontaneously. Now, she complains of bloody vaginal discharge with no other signs. O/E you notice a sweetish odor bloody discharge on the vaginal walls and introitus. Sterile pelvic examination shows a soft nontender uterus. Her P/R—78/min, B/P—110/76 mm Hg, temperature—37°C, and R/R—16/min. Her WBC count = 10,000 with predominant granulocytes. What is the most appropriate step?**
    a. Curettage
    b. Oral antibiotics
    c. Reassurance
    d. Vaginal culture

20. **What is the main aim of postpartum perineal care during the puerperium?**
    a. Preventing urinary tract infections
    b. Reducing perineal pain and swelling
    c. Promoting healing of perineal tears or episiotomy
    d. All of the above

ANSWERS

1. **a.** Lochia is the vaginal discharge for the first fortnight during puerperium.

   The discharge originates from the uterine body, cervix, and vagina. It has got a peculiar offensive fishy smell. Its reaction is alkaline tending to become acid toward the end.

   Depending upon the variation of the color of the discharge, it is named as:
   - Lochia rubra (red) 1-4 days
   - Lochia serosa (5-9 days): The color is yellowish or pink or pale brownish.
   - Lochia alba (pale white): 10-15 days

2. **a.**

3. **a.** 100 g
   Weight of uterus:
   - Immediately after delivery—1,000 g
   - At the end of 1 week—500 g
   - At the end of 2 weeks—300 g
   - At the end of 4 weeks—100 g (pre-pregnant state)

4. **a.** Protein
   Colostrum is a deep yellow serous fluid secreted from breasts starting from pregnancy and for 2-3 days after delivery.

   Composition: It has higher specific gravity and higher protein, vitamin A, D, E, K, immunoglobulin, sodium and chloride content than mature breast milk. It has lower carbohydrate, fat, and potassium than mature milk.

   Advantages: Antibodies (IgA, IgG, and IgM) and humoral factor (lactoferrin) provide immunological defense to the newborn.

   Laxative action due to fat globules
   It is an ideal natural starter food.

5. **d.** Can lead to abscess formation for which I and D may be required.

6. **b.** Progesterone only pill
   According to the American College of Obstetrics and Gynecologist (2000), progestin only contraceptives are the preferred choice in most of the cases. In addition, intrauterine devices (IUDs) may be recommended for the lactating sexually active woman after uterine involution.

7. **b.** Direct invasion
   Puerperal pyrexia—is defined as a rise of temperature reaching 100.4°F (38°C) or more (measured orally) on two separate occasions at 24 hours apart (excluding first 24 hours) within first 10 days following delivery.
   Any infection of genital tract which occurs as a complication of delivery is called as puerperal sepsis.
   Most common site of puerperal infection—placental site in vaginal delivery and uterine incision in cesarean section
   Most common manifestation of puerperal infection—endometritis
   Most common cause of puerperal sepsis—*Streptococcus*
   Most common route of infection—direct spread
   Single most significant risk factor for development of puerperal sepsis (uterine infection) = Route of delivery (It is M/C in cesarean delivery than vaginal delivery)
   Management: Clindamycin + Gentamicin ± Ampicillin

8. **d.** Decreased estrogen and progesterone
   Puerperal blues/3 days blues/baby blues
   It is transient state of mental illness observed 4-5 days after delivery in nearly 50% of postpartum women.
   Postpartum blues occurs at the height of hormonal change.
   Patients present with depression, anxiety, fearfulness, insomnia, helplessness, and negative feelings toward infant.
   It may last from a few days to 2-3 weeks.
   Generally self-limited, 20% of women may develop depression in the first postpartum year.

   Treatment: Reassurance and psychological support of family members
   Postpartum depression
   It is observed in 10-20% of mothers.
   It is more gradual in onset over the first 4-6 months following delivery or abortion.
   Changes in hypothalamic-pituitary-adrenal axis may be a cause.
   Manifested by loss of energy and appetite, insomnia, social withdrawal, irritability, and even suicidal attitude
   Risk of recurrence 50-100% in subsequent pregnancies

   Treatment: Should be started early. Fluoxetine or paroxetine is effective and has fewer side effects.

9. **d.** Vitamin K deficiency
   Formula feeds contain a host of vitamin and minerals, as well as trace elements (zinc, manganese, copper, and iodine) and electrolytes. In formula feeds, vitamin K is added in higher levels than in breast milk to reduce the risk of hemorrhagic diseases in newborn. So, vitamin K deficiency can never be a complication of formula fed babies.

10. **a.** IgA
    Composition of breast milk:
    - *Carbohydrate:* Lactose is present in high concentration in breast milk.
    - Protein content is low, as the baby cannot metabolize a high-protein diet. The proteins are mainly lactalbumin and lactoglobulin, which are easily digestible. It is also rich in the amino acids taurine and cysteine, which are necessary for neurotransmission and neuromodulation.
    - *Fats:* Breast milk is rich in polyunsaturated fatty acids (PUFA) needed for myelination.
    - *Water and electrolytes:* The water content is 86-87%.
    - *Immunological superiority:* Breast milk contains immunoglobulins, especially IgA and IgM, lysozyme, lactoferrin (which protects against enterobacteria), bifidus factor (to protect against *Escherichia coli*), PABA (which protects from malaria).

    "Breast milk has a high concentration of secretory IgA and IgM." "Colostrum contains antibody IgA produced locally".

11. **a.** 10-12 days
    Dutta says: Just after delivery, uterus is 13.5 cm above pubic symphysis and thereafter its size decreases by 1.25 cm/day which means by 10-12 days, it will be

an intrapelvic organ (i.e., below the level of pubic symphysis).

12. **b.** 6–8 weeks
Women not breastfeeding have return of menses usually within 6–8 weeks.

13. **d.** Retention of urine and constipation

14. **d.** All of the above. Oxytocin, prolactin, and HPL help in initiation of lactation.

15. **d.** All of the above lead to decrease in lactation.

16. **a.** A postpartum lady coming with h/o pain in breast and fever and nipples being warm, red, swollen, with no induration, fluctuance, and no pus extruding from them—leaves no doubt that the patient is having mastitis. Mastitis is not a contraindication for breastfeeding. She should continue feeding from both the breasts.

17. **b.** Lateral cutaneous femoral N
Obstetrical neuropathies:
- *M/C nerve injured during vaginal delivery:* Lateral femoral cutaneous nerve followed by femoral nerve
- *Risk factors:* Nulliparity, prolonged second stage of labor, pushing for a longer period in semifowler position
- *M/C nerves injured during cesarean section:* Iliohypogastric N and ilioinguinal N

18. **c.** Administration of single dose of ampicillin or first-generation cephalosporin at the time of cesarean.

The only proven way of decreasing uterine infection following cesarean section is administering a single dose of ampicillin or first-generation cephalosporin at the time of cesarean delivery. Rest none of the steps like double-layer closure of uterus, closure of peritoneum, use of stapler to close skin incision instead of sutures, etc. are not proven to have any benefits as far as incidence of infection is considered following surgery.

19. **c.** Reassurance
This patient is a puerperal female who is complaining of bloody vaginal discharge with no other significant abnormal signs. On examination, there is a sweetish odor bloody discharge on the vaginal walls and introitus. Her vitals are normal suggesting that this cannot be PPH (the most common cause of secondary PPH is retained bits of placenta for which curettage is done, but here it is not required).

Slight amount of bloody discharge called as lochia is absolutely normal for the first 15 days after delivery and does not require any treatment, so we will reassure the patient and do nothing.

Do not get confused with the finding of WBC count—10,000 with predominant granulocytes as this is a normal finding in the puerperal period. *Note:* leukocytes can rise to as high as 25,000 during puerperium probably as a response to the stress of labor). Since lochia has no foul smell, it means no infection and so no need for culture or antibiotics.

20. **d.** All of the above

Chapter 15: Abnormalities of the Puerperium: Part 1

Deepa Kala

1. **True about involution of uterus during puerperium is____.**
   a. Uterus regains nonpregnant size by 2 weeks.
   b. Endometrium is restored over placental site within a week.
   c. Involution of placental site is by absorption in situ.
   d. Involution of placental site is by process of exfoliation.

2. **Surgical site infection occurring in the first 2 days is usually due to:**
   a. Group A or B *streptococci*
   b. *Staphylococcus*
   c. Mycobacterium
   d. *Escherichia coli*

3. **Gram-positive aerobes most commonly involved in postpartum uterine infection:**
   a. Group B *Streptococci*
   b. *E. coli*
   c. *Clostridium* species
   d. Chlamydia trachomatis

4. **Chlamydial endometritis usually sets in on which day postpartum?**
   a. Day 2   b. Day 7
   c. Day 15   d. Day 4

5. **Puerperal pyrexia has all these features, *except*:**
   a. Temperature of >38°C or higher
   b. At least two episodes 6 hours apart
   c. One episode within first 24 hours of delivery
   d. Standard technique of taking oral temperature every 4 hourly should be followed.

6. **The organism responsible for toxic shock like syndrome is:**
   a. *Proteus* species   b. *Klebsiella*
   c. *Mycoplasma hominis* d. *Staphylococcus aureus*

7. **The most common cause of puerperal fever is:**
   a. Mastitis   b. Metritis
   c. Pyelonephritis d. Thrombophlebitis

8. **The chance of postpartum metritis is highest after:**
   a. Normal vaginal delivery
   b. Elective cesarean section
   c. Spontaneous abortion at 6 weeks
   d. Cesarean section after 14 hours of labor

9. **"Enigmatic fever" was name coined for clinical picture due to _____ in puerperal fever.**
   a. Fever due to pelvic abscess
   b. Fever due to thrombophlebitis
   c. Fever due to urinary tract infection
   d. Fever due to episiotomy infection

10. **A parametrial phlegmon:**
    a. Is responsible for persistent puerperal fever
    b. Is an area of induration in the parametrium due to intensive cellulitis
    c. May lead to pelvic abscess
    d. All of the above are true

11. **The most common urinary problem occurring in the postpartum period is:**
    a. Detrusor instability   b. Urinary tract infection
    c. Stress incontinence   d. Vesicovaginal fistula

12. **A 30-year-old P1L1 comes on D7 of lower segment cesarean section (LSCS) with right-sided chest pain and breathlessness.**
    She was a case of severe hypertension and has persistent edema of the feet. On examination, her vitals were:
    P—110/min; BP—130/80 mm Hg; SpO$_2$—94% ON RA
    What is the most likely diagnosis?
    a. Anemia   b. Myocardial infarction
    c. Pneumonia   d. Pulmonary embolism

13. Mrs D comes to the OPD with breast pain and discomfort, she is a Para-1 Living-1, 2-month post delivery. You establish a diagnosis of cracked nipple. All of the following are treatment options, *except*:
    a. Analgesics
    b. Stop breastfeeding
    c. Gentle hand expression to promote drainage
    d. Nipple shield
14. Sheehan's syndrome includes:
    a. Normal lactation
    b. Hyperthyroidism
    c. Amenorrhea
    d. Subinvolution of uterus
15. In Sheehan's syndrome, what is correct order of affection of secretion of the hormones:
    1. Prolactin
    2. Growth hormone
    3. TSH
    4. FSH
    a. 1, 2, 3, 4
    b. 1, 2, 4, 3
    c. 2, 1, 3, 4
    d. 2, 1, 4, 3
16. Appearance of severe perineal pain accompanied by difficulty in voiding and sudden appearance of a tense fluctuant and sensitive tumor point to diagnosis of:
    a. Acute cystitis
    b. Sphincter injury
    c. Vulval hematoma
    d. Cervical tear
17. P1L1 day 1 of full-term normal delivery complains of difficulty in wearing slippers in the right foot and walking. What is the most likely diagnosis?
    a. Thrombosis of right femoral vein
    b. Pelvic hematoma
    c. Foot drop
    d. Eclampsia
18. Which one of the following statement is correct in relation to postpartum depression?
    a. Antidepressants are contraindicated if breastfeeding.
    b. Postpartum depression may occur in the 12 months following delivery.
    c. Postpartum blues start 10 days after delivery.
    d. Women with postpartum blues commonly think of committing suicide.
19. True about postpartum depression is:
    a. Patient will have malformed infant.
    b. Hallucination may be present.
    c. There is loss of appetite and weight.
    d. It resolves in 2 weeks.
20. True about anticoagulation therapy for acute venous thromboembolism (VTE) during pregnancy and puerperium is____
    a. Can be stopped immediately after delivery
    b. Routine measurement of anti-Xa activity should be done for patients on low molecular weight heparin (LMWH) for treatment of acute VTE in pregnancy and puerperium.
    c. Wound drains for cesarean section and skin closure with mattress sutures is recommended in patients on LMWH.
    d. Thrombophilia screen should be done before initiating anticoagulant therapy.
21. The most common site of septic pelvic thrombophlebitis is____
    a. Uterine vein
    b. Ovarian vein
    c. Common iliac vein
    d. Inferior vena cava
22. Which statement is true regarding antihypertensive treatment in the postnatal period?
    a. Antihypertensives are not secreted in the breast milk.
    b. Diuretics can be freely used in women in the postnatal period who are breastfeeding.
    c. 2–3 times dosing of drugs is better than once daily tablets.
    d. Maternal renal function should be monitored when giving enalapril to treat hypertension in the postnatal period.
23. Which can be a risk factor for persistent postnatal perineal pain?
    a. Cesarean delivery
    b. Having a birth companion
    c. Multiparity
    d. Episiotomy or labial or perineal tear
24. Which blood test is used as a marker for severe sepsis in a case of puerperal sepsis?
    a. Serum lactate >4 mmol/L
    b. CRP >160 mg/L
    c. ESR >100 mm/h
    d. WBC count >16,000
25. Hypotension in a case of severe sepsis is termed nonresponsive if:
    a. Mean arterial pressure (MAP) remains below 60 mm of Hg.
    b. Initial fluid resuscitation of 20 mL/kg with crystalloids fails to increase MAP.

c. Initial fluid resuscitation of 10 mL/kg with crystalloids fails to increase MAP.
   d. MAP remains above 65 mm of Hg.

26. **WHO recommendations for prevention and treatment of maternal peripartum infections include:**
    a. Routine vaginal cleansing with chlorhexidine during labor
    b. Intrapartum antibiotic administration to women with group B *Streptococcus* colonization
    c. Routine antibiotic prophylaxis for women with episiotomy
    d. Antibiotic prophylaxis after cord clamping during cesarean section

27. **A post LSCS patient is brought on day 12 of delivery to hospital with history of convulsion. There is a history of loose motions few days back after which the patient developed severe headache. Now she is disoriented and has right hemiparesis. Most likely diagnosis is:**
    a. Puerperal eclampsia
    b. Puerperal psychosis
    c. Cerebral venous thrombosis
    d. Epilepsy

ANSWERS

1. **d.** *(Reference: Williams Textbook of Obstetrics, 20th edition, Chapter 24)*

2. **a.** Infections occurring within the first two postoperative days are most commonly caused by group A or B *streptococci* other commonly isolated pathogens include ureaplasma urealyticum, *Enterococcus faecalis*, *Escherichia coli*, *Proteus mirabilis*, and *Staphylococcal* species.
   (Reference: Boushra M, Rahman O. NIH-National library of medicine StatPearls: Postpartum Infection)

3. **a.** Most common pathogens in endometritis are those normally associated with the reproductive and urinary tracts and include group B *Streptococci*, enterococci, *Escherichia coli*, and *Klebsiella pneumoniae*.
   (Reference: Boushra M, Rahman O. NIH-National library of medicine StatPearls: Postpartum Infection)

4. **b.** In endometritis presenting after 7 days postpartum and in high-risk populations such as women under age 25, *Chlamydia trachomatis* should be suspected as the cause.
   (Reference: Boushra M, Rahman O. NIH-National library of medicine StatPearls: Postpartum Infection)

5. **c.** Puerperal pyrexia is exclusive of first 24 hours. Rarely, a high spiking fever more 39°C may be associated with virulent pelvic infection.
   (Reference: Williams Textbook of Obstetrics, 20th edition, chapter 24)

6. **d.** 10% of pregnant women have vaginal colonization with *Staphylococcus aureus*. Treatment is supportive as in septic shock.
   (Reference: Williams Textbook of Obstetrics, 20th edition, chapter 24)

7. **b.** *(Reference: Williams Textbook of Obstetrics, 20th edition, chapter 24)*

8. **d.** *(Reference: Williams textbook of obstetrics, 20th edition, chapter 24)*

9. **b.** Patients with pelvic thrombophlebitis improve clinically but fever spikes do not stop.
   (Reference: Williams Textbook of Obstetrics, 20th edition, chapter 24)

10. **d.** *(Reference: Williams Textbook of Obstetrics, 20th edition, chapter 24)*

11. **c.** Incidence of SUI is 7% as against incident of UTI which is 2–4%.
    (Reference: Williams Textbook of Obstetrics, 20th edition, chapter 24)

12. **d.** VTE is 10 times more common in pregnancy but the puerperium is the time of highest risk. The symptoms may be low-grade fever, leg pain and swelling, dyspnea, chest pain and even hemoptysis or collapse.
    (Reference: RCOG Green-Top Guideline Number 37b)

13. **b.** Stopping of breastfeeding is indicated only in cases of breast abscess.

14. **c.** Sheehan syndrome occurs when the anterior pituitary gland is damaged due to significant blood loss, classically after delivery. Common symptoms are absence of lactation, amenorrhea, hypothyroidism, and hyperinvolution of the uterus. Adrenal insufficiency can also occur.
    (Reference: Schury MP, Adigun R. NIH-National library of medicine StatPearls-Sheehan Syndrome)

15. **d.** *(Reference: Schury MP, Adigun R. NIH-National library of medicine StatPearls-Sheehan Syndrome)*

16. **c.** *(Reference: DC Dutta's Textbook of Obstetrics Hiralal Konar, 8th edition)*

17. **c.** *(Reference: DC Dutta's Textbook of Obstetrics Hiralal Konar, 8th edition, Chapter 30, Page 511)*

18. **b.** *(Reference: Williams Textbook of Obstetrics, 20th edition, Chapter 24)*

19. **c.** *(Reference: Williams Textbook of Obstetrics, 20th edition, Chapter 24)*

20. **c.** *(Reference: RCOG Green-Top Guideline Number 37b)*

21. **b.** Ovarian vein is involved in 40% of the cases because sepsis starts at the placental site which is usually in the upper part of the uterus. This region drains into the ovarian vein.
    (Reference: Williams Textbook of Obstetrics, 20th edition, Chapter 24)

22. **d.** *(Reference: https://www.nice.org.uk/guidance/cg107/chappter/1-Guidance)*

23. **d.**

24. **a.** Serum lactate ≥4 mmol/L is indicative of tissue hypoperfusion. It should be measured within 6 hours of the suspicion of severe sepsis to guide management.
    (Reference: Bacteria Sepsis in Pregnancy, Green Top Guideline_64a)

25. **b.** *(Reference: Bacteria sepsis in pregnancy, Green Top Guideline_64a)*

26. **b.** In women with group B *Streptococcus* colonization, antibiotic is needed to prevent early neonatal GBS infection. Antibiotic prophylaxis during cesarean section should be given before the skin incision.
    (Reference: WHO recommendations for prevention and treatment of maternal peripartum infections)

27. **c.** Obesity, bed rest, anemia, PIH, dehydration, and infection are contributory factors for cerebral venous thrombosis. Already there is a hypercoagulable state during pregnancy and postpartum.
    (Reference: WHO recommendations for prevention and treatment of maternal peripartum infections)

Chapter 16: Abnormalities of Puerperium: Part 2

Deepali Kapote, Madhura Mandlik

QUESTIONS

1. You are called to review a postnatal day 1 patient, who has had a normal vaginal delivery, which of the following finding would be of the most concern?
   a. Fever of 99°F
   b. Proteinuria
   c. Pain at episiotomy site
   d. Abdominal rigidity

2. Puerperal fever is persistent increase in temperature above:
   a. 99.8°F
   b. 100.4°F
   c. 98.4°F
   d. 101°F

3. Which of the following mode of delivery have the highest rate on endometriosis?
   a. Normal vaginal delivery
   b. Vacuum-assisted delivery
   c. Outlet forceps delivery
   d. Cesarean delivery

4. Which is not an increased risk factor for puerperal infection after surgery?
   a. Prolonged rupture of membranes
   b. Repeated vaginal examination
   c. External fetal monitoring
   d. Prolonged labor

5. Toxic shock syndrome in the puerperal period is most commonly caused by:
   a. Group A beta hemolytic *Streptococcus*
   b. Group B beta hemolytic *Streptococcus*
   c. Actinomycete
   d. *Staphylococcus*

6. Which of the following is not correct?
   a. Routine vaginal swab helps in reducing chances of infection
   b. Perioperative prophylaxis is recommended
   c. Obesity is a risk factor for abdominal wound dehiscence
   d. Repeated vaginal examination increases risk of infection

7. American College of Obstetricians and Gynecologists (ACOG) recommends the following for perioperative prophylaxis for cesarean delivery:
   a. 2G Ampicillin after delivery of baby
   b. 2G Ampicillin before skin incision
   c. 2G Ampicillin and metronidazole before skin incision
   d. 2G Ampicillin and metronidazole after placental delivery

8. Which of the following is not a risk factor for abdominal incision infection?
   a. Hypertension
   b. Obesity
   c. Anemia
   d. Prolonged rupture of membranes

9. A 30-year-old patient (gravida 2, para 2) has just delivered vaginally an infant weighing 4 kg after a spontaneous uncomplicated labor. She has had no problems during the pregnancy and labor. The placenta delivers spontaneously. There is immediate brisk vaginal bleeding of greater than 500 cc. After a significant period of hypovolemic shock, the bleeding was controlled and the vascular volume replaced. Estimates of blood loss were over 2,500 cc. The patient apparently recovered well. However, she was unable to breastfeed and gradually noted breast atrophy and no resumption of menses. Later, she developed constipation, slurred speech, and moderate nonpitting edema. Which of the following is the most likely diagnosis?
   a. Acute kidney injury
   b. Sheehan syndrome
   c. Asherman syndrome
   d. Amenorrhea–galactorrhea syndrome

10. A 20-year-old patient had an operative vaginal delivery with a second-degree perineal tear which was sutured. She also had a prolonged labor. In her antenatal period, she had anemia, and BMI was 30 kg/m². She develops a persistent fever of 101°F on the 3rd day postpartum. What is the most likely cause?
    a. Mastitis
    b. Endometritis
    c. Pneumonia
    d. Urinary tract infection

11. A patient presents 10 days post her normal vaginal delivery with complaints of her left breast being engorged, hot, red, and painful. She reports a fever of 101°F. If her breasts were cultured, which of the following is the most likely organism to be found?
    a. *Escherichia coli*
    b. *Streptococcus pyogenes*
    c. *Staphylococcus aureus*
    d. *Anaerobes*

12. Septic pelvic thrombophlebitis is best diagnosed using:
    a. Duplex ultrasound
    b. Clinical sign
    c. Vaginal swab
    d. CT

13. Which of the following can be attributed as not a finding in abnormal puerperium?
    a. Retention of urine and constipation
    b. Tachycardia and weight gain
    c. Retention of urine, constipation, and weight gain
    d. Constipation, tachycardia, and retention of urine

14. Royal College of Obstetricians and Gynecologists (RCOG) recommends closure of subcutaneous tissue to prevent wound infection if subcutaneous fat is:
    a. 3.5 cm
    b. 3 cm
    c. 2.5 cm
    d. 2 cm

15. A 32-year-old woman (gravida 2) has just delivered. After expression of the placenta, a red, raw surface is seen at the vaginal introitus. Simultaneously, the nurse states that the patient is pale and her BP is 70/40 mm Hg. External bleeding has been of normal amount. Which of the following would be the most likely diagnosis?
    a. Retained placental lobe
    b. Ruptured uterus
    c. Vaginal rupture
    d. Uterine inversion

16. Most common nerve injured during vaginal delivery is:
    a. Femoral nerve
    b. Lateral femoral cutaneous nerve
    c. Ilioinguinal nerve
    d. Iliohypogastric nerve

17. A 25-year-old patient finally delivered a 3.2 kg baby vaginally. Her prenatal course was complicated by anemia, poor weight gain, and maternal obesity. Her labor was protracted, including a 3-hour second stage, a mid-forceps delivery with a sulcus laceration, and a third-degree episiotomy. Which of the following is the most common route that results in serious complication of a septic thrombophlebitis?
    a. Arterial
    b. Venous
    c. Direct spread
    d. Lymphatic

18. A patient had a vaginal delivery after a prolonged second stage. She is now unable to void urine. Each of the following could be a reason and can be initially treated with Foley placement. Which of the following can represent a most serious etiology of inability to void in the immediate postpartum period?
    a. Overdistension of bladder
    b. Anesthesia
    c. Pain
    d. Hematoma

19. The cause of postpartum blues is:
    a. Decreased estrogen and progesterone
    b. Increased prolactin
    c. Decreased estrogen
    d. Decreased progesterone

20. A patient who is a known case of GDM delivers at term. It is important to check her blood sugar levels immediately postpartum, since there may be a decrease in the insulin requirements of diabetic patients. This can be partly explained by which of the following?
    a. Decreased human placental lactogen
    b. Decreased activity
    c. Increased insulin secretion
    d. Decrease in plasma estrogen

21. Which of the following is most appropriate for breast infection?
    a. *Streptococcus* is the only pathogen
    b. Due to pathogen from infant's gastrointestinal tract (GIT)

c. Mastitis does not affect neonate
d. Can lead to abscess and may warrant I and D

22. A 24-year-old P1L1 day 5 post normal vaginal delivery, placental separation was spontaneous, no complications in postnatal delivered, came with complain of bloody vaginal discharge. On examination, uterus is soft and nontender, discharge has a sweetish odor. Pulse is 87 bpm, she is a febrile and total leukocyte count is 12,000 with predominant granulocytes. What is the most appropriate management?
    a. Curettage
    b. IV antibiotics
    c. Reassurance
    d. Vaginal culture

23. A patient calls your clinic complaining of continued heavy vaginal bleeding. She had an "uncomplicated" vaginal birth 2 weeks ago of her second child. What is the most likely diagnosis from the following differentials?
    a. Uterine atony
    b. Retained placenta
    c. Uterine rupture
    d. Coagulopathies

24. A previously energetic woman complains of crying, loss of appetite, difficulty in sleeping, and feeling of low self-worth, beginning approximately 3 days after a normal vaginal delivery. These feelings persisted for approximately 1 week and then progressively diminished. Which of the following is the best term to describe her symptoms postpartum?
    a. Neuroses
    b. Psychoses
    c. Blues
    d. Depression

25. At delivery, a perineal laceration tore through the skin of the fourchette, vaginal mucous membrane, and the fascia and perineal muscles of the perineal body but not the anal sphincter or mucosa. This should be recorded in the medical record as what type of laceration?
    a. First degree
    b. Second degree
    c. Third degree
    d. Fourth degree

26. A 32-year-old P2L2 postcesarean delivery, developed deep venous thrombosis, she is on warfarin and asks you if she can breastfeed her baby:
    a. Stop warfarin and convert to low molecular weight heparin (LMWH)
    b. Breastfeed after 6 hours of taking warfarin
    c. Warfarin is not a contraindication for breastfeeding
    d. She will have to topfeed the baby

27. Common route of spread of puerperal sepsis is:
    a. Direct spread
    b. Hematogenous
    c. Lymphatics
    d. Retrograde flow

28. P1L1 day 2 post lower segment cesarean section, with BMI of 30 kg/m², develops pain in her right calf, which becomes swollen and tender. You have a clinical suspicion of deep vein thrombosis. Which of the following would be the most appropriate first mode on investigation for this patient?
    a. MRI
    b. Duplex ultrasonography
    c. CT scan
    d. X-ray

29. Formula fed infants have increased risk:
    a. Vitamin K deficiency
    b. Necrotizing enterocolitis
    c. Hair loss
    d. Hearing loss

30. A 20-year-old anemic patient delivered a baby by instrumental delivery. On day 5 postdelivery, she complained of discharge from episiotomy site. On assessing, she had an episiotomy gap. She was treated with dressing and secondary closure was done eventually. What would you advise for her postoperative care?
    a. Only liquid diet
    b. Wound care, stool softener
    c. Enema
    d. No special care needed

ANSWERS

1. **d.** Abdominal rigidity after a vaginal delivery could be indicative of a serious condition such as uterine rupture or internal bleeding. This requires immediate attention and further investigation to rule out any complications. The other findings mentioned, such as leukocytosis, proteinuria, a pulse rate of 60, and a single temperature of 100.4°F, are relatively common and may not be as concerning as abdominal rigidity in this context.

2. **b.** Several infective and noninfective factors can cause puerperal fever—a temperature of 38.0°C (100.4°F) or higher. Most persistent fevers after childbirth are caused by genital tract infection.

3. **d.** In the French Confidential Enquiry on Maternal Deaths, Deneux-Tharaux and coworkers (2006) cited

a nearly 25-fold increased infection-related mortality rate with cesarean versus vaginal delivery.

4. **c.** Important risk factors for infection following surgery included prolonged labor, membrane rupture, multiple cervical examinations, and internal fetal monitoring.

5. **a.** Over the past 25 years, there have been reports of group A β-hemolytic *Streptococcus* causing toxic shock-like syndrome and life-threatening infection (Castagnola, 2008; Nathan, 1994). In the past 10 years, skin and soft-tissue infections due to community-acquired methicillin-resistant *Staphylococcus aureus* (CA-MRSA) have become common. Although this variant is not a frequent cause of puerperal metritis, it is often implicated in abdominal incisional infections (Anderson, 2007; Patel, 2007).

6. **a.** Routine genital swabs are not recommended and do not help in decreasing risk of infection.

7. **b.** Single-dose prophylaxis with a 2-g dose of ampicillin or a first-generation cephalosporin is ideal. It is controversial whether the infection rate is lowered further if the antimicrobial is given before the skin incision compared with after umbilical cord clamping (Baaqeel, 2013; Macones, 2012; Sun, 2013). The American College of Obstetricians and Gynecologists (2016b) has concluded that the evidence favors predelivery administration.

8. **d.** Incisional infection risk factors include obesity, diabetes, corticosteroid therapy, immunosuppression, anemia, hypertension, and inadequate hemostasis with hematoma formation.

9. **b.** The most likely diagnosis is Sheehan's syndrome (pituitary necrosis). This is supported by the patient's history of significant postpartum bleeding and hypovolemic shock, which can lead to ischemic necrosis of the pituitary gland. The symptoms of breast atrophy, amenorrhea, and hormonal imbalances are consistent with pituitary dysfunction. Additionally, the development of constipation, slurred speech, and nonpitting edema can be attributed to the hormonal deficiencies caused by pituitary necrosis. Most common presentation of Sheehan syndrome is failure of lactation and amenorrhea.

10. **b.** The most likely etiology for the patient's persistent fever on the 3rd day postpartum is endometritis. Endometritis is an infection of the lining of the uterus, which commonly occurs after childbirth. The patient's complicated prenatal course, prolonged labor, and delivery with laceration and episiotomy increase the risk of developing endometritis. Symptoms of endometritis include fever, abdominal pain, and foul-smelling vaginal discharge. Prompt diagnosis and treatment with antibiotics are necessary to prevent complications.

11. **c.** *Staphylococcus aureus*, especially MRSA, is the most commonly isolated organism in breast infections.

12. **d.** The incidence of septic phlebitis has varied in several reports. In a 5-year survey of 45,000 women who were delivered at Parkland Hospital, Brown and associates (1999) found an incidence of septic pelvic thrombophlebitis in 1 per 9,000 gravidas following vaginal delivery and 1 per 800 after cesarean delivery. CT or MRI is most commonly used for diagnosis.

13. **a.** Retention in urine is common. Encourage patient to pass urine. Intestinal paresis causes constipation.

14. **d.** Women who have more than 2 cm subcutaneous fat should have suturing of subcutaneous space to decrease chances of wound infection and wound separation.
(Reference: Green-top guideline 72).

15. **d.** The most likely diagnosis in this scenario is uterine inversion. Uterine inversion occurs when the uterus turns inside out and protrudes through the cervix into the vagina. This can result in a red, raw surface at the vaginal introitus. The patient's pale appearance and low blood pressure indicate hypovolemia, which can be caused by uterine inversion due to excessive bleeding. The normal amount of external bleeding suggests that the bleeding is occurring internally, further supporting the diagnosis of uterine inversion.

16. **b.** Lateral femoral cutaneous nerve is the most common nerve to be injured followed by femoral nerve.

17. **b.** Septic thrombophlebitis is a serious complication of puerperal infection. It is most commonly spread through the venous route. The infection originates in the veins and spreads through the bloodstream, causing inflammation and blood clot formation. In this case, the patient had multiple risk factors for infection, including a complicated labor and delivery, which may have contributed to the development of septic thrombophlebitis through the venous route.

CHAPTER 16: Abnormalities of Puerperium: Part 2

18. **d.** A hematoma can represent a serious etiology of inability to void in the immediate postpartum period. Hematomas can occur due to trauma during delivery and can compress the urethra or bladder, leading to urinary retention. This can be initially treated with Foley placement to relieve the obstruction caused by the hematoma.

19. **a.** 50% postpartum women have postpartum blues. It occurs due to decrease in estrogen and progesterone. It usually occurs 4–5 days after delivery.

20. **a.** After delivery, the levels of chorionic somatomammotropin (hCS or hPL) decrease. It is produced by the placenta during pregnancy and acts as an antagonist to insulin, causing insulin resistance. So, a decrease in hPL levels postpartum would result in a decrease in insulin resistance and a subsequent decrease in insulin requirements for diabetic patients.

21. **d.** Mastitis is infection of breast parenchyma. Most common organism *Staphylococcus aureus* is the most common organism. Most commonly, the source of organism is infant's nose and throat.

22. **c.** Early in the puerperium, sloughing of decidual tissue results in a vaginal discharge of variable quantity. The discharge is termed lochia and contains erythrocytes, shredded decidua, epithelial cells, and bacteria. For the first few days after delivery, there is blood sufficient to color it red—lochia rubra. After 3 or 4 days, lochia becomes progressively pale in color—lochia serosa. After approximately the 10th day, because of an admixture of leukocytes and reduced fluid content, lochia assumes a white or yellow–white color—lochia alba. The average duration of lochial discharge ranges from 24 to 36 days (Fletcher, 2012). As patient is vitally stable, PPH is ruled out. Hence, reassurance is the right management.

23. **b.** Heavy vaginal bleeding after childbirth can be a sign of retained placental tissue in the uterus. When the placenta does not detach completely from the uterine wall, it can lead to persistent bleeding. Other differentials such as coagulopathies, uterine atony, uterine rupture, and vaginal lacerations may also cause bleeding, but in this scenario, retained placental fragments are the most likely cause based on the patient's history of an uncomplicated vaginal birth.

24. **c.** The term "blues" is the best term to describe the woman's symptoms postpartum. The symptoms of crying, loss of appetite, difficulty in sleeping, and feeling of low self-worth are consistent with the postpartum blues, also called baby blues. A common condition that affects women after giving birth and is characterized by mood swings, emotional instability, and sadness. The symptoms usually start within the first few days after delivery and mostly resolve in 1 or 2 weeks.

25. **b.** *Perineal tears are classified as follows:*
    - *First-degree tear:* Injury to perineal skin and/or vaginal mucosa
    - *Second-degree tear:* Injury to perineum involving perineal muscles but not involving the anal sphincter
    - *Third-degree tear:* Injury to perineum involving the anal sphincter complete
    - *Grade 3a tear:* Less than 50% of external anal sphincter (EAS) thickness torn
    - *Grade 3b tear:* More than 50% of EAS thickness torn
    - *Grade 3c tear:* Both EAS and internal anal sphincter (IAS) torn
    - *Fourth-degree tear:* Injury to perineum involving the anal sphincter and anorectal mucosa

26. **c.** Warfarin is not a contraindication for breastfeeding. It is excreted in very small amounts in breast milk and can be used safely during lactation. Warfarin is contraindicated in the first trimester of pregnancy and causes warfarin embryopathy. This entails microcephaly, nasal hypoplasia, optic atrophy, and chondrodysplasia punctata.

27. **a.** Most common route of spread of puerperal infection is direct spread.

28. **c.** Duplex ultrasonography should be done for suspected cases of deep vein thrombosis (DVT). In case the scan is negative and there is a strong suspicion, repeat the scan on day 3 and day 7.

29. **b.** Breast milk protects against NEC. Most of the neonates developing NEC are formula fed.

30. **b.** Secondary closure of the episiotomy is accomplished in layers, as described for primary episiotomy closure. Postoperative care includes local wound care, stool softeners, and nothing per vagina or rectum until healed.

Chapter 17: Bleeding in Early Pregnancy

Kunjal Bathija

QUESTIONS

1. A woman with 20 weeks pregnancy presents with bleeding per vaginum. On speculum examination, the os is open but no products have come out. The diagnosis is:
   a. Missed abortion
   b. Incomplete abortion
   c. Inevitable abortion
   d. Complete abortion

2. A 25-year-old female reports in the casualty with history of amenorrhea for two and half months and abdominal pain and bleeding per vaginum for 1 day. On examination, vital parameters and other systems are normal. On speculum examination, bleeding is found to come from os. On bimanual examination, uterus is of 10 weeks size, soft and os admits one finger. The most likely diagnosis is:
   a. Threatened abortion
   b. Missed abortion
   c. Inevitable abortion
   d. Incomplete abortion

3. A 28-year-old female with a history of 8 weeks amenorrhea complains of vaginal bleeding and lower abdominal pain. On USG examination, there is gestational sac with absent fetal parts. The diagnosis is:
   a. Ectopic pregnancy
   b. Incarcerated abortion
   c. Threatened abortion
   d. Corpus luteum cyst

4. A 28-year-old female with a history of 6 weeks of amenorrhea presents with pain in abdomen; USG shows fluid in pouch of Douglas. Aspiration yields dark color blood that fails to clot. Most probable diagnosis is:
   a. Ruptured ovarian cyst
   b. Ruptured ectopic pregnancy
   c. Red degeneration of fibroid
   d. Pelvic abscess

5. Most common manifestation of ectopic pregnancy is:
   a. Vomiting
   b. Bleeding
   c. Pain abdomen
   d. Shock

6. What is the typical pattern of bleeding in a threatened miscarriage?
   a. Heavy bleeding with severe abdominal pain
   b. Light spotting that resolves on its own
   c. Intermittent bleeding with cramping
   d. Prolonged heavy bleeding for several days

7. What diagnostic tool is commonly used to assess the viability of a pregnancy following bleeding in early pregnancy?
   a. Ultrasound
   b. Blood test
   c. Urine analysis
   d. Hysteroscopy

8. What is the recommended management for a confirmed miscarriage with heavy bleeding?
   a. Immediate surgical intervention
   b. Bed rest until the bleeding stops
   c. Expectant management or medication to induce miscarriage
   d. No intervention is necessary; bleeding will stop on its own

9. Which of the following is a potential sign of an ectopic pregnancy?
   a. Heavy bleeding with blood clots
   b. Severe lower abdominal pain on one side
   c. Absence of pregnancy symptoms
   d. Rapid weight gain

10. Which of the following is *not* a potential cause of bleeding in early pregnancy?
    a. Cervical polyps
    b. Infection
    c. Sexual intercourse
    d. Normal hormonal changes

11. A 36-year-old G1P0 woman presents for her first prenatal visit late in her first trimester of pregnancy; she complains of persistent vaginal bleeding, nausea, and pelvic pain. Physical examination is notable for a gravid uterus larger than expected for gestational age. Fetal heart tones are absent. Which of the following is most likely to be true?
    a. B-hCG levels will be higher than normal
    b. B-hCG levels will be lower than normal
    c. Uterus will be of normal levels
    d. TSH levels will be increased

12. A 34-year-old G1P0 woman at 29 weeks' gestation presents to the emergency department complaining of 2 hours of vaginal bleeding. The bleeding recently stopped, but she was diagnosed earlier with placenta previa by ultrasound. She denies any abdominal pain, cramping, or contractions associated with the bleeding. Her temperature is 36.8°C (98.2°F), blood pressure is 118/72 mm Hg, pulse is 75/min, and respiratory rate is 13/min. She reports she is Rh-positive, her hemoglobin is 11.1 g/dL, and coagulation tests, fibrinogen, and D-dimer levels are all normal. On examination, her gravid abdomen is nontender. Fetal heart monitoring is reassuring, with a heart rate of 155/min, variable accelerations, and no decelerations. Two large-bore peripheral intravenous lines are inserted and two units of blood are typed and crossed. What is the most appropriate next step in management?
    a. Admit to antenatal unit for bed rest and betamethasone
    b. Admit to antenatal unit for bed rest and blood transfusion
    c. Induction of labor
    d. Perform emergency cesarean section

13. All of the following can cause DIC during pregnancy, *except:*
    a. Diabetes mellitus
    b. Amniotic fluid embolism
    c. Intrauterine death
    d. Abruptio placentae

14. Which test differentiates maternal and fetal blood cell?
    a. APT test
    b. Kleihauer test
    c. Bubble test
    d. Lilly's test

15. Which of the following is not used in DIC?
    a. Heparin
    b. Epsilon aminocaproic acid
    c. Blood transfusion
    d. Intravenous fluids

16. In accidental hemorrhage, TOC:
    a. Induction of labor
    b. Treatment of hypofibrinogenemia then blood transfusion
    c. Simultaneous emptying of uterus and blood transfusion
    d. Wait and watch

17. In a nulliparous woman, the treatment of choice in ruptured ectopic pregnancy is:
    a. Salpingectomy
    b. Salpingo-oophorectomy
    c. Wait and watch
    d. Linear salpingostomy

18. A young lady presents with acute abdominal pain and history of 1½ months amenorrhea, on USG examination, there is collection of fluid in the pouch of Douglas and empty gestational sac. Diagnosis is:
    a. Ectopic pregnancy   b. Pelvic hematocele
    c. Threatened abortion   d. Twisted ovarian cyst

19. Most common cause of first trimester abortion is:
    a. Chromosomal abnormalities
    b. Syphilis
    c. Rhesus isoimmunization
    d. Cervical incompetence

20. All of the following are known causes of recurrent abortion, *except:*
    a. TORCH infections   b. SLE
    c. Rh incompatibility   d. Syphilis

ANSWERS

1. **c.** Inevitable abortion

2. **c.** Inevitable abortion—clinical picture—inevitable bleeding and pain, shock, size of uterus—equal or less, os—open with products felt, USG—dead fetus

3. **b.** Incarcerated abortion is a variant of missed abortion.
   Points in favor: Amenorrhea of 8 weeks (incarcerated abortion is seen in fetus before 12 weeks).
   USG showing gestational sac with no fetal part

In incarcerated abortion—small repeated hemorrhage occurs in the choriodecidual space, disrupting the villi from its attachment. The clotted blood with the contained ovum in called as blood mole. The ovum is dead and is either absorbed or remains as a rudimentary structure. So on USG—although gestational sac is seen, no fetal parts are seen.

4. **b.** *Ruptured ectopic pregnancy, Symptoms:* In ectopic pregnancy triad of: Amenorrhea (seen in 75% cases) followed by abdominal pain (seen in 100% cases, it is the most consistent symptom of ectopic pregnancy). Appearance of vaginal bleeding is seen: The above triad may be accompanied by nausea, vomiting, fainting attacks, or syncope. Patient may present in shock with pallor, tachycardia, hypotension, and cold clammy extremities, if ectopic pregnancy has ruptured.

5. **c.** Pain in abdomen. Most common and the most consistent symptom of ectopic pregnancy (undisturbed) is abdominal pain. It is seen in 95-100% cases. Pain is located in the lower abdomen/pelvic region. It can be unilateral or bilateral. In case of ruptured ectopic pregnancy: pain is due to hemoperitoneum and when internal hemorrhage floods the peritoneal cavity and irritates the undersurface of diaphragm and phrenic nerve, the patient also complains of shoulder tip and epigastric pain.

6. **c.** Intermittent bleeding with cramping

7. **a.** Ultrasound

8. **c.** Expectant management or medication to induce miscarriage

9. **b.** Severe lower abdominal pain on one side

10. **b.** Infection

11. **a.** B-hCG levels will be higher than normal. Patient complaining of extremes of nausea, vomiting + bleeding in first trimester + size of uterus more than the period of amenorrhea – think of molar pregnancy.

12. **a.** Admit to antenatal unit for bed rest and betamethasone.

    G1P0 woman at 29 weeks' gestation presents to the emergency department complaining of 2 hours of vaginal bleeding, the bleeding recently stopped, her vitals are stable [temperature is 36.8°C (98.2°F), blood pressure is 118/72 mm Hg, pulse is 75/min, and respiratory rate is 13/min], FHS are present and reassuring, i.e., there is no fetal distress.

    All this means we will manage this patient expectantly and there is no need to immediately terminate her pregnancy ruling out options **c** and **d**.
    So now, we have to choose between options:
    Admit to antenatal unit for bed rest and betamethasone.
    Admit to antenatal unit for bed rest and blood transfusion.
    The patient's Hb is 11.1, there is no need for immediate blood transfusion (ruling out option b), just cross-match and arrange blood and give betamethasone for hastening lung maturity.

13. **a.** Diabetes mellitus. DIC is a pathological condition associated with inappropriate activation of coagulation and fibrinolytic system. It is a secondary phenomenon resulting from an underlying disease state.
    More common causes of DIC:
    - Intrauterine fetal death
    - Amniotic fluid embolism
    - Preeclampsia-eclampsia
    - HELLP syndrome
    - Placenta abruption
    - Septic abortion

14. **a.** APT test—both Apt test and Kleihauer-Betke test can be used to detect the presence of fetal blood within a sample.
    Apt Test/Singers alkali denaturation test:
    Used to detect the presence or absence of fetal blood (qualitative) in a vaginal discharge to rule out vasa previa late in pregnancy or to detect the origin of a neonatal blood vomiting, whether it is a genuine upper GI hemorrhage/hemoptysis or simply swallowed maternal blood during delivery or from cracked nipple
    Kleihauer-Betke test:
    The sample is maternal peripheral smear and is used to see how much of fetal blood (quantitative) has been transfused into the maternal serum in order to assess the risk of isoimmunization and then the risk of hemolytic disease of newborn.
    Both of them rely on the fact that HbF is resistant to alkali (Apt) and acids (Kleihauer-Betke) and so the HbA-containing RBCs (maternal) will be hemolyzed but not the fetal RBCs as they have the HbF. *Correct*

answer: (a) Ritodrine. It is a beta-2 adrenergic receptor agonist—a class of medication used for smooth muscle relaxation. Since ritodrine has a bulky N-substituent, it has high β2-selectivity. Most side effects of beta-2 agonists result from their concurrent beta-1 activity, and include increase in heart rate, rise in systolic pressure, decrease in diastolic pressure, chest pain secondary to MI, and arrhythmia. Beta-agonists may also cause fluid retention secondary to a decrease in water clearance, which, when added to the tachycardia and increased myocardial work, may result in cardiac failure.

15. **b.** Epsilon aminocaproic acid
 Management of DIC:
 The most important step is to terminate the pregnancy—vaginal delivery without episiotomy is preferred to cesarean section.
   Volume replacement by crystalloids or colloids will reduce the amount of whole blood needed to restore the blood volume.
   500 mL of fresh blood raises the fibrinogen level approximately by 12.5 mg/100 mL and platelets by 10,000–15,000 mm^3.
   Fresh blood—helps in flushing out fibrin degradation product and improving the microcirculation.
 To replace fibrinogen: Fresh frozen plasma should be given:
   Fresh frozen plasma (FFP) is extracted from whole blood. It contains fibrinogen, anti-thrombin III, clotting factors V, XI, XII. FFP transfusion provides both volume replacement and coagulation factors. One unit of FFP (250 mL) raises the fibrinogen by 5–10 mg/dL. FFP does not need to be ABO or Rh compatible.
   Cryoprecipitate is obtained from thawed FFP. It is rich in fibrinogen, factor VIII, Von Willebrand's factor, and XIII.
   Cryoprecipitate provides less volume (40 mL) compared to FFP (250 mL). So it should not be used for volume replacement. One unit of cryoprecipitate increases the fibrinogen level by 5–10 mg/dL.
   In case of active bleeding with platelet counts <50,000/mL or prophylactically with platelet count 20–30,000/mL—platelet replacement should be done. Platelet should ABO and Rh specific. 1 units (50 mL) raises the platelet count by 7,500/mL
   Recombinant activated factors VIIA: (60–100 μg/kg IV) can reverse DIC within 10 minute, as it is a precursor for extrinsic clotting cascade which is replaced.
 Role of heparin:
 According to Williams Obstetrics, "Heparin is not used in DIC."

16. **c.** Simultaneous emptying of uterus and blood transfusion.
 The basic principle in the management of abruptio is termination of pregnancy along with correction of hypovolemia and restoration of blood loss.
   "With massive external bleeding, intensive resuscitation with blood plus crystalloids and prompt delivery to control hemorrhage are life saving for mother and hopefully fetus.
   This means option **c** is correct.
   "Expectant management of suspected placental abruption is the exception, not the rule. This management pathway should be attempted only with careful observation of the patient and a clear clinical picture."
   Correction of hypofibrinogenemia.
   "A rational approach (in abruptio) should be to withhold any specific therapy to rectify the coagulation disorders except in the circumstances such as overt bleeding or clinically evaluated thromboembolic process".

17. **a.** Salpingectomy
 In the question, the patient is presenting with ruptured ectopic pregnancy therefore surgical management is a must and we have to do laparotomy.
   In ruptured ectopic pregnancy, the tube is already damaged so the only surgery which has to be done is salpingectomy, whether the patient is a young/old or whether she is nulliparous or multiparous. Their is no role of salpingostomy. As discussed in previous question in case of ectopic pregnancy, salpingo-oophorectomy is never done.

18. **a.** Ectopic pregnancy
 Young lady presenting with history of:
 - Amenorrhea
 - Abdominal pain
 On USG:
 - Collection of fluid in pouch of Douglas
 - Empty gestational sac
 Indicate:
 - Ectopic pregnancy

19. **a.** Chromosomal abnormalities.

Abortion is spontaneous termination of pregnancy before 22 weeks or weight of fetus <500 g.

Incidence: About 15% of all conceptions end up in spontaneous abortions. Out of these, 80% occur before 12 weeks, i.e., in 1st trimester and among these 50–75% are due to chromosomal anomalies (Germplasm defect).

20. **a.** TORCH infection

As discussed in previous question, TORCH infection does not lead to recurrent abortion.

SLE is an established cause for recurrent abortion.

SLE is associated with antiphospholipid syndrome (anticardiolipin antibodies) and is known to cause recurrent abortions.

RH incompatibility is a known cause for spontaneous abortion and may lead to recurrent abortions if it remains unrecognized.

Syphilis also does not lead to recurrent abortions but if you have to rule out one option between TORCH infection and syphilis go for TORCH infection.

REFERENCES

1. Williams Obstetrics, 23rd edition, page 215
2. Williams Obstetrics, 23rd edition, p 1152
3. Williams Obstetrics, 22nd edition, pages 258, 259, 254
4. Williams Obstetrics, 23rd edition, pages 242, 243, 239
5. Dutta Obstetrics, 7th edition, pages 161, 162
6. Dutta Obstetrics, 7th edition, page 163
7. Dutta Obstetrics, 7th edition, page 182

Chapter 18

Vomiting in Early Pregnancy

Kunjal Bathija

QUESTIONS

1. Thiamine (vitamin B_1) deficiency results in which potential maternal complication of hyperemesis gravidarum?
   a. Renal failure
   b. Esophageal rupture
   c. Wernicke encephalopathy
   d. Osmotic demyelination syndrome

2. Which of the following gestational hormones is hypothesized to be correlated with hyperemesis gravidarum?
   a. Estrogen
   b. Testosterone
   c. Human placental lactogen (HPL)
   d. Human chorionic gonadotropin (hCG)

3. Which of the following dietary recommendations are effective in the management of hyperemesis gravidarum?
   a. Eating high-fat foods
   b. Drinking fluids with meals
   c. Removing salt from the diet
   d. Eating small, frequent meals

4. Thiamine replacement is essential prior to initiating hydration therapy in the patient with hyperemesis gravidarum because:
   a. Severe anemia may occur
   b. Vomiting may be exacerbated
   c. It may result in overhydration
   d. Dextrose causes the body to metabolize thiamine stores, which may result in Wernicke encephalopathy

5. Which of the following signs and symptoms is expected in a patient with hyperemesis gravidarum?
   a. Elevated pulse
   b. Ketotic breath smells
   c. Dry mucous membranes
   d. All of the above

6. Which of the following is seen in a urine dipstick analysis in the patient with hyperemesis gravidarum?
   a. Ketonuria
   b. Glycosuria
   c. Proteinuria
   d. Albuminuria

7. The diagnosis of impaired tissue integrity, especially in the oral mucous membranes, is due to
   a. Vitamin E deficiency
   b. Dehydration and vomiting
   c. Breathing through the mouth
   d. Increased vitamin consumption

8. Which of the following conditions increases the risk of hyperemesis gravidarum?
   a. Multiparity
   b. Cigarette smoking
   c. High pre-pregnancy body weight
   d. Maternal age older than 35 years

9. Primigravida with full-term complains of faintness on lying down and she feels well when turns to side or sitting position. This is due to:
   a. Increased vomiting during pregnancy
   b. IVC compression
   c. Increased intracranial pressure
   d. After heavy lunch

10. Which of the following factors is *not* associated with an increased risk of developing severe vomiting in pregnancy?
    a. Multiple pregnancies (twins, triplets, etc.)
    b. Young maternal age <20 years
    c. Obesity
    d. History of motion sickness

11. What is the typical timeframe for morning sickness to occur during pregnancy?
    a. First trimester
    b. Second trimester
    c. Third trimester
    d. Throughout the entire pregnancy

12. Which of the following conditions is *not* commonly associated with hyperemesis gravidarum?
    a. Electrolyte imbalances   b. Dehydration
    c. Preterm labor   d. Fetal abnormalities

13. What is the recommended treatment approach for mild-to-moderate vomiting in pregnancy?
    a. Prescription medications
    b. Hospitalization
    c. Lifestyle modifications
    d. Surgical intervention

14. Which medication is commonly prescribed to manage severe cases of vomiting in pregnancy?
    a. Acetaminophen   b. Ibuprofen
    c. Ondansetron   d. Diphenhydramine

15. When should a pregnant woman seek medical attention for vomiting during pregnancy?
    a. If she vomits more than twice a day
    b. If she is unable to keep any food or fluids down
    c. If she experiences weight loss
    d. All of the above

ANSWERS

1. **c.** Wernicke encephalopathy results from a deficiency of thiamine (vitamin B_1) and is manifested by confusion, gait ataxia, ophthalmoplegia (paralysis of the eye muscles), or convulsions. Typically, thiamine is initially lost by prolonged vomiting. When intravenous fluid replacement containing dextrose is given, the body's metabolism of the dextrose quickly consumes the remaining thiamine. Therefore, the cause is usually not the hyperemesis itself but is instead due to fluid replacement without thiamine supplementation. Although the condition is very rare, it is associated with a high mortality rate (20%).

2. **d.** Human chorionic gonadotropin has been suspected as the cause of hyperemesis gravidarum based chiefly on the observation that its peak concentration in pregnancy coincides with the peak of nausea and vomiting. Another suggestion for the causative role of hCG in persistent nausea and vomiting is the association between increased hCG concentrations and hyperemesis gravidarum in cases of twin and molar pregnancies.

3. **d.** Specific suggestions are to eat bread or crackers before getting out of bed in the morning, when nauseated, and before retiring for the night. Experts also recommend eating small meals every 2–3 hours; drinking liquids between meals rather than with meals to avoid gastric distention; eating low-fat, high-protein foods; avoiding fried foods; and salting food to taste.

4. **d.** Thiamine stores must be restored before intravenous therapy begins, as the dextrose in the solution causes the body to metabolize thiamine. As previously mentioned, thiamine deficiency can lead to Wernicke encephalopathy. Signs and symptoms of Wernicke encephalopathy include visual disturbances, such as diplopia or nystagmus, as well as disorientation, delusion, and gait ataxia. While there is no specific treatment regimen, some experts recommend parenteral thiamine 100–500 mg daily for 3 days and 2–3 mg per day thereafter.

5. **d.** On physical examination, the patient may appear weak, pale, and with dry mucous membranes. A ketotic breath smell may be noted. Infrequently, jaundice might be noted. A weight check may reveal weight loss, as much as 5 pounds in a week. Blood pressure may manifest orthostatic changes, and pulse may be elevated secondary to dehydration.

6. **a.** A urine dipstick analysis should be performed, with particular attention to the presence of ketones. Specific gravity will be increased.

7. **b.** This diagnosis includes impaired oral mucous membrane integrity, due to both dehydration and vomiting. Assessments might reveal a complaint of dry mouth, bad taste, or even excessive salivation. Inspection may reveal dry or cracked mucous membranes, pallor, ulcerations, edema, coated tongue, or hemangiomas (a network of small blood-filled capillaries near the surface of the skin).

8. **c.** High pre-pregnancy body weight and nulliparity (having not given birth to a child) have been cited as risk factors for hyperemesis, and as discussed, a high-fat diet has been found to greatly increase the odds. Maternal age younger than 20 years and twin gestation are also noted as risk factors. The condition can repeat itself in subsequent pregnancies and is more common in women with a history of spontaneous abortions. Trogstad et al. found that if a woman experienced hyperemesis in her first pregnancy, there was a 15.2% risk that she would experience it in subsequent pregnancies. Those never having suffered from the condition have a 0.7% risk in later pregnancies.

9. **b.** *Supine hypotension syndrome (postural hypotension):* During late pregnancy, the gravid uterus produces a compression effect on the inferior vena cava when the patient is in supine position. In 90% cases, this, however, results in opening up of the collateral circulation by means of paravertebral and azygos veins. In some cases (10%), when the collateral circulation fails to open up, the venous return of the heart may be seriously curtailed. This results in production of hypotension, tachycardia, and syncope called as supine hypotensive syndrome. The normal blood pressure is quickly restored by turning the patient to lateral position. That is why pregnant females are advised to lie in lateral positions best being left lateral.

10. **b.** Maternal age below 20 years
    Maternal age below 20 years is not associated with an increased risk of experiencing severe vomiting during pregnancy. However, multiple pregnancies, a history of motion sickness, and personal or family history of hyperemesis gravidarum are known risk factors.

11. **a.** First trimester
    Morning sickness typically occurs during the first trimester of pregnancy, usually starting around the 6th week and subsiding by the 12th to 14th week. However, it can vary from woman to woman, and some may experience it throughout their pregnancy.

12. **d.** Fetal abnormalities
    Hyperemesis gravidarum is typically not associated.

13. **c.** Lifestyle modifications
    Lifestyle modifications, such as dietary changes and adequate hydration, are usually the recommended treatment approach for mild-to-moderate vomiting in pregnancy.

14. **c.** Ondansetron
    Ondansetron is commonly prescribed to manage severe cases of vomiting in pregnancy when lifestyle modifications alone are ineffective.

15. **d.** All of the above
    Persistent vomiting, inability to keep any food or fluids down, and weight loss are signs that require medical attention during pregnancy.

Chapter 19: Gestational Trophoblastic Neoplasia

Jayashree V Kanavi

QUESTIONS

1. Patients with complete or partial moles should be reassured that they are generally at no increased risk of complications in later gestations.
    a. True
    b. False

2. After one molar pregnancy, the risk of having molar diseases in a future gestation is about ____
    a. 1–1.5%
    b. 2–2.5%
    c. 3–3.5%
    d. 4–4.5%

3. Patient with gestational trophoblastic neoplasia (GTN) who is treated successfully with chemotherapy can expect natural reproduction in the future.
    a. True
    b. False

4. β-hCG measurement 6 weeks after delivery of the subsequent pregnancy after molar pregnancy, to exclude occult trophoblastic neoplasia.
    a. True
    b. False

5. After normal β-hCG level is attained, how many more additional courses of chemotherapy are administered to reduce the risk of relapse of GTN?
    a. 1
    b. 2
    c. 3
    d. 4

6. In a case of GTN, EMA-Co regimen is the preferred primary treatment in patients with a high-risk prognostic score.
    a. >3
    b. >6
    c. <3
    d. <6

7. Single agent chemotherapy (8-day regimen) is administered every:
    a. 1 week
    b. 2 weeks
    c. 3 weeks
    d. 4 weeks

8. GTN stage 2, high risk category is treated initially with:
    a. Single agent chemotherapy
    b. Combination chemotherapy
    c. Second-line combination chemotherapy
    d. All the above

9. Hysterectomy is preferred treatment in all patients with stage 1—PSTT and ETT.
    a. True
    b. False

10. In a case of GTN, adjuvant chemotherapy is administered:
    1. To reduce the likelihood of disseminating viable tumor cells at surgery
    2. To maintain a cytotoxic level of chemotherapy in the bloodstream and tissues in case viable tumor cells are disseminated at surgery
    3. To occult metastasis that may be present at the time of surgery
    4. Not required for the cases of stage 1, for whom hysterectomy is being done
    a. 1 and 2
    b. 1, 2, and 3
    c. 1 and 3
    d. 1, 2, and 4

11. Human chorionic gonadotropin (10^3–10^4 IU/L) at the time of GTN diagnosis gets a score of:
    a. 0
    b. 1
    c. 2
    d. 4

12. In GTN, largest tumor size including uterus of >5 cm gets a score of:
    a. 0
    b. 1
    c. 2
    d. 4

13. Metastasis of GI tract of GTN gets a score of:
    a. 0
    b. 1
    c. 2
    d. 4

14. To categorize a GTN disease as high risk, prognostic score should be:
    a. Higher than 2
    b. Higher than 4
    c. Higher than 6
    d. Higher than 8

15. According to International Federation of Gynecology and Obstetrics (FIGO) staging of gestational trophoblastic tumors GTN extending to lungs with or without genital trait involvement belongs to:
    a. Stage 1
    b. Stage 2
    c. Stage 3
    d. Stage 4

16. In cases of gestational trophoblastic tumor, chance of vaginal metastasis is lesser compared to liver metastasis.
    a. True
    b. False

17. Metastatic GTN occurs in about _____ of patients after evaluation of a complete mole.
    a. 2%
    b. 4%
    c. 8%
    d. 10%

18. Which of the following statement is correct?
    The most common sites of metastasis of GTN are:
    a. Lungs (80%), vagina (30%), liver (12%)
    b. Lungs (10%), liver (10%), pelvis (10%)
    c. Lungs (50%), liver (30%), vagina (10%)
    d. Pelvis (80%), liver (10%), lungs (90%)

19. The principle pulmonary patterns produced by GTN are:
    1. Consolidation of the lobe
    2. Collapse of the lobe
    3. Discrete rounded densities
    4. An embolic pattern caused by pulmonary arterial occlusion
    a. 1 and 2
    b. 2 and 3
    c. 3 and 4
    d. 1 and 4

20. Which of the statements regarding follow-up after molar evaluation is correct?
    a. After molar evaluation, patients should be monitored with weekly determinations of β-hCG levels until the level is normal for three consecutive weeks
    b. After molar evaluation, patients should be monitored with weekly determinations of β-hCG levels until the level is normal, then every month for 3 months
    c. After molar evaluation, patients should be monitored with daily determinations of β-hCG for a week or until it normalizes, then weekly for three consecutive weeks
    d. After molar evaluation, patients should be monitored with monthly determinations of β-hCG until the levels are normal, then every 6 months for 2 years

21. Placental-site trophoblastic tumors consist predominantly:
    a. Intermediate trophoblast
    b. Syncytiotrophoblast
    c. Cytotrophoblast
    d. Extra villous trophoblast

22. In contrast to other trophoblastic tumor, placental-site trophoblastic tumor and epithelioid trophoblastic tumor are relatively insensitive to chemotherapy.
    a. True
    b. False

23. Prophylactic chemotherapy at the time of molar evacuation:
    1. Not required as the risk of developing persistent tumor is only 20%
    2. Should be considered in all the cases, post-evaluation
    3. After single course of prophylactic chemotherapy post molar evaluation, follow up is not required
    4. Prophylactic chemotherapy useful in the management of high risk complete molar pregnancy, especially when beta-hCG assessments for follow-up are unavailable or unreliable
    a. 1 and 2
    b. 2 and 3
    c. 3 and 4
    d. 1 and 4

24. Trophoblastic hyperplasia is diffuse in a case of complete mole.
    a. True
    b. False

25. Marked villous scalloping is seen in case of partial molar.
    a. True
    b. False

26. The molar chromosomes are entirely of paternal origin, with mitochondrial DNA of maternal origin.
    a. True
    b. False

27. The definitive diagnosis of a molar pregnancy is made by:
    a. Histological examinations
    b. Serum β-hCG
    c. Ultrasound examinations
    d. Physical examinations

28. Anti-D prophylaxis is not routinely recommended in a case of complete molar pregnancy as chorionic villi do not express RH factor.
    a. True
    b. False

29. Complications associated with molar pregnancy are, *except:*
    a. Hyperemesis gravidarum
    b. Preeclampsia
    c. Vaginal bleeding
    d. Gestational diabetes

30. Which is the most common symptom causing the patients to seek treatment for complete molar pregnancy?
    a. Vaginal bleeding
    b. Excessive vomiting
    c. Excessive uterine enlargement
    d. Preeclampsia

ANSWERS

1. **a.** True—although data regarding pregnancies after a partial mole are limited the information is reassuring
2. **a.** 1–1.5%
3. **a.** True
4. **a.** True
5. **c.** 3
6. **c.** >3
7. **b.** 2 weeks
8. **b.** Combination chemotherapy
9. **a.** True
10. **b.** 1, 2, and 3
11. **b.** 10^3–10^4 score 1
12. **c.** Score of 2—tumors more the 5 cm get scored of 2
13. **c.** GI tract metastasis of GTN gets a score of 2
14. **c.** Higher than 6
15. **c.** Stage III
16. **b.** False
17. **b.** 4%—metastatic GTN occurs in 4% of patients after evacuation of a complete mole but it is seen more often when GTN develops after nonmolar pregnancies
18. **a.** Lungs 80%, vagina 30%, liver 10%
19. **c.** GTN may produce four principal pulmonary patterns:
    a. An alveolar or "snow storm" pattern
    b. Discrete rounded densities
    c. Pleural effusion
    d. An embolic pattern caused by pulmonary arterial occlusion
20. **a.**
21. **a.** Intermediate trophoblast
22. **a.** True
23. **d.** 1 and 4
24. **a.** True
25. **a.** True
26. **a.** True
27. **a.** RCOG guidelines
28. **b.** Because trophoblast cells express the RhD factor, patients who are Rh–ve should receive Rh immunoglobulin
29. **d.** Preeclampsia was observed in 27% of patients with a complete hydatidiform mole. Hyperemesis requiring antiemetic or intravenous (IV) replacement therapy occurred in one-fourth of patients with complete mole. Vaginal bleeding is the most common symptoms causing patient to seek treatment for complete molar pregnancy. Gestational diabetes is not a complication of molar pregnancy.
30. **a.** Vaginal bleeding. It is reported to occur in 46% of patients. Molar tissues may separate from the decidua and disrupt maternal vessels and large volumes of retained blood may distend the endometrial cavity.

REFERENCES

1. Howkins & Bourne—Shaw's Textbook of Gynaecology, 18th edition, 2022.
2. Berek & Novak's Gynecology, 16th edition, 2019.
3. RCOG guidelines—Gestational Trophoblastic Disease Green top guideline 38.
4. ACOG guidelines Bulletin #53 diagnosis and treatment of gestational trophoblastic disease.

Chapter 20: Recurrent Abortions

Jyothi GS, Sahana Girish

QUESTIONS

1. A couple comes with a karyotype report of previous abortion. Among the causes of recurrent pregnancy loss (RPL), the following genetic cause is not associated with RPL:
   a. Balanced
   b. Reciprocal
   c. Robertsonian translocations
   d. Triploidy

2. A patient comes to outpatient department (OPD) with history of recent miscarriage at 4 months of gestation. She tells she has had previous two similar incidents in the past where she has aborted between 3 and 4 months of gestation. She also reports that there is some abnormality in her uterus, the details of which is unknown to her. The following are the recommended tests for assessment of the uterine anomalies in the nonpregnant state, *except*:
   a. Pelvic ultrasound
   b. Saline infusion sonohysterography
   c. Hysterosalpingogram
   d. Hysterolaparoscopy

3. Recurrent pregnancy loss is defined as two or more failed pregnancies confirmed by:
   a. Sonography
   b. Histopathology
   c. Both a and b
   d. a or b

4. A 31-year-old female and 33-year-old male married for 7 years with history of previous three abortions randomly happening at 7 weeks, 16 weeks, and 20 weeks. They are anxious to know the cause for pregnancy loss. The most common cause of RPL among the following options:
   a. Genetic
   b. Infections
   c. Uterine anomaly
   d. Endocrine causes

5. A 28-year-old P0L0A2 patient comes to OPD and says that she is anxious about conceiving as she has had previous two abortions. After ruling out other causes of RPL you think of some immunological causes as given below. All of these can be one of the causes, *except*:
   a. Systemic lupus erythematosus (SLE)
   b. Antiphospholipid antibody (APLA)
   c. Human leukocyte antigen (HLA) compatibility
   d. Antinuclear antibody (ANA)

6. A 28-year-old lady comes with history of previous pregnancy loss due occurring at 24 weeks of gestation. According to recommendation, screening of cervical length should be done for all women with:
   a. Prior one pregnancy loss
   b. Prior preterm birth
   c. Uterine anomaly
   d. Previous dilatation and curettage

7. A 30-year-old G3A2 pregnant woman comes to you with history of abortions where there was painless expulsion of products of conception in the second trimesters. You assess the patient and decide that cerclage is a good option for the present pregnancy. All of the following are contraindications for cerclage, *except*:
   a. Bleeding
   b. Pain
   c. Cervical length of 1.5 cm on ultrasound
   d. Ruptured membranes

8. Antiphospholipid antibody diagnosis includes:
   a. One or more unexplained deaths before 8 weeks
   b. History of previous pre-eclampsia delivered after 36 weeks

c. Presence of lupus anticoagulant (LA) according to guidelines of International Society on Thrombosis and Hemostasis
d. Decrease in immunoglobulin G (IgG) and IgM titers of anticardiolipin antibody (ACLA)

9. Most common cause of inherited thrombophilia leading to recurrent miscarriage (RM) is:
   a. Protein C deficiency
   b. Protein S deficiency
   c. Antithrombin III deficiency
   d. Factor V Leiden mutation

10. Recurrent pregnancy loss clinic is one of the recommendations for having a multidisciplinary approach to management of RPL. In one such discussion, the immunologist was explaining about immunological aspects of RPL. Role of histocompatibility in recurrent pregnancy loss is because of one of the following:
    a. Extravillous cytotrophoblasts express nonclassical class I HLA-G and-E molecules with increased expression of HLA-C antigens
    b. Reduced activity of T helper-1 (Th-1) cytokines and natural killer (NK) cells
    c. HLA-C can also regulate T cells
    d. The soluble HLA-G1 isoform downregulates both $CD8^+$ and $CD4^+$ T cell

11. A 35-year-old G4P1L1A2 with 20 weeks' gestation came to emergency room (ER) with complaints of (c/o) dull aching pain in lower abdomen. On examination, uterus was corresponding to 20 weeks of gestation with good fetal heart rate (FHR). Speculum examination revealed bulging membranes and cervical dilation. The lady was counseled for rescue cerclage and the risks were explained. Most common risk of rescue cerclage is:
    a. Rupture of membranes b. Tissue injury
    c. Infection   d. Hemorrhage

12. In the case explained in Q11 unfortunately the patient had miscarriage in spite of the cerclage. She now comes back in the next pregnancy at 12 weeks of gestation. Of all the recommendations for cervical cerclage, the best recommendation with good outcomes is:
    a. Ultrasound indicated
    b. History indicated
    c. Rescue cerclage
    d. Abdominal cerclage

13. A 35-year-old woman has come with history of thrombosis. In this woman, recommendation for screening include all of the following, *except*:
    a. MTFHR gene mutation
    b. Factor V Leiden
    c. Plasminogen activator inhibitor 1 (PAI-1)
    d. Vascular endothelial growth factor (VEGF)

14. G3A2 with 15 weeks of gestation is posted for prophylactic cerclage. Adjuvant therapies advocated before or at the time of cerclage are all, *except*:
    a. Tocolysis   b. Antibiotics
    c. Amnioreduction   d. Progesterone

15. A. Ultrasound indicated cervical encerclage is recommended for cervical length_____
    B. In twins, the minimum length for the indication for stitch_____
    C. Definition for failed cerclage for which abdominal cerclage can be offered delivery before_____ after a history or ultrasound-indicated [but not rescue] cerclage
    D. Type of cervical cerclage which has good outcome_____
    a. <2.5 cm, <1.5 cm, 28 weeks, both Shirodkar and McDonald have similar outcomes
    b. 2.5 cm, <1.5 cm, 24 weeks, Shirodkar is better
    c. 2.5 cm, 1.5 cm, 28 weeks, McDonald is better
    d. <2.5 cm, 1.5 cm, 24 weeks, both Shirodkar and McDonald have similar outcomes

16. Causes of RPL in ascending order of their occurrence:
    a. Chromosome abnormalities in the parents
    b. Uterine alterations
    c. Infections
    d. Endocrinological disorders
    e. Autoimmune diseases
    f. Unexplained

17. A 33-year-old lady and 35-year-old male married for 8 years with history of previous four abortions were evaluated for all the possible causes of RPL. Male factors resulting in idiopathic RPL include all, *except*:
    a. DNA fragmentation index (DFI) of 35%
    b. Y chromosome microdeletion
    c. DNA fragmentation index of 20%
    d. Sperm aneuploidy

18. A couple with history of previous three miscarriages and male karyotype showing 46XY9qh came for consultation. The testing recommended for detecting chromosomal abnormality in the embryo are all, *except:*
    a. Blastomere biopsy
    b. Trophectoderm biopsy
    c. Noninvasive preimplantation genetic testing (NIPGT)
    d. PGT-M

19. A 28-year-old lady with previous two miscarriages due to uterine anomaly comes to OPD for preconceptional counseling. Of all the causes of RPL due to uterine anomaly, correction of which of the anomaly is recommended for management of RPL:
    a. Septate uterus
    b. Bicornuate uterus
    c. Uterine didelphys
    d. Arcuate uterus

20. The results of PROMISE trial are all, *except:*
    a. *Main outcomes measured:* Live birth beyond 24 completed weeks of gestation (primary outcome), clinical pregnancy at 6–8 weeks, ongoing pregnancy at 12 weeks, miscarriage, and gestation at delivery
    b. There is no evidence that first trimester progesterone therapy improves outcomes in women with a history of unexplained RM
    c. This study explored the effect of treatment with other progesterone preparations during the luteal phase of the menstrual cycle
    d. Women received either micronized progesterone at a dose of 400 mg (two vaginal capsules of 200 mg) or placebo vaginal capsules twice daily

21. A 29-year-old lady and 40-year-old male came to OPD with history of secondary infertility of 1.5 year duration. She had previous four miscarriages in the first trimester. Husband was a known case of diabetes for the last 3 years on oral hypoglycemic agents (OHA). Semen analysis showed normozoospermia. Treatment option recommended for male factor resulting in RPL:
    a. PICSI
    b. Antioxidants
    c. Lifestyle modification
    d. Gene correction

22. A 31-year-old lady with menstrual irregularities and with history of RPL came to you with her abdominal scan reports. Correction of which of the acquired uterine anomaly is recommended in cases of RPL:
    a. Submucous fibroid   b. Endometrial polyp
    c. Intrauterine adhesions   d. Intramural fibroid

23. A 28-year-old with history of previous three abortions comes to you in an anxious state to conceive. You advise her to get evaluated for the same. Recommended investigations after two pregnancy loss are all, *except:*
    a. Karyotyping of parents
    b. Karyotyping of products of conception (POC)
    c. Two-dimensional (2D) ultrasound
    d. TORCH screening

24. A lady with RPL attends RPL clinic. Endocrinologist in the clinic explained to her that she might have endocrine issue after ruling out the other issues. Endocrine causes of RPL are all, *except:*
    a. Hyperprolactinemia
    b. Luteal phase defect (LPD)
    c. Diabetes mellitus
    d. Hyperthyroidism

25. Causes of RPL in anatomic abnormalities are all, *except:*
    a. Abnormal ovary   b. Abnormal vasculature
    c. Abnormal placentation   d. Intrauterine adhesions

26. A 30-year-old lady with fibroid uterus and with history of RPL has been advised to undergo myomectomy. The criteria to be considered for myomectomy would be:
    a. Any fibroids larger than 5 cm
    b. Submucous fibroids
    c. Intramural fibroid of <5 cm
    d. Cervical fibroid

27. A 28-year-old lady presented with history of secondary infertility with no living child. On further investigations, she was diagnosed with LPD. Diagnosis of LPD is by all of the following, *except:*
    a. Serum progesterone >10 mg/mL
    b. Endometrial biopsy showing out of phase of endometrium
    c. Decrease in integrated luteal phase levels of inhibin
    d. Decrease in mean luteinizing hormone (LH) biolevels

28. In the case described in Question 27, the first recommended treatment for luteal phase defect is:
   a. Progesterone
   b. Clomiphene citrate
   c. Human menopausal gonadotropin
   d. Bromocriptine

29. A 32-year-old lady with body mass index (BMI) of 34 with menstrual irregularities and USG features suggestive of PCO with history of RPL comes for preconceptional counseling hypothesis for RPL in PCO are all, *except*:
   a. Insulin resistance
   b. Obesity
   c. Hyperhomocysteinemia
   d. Increased LH

30. *Assertion:* Membrane rupture during or within 48 hours following cervical cerclage is considered as an indication for removal of cerclage
   Reason: Increased likelihood of fetal and maternal infection
   a. Assertion is correct, reason is wrong
   b. Assertion and reason are correct but reason is not appropriate for the assertion
   c. Assertion and reason are correct and reason is appropriate for the assertion
   d. Assertion and reason are wrong

ANSWERS

1. **d.** Triploidy
   Risk of RPL in couples with balanced translocation is >25% as per many reports. However, triploidy as a cause is not to be found.
   [Reference: Royal College of Obstetricians and Gynaecologists. (2014). Umbilical Cord Prolapse Green-top Guideline No. 50. (online) Available from: https://www.rcog.org.uk/media/3wykswng/gtg-50-umbilicalcordprolapse-2014.pdf (Last accessed December, 2023)]

2. **d.** Hysterolaparoscopy
   Diagnostic hysterolaparoscopy is an effective diagnostic and therapeutic modality for certain significant and correctable abnormalities in pelvis, tubes, and uterus which are missed by other imaging modalities.
   [Reference: Royal College of Obstetricians and Gynaecologists. (2014). Umbilical Cord Prolapse Green-top Guideline No. 50. [online] Available from: https://www.rcog.org.uk/media/3wykswng/gtg-50-umbilicalcordprolapse-2014.pdf (Last accessed December, 2023)]

3. **a or b.** Recurrent pregnancy loss is defined as two or more failed pregnancies confirmed by sonography or histopathology before 20 weeks of gestation or three or more miscarriages before 24 weeks of gestation irrespective of sonography or histopathology report (RCOG, ESHRE).
   (Reference: Williams Obstetrics, 25th Edition, page 9/38)

4. **a, c, and d.**
   - *Genetic causes:* 2–4%
   - *Infections:* Not a common cause
   - *Uterine anomaly:* 15%
   - *Endocrine causes:* 8–12%
   (Reference: Williams Obstetrics, 25th Edition, page 11/38)

5. **d.** ANA
   Immunologic mechanisms have been proposed as part of the pathogenesis mechanisms involved in RPL. Presence of positive ANAs is regarded as a typical feature of autoimmunity. Many studies had tried to clarify the association of ANA with RPL, but the conclusions were controversial.
   (Reference: Kwak-Kim J, Park JC, Ahn HK, Kim JW, Gilman-Sachs A. Immunological modes of pregnancy loss. Am J Reprod Immunol. 2010;63(6):611-23)

6. **b.** Prior preterm birth
   Prior preterm birth is a criteria for screening of cervical length when a patient presents with history of previous pregnancy loss.
   (Reference: Williams Obstetrics, 25th Edition, page 12/38)

7. **c.** Cervical length of 1.5 cm on ultrasound
   Contraindications to cerclage usually include bleeding, contractions, or ruptured membranes, which substantially raises the likelihood of failure. Thus, prophylactic cerclage before dilatation is preferable. Short cervical length is an indication for prophylactic cerclage.
   (Reference: Williams Obstetrics, 25th Edition, page 12/38)

8. **c.** Presence of lupus anticoagulant (LA) according to guidelines of International Society on Thrombosis and Hemostasis
   (Reference: Williams Obstetrics, 25th Edition, page 10/38)

9. **d.** Factor V Leiden mutation
   It has been suggested that women with thrombophilia have an increased risk of pregnancy loss and other adverse pregnancy outcomes. Thrombophilia is an important predisposition to blood clot formation and is considered as a significant risk factor for RPL. The inherited predisposition to thrombophilia is most often associated with factor V Leiden mutation
   (Reference: DC Dutta's Textbook of Gynecology, 8th Edition, page 196)

10. **d.** The soluble HLA-G1 isoform downregulates both $CD8^+$ and $CD4^+$ T cell
    Role of histocompatibility in recurrent pregnancy loss is because the soluble HLA-G1 isoform downregulates both $CD8^+$ and $CD4^+$ T cell.
    (Reference: Kwak-Kim J, Park JC, Ahn HK, Kim JW, Gilman-Sachs A. Immunological modes of pregnancy loss. Am J Reprod Immunol. 2010;63(6):611-23.)

11. **a.** Rupture of membranes
    Rescue cerclage with a thinned dilated cervix is more difficult and risks tissue tearing and membrane puncture. Replacement of the prolapsed amniotic sac back into the uterus will usually aid suturing (Locatelli, 1999). Options include steep Trendelenburg or filling the bladder with 600 mL of saline through an indwelling Foley catheter.
    (Reference: Williams Obstetrics, 25th Edition, page 14/38)

12. **a.** Ultrasound indicated
    Ultrasound indicated encerclage is the best recommendation with good outcomes in a patient with previous pregnancy loss according to the International Federation of Gynecology and Obstetrics (FIGO) guidelines.
    (Reference: FIGO practice guidelines, 2021)

13. **d.** VEGF. Not recommended for screening.
    Vascular endothelial growth factor (VEGF) is essential for implantation, development of embryo, and placental angiogenesis. Women with low VEGF level are believed to be at higher risk of RPL.
    [Reference: Arias-Sosa LA, Acosta ID, Lucena-Quevedo E, Moreno-Ortiz H, Esteban-Pérez C, Forero-Castro M. Genetic and epigenetic variations associated with idiopathic recurrent pregnancy loss. J Assist Reprod Genet. 2018;35(3):355-66.]

14. **d.** Progesterone
    Use of progesterone as adjuvant with prophylactic cervical cerclage is advocated. Vaginal progesterone may improve outcomes in pregnancies with a short cervix despite cervical cerclage including prolonged pregnancy and higher birthweight, compared to treatment with cerclage alone.
    [Reference: Koskas M, Amant F, Mirza MR, Creutzberg CL. Cancer of the corpus uteri: 2021 update. Int J Gynaecol Obstet. 2021;155 Suppl 1(Suppl 1):45-60. Special section: FIGO Working Group for Preterm Birth – Good Practice Recommendations. Int J Gynaecol Obstet. 2021;1-e4, 1-165]

15. **a.** <2.5 cm, <1.5 cm, 28 weeks, both Shirodkar and McDonald have similar outcomes.
    Ultrasound indicated cervical cerclage is recommended for cervical length <2.5 cm. In twins, minimum length for cervical cerclage is <1.5 cm. Definition for failed cerclage for which abdominal cerclage can be offered delivery before 28 weeks after a history or ultrasound-indicated [but not rescue] cerclage. Both Shirodkar and McDonald cervical cerclage have good outcome.
    [Reference: International Journal of Gynecology & Obstetrics Volume 155, Issue 1: Special section: FIGO Working Group for Preterm Birth – Good Practice Recommendations Oct 2021 Pagese 1-e4, 1-165]

16. **c, a, b, d, e, and f.**
    - 2–5%
    - 10–15%
    - 0.5–5%
    - 17–20%
    - 20%
    - 50%

    [Reference: Arias-Sosa LA, Acosta ID, Lucena-Quevedo E, Moreno-Ortiz H, Esteban-Pérez C, Forero-Castro M. Genetic and epigenetic variations associated with idiopathic recurrent pregnancy loss. J Assist Reprod Genet. 2018;35(3):355-66.]

17. **c.** DFI of 20%
    In recent years, there has been a growing focus on the role of male factors in inducing RPL since the integrity of the sperm genome is critical for the start and continuation of a successful pregnancy. Male factors resulting in idiopathic RPL are DFI of 20%, sperm aneuploidy, and Y chromosome microdeletion.

[Reference: Arias-Sosa LA, Acosta ID, Lucena-Quevedo E, Moreno-Ortiz H, Esteban-Pérez C, Forero-Castro M. Genetic and epigenetic variations associated with idiopathic recurrent pregnancy loss. J Assist Reprod Genet. 2018;35(3):355-66.]

18. **d.** PGT-M
Testing recommended for detecting chromosomal abnormalities in the embryo are blastomere biopsy, trophectoderm biopsy, NIPGT. More advanced platforms, such as next-generation sequencing (NGS) and microarray comparative genomic hybridization (aCGH), require optimum DNA from several cells for amplification are appropriate for blastocyst biopsy.
[Reference: Aoyama N, Kato K. Trophectoderm biopsy for preimplantation genetic test and technical tips: A review. Reprod Med Biol. 2020;19(3):222-31.]

19. **a.** Septate uterus
Even if proof of efficacy of surgical management of certain uterine anomalies is often lacking for managing RPLs, surgery should be encouraged in certain circumstances for improving subsequent pregnancy outcome. Uterine anomalies, such as uterine septa and intrauterine adhesions are the primary surgical indications for managing RPLs.
(Reference: ESHRE guidelines, page 125)

20. **c.** This study explored the effect of treatment with other progesterone preparations during the luteal phase of the menstrual cycle
Progesterone is essential to maintain a healthy pregnancy. Guidance from the Royal College of Obstetricians and Gynecologists and a Cochrane review called for a definitive trial to test whether or not progesterone therapy in the first trimester could reduce the risk of miscarriage in women with a history of unexplained RM. The PROMISE trial was conducted to answer this question. A concurrent cost-effectiveness analysis was conducted.
[Reference: Coomarasamy A, Williams H, Truchanowicz E, Seed PT, Small R, Quenby S, et al. PROMISE: first-trimester progesterone therapy in women with a history of unexplained recurrent miscarriages - a randomised, double-blind, placebo-controlled, international multicentre trial and economic evaluation. Health Technol Assess. 2016 May;20(41):1-92.]

21. **c.** Lifestyle modification
Physiological intracytoplasmic sperm injection (PICSI) is used in severe sodium-dependent organic anion transporter (SOAT), antioxidants have not been proven to improve the condition, gene correction is not helpful.
(Reference: ESHRE guidelines, page 134)

22. **c.** Intrauterine adhesions
Even if proof of efficacy of surgical management of certain uterine anomalies is often lacking for managing RPLs, surgery should be encouraged in certain circumstances for improving subsequent pregnancy outcome. Uterine anomalies such as uterine septa and intrauterine adhesions are the primary surgical indications for managing RPLs.
(Reference: ESHRE guidelines, page 128)

23. **d.** TORCH screening
Recommended investigations after two pregnancy loss are karyotyping of parents, karyotyping of POC and TORCH screening. 2D ultrasound is not one of the recommended investigations according to ESHRE guidelines-103.
(Reference: ESHRE guidelines-103)

24. **d.** Hyperthyroidism
Endocrine factors may contribute to 8–12% of recurrent pregnancy loss. Therefore, an endocrine evaluation is a critical component of the RPL workup. Hyperprolactinemia, LPD, diabetes mellitus (DM), and hypothyroidism are a few endocrine causes.
[Reference: Ford HB, Schust DJ. Recurrent pregnancy loss: etiology, diagnosis, and therapy. Rev Obstet Gynecol. 2009;2(2):76-83.]

25. **a.** Abnormal ovary
Anatomic abnormalities account for 10–15% of cases of RPL and are generally thought to cause miscarriage by interrupting the vasculature of the endometrium, prompting abnormal and inadequate placentation.
[Reference: Ford HB, Schust DJ. Recurrent pregnancy loss: etiology, diagnosis, and therapy. Rev Obstet Gynecol. 2009;2(2):76-83.]

26. **a.** Any fibroids larger than 5 cm
Myomectomy should be considered in cases of submucosal fibroids or any type fibroids larger than 5 cm. Resection has been shown to significantly improve live birth rates from 57 to 93%. Myomectomy can be performed via open laparotomy, laparoscopy, or hysteroscopy.

[Reference: Ford HB, Schust DJ. Recurrent pregnancy loss: etiology, diagnosis, and therapy. Rev Obstet Gynecol. 2009;2(2):76-83.]

27. **a.** Serum progesterone >10 mg/mL
Diagnosis of LPD is by endometrial biopsy showing out of phase of endometrium, decrease in integrated luteal phase levels of inhibin and decrease in mean LH-bio levels.
[Reference: Soules MR, McLachlan RI, Ek M, Dahl KD, Cohen NL, Bremner WJ. Luteal phase deficiency: characterization of reproductive hormones over the menstrual cycle. J Clin Endocrinol Metab. 1989;69(4):804-12.]

28. **b.** Clomiphene citrate
First recommended treatment for LPD is clomiphene citrate. It triggers your ovaries to make more follicles, which release eggs.
[Reference: Bopp B, Shoupe D. Luteal phase defects. J Reprod Med. 1993;38(5):348-56.]

29. **d.** Increased LH
Hypothesis for RPL in PCO is insulin resistance, obesity, and hyperhomocysteinemia.
[Reference: Chakraborty P, Goswami SK, Rajani S, Sharma S, Kabir SN, Chakravarty B, et al. Recurrent pregnancy loss in polycystic ovary syndrome: role of hyperhomocysteinemia and insulin resistance. PLoS One. 2013;8(5):e64446.]

30. **c.** Assertion and reason are correct and reason is appropriate for the assertion.

Membrane rupture during suture placement or within the first 48 hours following surgery is considered by some to be an indication for cerclage removal because of the likelihood of serious fetal or maternal infection. That said, the range of management options includes observation, removal of the cerclage and observation, or removal of the cerclage and labor induction.
(Reference: William's Textbook, 25th Edition. page 16/38)

Chapter 21: Spontaneous Abortion, Ultrasound Findings, and Septic Abortion

Radhika Chetan, Ananya Girish

QUESTIONS

1. As per the World Health Organization (WHO), abortion is defined as an expulsion of products of conception before ____ weeks of gestational age.
   a. 20 weeks
   b. 22 weeks
   c. 24 weeks
   d. 28 weeks

2. Miscarriage risk in clinically recognized pregnancy is about:
   a. 15–20%
   b. 25–30%
   c. 35–40%
   d. 50%

3. Abortion and chromosomal anomaly rates decrease with:
   a. Advanced maternal age
   b. Advanced paternal age
   c. Advanced gestational age
   d. Teenage pregnancy

4. Most common chromosomal abnormality in abortion fetuses is:
   a. Monosomy
   b. Translocation
   c. Triploidy
   d. Trisomy

5. Adverse outcomes associated with threated abortion include all, *except*:
   a. Placenta previa
   b. Placental polyp
   c. Abruptio placenta
   d. Manual removal of placenta

6. Nonviable pregnancy is diagnosed:
   a. When gestational sac is >25 mm with absent embryo
   b. When gestational sac is >20 mm with absent embryo
   c. When CRL (crown–rump length) is ≥5 mm with absent cardiac activity
   d. None of the above

7. Unfavorable outcome is expected when early pregnancy scan has:
   a. Yolk sac diameter of >7 mm in <10 weeks pregnancy
   b. Fetal heart rate (FHR) of 100 at 6 weeks of pregnancy
   c. Subchorionic hematoma sized about 15% of gestational sac
   d. Difference between mean sac diameter (MSD) and CRL is >5 mm

8. Which of the following sentences is true?
   a. Transabdominal ultrasound is preferred over transvaginal scan for early pregnancy diagnosis
   b. Doppler ultrasound is required to evaluate embryo
   c. M-mode imaging is used to document heartbeat
   d. All of the above

9. Cervical shock refers to:
   a. Shock features due to incomplete abortion, products in cervical canal
   b. Shock features due to inadvertent paracervical block
   c. Shock features due to cervical hemorrhage after complete abortion
   d. None of the above

10. Serum progesterone level of <15 nmol/L in early pregnancy suggests:
    a. Discriminatory threshold for visualizing gestational sac
    b. Nonviable pregnancy
    c. Serial values are more important than a single cut-off value
    d. Threatened abortion

11. Features of abnormal yolk sac include all, *except*:
    a. Calcified sac
    b. Irregular sac
    c. Free-floating sac
    d. None of the above

12. A 26-year-old Mrs Rita, married for 5 years, had amenorrhea of 2 months and no other symptoms. She did urine pregnancy test at home, which was positive. She reported to scanning center and transvaginal ultrasound showed embryo, with CRL of 9 mm and absent heartbeat. What is your course of action?
    a. Check serial β-human chorionic gonadotropin (β-HCG) values, look for doubling
    b. Repeat transvaginal ultrasound after 10 days
    c. Missed miscarriage—offer termination
    d. Blighted ovum—offer misoprostol for termination

13. Mrs Prema, G3P1L1, with past history of molar pregnancy, got her scanning done at 2 months of pregnancy. Transvaginal ultrasound showed gestational sac with yolk sac. MSD is 20 mm and nonvisualization of embryo and cardiac activity. How do you manage this case?
    a. Check serial β-hCG values
    b. Repeat transvaginal ultrasound after 10 days
    c. Missed abortion—offer termination
    d. Blighted ovum—offer termination

14. Mrs Sonu came for transvaginal scan and her report included presence of gestational sac and amniotic sac with no visible embryo. How do you counsel her?
    a. Check serial β-hCG values, look for doubling
    b. Repeat transvaginal ultrasound after 10 days
    c. Missed abortion—offer termination
    d. An embryonic pregnancy—offer termination

15. Mrs Ratna with history of recurrent miscarriage reported for transvaginal ultrasound at 2 months of pregnancy. Her scanning report showed single intrauterine gestational sac with embryo corresponding to 7 weeks of pregnancy and FHR of 90 per minute. How do you counsel her?
    a. Poor prognosis and offer termination of pregnancy
    b. Repeat scanning in 1–2 weeks in view of bradycardia
    c. Check serial β-hCG values, look for doubling
    d. Presence of cardiac activity is good prognostic indicator irrespective of heart rate

16. A 28-year-old primigravida, presents with abdominal pain and bleeding per vagina, soaking two pads. Examination revealed stable vitals, bulky uterus, and closed cervical os. Ultrasound showed 8 weeks embryo with good cardiac activity. What is your diagnosis?
    a. Threatened abortion
    b. Inevitable abortion
    c. Subchorionic hematoma
    d. Luteal phase defect

17. Mrs Neelam, with 3 months of pregnancy, gives history of passage of clots and continuous bleeding per vagina. Examination revealed stable vitals, bulky uterus with closed cervical os and absent bleeding. Ultrasound scanning showed bulky uterus with thickened endometrium of 14 mm. How do you proceed?
    a. Threatened abortion, offer progesterone
    b. Complete abortion, no further interventions
    c. Incomplete abortion, offer misoprostol
    d. Inevitable abortion, wait for complete expulsion

18. A 23-year-old lady who had taken abortion pill for missed abortion came with complaints of excessive bleeding per vagina on 3rd day. She was changing two pads for every 2 hours, excessive fatigue and giddiness. On examination, she is conscious and well oriented. Her pulse is 120 bpm and blood pressure is 100/70 mm Hg. Abdomen examination was unremarkable. Pelvic examination revealed 8 weeks uterus with cervical os open, products of conception in cervical canal. Which one of the options is best in management of this case?
    a. Incomplete abortion—offer manual vacuum aspiration
    b. Incomplete abortion—offer misoprostol
    c. Allow for spontaneous expulsion as already taken pills
    d. None of the above

19. Mrs Neha, a 32-year-old lady, came with complaints of fever, foul smelling discharge per vagina and history of abortion 1 week ago. Examination revealed temperature of 36°, tachycardia, and hypotension. Abdomen examination is unremarkable. On pelvic examination, uterus is bulky and os-closed with minimal foul smelling discharge. Ultrasound revealed bulky uterus with 80 cc retained products of conception. What is the diagnosis and sequence of action?
    a. Septic abortion, managed as antibiotics—fluid management—evacuation
    b. Septic abortion, managed as fluid management—evacuation—antibiotics
    c. Septic abortion managed as antibiotics—evacuation—fluid management
    d. Incomplete abortion—gives misoprostol

20. Mrs Sneha, a 30-year-old lady, came with complaints of fever, foul smelling discharge per vagina, vomiting, and history of abortion 1 week ago. She is conscious, drowsy responds to verbal commands. Examination revealed temperature of 36°, tachycardia, and hypotension. On examination, abdomen is distended with guarding and rigidity and absent bowel sounds. On pelvic examination, uterus is bulky and os-closed with minimal foul smelling discharge. Ultrasound revealed bulky uterus with 80 cc retained products of conception and collection in pelvic and paracolic gutters suggestive of multiple abscess in peritoneal cavity. What is your diagnosis?
    a. Septic abortion—grade 1
    b. Septic abortion—grade 2
    c. Septic abortion—grade 3
    d. Septic abortion—grade 4

21. Which of the following complication is *not* caused by retained products of conception?
    a. Hemorrhage
    b. Sepsis
    c. Placental polyp
    d. None of the above

22. Feature of endotoxic shock in septic abortion include all, *except*:
    a. Hypothermia
    b. Hyperthermia
    c. Hypertension
    d. Tachycardia

23. Ultrasonogram features suggestive of suspicious failed pregnancy include all, *except*:
    a. Crown-rump length <7 mm and no cardiac activity
    b. Mean gestational sac diameter of 16–24 mm with absent embryo
    c. Empty amnion with absent embryo
    d. Subchorionic hematoma >60 mL

24. All these are risk factors for spontaneous abortion, *except*:
    a. Age >40 years
    b. Excessive caffeine consumption
    c. Maternal underweight
    d. Viral infections

25. Radiation threshold for development of congenital malformations, fetal death in early pregnancy is:
    a. 0.1–0.2 Gy   b. 0.4–0.5 Gy
    c. 120 rads   d. 110 rads

26. Environmental and occupational factors associated with abortion include all, *except*:
    a. Phthalates
    b. Polypropylene
    c. Dichlorodiphenyltrichloroethane (DDT)
    d. Bisphenol A

27. Sequence of events on transvaginal scan in normal intrauterine pregnancy include:
    a. Gestational sac—yolk sac—embryo—amnion
    b. Gestational sac—yolk sac—amnion—embryo
    c. Gestational sac—embryo—yolk sac—amnion
    d. Yolk sac—gestational sac—amnion—embryo

28. Features of subchorionic hematoma include:
    a. Crescent shape   b. Internal echoes
    c. Septae   d. All of the above

29. Abnormally small gestational sac is diagnosed when difference between MSD and CRL length is?
    a. Less than 5 mm   b. Less than 10 mm
    c. More than 5 mm   d. More than 10 mm

30. Size of yolk sac associated with poor outcome in first trimester ultrasound is:
    a. More than 4 mm   b. Less than 4 mm
    c. More than 7 mm   d. Less than 7 mm

ANSWERS

1. **a.** 20 weeks
   Both WHO and CDC define gestational age for abortion as 20 weeks, or conceptus weight <500 g for uniformity across countries. Period of salvageability can vary across many places based on levels neonatal intensive care unit (NICU) care, definitions for defining abortion is taken as 20 weeks.
   [Reference: Cunningham FG, Leveno KJ, Dashe JS, Hoffman BL, Spong CY (Eds). Williams Obstetrics, 26th edition. New York: McGraw Hill/Medical; 2022]

2. **a.** 15–20%
   Loss of pregnancy before missed period (clinically unrecognized) can be as high as 30–40%. In clinically recognized pregnancy it is about 15–20%.
   (Reference: James High Risk Pregnancy, 5th edition.)

3. **c.** Advanced gestational age
   Abortion and chromosomal anomaly rates increase in early pregnancy and as maternal age, paternal age increase and also in teenage pregnancy. Chromosomal anomalies and abortion rates decrease as the gestational age advances.

[Reference: Cunningham FG, Leveno KJ, Dashe JS, Hoffman BL, Spong CY (Eds). Chapter 66: Williams Obstetrics, 26th edition. New York: McGraw Hill/Medical; 2022]

4. **d.** Trisomy
   More than half of early pregnancy miscarriages are associated with chromosomal abnormalities. 50-60% are trisomy, 9-13% are monosomy and triploidy in 11-12%.
   [Reference: Cunningham FG, Leveno KJ, Dashe JS, Hoffman BL, Spong CY (Eds). Williams Obstetrics, 26th edition. New York: McGraw Hill/Medical; 2022]

5. **b.** Placental polyp
   Threatened miscarriage is associated with increased risks of antepartum hemorrhage (placenta previa and abruption) and preterm labor. Placental polyp presents after incomplete abortion or after delivery due to retained products of conception.
   (Reference: William's Obstetrics, 25th and 26th edition)

6. **a.** When gestational sac is >25 mm with absent embryo
   Criteria for nonviable pregnancy include gestational sac >25 mm without embryo and CRL of 7 mm without cardiac activity.
   (Reference: William's Obstetrics, 25th edition)

7. **a.** Yolk sac diameters of >7 mm in <10 weeks pregnancy
   Unfavorable outcome is expected when early pregnancy scan has yolk sac diameter of >7 mm in <10 weeks pregnancy, FHR of <90 at 6 weeks of pregnancy, subchorionic hematoma sized about two-thirds of gestational sac and difference between MSD and CRL is <5 mm.
   (Reference: Callen's Ultrasonography in Obstetrics and Gynaecology, 6th edition)

8. **c.** M-mode imaging is used to document heartbeat
   Transvaginal ultrasound is preferred for early pregnancy diagnosis. And Doppler ultrasound is avoided in early pregnancy to reduce the risk of exposure. M-mode imaging is used to calculate heartbeat in pregnancy.
   [Reference: Cunningham FG, Leveno KJ, Dashe JS, Hoffman BL, Spong CY (Eds). Williams Obstetrics, 26th edition. New York: McGraw Hill/Medical; 2022]

9. **a.** Shock features due to incomplete abortion, products in cervical canal
   Cervical shock refers to sudden onset shock features due to instrumentation on cervix (holding with vulsellum) or due to stretching of cervix due to products in cervical canal. Inadvertent injection of paracervical block results in convulsions due to vascular injection. Shock features due to hemorrhage after complete or incomplete abortion is called hemorrhagic/hypovolemic shock.
   (Reference: James High-risk Pregnancy, 5th edition)

10. **b.** Nonviable pregnancy
    Serum progesterone level of >80 nmol/L in early pregnancy suggests good outcome. However, values <15 nmol/L suggest nonviable pregnancy. Serial values are important while measuring β-hCG values, not for serum progesterone. β-hCG values of 2,000 are used as discriminatory zone for visualization of gestational sac in ultrasound. Progesterone value is not relevant as discriminatory zone.
    (Reference: James High-risk Pregnancy, 5th edition, page 89)

11. **d.** None of the above
    Features of abnormal yolk sac include all large yolk sac of >7mm, calcified sac, irregular sac, and free-floating sac. They are associated with pregnancy failures.
    (References: Callen's Ultrasonography in Obstetrics and Gynaecology, 6th edition and Essentials of Obstetrics by Lakshmi Seshadri)

12. **c.** Missed miscarriage—offer termination
    Absence of cardiac activity with CRL of 7 mm suggests pregnancy failure. Miscarriage word is preferred over other terminologies. Blighted ovum generally refers to gestational sac with absent embryo. Presence of CRL means presence of embryo. As there is absent cardiac activity, preferred treatment in this case is to offer termination.
    (Reference: Callen's Ultrasonography in Obstetrics and Gynaecology, 6th edition)

13. **b.** Repeat transvaginal ultrasound after 10 days
    Absent embryo after MSD of 25 mm, suggests failure of pregnancy. As the gestational sac diameter is 20 mm, best option would be to repeat ultrasound after 10-14 days, Serial β-hCG is more helpful when suspicion of extrauterine pregnancy is there or to support diagnosis of failed intrauterine pregnancy.
    (Reference: Callen's Ultrasonography in Obstetrics and Gynaecology, 6th edition)

14. **b.** Repeat transvaginal ultrasound after 10 days
    Generally, amnion appears after embryo. Presence of only amnion refers to empty amnion syndrome. However, as there can be possibility of twin gestational sacs appearing as gestational sac and amnion, best option would be to repeat ultrasound after 10–14 days to confirm absence of embryo.
    (Reference: Callen's Ultrasonography in Obstetrics and Gynaecology, 6th edition)

15. **b.** Repeat scanning in 1–2 weeks in view of bradycardia.
    The mean FHR is 100–110/min at 6 weeks and 150/min around 8–9 weeks. Slow fetal heart suggests high risk of abortion and/or fetal malformation. They need to be followed up in 1–2 weeks to check if bradycardia is persistent.
    (Reference: Callen's Ultrasonography in Obstetrics and Gynaecology, 6th edition)

16. **a.** Threatened abortion
    By definition, threatened miscarriage includes complaints of bleeding per vagina, closed cervical os, and ultrasound features of live pregnancy.
    [Reference: Cunningham FG, Leveno KJ, Dashe JS, Hoffman BL, Spong CY (Eds). Williams Obstetrics, 26th edition. New York: McGraw Hill/Medical; 2022]

17. **b.** Complete abortion, no further interventions
    Three months of pregnancy with passage of clots, closed cervical os with absent active bleeding, and ultrasound features of absent products suggest complete abortion. Endometrium up to 15 mm thickness with absent bleeding clinically correlates with complete abortion.
    [References: Cunningham FG, Leveno KJ, Dashe JS, Hoffman BL, Spong CY (Eds). Williams Obstetrics, 26th edition. New York: McGraw Hill/Medical; 2022. And Konar H. D C Dutta's Textbook of Obstetrics, 10th edition. New Delhi: Jaypee Brothers Medical Publishers (P) Ltd.; 2022]

18. **a.** Incomplete abortion—offer manual vacuum aspiration
    Complaints of bleeding per vagina in early pregnancy, clinical features suggestive of products in cervical canal suggest incomplete abortion. Vacuum aspiration is preferred treatment over curettage. When patient is early, features of shock surgical evacuation is preferred over medical methods.
    [Reference: Comprehensive abortion care training and service guidelines by NHM 2018]

19. **a.** Septic abortion, managed as antibiotics—fluid management—evacuation
    Surviving sepsis guidelines 2021 recommend administration of antibiotics within 1 hour of diagnosis followed by volume expansion using intravenous fluid therapy. Every hour of delay in administration of antibiotics lead to increase in mortality rates. Evacuation is planned after antibiotic administration and patient is stabilized unless there is life-threatening hemorrhage.
    (References: Comprehensive abortion care training and service guidelines by NHM 2018 and surviving sepsis campaign guidelines 2021)

20. **d.** Septic abortion grade 4
    There are three grades of septic abortion. Grade 1 sepsis is when the infection is confined to uterus, grade 2 is when confined to pelvis and grade 3 is when infection spreads beyond pelvis and involves systemic signs (guarding-rigidity) and features of end-organ dysfunction.
    (Reference: Konar H. D C Dutta's Textbook of Obstetrics, 10th edition. New Delhi: Jaypee Brothers Medical Publishers (P) Ltd.; 2022)

21. **d.** None of the above
    Complications retained products of conception include hemorrhage, sepsis, and formation of organized mass called placental polyp.
    [Reference: Konar H. D C Dutta's Textbook of Obstetrics, 10th edition. New Delhi: Jaypee Brothers Medical Publishers (P) Ltd.; 2022]

22. **c.** Hypertension
    Endotoxic shock (gram-negative sepsis) in septic abortion may present with hypothermia, hyperthermia (fever), hypotension, tachycardia, and tachypnea. Hypertension is not a feature of gram-negative sepsis.
    [Reference: Konar H. D C Dutta's Textbook of Obstetrics, 10th edition. New Delhi: Jaypee Brothers Medical Publishers (P) Ltd.; 2022]

23. **d.** Subchorionic hematoma >60 mL
    Ultrasound features are different for:
    - Pregnancy failure
    - Suspicion of pregnancy failure
    - Impending pregnancy failure

    Ultrasonogram features suggestive of suspicious failed pregnancy include CRL <7 mm and no cardiac activity, gestation sac 16–24 mm, enlarged yolk sac (>7mm), and empty amnion.

Risk factors for impending failure include slow embryonic heart rate, subchorionic hematoma >60 mL, and difference in MSD and CRL is <5 mm.
(Reference: Callen's Ultrasonography in Obstetrics and Gynaecology, 6th edition)

24. **c.** Maternal underweight
Risk factors for spontaneous abortion include age >40 years, obesity, excessive caffeine consumption (>200 mg/day), viral infections, diabetes, and thyroid disorders.

Maternal underweight is not associated with increased risk of abortion.
[Reference: Cunningham FG, Leveno KJ, Dashe JS, Hoffman BL, Spong CY (Eds). Williams Obstetrics, 26th edition. New York: McGraw Hill/Medical; 2022]

25. **a.** 0.1–0.2 Gy
Radiation exposure of 0.1–0.2 Gy in the first 2 weeks of pregnancy results in embryonic death, congenital malformations if exposed between 2 and 8 weeks of pregnancy, intellectual disability between 16 and 25 weeks of pregnancy.
[Reference: Cunningham FG, Leveno KJ, Dashe JS, Hoffman BL, Spong CY (Eds). Chapter 66: Williams Obstetrics, 26th edition. New York: McGraw Hill/Medical; 2022]

26. **b.** Polypropylene
Environmental and occupational factors associated with abortion include phthalates, nitrous oxide, bisphenol A, polychlorinated biphenyl, and DDT. Polypropylene is a suture material, not teratogenic.
[Reference: Cunningham FG, Leveno KJ, Dashe JS, Hoffman BL, Spong CY (Eds). Williams Obstetrics, 26th edition. New York: McGraw Hill/Medical; 2022]

27. **a.** Gestational sac—yolk sac—embryo—amnion
The normal order of appearance in early pregnancy ultrasound are gestational sac—yolk sac—embryo—cardiac activity and then amnion. Thus, it is normal to see embryo without amnion. Appearance of amnion with no embryo is termed as empty amnion sign.
(Reference: Callen's Ultrasonography in Obstetrics and Gynaecology, 6th edition)

28. **d.** All of the above
Subchorionic hematoma may be rounded, irregular or crescent shape, anechoic or may have internal echoes and may have septation.
(Reference: Callen's Ultrasonography in Obstetrics and Gynaecology, 6th edition)

29. **a.** <5 mm
Gestational sac is normally larger than the embryo. Sac is considered as small if MSD and CRL is <5 mm and normal if 5 mm or greater. Small sac diameter is associated with poor prognosis in terms of pregnancy failure.
(Reference: Callen's Ultrasonography in Obstetrics and Gynaecology, 6th edition)

30. **c.** >7 mm
The normal yolk sac diameter measures approximately 4.5 mm (inner-inner) and 6 mm (outer-outer) in the early pregnancy. Unfavorable outcome is expected when early pregnancy scan has yolk sac diameter of >7 mm in <10 weeks pregnancy.
(Reference: Callen's Ultrasonography in Obstetrics and Gynaecology, 6th edition)

Chapter 22

Ectopic Pregnancy

Priyanka Rai, Swapnil Bala

QUESTIONS

1. Percentage of first trimester pregnancies in developed countries is ectopically located.
   a. 0.1–0.5%
   b. 0.2–1.0%
   c. 0.5–1.5%
   d. 1.0–2.0%

2. What percentage of ectopic pregnancies demonstrates appropriately rising β-human chorionic gonadotropin (β-HCG) levels?
   a. 15%
   b. 20.8%
   c. 48%
   d. 25%

3. A pregnant woman came for routine antenatal USG at 8 weeks of gestation. Which of the following features is suggestive of a pseudogestational sac?
   a. Presence of yolk sac
   b. Intradecidual sac sign
   c. Central location
   d. Double decidual sign

4. Which type of tubal pregnancy ruptures at a later stage?
   a. Ampullary
   b. Interstitial
   c. Fimbrial
   d. Isthmic

5. Which of the following clinical features is not seen in a patient of ruptured ectopic pregnancy?
   a. Shoulder tip pain
   b. Decidual cast
   c. Vertigo and syncope
   d. Shock index of 0.7

6. In ectopic pregnancies, the absence of which tissue layer of the fallopian tube facilitates rapid invasion of proliferating trophoblasts into muscularis.
   a. Connective tissue
   b. Serosa
   c. Epithelium
   d. Submucosa

7. Women having pregnancy while using contraceptive measure, maximum number of ectopic pregnancies seen with the use of:
   a. OCPs
   b. POPs
   c. NuvaRing
   d. Progestin releasing intrauterine device (IUD)

8. A third para gravida got admitted with a history of sudden onset of right-sided lower abdominal pain and bleeding per vagina after a period of amenorrhea of 5 weeks. Her BP is 80/50 mm Hg and her pulse rate is 138 bpm. Transvaginal ultrasound (TVS) reveals the presence of a large amount of free fluid in the pelvis and the absence of an intrauterine gestational sac. What is the most appropriate management?
   a. Perform laparoscopic salpingectomy
   b. Laparotomy followed by salpingectomy
   c. Laparoscopic salpingo-oophorectomy
   d. Treat with intramuscular methotrexate (MTX)

9. Selection criteria for medical management of ectopic pregnancy are, *except:*
   a. Unruptured tubal ectopic pregnancy
   b. Patient hemodynamically stable
   c. Serum HCG <3,000 IU/L
   d. Presence of fetal cardiac activity

10. A 27-year-old nulligravida presents with an ectopic pregnancy at the ampullary end of the tube with a damaged opposite tube. The patient is hemodynamically stable. The best mode of treatment will be:
    a. Salpingectomy at laparotomy
    b. Linear salpingectomy at laparotomy
    c. Laparoscopic linear salpingostomy
    d. Laparoscopic tubal segmental resection and end-to-end anastomosis

11. Mrs X, 6 weeks of gestation, conceived by in vitro fertilization is diagnosed to have heterotopic pregnancy. The management of ectopic pregnancy is:
    a. Medical management with MTX
    b. Laparoscopic salpingectomy
    c. Abort the intrauterine pregnancy, then give MTX
    d. Management with systemic prostaglandin F2α (PGF2α)

12. The most common infection resulting in ectopic pregnancy is:
    a. Chlamydia   b. Gonococci
    c. Candida   d. Syphilis

13. Arias-Stella reaction: All are true, *except:*
    a. Presence of hyperchromatic nuclei
    b. Specific to ectopic pregnancy
    c. Progesterone-influenced event
    d. Adenomatous change of endometrial glands

14. A 25-year-old female comes with amenorrhea for 2 months and bleeding per vaginum for the past 15 days (spotting). She has done her pregnancy test at home which was positive. On pelvic examination, there is slight bleeding through the external os, and the internal os is closed, you will manage this case by:
    a. USG + conservative management
    b. USG + immediate laparoscopy
    c. D&C
    d. Suction evacuation

15. A 22-year-old primigravida presents with 40 days of amenorrhea positive and β-hCG of >1,000 units. No gestational sac is seen in the uterus. What is the further management?
    a. Observation
    b. Repeat β-hCG after 48 hours
    c. Repeat β-hCG after 1 week
    d. Medical management

16. "Lithopedion" is a complication related to:
    a. Ovarian pregnancy
    b. Tubal pregnancy
    c. Abdominal pregnancy
    d. None of the above

17. Most common endometrial reaction in ectopic pregnancy is:
    a. Decidual reaction with chorionic villi
    b. Decidual reaction without chorionic villi
    c. Arias-Stella reaction
    d. Secretory change

18. The general surgeons have operated on a woman to rule out appendicitis and the signs of an abdominal pregnancy with around 18–20 weeks fetus and placenta attached to the omentum. The best course of action in this case is:
    a. Removal of both fetus and placenta
    b. Removal of the fetus only
    c. Laparoscopic ligation of umbilical cord
    d. Closely follow until viability and then deliver by laparotomy

19. Which of the following is not true regarding salpingostomy performed for an ectopic pregnancy?
    a. Up to 15% have persistence of trophoblastic tissue
    b. Procedure of choice for ruptured ectopic pregnancies
    c. Subsequent pregnancy rates are comparable to those for ectopic managed by salpingectomy
    d. Mean resolution time to a negative β-hCG is 20 days following surgery

20. A 33-year-old G4P2 at 5–6 weeks of gestation by last menstrual period (LMP) presents with severe abdominal pain, giddiness, and weakness. On TVS, she is diagnosed to have a complex left adnexal mass with free fluid in Morrison's pouch. What is the minimum amount of accumulated hemoperitoneum which would be expected at the time of surgery?
    a. 100–200 mL
    b. 200–300 mL
    c. 300–400 mL
    d. 400–500 mL

21. Why do we perform dilatation and curettage prior to administering MTX in cases of ectopic pregnancy?
    a. To assess for endometrial decidualization
    b. To confirm the absence of trophoblastic tissue
    c. To confirm a secretory endometrium
    d. None of the above

22. What percentage of women treated with single-dose MTX therapy requires an additional dose of medication for an inadequate clinical response?
    a. 2–5%
    b. 5–10%
    c. 25–30%
    d. 15–20%

23. A woman attends the antenatal clinic at POA 5 weeks having no complaints. Her periods are regular and she is sure of dates. Urinary hCG is positive. TVS does not reveal any intrauterine or ectopic pregnancy. Serum β-hCG doubles from 1,000 to 2,000 IU/L after 48 hours. What is the next step in management?
    a. Give a single dose of MTX
    b. Perform laparoscopy
    c. Repeat TVS after 3 days
    d. Perform serum β-hCG after 1 week

24. Selection criteria for medical management of ectopic pregnancy are, *except*:
    a. Unruptured tubal ectopic pregnancy
    b. Hemodynamic stable patient
    c. Serum hCG <3,000 IU/L
    d. Presence of fetal cardiac activity

25. A female has a history of infertility treatment and 6 weeks of amenorrhea, serum β-hCG is 1,000 IU and USG shows an empty sac in the uterus. Next step in the management is:
    a. Expectant management
    b. Medical management
    c. Repeat β-hCG after 48 hours
    d. Repeat β-hCG after 7 days

26. True statement regarding ectopic pregnancy, *except*:
    a. Serum progesterone >25 ng/mL exclude ectopic
    b. β-hCG levels should be >1,000 mIU/mL for earliest detection by TVS
    c. β-hCG doubles in 48 hours
    d. Actinomycin D may be used for treatment

27. A hemodynamically stable nulliparous patient with ectopic pregnancy has an adnexal mass of 2.5 × 3.5 cm and a β-hCG titer of 1,800 IU/mL. What modality of treatment is suitable for her?
    a. Conservative management
    b. Medical management
    c. Laparoscopic surgery
    d. Laparotomy

28. A 38-year-old G3P2 presents at 6–7 weeks gestation complaining of mild lower abdominal pain and spotting and is found to have a 3.5-cm left ectopic pregnancy. She has a history of severe persistent asthma and was treated for an asthma exacerbation 3 days ago. She also has a history of a prior ectopic pregnancy treated with salpingectomy, chronic hypertension for which she takes labetalol, and type 2 diabetes managed with insulin. What aspect of her history would preclude treatment with MTX?
    a. Type 2 diabetes
    b. Chronic hypertension
    c. Severe persistent asthma with recent exacerbation
    d. History of a prior ectopic pregnancy treated with salpingectomy

29. What is the ectopic resolution rate following MTX administration?
    a. 66%   b. 90%
    c. 80%   d. 33%

30. A 33-year-old G3P1 presents at 6 weeks gestation by LMP complaining of pelvic pain and nausea. Her β-HCG is 3,000 mIU/mL and no intrauterine pregnancy is seen on ultrasound. No adnexal masses or free fluid are visualized. What is the best management strategy?
    a. No intervention
    b. Surgical therapy
    c. Methotrexate injection
    d. Expectant management with 48-hour follow-up

ANSWERS

1. **c.** 0.5–1.5%
Following fertilization and fallopian tube transit, the blastocyst normally implants in the endometrial lining of the uterine cavity. Implantation elsewhere is considered ectopic. In the United States, numbers from an insurance database and from Medicaid claims showed ectopic pregnancy rates of 1.54% and 1.38%, respectively, in 2013.
[References: Cunningham FG, Leveno KJ, Dashe JS, Hoffman BL, Spong CY, Casey BM. Williams Obstetrics, 26th edition. New York: McGraw Hill; 2022. p. 574; Tao G, Patel C, Hoover KW. Updated Estimates of Ectopic Pregnancy among Commercially and Medicaid-Insured Women in the United States, 2002-2013. South Med J. 2017;110(1):18-24.]

2. **b.** 20.8%
[Reference: Silva C, Sammel MD, Zhou L, Gracia C, Hummel AC, Barnhart K. Human chorionic gonadotropin profile for women with ectopic pregnancy. Obstet Gynecol. 2006;107(3):605-10]

3. **c.** Central location
   It is a feature of the pseudogestational sac seen in ectopic pregnancies. Pseudogestational sac is a collection of fluid between the endometrial layers, surrounded by a thick decidua. Its presence increases the suspicion of ectopic pregnancy.
   [Reference: Fylstra DL. Avoiding misdiagnosing an early intrauterine pregnancy as an ectopic pregnancy. World J Obstet Gynecol. 2015;4(3):58-63.]

4. **b.** Interstitial
   Interstitial tubal pregnancy ruptures at a later stage, i.e., at 12-16 weeks. This is because pregnancy at this site is closer to the uterine myometrium which provides support as pregnancy advances. Isthmic and ampullary pregnancies terminate by tubal rupture. However, isthmic pregnancy ruptures earlier. Ampullary and infundibular pregnancy can terminate by tubal abortion as well.
   [Reference: Tulandi T, Al-Jaroudi D. Interstitial pregnancy: results generated from the Society of Reproductive Surgeons Registry. Obstet Gynecol. 2004; 103(1):47-50.]

5. **d.** Shock index
   Shock index is calculated as heart rate/systolic blood pressure (HR/SBP). The range of values for SI for patients being evaluated for pain and/or vaginal bleeding within the first trimester of pregnancy, who do not have a ruptured ectopic pregnancy, are within the previously reported range of 0.5-0.7 for nonpregnant patients. A SI >0.85 made the diagnosis of ruptured ectopic pregnancy 15.0 (95% confidence interval (CI): 5.6-40.4) times more likely.
   [Reference: Birkhahn RH, Gaeta TJ, Bei R, Bove JJ. Shock index in the first trimester of pregnancy and its relationship to ruptured ectopic pregnancy. Acad Emer Med. 2002;9(2):115-9.]

6. **d.** Submucosa
   With tubal pregnancy, because the fallopian tube lacks a submucosal layer, the fertilized ovum promptly burrows through the epithelium. The zygote comes to lie near or within the muscularis, which is invaded by a rapidly proliferating trophoblast. The embryo or fetus in an ectopic pregnancy is often absent or stunted.
   (Reference: Cunningham FG, Leveno KJ, Dashe JS, Hoffman BL, Spong CY, Casey BM. Williams Obstetrics, 26th edition. New York: McGraw Hill; 2022. p. 576.)

7. **d.** Progestin-releasing IUD
   With any form of contraception, the absolute number of ectopic pregnancies is decreased because pregnancy occurs less often. However, with some contraceptive method failures, the relative number of ectopic pregnancies is increased. Examples include tubal sterilization, copper and progestin-releasing intrauterine devices (IUDs), and progestin-only contraceptives.
   (Reference: Cunningham FG, Leveno KJ, Dashe JS, Hoffman BL, Spong CY, Casey BM. Williams Obstetrics, 26th edition. New York: McGraw Hill; 2022. p. 576.)

8. **b.** Laparotomy followed by salpingectomy
   This is a case of ruptured ectopic pregnancy as indicated by a large amount of free fluid in the pelvis on TVS and vitals suggestive of the hemodynamically unstable condition of the patient. So, the appropriate management in this case is salpingectomy via laparotomy.
   [Reference: Hajenius PJ, Mol F, Mol BW, Bossuyt PM, Ankum WM, van der Veen F. Interventions for tubal ectopic pregnancy. Cochrane Database Syst Rev. 2007;2007(1):CD000324.]

9. **d.** Presence of fetal cardiac activity
   The best candidate for medical therapy is a woman who is asymptomatic, motivated, and compliant. With medical therapy, some classic predictors of success include a low initial serum β-hCG level, small ectopic pregnancy size, and absent fetal cardiac activity. Of these, initial serum β-hCG level is the best prognostic indicator with single-dose MTX.
   (Reference: Cunningham FG, Leveno KJ, Dashe JS, Hoffman BL, Spong CY, Casey BM. Williams Obstetrics, 26th edition. New York: McGraw Hill; 2022. p. 589.)

10. **c.** Laparoscopic linear salpingostomy
    Since the patient is nulligravida and is hemodynamically stable, laparoscopy can be performed. A linear incision is made in the intact tube and forceps are used to remove the products of conception.
    [Reference: Hajenius PJ, Mol F, Mol BW, Bossuyt PM, Ankum WM, van der Veen F. Interventions for tubal ectopic pregnancy. Cochrane Database Syst Rev. 2007; 2007(1):CD000324.]

11. **b.** Laparoscopic salpingectomy
    Heterotopic pregnancy treatment needs laparoscopy and, most often, a salpingectomy or salpingostomy.

However, in hemodynamically unstable cases, laparotomy may be needed. Systemic MTX has no role in the management of heterotopic pregnancy due to the presence of a viable intrauterine pregnancy. Some literature described the use of local injection of potassium chloride and MTX, but the success rate is controversial.
[Reference: Ali T, Tawab MA, ElHariri MAG, Ayad AA. Heterotopic pregnancy: a case report. Egypt J Radiol Nucl Med. 2020;51(1): 1-4.]

12. **a.** *Chlamydia*
Chlamydia trachomatis infection results in the production of interleukin-1 by tubal epithelial cells; this happens to be a vital indicator for embryo implantation within the endometrium. Interleukin-1 also has a role in downstream neutrophil recruitment which would further contribute to fallopian tubal damage.
[Reference: Mummert T, Gnugnoli DM. Ectopic Pregnancy. In: StatPearls [Internet]. Treasure Island (FL): StatPearls Publishing; 2023.]

13. **b.** Specific to ectopic pregnancy
The reactive and benign phenomenon of the endometrium induced by hormonal stimulation and characterized by cytomegaly and nuclear enlargement of endometrial glands; typically associated with intrauterine or two extrauterine pregnancies or with gestational trophoblastic disease.
Reference: Ardighieri L. (2023). Uterus: Nontumor—Arias-Stella reaction. [online] Available from https://www.pathologyoutlines.com/topic/uterusariasstella.html [Last accessed December, 2023].

14. **a.** USG + conservative management
This case should be managed conservatively because on USG there will be localization of pregnancy and further serial serum β-hCG will be done. We will have to rule out the possibility of abortion like threatened or missed abortion.
[References: Cunningham FG, Leveno KJ, Dashe JS, Hoffman BL, Spong CY, Casey BM. Williams Obstetrics, 26th edition. New York: McGraw Hill; 2022. p. 589; Everett C. Incidence and outcome of bleeding before the 20th week of pregnancy: prospective study from general practice. BMJ. 1997;315(7099):32-4.]

15. **b.** Repeat β-hCG after 48 hours
The management of this case of ectopic pregnancy requires repeat serum β-hCG after 48 hours to see its doubling time which is further required for decision-making whether this case has to be managed conservatively or any medical and surgical intervention is required.
(Reference: Cunningham FG, Leveno KJ, Dashe JS, Hoffman BL, Spong CY, Casey BM. Williams Obstetrics, 26th edition, New York: McGraw Hill; 2022. p. 580.)

16. **c.** Abdominal pregnancy
A very rare incidence is reported when the fetus dies during abdominal pregnancy and it is too large to reabsorb, it calcifies and remains a lithopedion (known as stone baby) for many years.
[Reference: Fagan CJ, Schreiber MH, Amparo EG. Lithopedion: stone baby. Arch Surg. 1980;115(6):764-6.]

17. **b.** Decidual reaction without chorionic villi
Identification of decidua without villus structure is most suggestive of ectopic pregnancy. Chorionic villi that float in normal saline as lacy fronds are very much suggestive of intrauterine pregnancy.
[Reference: Lopez HB, Micheelsen U, Berendtsen H, Kock K. Ectopic pregnancy and its associated endometrial changes. Gynecol Obstet Invest. 1994;38(2):104-6.]

18. **b.** Removal of the fetus only
The ideal surgery is to remove the entire sac, fetus, placenta, and membrane. This can be done if the placenta is attached to a removable organ like the uterus or broad ligament. Here the placenta is attached to the omentum, so it is better to take out the fetus and leave behind the placenta and the sac after tying and cutting the cord with its placental attachment. Absorption of the placenta will occur by aseptic autolysis.
[References: Cunningham FG, Leveno KJ, Dashe JS, Hoffman BL, Spong CY, Casey BM. Williams Obstetrics, 26th edition. New York: McGraw Hill; 2022. p. 603; Harirah HM, Smith JM, Dixon CL, Hankins GD. Conservative Management and Planned Surgery for Periviable Advanced Extrauterine Abdominal Pregnancy with Favorable Outcome: Report of Two Cases. AJP Rep. 2016;6(3):e301-8.]

19. **b.** Procedure of choice for ruptured ectopic pregnancies
[Reference: Tulandi T, Guralnick M. Treatment of tubal ectopic pregnancy by salpingotomy with or without tubal suturing and salpingectomy. Fertil Steril. 1991;55(1):53-5. Erratum in: Fertil Steril. 1991; 55(6):1213-4.]

20. **d.** 400–500 mL
A small amount of peritoneal fluid is physiologically normal. However, with hemoperitoneum, anechoic or hypoechoic fluid initially collects in the dependent retrouterine cul-de-sac. It then additionally surrounds the uterus as blood fills the pelvis. With significant intra-abdominal hemorrhage, blood will track up the pericolic gutters to fill the Morison pouch near the liver. Free fluid in this pouch typically is not seen until accumulated volumes reach 400–600 mL.
[References: Cunningham FG, Leveno KJ, Dashe JS, Hoffman BL, Spong CY, Casey BM. Williams Obstetrics, 26th edition. New York: McGraw Hill; 2022. p. 585; Branney SW, Wolfe RE, Moore EE, Albert NP, Heinig M, Mestek M, et al. Quantitative sensitivity of ultrasound in detecting free intraperitoneal fluid. J Trauma. 1995; 39(2):375-80.]

21. **b.** To confirm the absence of trophoblastic tissue
[Reference: Chung K, Chandavarkar U, Opper N, Barnhart K. Reevaluating the role of dilation and curettage in the diagnosis of pregnancy of unknown location. Fertil Steril. 2011;96(3):659-62.]

22. **d.** 15–20%
After single-dose MTX, mean serum β-hCG levels may rise or fall during the first 4 days and then should gradually decline. If the level fails to drop by ≥15% between days 4 and 7, a second MTX dose is recommended. This is necessary for 20% of women treated with single-dose therapy (Cohen, 2014). In such cases, a complete blood count (CBC), creatinine level, and liver function tests (LFTs) are rechecked. If these surveillance tests are normal, a second equivalent dose is administered. The date of this second injection will become the new day 1, and the protocol is restarted.
[References: Cunningham FG, Leveno KJ, Dashe JS, Hoffman BL, Spong CY, Casey BM. Williams Obstetrics, 26th edition. New York: MCGRAW-HILL; 2022. p. 590; Cohen A, Bibi G, Almog B, Tsafrir Z, Levin I. Second-dose methotrexate in ectopic pregnancies: the role of beta human chorionic gonadotropin. Fertil Steril. 2014;102(6):1646-9.]

23. **c.** Repeat TVS after 3 days
This woman has positive urine pregnancy test (UPT), but the TVS does not reveal an intrauterine pregnancy or an ectopic pregnancy. Therefore, her period of gestation could be <5 weeks, or she could be having a pregnancy in an unknown location. Serum β-hCG doubled up to 2,000 IU/L in 48 hours. She is likely to have a developing early intrauterine pregnancy with the wrong dates, but the possibility of an ectopic pregnancy cannot be excluded as there was no visible intrauterine pregnancy on TVS. So, a scan should be performed after 3 days, as the serum β-hCG is >1,500 IU//L and there is always the risk of rupture if it is a case of tubal pregnancy.
[Reference: Cunningham FG, Leveno KJ, Dashe JS, Hoffman BL, Spong CY, Casey BM. Williams Obstetrics, 26th edition. New York: MCGRAW-HILL; 2022. p. 581.]

24. **d.** Presence of fetal cardiac activity
The presence of fetal cardiac activity is not a contraindication for medical management but the high failure rate of medical management in case of high β-HCG concentrations and the presence of embryonic heart activity.
[Reference: Taylor HS, Pal L, Sell E. Speroff's Clinical Gynecologic Endocrinology and Infertility, 9th edition. Philadelphia: Wolters Kluwer Health; 2019. p. 3330.]

25. **a.** Expectant management
This is a case of early intrauterine pregnancy, there is a gestational sac inside the uterine cavity and the next structure to appear is a yolk sac followed by an embryo and further cardiac activity. For cases in which a gestational sac has no embryo or yolk sac, additional time and repeat TVS are recommended. M-mode should be used to document cardiac activity and measure the rate.
[Reference: Expert Panel on Women's Imaging; Brown DL, Packard A, Maturen KE, Deshmukh SP, Dudiak KM, et al. ACR Appropriateness Criteria® First Trimester Vaginal Bleeding. J Am Coll Radiol. 2018;15(5S):S69-S77.]

26. **c.** β-hCG doubles in 48 hours
(Reference: Cunningham FG, Leveno KJ, Dashe JS, Hoffman BL, Spong CY, Casey BM. Williams Obstetrics, 26th edition. New York: McGraw Hill; 2022. pp. 580-86.)

27. **b.** Medical management
The ideal candidate has the following characteristics:
- *Absolute characteristics:* Hemodynamic stability, no evidence of tubal rupture, or acute intra-abdominal bleeding. Reliable commitment to comply with

required follow-up care, no contraindications to MTX treatment.
- *Preferred characteristics:* Absent or minimal symptoms (pain), serum β-hCG concentration <5,000 IU/L, absent embryonic heart activity, ectopic mass measuring <4 cm in diameter, willing to accept blood products in case of emergency, easy access to the healthcare system

[Reference: Taylor HS, Pal L, Sell E. Speroff's Clinical Gynecologic Endocrinology and Infertility, 9th edition. Philadelphia: Lippincott Williams & Wilkins (LWW); 2020. p. 3331.]

28. **c.** Severe persistent asthma with recent exacerbation
Severe persistent asthma is a contraindication to MTX treatment others are viable and desired intrauterine pregnancy, breastfeeding, immunodeficiency states, and hematologic abnormalities (severe anemia, leukopenia, and thrombocytopenia), known sensitivity to MTX, active pulmonary disease, active peptic ulcer disease, alcoholism, clinically important hepatic, or renal dysfunction

[Reference: Taylor HS, Pal L, Sell E. Speroff's Clinical Gynecologic Endocrinology and Infertility, 9th edition. Philadelphia: Lippincott Williams & Wilkins (LWW); 2019. p. 3332.]

29. **b.** 90%

[References: Cunningham FG, Leveno KJ, Dashe JS, Hoffman BL, Spong CY, Casey BM. Williams Obstetrics, 26th edition. New York: McGraw Hill; 2022. p. 588; Barnhart KT, Gosman G, Ashby R, Sammel M. The medical management of ectopic pregnancy: a meta-analysis comparing "single dose" and "multidose" regimens. Obstet Gynecol. 2003;101(4):778-84.]

30. **d.** Expectant management with 48-hour follow-up

[References: Cunningham FG, Leveno KJ, Dashe JS, Hoffman BL, Spong CY, Casey BM. Williams Obstetrics, 26th edition. New York: McGraw Hill; 2022. p. 593; Helmy S, Sawyer E, Ofili-Yebovi D, Yazbek J, Ben Nagi J, Jurkovic D. Fertility outcomes following expectant management of tubal ectopic pregnancy. Ultrasound Obstet Gynecol. 2007;30(7):988-93.]

Chapter 23

Multifetal Gestation

Pavika Lal, Garima Gupta

QUESTIONS

1. **Regarding types of multiple pregnancies, which of the following is true?**
   a. Monozygotic twins result from mitotic division of a single zygote into "identical" twins
   b. Dichorionic (DC) twins result from division at 9–13 days
   c. Division before day 3 leads to twins with a shared placenta but separate amnions, monochorionic diamniotic (MCDA).
   d. All DC twins are nonidentical.

2. **Which of the following is not an important factor affecting dizygotic twins?**
   a. In vitro fertilization (IVF)
   b. Genetic factors
   c. Increasing maternal age
   d. Body mass index

3. **All maternal complications in multifetal pregnancy are increased as compared to singleton pregnancy, *except*:**
   a. PPH
   b. Hypertensive disorders of pregnancy
   c. Gestational diabetes
   d. Hypothyroidism

4. **All fetal complications in multifetal pregnancy are increased as compared to singleton pregnancy, *except*:**
   a. Congenital fetal anomalies
   b. Still birth
   c. Congenital fetal infections
   d. Fetal asphyxia

5. **Most common cause of preterm birth in twin pregnancy is:**
   a. Preterm premature rupture of membranes (PPROM)
   b. Iatrogenic
   c. Spontaneous
   d. Bacterial vaginosis

6. **Which of the following ovulation induction drug has the highest risk for multiple pregnancies?**
   a. Clomiphene citrate
   b. Letrozole
   c. Clomiphene citrate+ metformin
   d. Gonadotropins

7. **Most powerful predictor of twin-to-twin transfusion syndrome (TTTS) on first trimester USG is:**
   a. Reversal or absence of ductus venosus a wave
   b. Intertwin nuchal translucency (NT) discrepancy
   c. Intertwin crown–rump length (CRL) discrepancy
   d. Membrane folding

8. **All are cardiac dysfunctions in recipient twin in TTTS, *except*:**
   a. Myocardial hypertrophy
   b. Valvular regurgitant lesions
   c. Impaired diastolic function
   d. Coarctation of aortic isthmus

9. **All are true for discordant growth in twins, *except*:**
   a. Calculated by the formula = larger estimated or actual weight—smaller estimated or actual weight divided by larger estimate or actual weight × 100
   b. Clinically significant weight difference of 10–15% is important to diagnose discordancy
   c. Abdominal circumference can be used reliably for estimation of discordancy in twins
   d. Possibility of chromosomal anomalies, genetic syndromes, and fetal congenital infections should be considered while workup of discordancy among twins

10. **In twin reversed arterial perfusion (TRAP), all are true, *except*:**
    a. Diagnosis can be made in first trimester
    b. In TRAP, blood flows via the umbilical artery of the pump twin in reverse direction into the umbilical artery of the co-twin via artery to artery anastomosis
    c. Associated with long-term neurological sequel for pumped twin due to chronic hypoxemia
    d. It is an abnormality unique to monochorionic (MC) twins in 10% of cases

11. **All are true for twin anemia polycythemia sequence (TAPS) syndrome, *except*:**
    a. Represent a true, very slow intertwin transfusion imbalance
    b. Gross morphology of placenta shows small unidirectional arteriovenous (AV) anastomosis with no compensatory artery to artery anastomosis
    c. Prenatal diagnosis is made by decrease in middle cerebral artery-peak systolic velocity (MCA-PSV) in donor twin and increase in MCA-PSV in recipient twin
    d. Postnatal diagnosis is made by intertwin hemoglobin difference of >8 g/dL

12. **The most common cause of TAPS is:**
    a. Occurs spontaneously in MC twins
    b. Due to presence of minute residual anastomosis after fetoscopic laser ablation for TTTS
    c. As a result of genetic syndrome in the one of the fetus
    d. Fetal congenital infections

13. **In TAPS, both the donor and the recipient twin remains euvolemic due to:**
    a. Absence of artery to artery anastomosis
    b. Redistribution of placental blood flow through anastomosis
    c. Effectiveness of renin-angiotensin-aldosterone system
    d. both a and b

14. **The definitive treatment of TAPS is:**
    a. Fetoscopic laser surgery
    b. Expectant/conservative management as spontaneous resolution occurs
    c. Careful monitoring and repeated fetal blood transfusions
    d. To convert it into twin oligopoly sequence by amnioinfusion in one sac and amniodrainage of the other sac

15. **The most common type of Siamese twins is:**
    a. Thoracopagus   b. Pygopagus
    c. Ischiopagus   d. Craniopagus

16. **All of the following statements about single intrauterine fetal demise (sIUFD) are correct, *except*:**
    a. Timing and chorionicity are important factors in determining the outcome of a co-twin
    b. Monochorionic survivor twins are at five times higher risk of death after sIUFD compared with dichorionic (DC) survivor twins
    c. The risk of fetal death in DC twin pregnancies with selective intrauterine growth restriction (IUGR) doubles that of IUGR in singleton pregnancies
    d. Among the types of selective IUGR in monochorionic (MC) twin pregnancies, type II has the highest rate of severe fetal deterioration

17. **All are true regarding selective termination, *except*:**
    a. This procedure is done in presence of an abnormal fetus with a normal fetus
    b. It improves prognosis of normal fetus
    c. 0.2–0.5 mL 15% KCl is injected into the heart of abnormal fetus
    d. Done at 14–16 weeks

18. **A monochorionic (MC) twin pregnancy showed a discordant CRL at 12 weeks gestation, and a discordant amniotic fluid volume at 15 weeks with a deepest vertical pocket of 1.8 cm in the smaller twin and 6.3 cm in the larger twin. Both bladders are visible.**

    Which of the following is the likely diagnosis?
    a. Unequal placental sharing
    b. Twin-to-twin transfusion syndrome
    c. Complicated MC twin pregnancy, suspected to develop either selective fetal growth restriction or TTTS
    d. Physiological variation

19. **In MC twins with discordant growth, measuring the blood flow waveforms by Doppler plays an important role in both identifying the cause and predicting the outcome. Which description of how to measure these waveforms is correct?**
    a. The Doppler sample volume should be placed in the intrafetal part of the umbilical artery, close to the bladder
    b. The Doppler sample volume should be enlarged to capture both arteries in one image

c. The Doppler sample volume should be placed in the umbilical artery at a zero degree angle, assisted by color, close to the placental surface
d. The Doppler sample volume should be placed in a free loop of the cord, about half way between the fetus and the placenta, at 90°

20. **Which of the following is true about prediction and prevention of preterm labor in multifetal pregnancies?**
    a. Women should be advised to abstain from sexual intercourse
    b. A cervical length of <25 mm in a twin pregnancy at 20–24 weeks gestation is a good predictor of preterm labor and delivery
    c. Bed rest in hospital is more effective at preventing preterm labor compared with bed rest at home
    d. Although cervical cerclage has been shown to be ineffective in preventing preterm labor in twin pregnancy, it has been shown to be effective in triplet pregnancy

21. **Which of the following is true about progesterone treatment in twin pregnancies?**
    a. Progesterone treatment prevents preterm delivery before 34 weeks in unselected twin pregnancies
    b. Progesterone treatment prevents preterm delivery before 34 weeks in high-risk twin pregnancies
    c. Results from progesterone treatment in singletons are likely to be even more effective in twins as the incidence of PTD is higher
    d. All are incorrect

22. **Which of the following statements is true about treatment with a cervical pessary in twin pregnancies?**
    a. The sole mechanism of action of a cervical pessary is to close the cervical canal
    b. Insertion of a cervical pessary in women with twin pregnancies increases gestational age at delivery
    c. Treatment of twin pregnant women with a cervical pessary has no effect on neonatal outcome
    d. Significant maternal adverse effects have been reported with cervical pessaries

23. **All are true regarding timing of delivery in twin gestation, *except:***
    a. Uncomplicated DC twins should be delivered at 38 weeks period of gestation (POG)
    b. Uncomplicated MC twins should be delivered at 37 weeks POG
    c. In case of uncomplicated triplet pregnancy, elective birth is recommended beyond 35 weeks after antenatal course of corticosteroids
    d. In case discordancy or anomalies in MC twins, timing of delivery is based on condition of uncompromised fetus

24. **All of the following are true about congenital anomalies which are considered unique to twin pregnancy, *except:***
    a. Midline structural defects
    b. Hip dislocation, foot deformity is due to overcrowding
    c. Microcephaly, renal dysplasia, and intestinal atresia resulting from vascular events
    d. Congenital diaphragmatic hernia

25. **For screening of trisomy 21 in twin pregnancy, all are true, *except:***
    a. For dizygotic pregnancy, the risk of chromosomal anomalies for each twin is same as that for singleton gestation
    b. For dizygotic, since two fetuses are present, the risk of one being affected is twice as high
    c. In monozygotic twins, the age-related risk of fetal Down syndrome is same as in singleton pregnancy although only one fetus will be affected
    d. There may be variation in phenotypic expression of aneuploidy in monozygotic twins

26. **All of the following hold true for determining the age in twin pregnancy, *except:***
    a. Twin pregnancy should be ideally dated when the CRL measures between 55 and 85 mm or 11+0 to 13+6 weeks
    b. Larger of two CRLs should be used
    c. Twin pregnancy via IVF should be dated according to oocyte retrieval date and adding 14 days
    d. Smaller twin is generally not used for dating to avoid false reassurance that it is growing appropriately

27. **All are true about pathophysiology of TTTS, *except:***
    a. Virtually all MCDA placentas have vascular connections, yet TTTS occurs in only 10–15% of MC twins
    b. Both artery-to-artery and vein-to-vein are superficially direct anastomosis connections allowing bidirectional flow whereas AV anastomosis is located deep within the placenta allowing unidirectional flow

c. Mortality is highest in absence of artery-to-artery anastomosis and lowest when these anastomoses are present
d. Complex interaction of renin-angiotensin-aldosterone pathway in twins may be involved in development of TTTS

28. **All are true for systemic labeling of twins,** *except:*
   a. It allows allocation for proper fetal growth during serial scan throughout the pregnancy to the same twin
   b. Provide an accurate system to ensure invasive prenatal diagnosis when screening for aneuploidies
   c. Each fetus within the twin pregnancy can be oriented at 11–14 weeks ultrasound assessment
   d. Lateral fetal orientation is associated with intertwin membrane running horizontally along the longitudinal axis of the uterus

29. **All are true for determination of chorionicity,** *except:*
   a. Best determined between 11 and 14 weeks POG
   b. Monochorionic twins can be diagnosed with the presence of T sign and DC twins with help of twin peak sign/lambda signs
   c. Both T and lambda are almost 80% sensitive for diagnosis of chorionicity
   d. Regression of chorion frondosum leads to gradual loss of lambda signs as pregnancy advances into the second trimester

30. **All are true for monoamniotic twins,** *except:*
   a. Cord entanglement is universally present in monochorionic monoamniotic (MCMA) twins and is used as a bad prognostic sign
   b. Monoamniotic twinning is due to splitting of bilaminar germ disk between 9 and 12 days
   c. Careful assessment at the detailed anomaly scan and follow-up 2 weekly for growth and liquor volume, and more intense surveillance from 26 weeks with Doppler should be done
   d. In uncomplicated monoamniotic twin, optimal timing of delivery is between 32 and 34 weeks of gestation

ANSWERS

1. **a.** Monozygotic twins result from mitotic division of a single zygote into "identical" twins
   Division of a single zygote before day 3 results in DC but monozygotic twins, which are therefore identical, but with separate placentas and amnions. All dizygotic twins are DC. Division at 9–13 days is rare and results in MCMA twins with a single amniotic sac and shared placenta. Division beyond 13 days results in conjoined twins. As MC twins are derived from a single zygote, they are always identical.

2. **d.** Body mass index
   Twenty percent of all IVF conceptions are multiple; 5–10% of conceptions with the ovulation-inducing drug clomiphene are multiple.

3. **d.** Hypothyroidism
   [Reference: Dias T, Bhide A. Multiple pregnancy. In: Bhide A, Arulkumaran S, Damania KR, Daftary SN (Eds). Arias' Practical Guide to High-Risk Pregnancy and Delivery: A South Asian Perspective, 5th edition. Gurugram: Elsevier-RELX India Pvt Ltd.; 2020. p. 158]

4. **d.** Fetal asphyxia
   [Reference: Dias T, Bhide A. Multiple pregnancy. In: Bhide A, Arulkumaran S, Damania KR, Daftary SN (Eds). Arias' Practical Guide to High-Risk Pregnancy and Delivery: A South Asian Perspective, 5th edition. Gurugram: Elsevier-RELX India Pvt Ltd.; 2020. p. 159]

5. **c.** Spontaneous
   [Reference: Dias T, Bhide A. Multiple pregnancy. In: Bhide A, Arulkumaran S, Damania KR, Daftary SN (Eds). Arias' Practical Guide to High-Risk Pregnancy and Delivery: A South Asian Perspective, 5th edition. Gurugram: Elsevier-RELX India Pvt Ltd.; 2020. p. 159]

6. **d.** Gonadotropins
   [Reference: Diamond MP, Mitwally M, Casper R, Ager J, Legro RS, Brzyski R, et al. Estimating rates of multiple gestation pregnancies: sample size calculation from the assessment of multiple intrauterine gestations from ovarian stimulation (AMIGOS) trial. Contemp Clin Trials. 2011;32(6):902-8]

7. **a.** Reversal or absence of ductus venosus "a wave"
   [Reference: Stagnati V, Zanardini C, Fichera A, Pagani G, Quintero RA, Bellocco R, Prefumo F. Early prediction of twin-to-twin transfusion syndrome: systematic review and meta-analysis. Ultrasound Obstet Gynecol. 2017;49(5):573-82]

8. **d.** Coarctation of aortic isthmus
   [Reference: Miller JL. Twin to twin transfusion syndrome. Transl Pediatr. 2021;10(5):1518-29]

9. **b.** Clinically significant weight difference of 10–15% is important to diagnose discordancy

Clinically significant weight difference of 25% is important to diagnose discordancy.
[Reference: Tamblyn J, Morris RK. Multiple pregnancy. In: James D, Steer PJ, Weiner CP, Gonik B, Robson SC (Eds). High-risk Pregnancy, 5th edition. United Kingdom: Cambridge University Press; 2017. p. 1586]

10. **d.** It is an abnormality unique to monochorionic (MC) twins in 10% of cases.
[Reference: Tamblyn J, Morris RK. Multiple pregnancy. In: James D, Steer PJ, Weiner CP, Gonik B, Robson SC (Eds). High-risk Pregnancy, 5th edition. United Kingdom: Cambridge University Press; 2017. p. 1589]

11. **c.** Prenatal diagnosis is made by decrease in middle cerebral artery-peak systolic velocity (MCA-PSV) in donor twin and increase in MCA-PSV in recipient twin
[Reference: Tamblyn J, Morris RK. Multiple pregnancy. In: James D, Steer PJ, Weiner CP, Gonik B, Robson SC (Eds). High-risk Pregnancy, 5th edition. United Kingdom: Cambridge University Press; 2017. p. 1591]

12. **b.** Due to presence of minute residual anastomosis after fetoscopic laser ablation for TTTS
[Reference: Tamblyn J, Morris RK. Multiple pregnancy. In: James D, Steer PJ, Weiner CP, Gonik B, Robson SC (Eds). High-risk Pregnancy, 5th edition. United Kingdom: Cambridge University Press; 2017. p. 1591]

13. **c.** Effectiveness of renin-angiotensin-aldosterone system
[Reference: Dias T, Bhide A. Multiple pregnancy. In: Bhide A, Arulkumaran S, Damania KR, Daftary SN (Eds). Arias' Practical Guide to High-Risk Pregnancy and Delivery: A South Asian Perspective, 5th edition. Gurugram: Elsevier-RELX India Pvt Ltd.; 2020. p. 161]

14. **a.** Fetoscopic laser surgery
[Reference: Dias T, Bhide A. Multiple pregnancy. In: Bhide A, Arulkumaran S, Damania KR, Daftary SN (Eds). Arias' Practical Guide to High-Risk Pregnancy and Delivery: A South Asian Perspective, 5th edition. Gurugram: Elsevier-RELX India Pvt Ltd.; 2020. p. 161]

15. **a.** Thoracopagus
[Reference: Tamblyn J, Morris RK. Multiple pregnancy. In: James D, Steer PJ, Weiner CP, Gonik B, Robson SC (Eds). High-risk Pregnancy, 5th edition. United Kingdom: Cambridge University Press; 2017. p. 1605]

16. **c.** The risk of fetal death in DC twin pregnancies with selective intrauterine growth restriction (IUGR) doubles that of IUGR in singleton pregnancies.
[Reference: Tamblyn J, Morris RK. Multiple pregnancy. In: James D, Steer PJ, Weiner CP, Gonik B, Robson SC (Eds). High-risk Pregnancy, 5th edition. United Kingdom: Cambridge University Press; 2017. p. 1586]

17. **d.** Done at 14–16 weeks
(Reference: Beriwal S, Impey L, Ioannou C. Multifetal pregnancy reduction and selective termination. Obstet Gynaecol. 2020;22:284-92)

18. **c.** Complicated MC twin pregnancy, suspected to develop either selective fetal growth restriction or TTTS
[Reference: Dias T, Bhide A. Multiple pregnancy. In: Bhide A, Arulkumaran S, Damania KR, Daftary SN (Eds). Arias' Practical Guide to High-Risk Pregnancy and Delivery: A South Asian Perspective, 5th edition. Gurugram: Elsevier-RELX India Pvt Ltd.; 2020. p. 160]

19. **c.** The Doppler sample volume should be placed in the umbilical artery at a zero degree angle, assisted by color, close to the placental surface.

In singletons, this way of measuring the umbilical artery pulsatility index is commonly performed and, in dichorionic (DC) twins, this is a way to make sure that the correct fetus is assessed. The typical Doppler patterns in monochorionic (MC) twins are caused by the vascular anastomoses, and the strongest effects are to be expected close to the placental surface. The angle should be as close to zero as possible as this increases the reliability of diagnosing absent end diastolic flow. An angle of >30° may falsely suggest the presence of absent end diastolic flow. A sample volume that is too large will distort the waveforms. The sample volume should just enclose the lumen of the artery.

20. **b.** A cervical length of <25 mm in a twin pregnancy at 20–24 weeks gestation is a good predictor of preterm labor and delivery.

No evidence has been published on the value of sexual abstinence in twin and triplet pregnancies. A systematic review of 21 studies concluded that transvaginal cervical length at 20–24 weeks' gestation is a good predictor of spontaneous preterm birth in asymptomatic women with twin pregnancies. A National Institute of Health and Clinical Excellence guideline reviewed all published literature on cervical length and prediction of preterm labor, and found that the best cut-off at 20–24 weeks in twin pregnancy was

25 mm. A Cochrane Systematic Review of seven RCTs evaluating hospitalization and bed rest in twin and triplet pregnancies to reduce preterm delivery found no evidence to support this intervention. A systematic review and meta-analysis of individual patient data of five RCTs of vaginal progesterone to prevent preterm delivery in pregnancy with a short cervix found that it reduced preterm delivery in singletons, but no such effect in twins. Cervical cerclage has not been found to be effective in twin or triplet pregnancies. https://obgyn.onlinelibrary.wiley.com/doi/10.1002/uog.9013

21. **d.** All are incorrect.

    Progesterone treatment in unselected twin pregnancies does not reduce the rate of preterm delivery before 34 weeks. In women with singleton pregnancies and a short cervical length at 20–23 weeks' gestation, treatment with vaginal progesterone had been found to reduce the risk of delivery before 33 weeks of gestation by about 45%. In women with singleton pregnancies and a history of previous preterm delivery, progesterone treatment also significantly reduced the rate of perinatal complications. Results from singleton pregnancies, however, cannot be directly transferred to multiple pregnancies. More than 10 randomized-controlled trials of progesterone treatment in twin pregnancies have now been published, and none of these trials have found any effect of progesterone. In fact, the odds ratio of delivery before 34 weeks in twin pregnancies was 1.0 [95% confidence interval (CI): 0.9–1.2]. High-risk twin pregnancies (i.e., with a history of prior preterm delivery or short cervical length) have been less extensively studied, but again progesterone treatment does not seem to increase gestational length. Progesterone does not reduce perinatal mortality or perinatal morbidity in unselected twin cohorts. In high-risk twin pregnancies (i.e., women with a short cervix before 24 weeks' gestation), there may be an effect on perinatal morbidity, but insufficient data are available to recommend this treatment outside randomized-controlled trials. https://pubmed.ncbi.nlm.nih.gov/19523680/

22. **c.** Treatment of twin pregnant women with a cervical pessary has no effect on neonatal outcome.

    A cervical pessary closes the cervical canal tightly, thus protecting the mucus plug, providing support to the cervix, and also changing the angle of the cervical canal to become more acute. If the cervical canal angle does not change with insertion of a pessary, as estimated by magnetic resonance imaging, this may be associated with preterm delivery. In a large randomized-controlled trial in singleton pregnancies, insertion of the Arabin pessary reduced the rate of preterm delivery from 27 to 6%. The effect has been investigated in several other randomized-controlled trials in singleton and twin gestations, but results are not yet available. The preliminary data from a Dutch, multicenter, randomized-controlled trial, however, showed no reduction in preterm delivery rate before 32 weeks (9% vs. 12%) nor before 37 weeks of gestation (54% vs. 57%). The cervical pessary may have a place in the treatment of women with a short cervical length, but this remains to be investigated in properly designed randomized-controlled trials. In the one randomized-controlled trial of twin pregnancies thus reported, no difference was found in the rate of adverse perinatal outcome between women treated with a cervical pessary and controls. In fact, 42 women (11%) in the pessary group and 42 women (11%) in the control group delivered at least one child with an adverse neonatal outcome. Again, in women with short cervical length at 16–20 weeks, there may be an effect as the rate of adverse neonatal outcome was 10% in the group treated with a pessary compared with 25% in the group without treatment. There do not appear to be any significant adverse maternal effects associated with cervical pessary use. https://pubmed.ncbi.nlm.nih.gov/33946019/

23. **d.** In case discordancy or anomalies in MC twins, timing of delivery is based on condition of uncompromised fetus.
    [Reference: Dias T, Bhide A. Multiple pregnancy. In: Bhide A, Arulkumaran S, Damania KR, Daftary SN (Eds). Arias' Practical Guide to High-Risk Pregnancy and Delivery: A South Asian Perspective, 5th edition. Gurugram: Elsevier-RELX India Pvt Ltd.; 2020. p. 166]

24. **d.** Congenital diaphragmatic hernia
    [Reference: Tamblyn J, Morris RK. Multiple pregnancy. In: James D, Steer PJ, Weiner CP, Gonik B, Robson SC (Eds). High-risk Pregnancy, 5th edition. United Kingdom: Cambridge University Press; 2017. p. 1585]

25. **c.** In monozygotic twins, the age-related risk of fetal Down syndrome is same as in singleton pregnancy although only one fetus will be affected.

[Reference: Tamblyn J, Morris RK. Multiple pregnancy. In: James D, Steer PJ, Weiner CP, Gonik B, Robson SC (Eds). High-risk Pregnancy, 5th edition. United Kingdom: Cambridge University Press; 2017. p. 1585]

26. **a.** Twin pregnancy should be ideally dated when the CRL measures between 55 and 85 mm or 11+0 to 13+6 weeks

[References: Tamblyn J, Morris RK. Multiple pregnancy. James D, Steer PJ, Weiner CP, Gonik B, Robson SC (Eds). High-risk Pregnancy, 5th edition. United Kingdom: Cambridge University Press; 2017. p. 1592; Dias T, Bhide A. Multiple pregnancy. In: Bhide A, Arulkumaran S, Damania KR, Daftary SN (Eds). Arias' Practical Guide to High-Risk Pregnancy and Delivery: A South Asian Perspective, 5th edition. Gurugram: Elsevier-RELX India Pvt Ltd.; 2020. p. 162; and Khalil A, Rodgers M, Baschat A, Bhide A, Gratacos E, Hecher K, et al. ISUOG guidelines: role of ultrasound in twin pregnancy. Ultrasound Obstet Gynecol. 2016;47(2):247-63]

27. **c.** Mortality is highest in absence of artery-to-artery anastomosis and lowest when these anastomoses are present.

[Reference: Galea P, Jain V, Fisk NM. Insights into the pathophysiology of twin-twin transfusion syndrome. Prenat Diagn. 2005;25(9):777-85]

28. **d.** Lateral fetal orientation is associated with intertwin membrane running horizontally along the longitudinal axis of the uterus.

[Reference: Dias T, Bhide A. Multiple pregnancy. In: Bhide A, Arulkumaran S, Damania KR, Daftary SN (Eds). Arias' Practical Guide to High-Risk Pregnancy and Delivery: A South Asian Perspective, 5th edition. Gurugram: Elsevier-RELX India Pvt Ltd.; 2020. pp. 162-3]

29. **c.** Both T and lambda are almost 80% sensitive for diagnosis of chorionicity.

[Reference: Dias T, Bhide A. Multiple pregnancy. In: Bhide A, Arulkumaran S, Damania KR, Daftary SN (Eds). Arias' Practical Guide to High-Risk Pregnancy and Delivery: A South Asian Perspective, 5th edition. Gurugram: Elsevier-RELX India Pvt Ltd.; 2020. p. 162]

30. **a.** Cord entanglement is universally present in monochorionic monoamniotic (MCMA) twins and is used as a bad prognostic sign.

[Reference: Dias T, Bhide A. Multiple pregnancy. In: Bhide A, Arulkumaran S, Damania KR, Daftary SN (Eds). Arias' Practical Guide to High-Risk Pregnancy and Delivery: A South Asian Perspective, 5th edition. Gurugram: Elsevier-RELX India Pvt Ltd.; 2020. p. 161]

Chapter 24: Oligohydramnios and Polyhydramnios

Pradnya Changede, Neha Khairnar, Rajat Agrawal

QUESTIONS

1. **Maternal intake of following drug is known to cause oligohydramnios:**
   a. Proton pump inhibitors
   b. Angiotensin-converting enzyme (ACE) inhibitors
   c. Penicillin
   d. Antihistaminic

2. **Oligohydramnios increases the risk of:**
   a. Umbilical cord compression
   b. Skeletal deformities
   c. Pulmonary hypoplasia
   d. All of the above

3. **What is the drug of choice in treatment of oligohydramnios?**
   a. Labetalol
   b. ACE inhibitor
   c. Vasopressin
   d. Oxytocin

4. **What is the normal range of amniotic fluid volume at term in mL?**
   a. 5–25
   b. 50–100
   c. 600–800
   d. 100–1,000

5. **The most suitable fluid for amnioinfusion is:**
   a. Normal saline
   b. Ringer's lactate
   c. Distilled water
   d. Dextrose solution

6. **L-arginine used in oligohydramnios to:**
   a. Decreases fetal urine output
   b. Increases uteroplacental flow
   c. Increases maternal urine output
   d. Increases fetal urine output

7. **Oligohydramnios is seen in all, *except*:**
   a. Twin-twin transfusion syndrome
   b. Rh incompatibility
   c. Intrauterine growth restriction (IUGR)
   d. Postmaturity

8. **Potter's syndrome includes all, *except*:**
   a. Polyhydramnios
   b. Pulmonary hypoplasia
   c. Renal agenesis
   d. Facial deformity

9. **Peak amniotic fluid volume is seen at __ weeks of gestation.**
   a. 30–34 weeks
   b. 18–22 weeks
   c. 40–42 weeks
   d. 8–12 weeks

10. **All are components of full biophysical profile (BPP), *except*:**
    a. Fetal breathing
    b. Amniotic fluid index (AFI)
    c. Single deepest vertical pocket (SDP) of amniotic fluid
    d. Fetal movement

11. **In pregnancies with oligohydramnios, __ is a better method of assessment of amniotic fluid.**
    a. AFI
    b. Single deepest vertical pocket of amniotic fluid
    c. Qualitative assessment
    d. Dye determination

12. **All of the following conditions result in oligohydramnios, *except*:**
    a. Posterior urethral valve
    b. Post-term pregnancy
    c. Esophageal atresia
    d. Preeclampsia

13. **Amniotic fluid is completely replaced over __ hours.**
    a. 6 hours
    b. 12 hours
    c. 18 hours
    d. 24 hours

14. **USG findings of few patients are given below, out of these which of the following patients have polyhydramnios?**
    a. AFI: 8 cm
    b. AFI: 22 cm
    c. SDP: 8.5 cm
    d. SDP: 5.6 cm

15. All of the following are maternal causes of polyhydramnios, *except:*
    a. Overt diabetes
    b. Gestational diabetes mellitus (GDM)
    c. Nonsteroidal anti-inflammatory drugs (NSAIDs)
    d. Liver failure

16. All of the following are fetal causes of polyhydramnios, *except:*
    a. Multiple gestation
    b. Neural tube defects
    c. Esophageal atresia
    d. Renal agenesis

17. A routine USG of a multigravida at 28 weeks revealed an AFI of 27 cm, which of the following cannot cause this condition?
    a. Diabetes mellitus   b. Preeclampsia
    c. Esophageal atresia   d. Open spina bifida

18. A 30-year-old g3p2l2 at 35 weeks is complaining of difficulty in breathing. On examination, flanks are full and abdominal girth is 160 cm. USG revealed that the SDP is 10 cm. What is the next step in management?
    a. Intravenous (IV) furosemide
    b. Indomethacin therapy
    c. Amniocentesis
    d. Artificial rupture of membranes

19. Which of the following is not a function of amniotic fluid?
    a. Maintain temperature
    b. Bacteriostatic property
    c. Provide nutrition in the form of fat and protein
    d. Prevent ascending infection to uterine cavity during labor

20. Mild polyhydramnios is defined as:
    a. AFI: 24-29.9 cm   b. AFI: 25-29.9 cm
    c. AFI: 30-34.9 cm   d. AFI: >35 cm

21. Most common cause of mild polyhydramnios is:
    a. Idiopathic
    b. Gastrointestinal (GI) anomaly
    c. Neural tube defect
    d. Renal anomaly

22. What contributes to the formation of amniotic fluid during early pregnancy?
    a. Fetal urine
    b. Fetal extracellular fluid
    c. Ultrafiltrate of maternal plasma
    d. Ultrafiltrate of fetal plasma

23. All of the following is expected in clinical examination of a term polyhydramnios patient, *except:*
    a. Fundal height > gestational age
    b. Feeble heart sound on Doppler
    c. Abdominal circumference < gestational age
    d. Tense abdominal wall

24. Drug used to treat polyhydramnios and its complications:
    a. Nitric oxide (NO)   b. Indomethacin
    c. Beta blockers   d. Arginine

25. Treatment of polyhydramnios includes all, *except:*
    a. Indomethacin   b. Amniocentesis
    c. Amnioinfusion   d. All of the above

26. Criteria for severe polyhydramnios include:
    a. AFI: 30-34.9   b. SDP >16 cm
    c. AFI: 25-29 cm   d. SDP: 12-15 cm

27. All is true about AFI, *except:*
    a. Calculated by dividing uterus in four quadrants
    b. Pocket should not contain cord or fetal extremity
    c. Sum of maximal vertical pocket of amniotic fluid /4
    d. Line through umbilicus for upper and lower division

28. During amniocentesis, the risk of abortion is ___.
    a. 0.5-1%   b. 0.1-0.3%
    c. 1-2%   d. 2-2.5%

29. Which dye is not used during amniocentesis of twins?
    a. Methylene blue   b. Indigo carmine
    c. Fluorescein   d. Indocyanine green

30. A 30-year-old g3p2l2 with multifetal pregnancy is diagnosed with polyhydramnios. What is amniotic fluid volume required to diagnose this condition?
    a. >1,000 mL   b. >1,500 mL
    c. >2,000 mL   d. >2,500 mL

ANSWERS

1. **b.** ACE inhibitors
   Intake of drugs like prostaglandin (PG) inhibitors, ACE inhibitors may cause oligohydramnios.
   (Reference: DC Dutta's Textbook of Obstetrics, 9th edition, page 203)

2. **d.** All of the above
   The perinatal outcome is worse when oligohydramnios is severe and prolonged, resulting in skeletal deformities and abnormal fetal heart patterns due to cord compression. The risk of pulmonary hypoplasia increases as the gestational age decreases at which membranes rupture and significant oligohydramnios occurs.
   (Reference: Ian Donald's Practical Obstetric Problems, 7th edition, page 383)

3. **c.** Vasopressin
   Maternal 1-deamino-[8-D-arginine] vasopressin and oral water administration can reduce and stabilize plasma osmolality and increase amniotic fluid volume. Vasopressin therapy has potential for the prevention and treatment of oligohydramnios.
   [Reference: Ross MG, Cedars L, Nijland MJ, Ogundipe A. Treatment of oligohydramnios with maternal 1-deamino-[8-D-arginine] vasopressin-induced plasma hypoosmolality. Am J Obstet Gynecol. 1996;174(5):1608-13.]

4. **c.** 600–800
   At term, the amniotic fluid volume measures about 600–800 mL.
   (Reference: DC Dutta's Textbook of Obstetrics, 9th edition, page 34)

5. **b.** Ringer's lactate
   The composition of Lactated Ringer's solution is similar to amniotic fluid for both electrolyte composition and pH. This infusion solution seems to be the most suitable choice for amnioinfusion.
   [Reference: Adama van Scheltema PN, In't Anker PS, Vereecken A, Vandenbussche FP, Deprest JA, Devlieger R. Biochemical composition of fluids for amnioinfusion during fetoscopy. Gynecol Obstet Invest. 2008;66(4):227-30]

6. **b.** Increases uteroplacental flow
   L-arginine promotes the intrauterine growth of the fetus by increasing bioavailability of endothelial NO production and improving the umbilical artery flow in fetal growth restriction (FGR) and hypertension.
   [Reference: Soni A, Garg S, Patel K, Patel Z. Role of L-arginine in Oligohydramnios. J Obstet Gynaecol India. 2016;66(Suppl 1):279-83.]

7. **b.** Rh incompatibility
   Rh isoimmunization presents with hydrops fetalis which includes ascites, pericardial effusion, subcutaneous and scalp edema, polyhydramnios, and placentomegaly.
   (Reference: Ian Donald's Practical Obstetric Problems, 7th edition, page 392)

8. **a.** Polyhydramnios
   Potter syndrome is a fetal congenital disorder characterized by the changes in physical appearance of neonate due to oligohydramnios caused by renal agenesis and impairment. It is incompatible with life as these neonates have pulmonary hypoplasia that leads to respiratory distress within an hour of birth.
   (Reference: Practical guide to high risk pregnancy and delivery—Arias, 3rd edition, page 88)

9. **a.** 30–34 weeks
   Peak amniotic fluid volume is seen at 30–34 weeks.
   (Reference: UpToDate (2022). Assessment of amniotic fluid volume. [online] Available from: https://www.uptodate.com/contents/assessment-of-amniotic-fluid-volume#:~:text=Amniotic%20fluid%20volume%20(AFV)%20is,AFV%20will%20be%20discussed%20here [Last accessed December, 2023]).

10. **b.** AFI
    Components of full biophysical profile (BPP) are nonstress test (NST), fetal movement, fetal breathing, fetal tone, and amniotic fluid (SDP).
    (Reference: Practical guide to high risk pregnancy and delivery—Arias, 3rd edition, page 121)

11. **b.** Single deepest vertical pocket of amniotic fluid
    Single deepest vertical pocket will perform better in pregnancy with oligohydramnios and AFI will perform better in polyhydramnios.
    (Reference: UpToDate (2022). Assessment of amniotic fluid volume. [online] Available from: https://www.uptodate.com/contents/assessment-of-amniotic-fluid-volume#:~:text=Amniotic%20fluid%20volume%20(AFV)%20is,AFV%20will%20be%20discussed%20here [Last accessed December, 2023]).

12. **c.** Esophageal atresia
    Esophageal atresia is a cause of polyhydramnios.
    (Reference: Practical guide to high risk pregnancy and delivery—Arias, 3rd edition, page 121)

13. **d.** 24 hours
    Amniotic fluid gets replaced completely in 24 hours.
    (Reference: UpToDate (2022). Assessment of amniotic fluid volume. [online] Available from: https://www.uptodate.com/contents/assessment-of-amniotic-fluid-

volume#:~:text=Amniotic%20fluid%20volume%20 (AFV)%20is,AFV%20will%20be%20discussed%20here [Last accessed December, 2023])

14. **c.** SDP: 8.5 cm
According to definition, SDP of >8 cm and AFI of >25 cm indicates polyhydramnios and SDP <2 cm and AFI >5 cm indicates oligohydramnios.
(References: William's Obstetrics, 24th edition, page 236 and Williams Obstetrics, 25th edition, page 230)

15. **c.** NSAIDs
NSAIDs are a maternal cause of oligohydramnios and not polyhydramnios.
Maternal causes of polyhydramnios are as follows:
- Overt diabetes
- GDM
- Liver failure
- Cardiac diseases

(References: William's Obstetrics, 24th edition, page 231 and Williams Obstetrics, 25th edition, page 225)

16. **d.** Renal agenesis
Renal agenesis is a fetal cause of oligohydramnios and not polyhydramnios.
(References: William's Obstetrics, 24th edition, page 231 and Williams Obstetrics, 25th edition, page 225)

17. **b.** Preeclampsia
The given clinical picture is suggestive of polyhydramnios. Preeclampsia is a cause for oligohydramnios and not polyhydramnios.
(References: Williams Obstetrics, 24th edition, page 235-36 and Williams Obstetrics, 25th edition, page 229-30)

18. **c.** Amniocentesis
The given clinical picture is suggestive of polyhydramnios associated with respiratory distress. In such cases, therapeutic amniocentesis termed amnioreduction is done.
Amnioreduction helps in polyhydramnios by:
- Relieving respiratory distress by reducing mechanical pressure on diaphragm.
- May improve obstructive uropathy
- May lower the preterm delivery risk

(References: Williams Obstetrics, 24th edition, page 220, 236, 247; Williams Obstetrics, 25th edition, page 871; and DC Dutta's Textbook of Obstetrics, 9th edition, page 487)

19. **c.** Provide nutrition in the form of fat and protein
The nutritive value of amniotic fluid is negligible because amniotic fluid is predominantly water. It contains the following:
- Water: 98–99%
- Solids: 1–2% (organic, inorganic, suspended particles)
- *Functions of amniotic fluid during pregnancy:*
  - Shock absorber
  - Temperature regulation
  - Growth and free movement of fetus
  - Bacteriostatic property
- *Functions of amniotic fluid during labor:*
  - Dilation of cervix
  - Aseptic action prevention ascending infection
  - Acts as a cushion between fetus and umbilical cord

(References: Williams Obstetrics, 24th edition, page 231 and Williams Obstetrics, 25th edition page 225)

20. **b.** AFI: 25–29.9 cm
Mild polyhydramnios is defined as AFI 25–29.9 cm and SDP 8–9.9 cm.
(Reference: Williams Obstetrics, 25th edition, page 228)

21. **a.** Idiopathic
40% of polyhydramnios is idiopathic.
(Reference: Williams Obstetrics, 25th edition, page 229)

22. **c.** Ultrafiltrate of maternal plasma
Ultrafiltrate of maternal plasma contributes to amniotic fluid in early pregnancy
Amniotic fluid is formed by:
- *Early pregnancy:* Ultrafiltrate of maternal plasma
- *Second trimester:* The extracellular fluid that diffuses through the fetal skin and thus reflects the composition of fetal plasma.
- *After 20 weeks:* Keratinization of fetal skin prevents diffusion across the skin. Hence fetal urine forms amniotic fluid.

(Reference: Williams Obstetrics, 24th edition, page 135)

23. **c.** Abdominal circumference < gestational age
Clinical examination of a term polyhydramnios patient has following features:
Fundal height > gestational age, feeble heart sound on Doppler, and tense abdominal wall.
(References: Williams Obstetrics, 24th edition, page 235 and Williams Obstetrics, 25th edition, page 229)

24. **b.** Indomethacin
    Indomethacin has been used to reduce amount of amniotic fluid. It acts by decreasing fetal urine output.
    (Reference: Practical guide to high risk pregnancy and delivery—Arias, 3rd edition, page 121)

25. **c.** Amnioinfusion
    Treatment of polyhydramnios includes indomethacin and therapeutic amniocentesis
    (Reference: UpToDate. Treatment of polyhydramnios)

26. **b.** SDP >16 cm
    Criteria of severe polyhydramnios include SDP >16 cm and AFI >35 cm
    (Reference: UpToDate. Criteria for mild, moderate, and severe polyhydramnios)

27. **c.** Sum of maximal vertical pocket of amniotic fluid /4
    Amniotic fluid index is calculated by dividing uterus in four quadrants by passing line through umbilicus for upper and lower division and through linea nigra for right and left division. Pocket should not contain cord or fetal extremity.
    (Reference: UpToDate. (2022). Assessment of amniotic fluid volume. [online] Available from: https://www.uptodate.com/contents/assessment-of-amniotic-fluid-volume#:~:text=Amniotic%20fluid%20volume%20(AFV)%20is,AFV%20will%20be%20discussed%20here [Last accessed December, 2023])

28. **b.** 0.1–0.3%
    During amniocentesis, the risk of abortion is 0.1–0.3% in skilled hands according to ACOG.
    (Reference: UpToDate. Amniocentesis)

29. **a.** Methylene blue
    Methylene blue has adverse fetal and neonatal effects.
    (Reference: UpToDate. Estimation of amniotic fluid volume)

30. **c.** >2,000 mL
    Polyhydramnios is an abnormal increase in amniotic fluid. It is defined as the presence of amniotic fluid volume >2,000 mL.
    (Reference: William's Obstetrics, 25th edition, page 225)

Chapter 25

Abnormalities of the Placenta and Umbilical Cord

Rajshree Dayanand Katke

QUESTIONS

1. **What is the most common placental abnormality?**
   a. Previa
   b. Abruption
   c. Retained placenta
   d. Placenta accreta

2. **Which of the following statements about placenta previa is true?**
   a. It is more common in primigravidas
   b. It is characterized by painless vaginal bleeding
   c. It does not require any intervention during pregnancy
   d. It occurs when the placenta partially separates from the uterus

3. **What is the main risk factor for placenta accreta?**
   a. Maternal age over 35 years
   b. Multiparity
   c. In vitro fertilization (IVF)
   d. Previous cesarean section

4. **Which type of placenta accreta is associated with the deepest invasion into the wall of the uterus?**
   a. Placenta accreta
   b. Placenta increta
   c. Placenta percreta
   d. Placenta previa

5. **Wharton's jelly of umbilical cord is derived from:**
   a. Ectoderm
   b. Endoderm
   c. Mesoderm
   d. Trophoblast

6. **What percentage of pregnancies is affected by umbilical cord abnormalities?**
   a. 2–5%
   b. 10–15%
   c. 25–30%
   d. 40–45%

7. **The folds of Hoboken are found in:**
   a. The placenta
   b. Uterus
   c. Umbilical cord
   d. The amnion

8. **What is the definition of a nuchal cord?**
   a. A cord that is wrapped around the fetal neck
   b. A cyst within the umbilical cord
   c. A cord that is shorter than normal
   d. A cord that is twisted on itself

9. **Which of the following is a potential complication of cord prolapse?**
   a. Fetal macrosomia
   b. Fetal distress
   c. Placenta previa
   d. Polyhydramnios

10. **What is the immediate management of a suspected cord prolapse?**
    a. Emergency cesarean section
    b. Digital vaginal examination to determine cord position
    c. Bed rest and continuous fetal monitoring
    d. Administering tocolytic medication

11. **Which of the following is not a potential cause of true umbilical cord knots?**
    a. Long umbilical cord
    b. Decreased amniotic fluid
    c. Maternal diabetes
    d. Fetal malpresentation

12. **What is the significance of a true umbilical cord knot?**
    a. It can lead to fetal growth restriction
    b. It can cause preterm labor
    c. It is usually harmless and asymptomatic
    d. It can lead to umbilical cord compression

13. **Which of the following is a potential risk factor for velamentous cord insertion?**
    a. Advanced maternal age
    b. Multiple gestations
    c. Maternal hypertension
    d. Preterm rupture of membranes

14. What is the main complication associated with velamentous cord insertion?
    a. Cord prolapse
    b. Placental abruption
    c. Fetal growth restriction
    d. Umbilical cord vessel rupture

15. What is the most common type of umbilical cord anomaly?
    a. Single umbilical artery   b. Accessory lobe
    c. Long umbilical cord   d. Knots

16. Following a normal vaginal delivery, the placenta delivered by controlled cord traction appeared as shown below. What is the condition known as?
    a. Bilobate placenta   b. Placenta succenturiata
    c. Placenta membranacea d. Placenta marginata

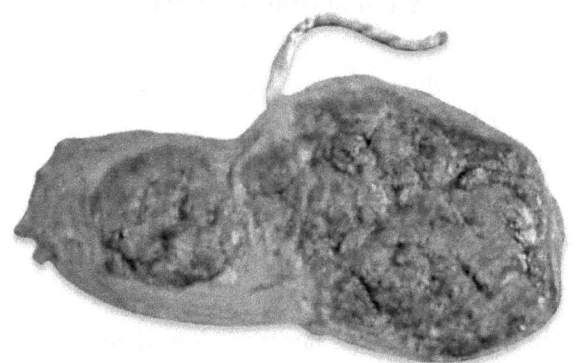

17. A primigravida delivered a baby at term with birth weight of 1.9 kg via normal vaginal delivery. The placenta delivered appears as shown in the image. What is the condition known as?
    a. Placenta succenturiata
    b. Placenta marginata
    c. Circumvallate placenta
    d. Circummarginate placenta

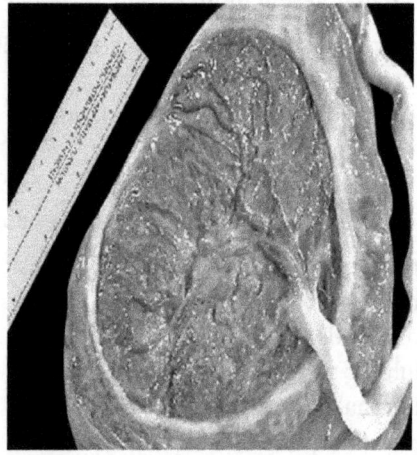

18. What imaging modality can be used to diagnose placenta accreta?
    a. Ultrasound
    b. Magnetic resonance imaging (MRI)
    c. Hysterosalpingography
    d. CT scan

19. Which of the following cannot cross placenta?
    1. Iron
    2. Albumin
    3. Immunoglobulin M
    4. Immunoglobulin G
    a. 1 and 2   b. Only 3
    c. 2 and 3   d. 3 and 4

20. What is the uteroplacental blood flow at term?
    a. 350–600 mL
    b. 250–450 mL
    c. 500–750 mL
    d. 800–1,050 mL

21. At what period of gestation are the weights of fetus and placenta equal?
    a. 14 weeks   b. 15 weeks
    c. 17 weeks   d. 21 weeks

22. Which of the following does not contribute to the prevention of rejection of fetus?
    a. Decidual natural killer cells
    b. Decidual stromal cells
    c. Trophoblasts
    d. Maternal leukopenia

23. USG of 24-year-old primigravida at 20 weeks of gestation shows the presence of a single umbilical artery. No other gross fetal anomalies were detected. Which of the following is true regarding this finding?
    a. It is an insignificant finding
    b. Occurs in 10% of newborn
    c. It is an indicator of increased risk of malformation of fetus
    d. Equally common in newborn of diabetic and nondiabetic mothers

24. What is the main function of the umbilical cord during pregnancy?
    a. Provides oxygen to the fetus
    b. Allows nutrients to pass from the mother to the fetus
    c. Removes waste products from the fetus
    d. All of the above

CHAPTER 25: Abnormalities of the Placenta and Umbilical Cord

25. What is the optimal number of vessels in the umbilical cord?
    a. One artery and one vein
    b. Two arteries and one vein
    c. Three arteries and two veins
    d. It may vary from pregnancy to pregnancy

26. What is the main diagnostic test for umbilical cord abnormalities?
    a. Ultrasound
    b. Doppler velocimetry
    c. Amniocentesis
    d. Chorionic villus sampling (CVS)

27. All are true regarding Duncan placental separation, *except:*
    a. Peripheral separation
    b. Maternal surface presents at vulva
    c. More blood loss
    d. Most common method of separation

28. What is the normal cord pH
    a. 7.1
    b. 7.2
    c. 6.1
    d. 6.2

29. How is normal placenta described?
    1. Discoid
    2. Hemochorial
    3. Deciduate
    a. 1 and 2
    b. 2 and 3
    c. 1 and 3
    d. 1, 2, and 3

30. What does a placental cotyledon compromise of?
    a. Portions of the basal plate divided by clefts
    b. Portions of the chorionic plate divided by clefts
    c. Area supplied by multiple truncal chorionic villi
    d. Area supplied by one spiral artery

ANSWERS

1. **a.** Previa
2. **b.** It is characterized by painless vaginal bleeding
3. **d.** Previous cesarean section
4. **c.** Placenta percreta
5. **c.** Mesoderm
6. **a.** 2-5%
7. **c.** Umbilical cord
8. **a.** A cord that is wrapped around the fetal neck
9. **b.** Fetal distress
10. **a.** Emergency cesarean section
11. **c.** Maternal diabetes
12. **d.** It can lead to umbilical cord compression
13. **b.** Multiple gestation
14. **c.** Fetal growth restriction
15. **a.** Single umbilical artery
16. **b.** Placenta succenturiate
17. **c.** Circumvallate placenta
18. **b.** Magnetic resonance imaging (MRI)
19. **c.** 2 and 3
20. **c.** 500-750 mL
21. **c.** 17 weeks
22. **a.** Maternal leukopenia
23. **c.** It is an indicator of increased risk of malformation of fetus
24. **d.** All of the above
25. **b.** Two arteries and one vein
26. **a.** Ultrasound
27. **d.** Most common method of separation
28. **b.** 7.2
29. **d.** 1, 2, and 3
30. **a.** Portions of the basal plate divided by clefts

Chapter 26: Hypertensive Disorders in Pregnancy

Shubhangi Nawarange, Rajshree Dayanand Katke

QUESTIONS

1. **Classification of hypertensive disorders of pregnancy includes:**
   a. Preeclampsia and eclampsia syndrome
   b. Chronic hypertension
   c. Preeclampsia superimposed on chronic hypertension
   d. All of the above

2. **Criteria required for diagnosis of pregnancy associated hypertension are as follows, *except*:**
   a. Blood pressure (BP) >140/90 mm Hg after 20 weeks in previous normotensive women
   b. Proteinuria >300 mg/24 hour
   c. Urine protein: creatinine ratio <0.3
   d. Serum transaminases levels twice normal

3. **Mechanisms for etiopathogenesis of preeclampsia are:**
   a. Placental implantation with abnormal trophoblastic invasion of uterine vessels
   b. Dysfunctional immunological tolerance between maternal and fetal tissues
   c. Genetic predisposition to genes and epigenetic influences
   d. All of the above

4. **Criteria for diagnosis of gestational hypertension are all, *except*:**
   a. Blood pressure >140/90 mm Hg for first time after midpregnancy
   b. Proteinuria
   c. 10% eclampsia seizures developed overt preeclampsia
   d. Blood pressure return to normal by 12 weeks postpartum

5. **Following are the features of severe preeclampsia syndrome with multiorgan involvement:**
   a. Renal dysfunction
   b. Pulmonary edema
   c. Hepatocellular necrosis
   d. All of the above

6. **What are the following indicators of severity of gestational hypertensive disorders?**
   a. Diastolic BP >110 mm Hg and systolic BP >160 mm Hg
   b. Proteinuria positive >1+, visual disturbance, headache
   c. Oliguria
   d. All of the above

7. **Which of the following women are at the highest risk for preeclampsia?**
   a. A patient with history of preeclampsia starting early in the third trimester of the pregnancy
   b. A patient with history of preterm delivery in her previous pregnancy
   c. Grand multipara
   d. A patient who has no family history of preeclampsia

8. **A patient with preeclampsia has diastolic blood pressure >110 mm Hg, proteinuria +1, she complaints of blurring of vision and upper abdominal pain. In which of the following grades of preeclampsia patient belongs to:**
   a. Preeclampsia
   b. Gestational hypertension (HTN)
   c. Eclampsia
   d. Severe preeclampsia with imminent eclampsia features

9. Which fetal condition is common in pregnancies accompanied by preeclampsia?
   a. Congenital malformation
   b. Heart failure due to hypertension (HTN)
   c. Hemorrhagic diseases of the newborn
   d. Intrauterine fetal growth restriction

10. Which of the following are features of HELLP syndrome, *except*?
    a. Raised bilirubin (>1.2 mg/dL)
    b. Low platelet (LP) count (<100,000)
    c. Low serum uric acid
    d. Impaired renal and liver function

11. Which of the following are risk factors of preeclampsia, *except*?
    a. Multiparity
    b. Advanced maternal age
    c. Family history
    d. History of disorders characterized by microvascular diseases

12. Which are the effects of preeclampsia complicating the fetal condition?
    a. Intrauterine growth restriction
    b. Intrauterine fetal death
    c. Birth asphyxia
    d. All of the above

13. Diagnostic criteria for essential hypertension in pregnancy are, *except*:
    a. Rise in blood pressure >140/90 mm Hg or more during pregnancy prior to 20 weeks
    b. Cardiac enlargement on chest radiograph and ECG
    c. On follow-up, it shows persistent rise of blood pressure even after 42 days following delivery
    d. Nonpresence of medical disorders

14. Posterior reversible encephalopathy syndrome characterized by:
    a. Presents with hypertension, headache, encephalopathy, seizures, cortical visual disturbance, or blindness
    b. Imaging shows (B/L) symmetrical vasogenic edema in occipital and posterior parietal lobes
    c. a + b
    d. None of the above

15. All of the following may be used in pregnancy associated hypertension, *except*:
    a. Nifedipine   b. Captopril
    c. Methyldopa   d. Hydralazine

16. Primigravida with 36 weeks of gestation presents with vomiting, nausea, epigastric pain, and right upper quadrant pain and elevated liver (EL) enzymes, thrombocytopenia and serum bilirubin >1.2 mg/dL, diagnosis is:
    a. Eclampsia
    b. Chronic hypertension
    c. HELLP syndrome
    d. Abruptio placenta

17. Which is a drug of choice for severe preeclampsia?
    a. Labetalol
    b. Metoprolol
    c. α-methyldopa
    d. Nifedipine

18. A 26-year-old primigravida with pregnancy-induced hypertension with blood pressure of 150/100 mm Hg at 32 weeks of gestation with no other complications, her blood pressure is controlled on treatment. If there are no complications, the pregnancy should be terminates at:
    a. 42 completed weeks
    b. 37 completed weeks
    c. 32 completed weeks
    d. 41 completed weeks

19. Which of the following is true regarding serum magnesium level in magnesium toxicity?
    a. Loss of deep tendon reflexes >7 mEq/L
    b. Respiratory depression <8 mEq/L
    c. Cardiac arrest >15 mEq/L
    d. All of the above

20. A 38-year-old women presents at 32 weeks of gestation in her first pregnancy with blood pressure 144/90 mm Hg with no proteinuria, previous BP at beginning of her pregnancy was 100/60 mm Hg with no headaches or visual disturbance. What is the diagnosis?
    a. Mild preeclampsia
    b. Imminent preeclampsia
    c. Gestational hypertension
    d. Eclampsia

21. What are the causes of maternal deaths in eclampsia?
    a. Cerebral hemorrhage
    b. Acute renal failure
    c. Aspiration pneumonia
    d. All of the above

22. A 24-year-old primigravida with severe preeclampsia at 36 weeks gestation is having a seizure on arrival in casualty with blood pressure 180/100 mm Hg, urine albumin is 3+, the woman is actively convulsing, what is the line of management?
    a. Put airway and suction and start on antihypertensive
    b. Intravenous MgSO$_4$
    c. Termination of pregnancy
    d. All of the above

23. Biochemical and laboratory findings in case of severe preeclampsia are as:
    a. Platelet count <100,000
    b. Marked elevated serum glutamic oxaloacetic transaminase (SGOT) and serum glutamic pyruvic transaminase (SGPT) levels
    c. Serum creatinine >1.1 mg/dL
    d. All of the above

24. Drugs used in the treatment of acute hypertensive *crisis* is:
    a. Intravenous labetalol
    b. Intravenous hydralazine
    c. Nitroglycerin infusion
    d. All of the above

25. What is the drug of choice for status eclampticus?
    a. Prostaglandin   b. Mannitol
    c. Thiopentone sodium   d. Carbamazepine

26. A 30-year-old woman presents at 34 weeks of gestation in her first pregnancy with BP 170/100 mm Hg with significant proteinuria >2+ on urinalysis, with blurring of vision, headache, and vomiting, how will you manage?
    a. Immediate admission to hospital
    b. Start on labetalol as antihypertensive
    c. Start intravenous MgSO$_4$
    d. All of the above

27. A 30-year-old patient with G3P1L1A1 came at 11 weeks of pregnancy. In her previous pregnancy, she had preterm delivery at 34 weeks in view of severe preeclampsia. What is the first step of treatment in this patient?
    a. Start on aspirin 75 mg
    b. Uterine artery Doppler at 20 weeks
    c. Plan for delivery at 37 weeks
    d. Start on labetalol

28. Signs of intravenous magnesium toxicity when using in imminent preeclampsia and eclampsia:
    a. Loss of deep tendon reflexes
    b. Decreased respiratory rate (<12 breaths/min)
    c. Urine output <30 mL/hour
    d. All of the above

29. What are the fetal complications of severe preeclampsia all below, *except*?
    a. Intrauterine fetal death
    b. Intrauterine growth restriction
    c. Birth asphyxia
    d. Neonatal jaundice at birth

30. What is true about positive roll over test?
    a. Prediction test for preeclampsia
    b. After resting in the left lateral position and returned to supine position includes a rise in diastolic pressure of >20 mm Hg or more is positive test
    c. a + b
    d. It is performed at 10–12 weeks of gestation

31. What are the findings on color Doppler velocimetry suggestive of fetal at risk in hypertensive disorders of pregnancy?
    a. Systolic/diastolic (S/D) ratio >2, persistence of diastolic notch after 23 weeks
    b. Absent or reversal of end-diastolic flow
    c. Extensive calcification of placenta
    d. All of the above

32. How can we do antenatal fetal surveillance in hypertensive disorder of pregnancy patients?
    a. Nonstress test and daily fetal movement count by mother
    b. Serial obstetrics ultrasound with color Doppler effect
    c. Biophysical profile
    d. All of the above

ANSWERS

1. **d.** All of the above
   Classification of hypertensive disorders of pregnancy involves four types: (1) preeclampsia and eclampsia syndrome, (2) chronic hypertension of any etiology, (3) preeclampsia superimposed on chronic hypertension, and (4) gestational hypertension in which hypertension resolves by 12 weeks postpartum.

2. **c.** *Urine protein:* Creatinine ratio <0.3
   Urine protein: Creatinine ratio <0.3. This is wrong because proteinuria characterized by:
   - Urine protein >300 mg /24 hours
   - Urine protein: creatinine ratio >0.3
   - Dipstick + persistent

3. **d.** All of the above
   Correct answer is all of the above. All are true regarding etiology of preeclampsia syndrome.

4. **b.** Proteinuria
   - Gestational hypertension (HTN): Blood pressure >140/90 mm Hg or greater for first time after 20 weeks but lack proteinuria in previously normotensive patient
   - Proteinuria is not a diagnostic feature of gestational hypertension.
   - Even though 10% of eclamptic seizures develop before overt proteinuria can be detected.

5. **d.** All of the above
   Multiorgan involvement in severe preeclampsia is reflected by thrombocytopenia, renal dysfunction, hepatocellular necrosis, central nervous system perturbations, or pulmonary edema.

6. **d.** All of the above
   Indicators of severity of gestational hypertensive disorder are diastolic blood pressure >110 mm Hg and systolic BP >160 mm Hg, proteinuria (>+), headache, visual disturbances, oliguria, convulsions, upper abdominal pain, increase in serum creatinine >1.1, thrombocytopenia <100,000, raised serum transaminases (twice the normal), pulmonary edema, and fetal growth restriction.

7. **a.** A patient with history of preeclampsia starting early in the third trimester of the pregnancy
   - There is 25% chance of recurrence of preeclampsia in subsequent pregnancies.
   - Risk of preeclampsia is more in young and nullipara.
   - Family history of preeclampsia on maternal side is also a risk factor.

8. **c.** Eclampsia
   Preeclampsia with severe features includes:
   - Systolic blood pressure ≥160 mm Hg or diastolic pressure ≥110 mm Hg
   - Proteinuria 1+ or >
   - Liver derangement with transaminitis; upper abdominal pain
   - Thrombocytopenia, renal insufficiency, pulmonary edema, new-onset headache, or visual changes

9. **d.** Intrauterine fetal growth restriction
   In preeclampsia, the normal endovascular invasion of cytotrophoblast into the spiral arteries fails to occur beyond decidua myometrial junction due to which musculoelastic media in the myometrial segment remains responsive to vasoconstrictor stimuli resulting in decrease blood flow which results in placental changes and causes chronic uteroplacental insufficiency which leads to intrauterine growth restriction (IUGR).

10. **d.** Impaired renal and liver function
    In HELLP syndrome, there is increased hemolysis and parenchymal necrosis of the liver causes elevation in hepatic enzyme levels—serum aspartate aminotransferase (AST), alanine aminotransferase (ALT) (twice the normal), lactate dehydrogenase (LDH) >600 IU/L and bilirubin (>1.2 mg/dL). Platelet aggregation is increased and reduced platelet levels may be indicative of impending HELLP syndrome.
    Uric acid although a poor predictor of HELLP syndrome but it is increased.

11. **a.** Multiparity
    Multiparity is not a risk factor, young and nulliparity are risk factors of preeclampsia advance maternal age >35 years, chronic hypertension, chronic renal diseases, autoimmune diseases, and multiple pregnancies are the risk factors and maternal family history are risk factors for preeclampsia.

12. **d.** All of the above
    The fetal risk is related to the severity of preeclampsia, duration of the disease, and degree of proteinuria. It causes:
    - Intrauterine death—due to spasm of uteroplacental circulation leading to accidental hemorrhage
    - Intrauterine growth restriction—due to chronic placental insufficiency
    - Asphyxia
    - Prematurity

13. **d.** Nonpresence of medical disorders
    The diagnostic criteria of essential hypertension are:
    - Rise of blood pressure to the extent of 140/90 mm Hg or more during pregnancy prior to the 20th week (molar pregnancy excluded)

- Cardiac enlargement on chest radiograph and ECG
- Presence of medical disorders
- Prospective follow-up shows persistent rise of blood pressure even after 42 days following delivery

14. c. a + b

Posterior reversible encephalopathy syndrome (PRES) is a transient neuroradiological entity characterized by the hypertension, generalized seizures, altered mental status, headache, and vision changes.

The hallmark of diagnosis is bilateral symmetrical vasogenic edema in the occipital and posterior parietal lobes.

15. b. Captopril

Because captopril is an angiotensin-converting-enzyme (ACE) inhibitor hence not used in treatment of pregnancy-associated hypertension as it causes fetal oliguria and fetal oligohydramnios leads to development congenital anomalies, bony deformities, respiratory distress syndrome, limb contractures, pulmonary hypoplasia, and neonatal death in fetus.

16. c. HELLP syndrome

In this patient, as patient is presented in the third trimester along with all clinical symptoms, such as vomiting, nausea, epigastric pain, and right upper quadrant pain and elevated liver enzymes, thrombocytopenia and serum bilirubin >1.2 mg/dL, all these features are suggestive of HELLP syndrome.

HELLP syndrome has hemolysis (H), elevated liver (EL) enzymes, and low platelet (LP) count (<100,000).

17. a. Labetalol
- Labetalol is an adrenoceptor antagonist (α + β-blocker).
- It is a drug of choice for acute severe hypertension in pregnancy as it lowers blood pressure more rapidly and causes less tachycardia as compared to other drugs.
- It is used because of its effectiveness and low incidence of side effects.

18. b. 37 completed weeks

This patient is a case of hypertension in pregnancy with no other complications and secondary to that there are chances of developing uteroplacental insufficiency which is more if pregnancy is continued till 40 weeks, as 37 weeks is the ideal time for termination as it is term and fetal lung maturity is also achieved.

19. a. Loss of deep tendon reflexes >7 mEq/L

Optimum serum magnesium level is 4.8–8.4 mg/dL (4–7 mEq/L) to be maintained.

Magnesium toxicity and high serum Mg level is seen as:
- Loss of deep tendon reflexes >7 mEq/L
- Respiratory depression >10 mEq/L
- Cardiac arrest >25 mEq/L

20. c. Gestational hypertension

This case is of gestational hypertension as there is no proteinuria and no any premonitory signs and symptoms of preeclampsia.

21. d. All of the above

Causes of maternal deaths in eclampsia are cerebral hemorrhage, pulmonary edema, aspiration pneumonia, cardiac failure, acute renal failure, cardiopulmonary arrest, and acute respiratory distress syndrome.

22. d. All of the above

This is a case of eclampsia, as a woman is actively convulsing first put an airway and suction to prevent trauma and aspiration and to maintain airway, breathing, and circulation, then start on antihypertensive and intravenous $MgSO_4$ followed by termination of pregnancy.

23. d. All of the above

Biochemical and laboratory findings in case of severe preeclampsia are as follows:
- Platelet count <100,000
- Elevated serum glutamic oxaloacetic transaminase (SGOT) and serum glutamic pyruvic transaminase (SGPT)
- Serum creatinine >1.1 mg/dL
- Blood uric acid level >4 mg/dL
- Protein creatinine ratio >0.3
- Abnormal coagulation profile

24. d. All of the above

Drugs used in the treatment of acute hypertensive crisis are:
- Intravenous labetalol
- Intravenous hydralazine
- Nitroglycerin infusion
- Nifedipine
- Sodium nitroprusside

25. **c.** Thiopentone sodium
 In status eclampticus, thiopentone sodium 0.5 mg dissolved in 20 mL of 5% of dextrose given IV slowly under supervision of anesthesiologist.

26. **d.** All of the above
 She is a case of severe preeclampsia with premonitory symptoms, hence patient needs to be admitted to hospital stat and start on antihypertensive drugs like labetalol and prophylactic IV $MgSO_4$ followed by termination of pregnancy which is the line of management.

27. **a.** Start on aspirin 75 mg
 As this patient is pregnant for 11 weeks and she had previous history of preterm delivery due to preeclampsia, hence she is at a high risk to develop preeclampsia during this pregnancy.
 Pregnant women who are at a high risk of preeclampsia should take 75–150 mg of aspirin daily from 12 weeks of gestation.

28. **d.** All of the above
 Following are signs of magnesium toxicity:
 - Loss of deep tendon reflexes
 - Decreased respiratory rate (<12 breaths/min)
 - Urine output <30 mL/hour
 - Chest pain and heart block

29. **d.** Neonatal jaundice at birth
 Fetal complications of severe preeclampsia are as follows:
 - Intrauterine death—due to spasm of uteroplacental circulation leading to accidental hemorrhage
 - Intrauterine growth restriction—due to chronic placental insufficiency
 - Asphyxia
 - Prematurity

30. **c.** a + b
 - It is predictive test for pregnancy-induced hypertension (PIH).
 - Roll over test: This screening test is done between 28 and 32 weeks.
 - Blood pressure is measured with the patient on her side first and then the patient is asked to roll on her back to check the blood pressure once again.
 - An increase of 20 mm Hg in diastolic pressure from side to back position indicates a positive "roll over test".
 - About 33% of women with positive "roll over test" developed hypertension later.

31. **d.** All of the above
 Color Doppler is one of the tests for prediction of pregnancy-induced hypertension.
 In uterine artery, Doppler flow velocimetry mean pulsatility index (PI) > 1.45 and if there is presence of bilateral (B/L) early diastolic notch which can give rise to adverse outcome in neonate and intrauterine fetal growth restriction.

32. **d.** All of the above
 Antepartum fetal surveillance in hypertensive disorders of pregnancy is very important to prevent intrauterine growth restriction and other fetal complications, following are the methods:
 - Daily fetal movement count and nonstress test
 - Serial obstetrics ultrasound and color Doppler
 - Biophysical profile (BPP) should be 8–10, it should be repeated weekly.
 - Biophysical profile <6 suspected chronic asphyxia, BPP <4 and below suspect asphyxia.

REFERENCES

1. Cunningham FG, Leveno KJ, Dashe JS, Hoffman BL, Spong CY, Casey BM (Eds). Williams Obstetrics, 26th edition. New York: McGraw Hill; 2022.
2. Konar H. D C Dutta's Textbook of Obstetrics, 10th edition. New Delhi: Jaypee Brothers Medical Publishers (P) Ltd.; 2022.

Chapter 27

Anemia in Pregnancy

Somya Suman, Sarita Bhalerao

QUESTIONS

1. Which of the following is the most effective parenteral iron preparation prescribed for postpartum women with iron deficiency anemia?
   a. Ferrous sucrose
   b. Ferrous bisglycinate
   c. Ferric carboxymaltose (FCM)
   d. Iron dextran

2. A pregnant woman with thalassemia major presents to the clinic at 24 weeks of gestation with fatigue and shortness of breath. Which of the following is true regarding the management of this condition?
   a. Parenteral iron therapy is the treatment of choice
   b. Oral iron therapy is indicated
   c. Breastfeeding is not safe after delivery
   d. Repeated transfusions are necessary to maintain hemoglobin (Hb) level above 10 g/dL

3. A pregnant woman was brought by her husband after fainting at home. He gave a history of her being clumsy and forgetful over the last few weeks. Investigation revealed high mean corpuscular volume (MCV) with hypersegmented neutrophils. How will you manage this patient?
   a. 100 µg of intramuscular (IM) cyanocobalamin
   b. 1,000 µg of intramuscular (IM) cyanocobalamin + folic acid
   c. 400 µg of folic acid
   d. 500 µg of oral cyanocobalamin

4. A woman at 36 weeks of gestation was brought to the clinic by her concerned husband. He mentioned that over the last few weeks he noticed her chewing on cardboard pieces and ice cream sticks on multiple occasions. On examinations, pallor was present and hemoglobin (Hb) was 8.6 g/dL. What is the most appropriate treatment regimen?
   a. Folic acid
   b. Red cell transfusion
   c. Ferric carboxymaltose
   d. Vitamin B_{12}

5. Which of the following is true regarding parenteral iron therapy for iron deficiency anemia in pregnant women?
   a. Can be given in first trimester
   b. Avoided in chronic liver disease
   c. Can be given alongside oral iron therapy
   d. Sensitivity test is mandatory

6. A pregnant woman presented to the clinic with complaints of dizziness. On examination, pallor was present. She will be considered severely anemic if her hemoglobin is less than:
   a. 4 g/dL
   b. 5 g/dL
   c. 7 g/dL
   d. 8 g/dL

7. What is the average maternal requirement of iron during a singleton pregnancy?
   a. 300 mg
   b. 1,000 mg
   c. 400 mg
   d. 800 mg

8. A pregnant woman at 10 weeks of gestation presented with insomnia due to a compulsive urge to keep moving her legs. Blood tests revealed a hemoglobin (Hb) value of 10.1 g/dL. Which of the following is the most sensitive indicator for her underlying condition?
   a. Serum iron level
   b. Serum ferritin
   c. Serum transferrin
   d. Serum erythropoietin

9. An anxious primigravida with sickle cell trait comes to you for her first antenatal checkup. Which of the following is correct that she is at a higher risk of developing during the course of this pregnancy?
   a. Preeclampsia
   b. Abortions
   c. Urinary tract infections
   d. Placental abruptions
   e. Preterm labor

10. Identify the correctly matched dose for folic acid supplementation that should be given in pregnant women suffering from sickle cell anemia.
    a. 5 mg
    b. 1 mg
    c. 500 µg
    d. 8 mg

11. Dose to start parenteral iron infusion for a woman at 38 weeks of gestation. We will use which formula?
    a. 2.4 × (target Hb − actual Hb) × body weight (kg)
    b. 2.4 × (target Hb − actual Hb) × body weight (kg) + 500 mg
    c. 2.4 × (target Hb − actual Hb) × body weight (kg) + 500 µg
    d. 2.4 × (target Hb − actual Hb) × body weight (kg) + 50 mg/kg

12. A pregnant woman presented with complaints of difficulty concentrating at work. Investigation revealed low mean corpuscular volume (MCV) with blood picture as shown, what is the likely diagnosis?

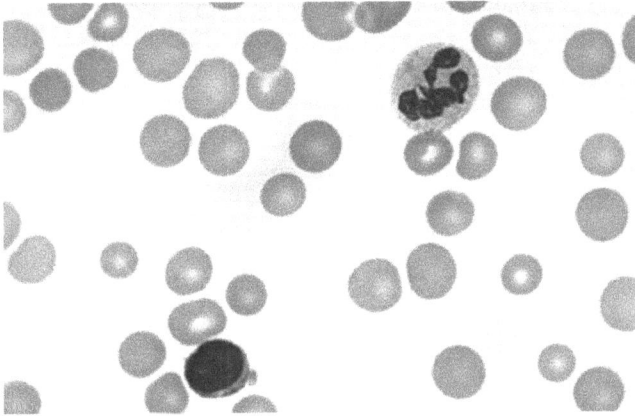

    a. Iron deficiency anemia
    b. Dimorphic anemia
    c. Sickle cell anemia
    d. Folic acid deficiency

13. A G3P2 female patient who is an agricultural laborer presents with complaints of fatigue at 39 weeks of gestation. On examination, pallor and mild pedal edema are present. Her hemoglobin (Hb) is 6.7 g/dL. How will you manage this patient?
    a. Iron sucrose infusion
    b. Ferric carboxymaltose infusion
    c. Packed cell transfusion
    d. Iron dextran infusion

14. Which of the following is the second most common pathological cause of anemia in pregnancy?
    a. Anemia associated with chronic disease
    b. Sickle cell anemia
    c. Iron deficiency anemia
    d. Megaloblastic anemia

15. A pregnant woman at 16 weeks pregnancy shows a hemoglobin (Hb) of 10.5 g%. The doctor suggests a peripheral blood smear to know the cause of anemia. The anemia in this patient can be considered physiological anemia. What would be blood picture of this patient?
    a. Microcytic and hypochromic
    b. Macrocytic and hyperchromic
    c. Normocytic and normochromic
    d. Microcytic and normochromic

16. Four patients are presented at an antenatal clinic. The first one has a 32-week pregnancy, second one has 17 weeks, and third one has 39 weeks pregnancy, and the fourth one is labor. All have a hemoglobin (Hb) of 8 g%. Which indicates parenteral iron therapy?
    a. 32 weeks
    b. 17 weeks
    c. In labor
    d. 38 weeks

17. According to World Health Organization (HO), anemia in pregnancy is diagnosed, when hemoglobin is less than:
    a. 10.0 g%
    b. 11.0 g%
    c. 12.0 g%
    d. 9.0 g%

18. Which of the following tests is most sensitive for the detection of iron depletion in pregnancy?
    a. Serum iron
    b. Serum ferritin
    c. Serum transferrin
    d. Serum iron-binding capacity

19. A 37-year-old multipara construction laborer has a blood picture showing hypochromic anisocytosis. This is most likely indicative of:
    a. Iron deficiency
    b. Folic acid deficiency
    c. Malnutrition
    d. Combined iron and folic acid deficiency

20. A pregnant female presents with fever. On laboratory investigation her hemoglobin (Hb) was decreased (7 g%). Total leukocyte count (TLC) was normal and platelet count was also decreased. Peripheral smear shows fragmented red blood cells (RBCs). Which is least probable diagnosis?
    a. Disseminated intravascular coagulation (DIC)
    b. Thrombotic thrombocytopenic purpura (TTP)
    c. HELLP syndrome
    d. Evans syndrome

21. The following are related to the treatment of thalassemia major, *except*:
    a. Blood transfusion
    b. Folic acid
    c. Routine iron therapy
    d. Deferoxamine improves pregnancy outcome

22. Tablet supplied by government of India includes:
    a. 60 mg elemental iron + 500 μg of folic acid
    b. 200 mg elemental iron + 1 mg of folic acid
    c. 100 mg elemental iron + 500 μg of folic acid
    d. 100 mg elemental iron + 5 mg of folic acid

23. With oral iron therapy, rise in Hb% can be seen after:
    a. 1 week   b. 3 weeks
    c. 4 weeks   d. 6 weeks

24. Site for maximum iron absorption of iron:
    a. Stomach   b. Duodenum
    c. Ileum   d. Large intestine

25. Which one is false regarding physiological changes in pregnancy?
    a. Hemoglobin (Hb) and hematocrit (Hct)—decrease
    b. Factor V, VII, VIII, X, XII and von Willebrand factor (vWF)—increase
    c. Fibrinogen—increase
    d. Antithrombin III and protein C—increase

26. In sickle cell anemia, life span of red blood cell is:
    a. 17 days   b. 40 days
    c. 76 days   d. 110 days

27. Which one is true regarding iron metabolism:
    a. Greater iron stores in women as compared to men
    b. Greater iron absorption from gastrointestinal (GI) tract during pregnancy
    c. Decreased iron absorption from the GI tract during pregnancy
    d. Greater iron requirements in early pregnancy as compared to late pregnancy
    e. Decreased absorption of iron in the presence of ascorbic acid

28. Which is false regarding contraception in sickle cell anemia:
    a. Oral pill
    b. Intrauterine contraceptive device (IUCD)
    c. Progestin-only pill or implant
    d. No contraceptives are used

29. Which is false regarding diagnosis of thalassemia:
    a. Low mean corpuscular volume (MCV), mean corpuscular hemoglobin (MCH), and normal mean corpuscular hemoglobin concentration (MCHC)
    b. Concentration of hemoglobin A2 (HbA2) and fetal hemoglobin (HbF) is raised
    c. Definitive diagnosis is made by globin chain and DNA synthesis
    d. Antenatal diagnosis by amniocentesis and chorionic villus sampling
    e. Preimplantation testing is not possible

30. Conditions leading to Hemolytic anemia ? Which one is true?
    a. Congenital red cell abnormality
    b. Antibodies directed against red cell membrane protein
    c. Can be due to primary disorder and sickle cell anemia and hereditary spherocytosis
    d. Can be secondary to underlying conditions like SLE or Pre-eclampsia
    e. Malignancy in Pregnancy leading to Microangiopathic hemolytic anemia
    1. a, b, c, d, e all are true
    2. a, b, c are true
    3. d and e are false
    4. a and e are only true

ANSWERS

1. **c.** Ferric carboxymaltose
   Ferric carboxymaltose (FCM) is considered superior to all the other parenteral iron supplementation, especially for iron deficiency anemia in postpartum women.
   Ferric carboxymaltose is a *dextran-free intravenous (IV) iron* preparation. It allows rapid administration of high doses of iron (up to *1,000 mg iron* in 15 minutes).
   It is *safe and effective* in improving the mean hemoglobin (Hb) level. It avoids the need for blood transfusions.
   (Reference: FOGSI - recommendation on management of iron deficiency anemia in pregnancy; Williams obstetrics 25th edition)

2. **a.** Parenteral iron therapy is the treatment of choice.
   In thalassemia major, both oral and parenteral iron preparations are avoided. This is because these patients are already in a state of iron overload due to multiple blood transfusions.

Pregnancy in patients with thalassemia major is very rare. In case pregnancy occurs, the following strategies are adopted:
- Iron chelating agents should be stopped.
- 5 mg folic acid supplementation should be given orally.
- Pneumococcal vaccination and boosters are advised prior to pregnancy.
- Repeated blood transfusions are given to maintain hemoglobin (Hb) levels above 10 g/dL.
- Breastfeeding is safe and iron chelation therapy can be resumed postdelivery.

(Reference: Arias practical guide to high-risk pregnancy and delivery)

3. **b.** 1,000 µg of intramuscular (IM) cyanocobalamin + folic acid

   The given scenario points to *vitamin B_{12} deficiency*. It is treated by *vitamin B_{12} injections* with folic acid supplementations. *1,000 µg of intramuscular (IM) cyanocobalamin* should be given initially every week for 6 weeks, following which it should be given once every month.

   Megaloblastic anemia caused by vitamin B_{12} deficiency should be identified and treated accordingly because folic acid supplementation alone will not help.

   Causes of vitamin B_{12} deficiency leading to anemia in pregnancy:
   - Gastric resection
   - Addisonian pernicious anemia
   - Crohn's disease
   - Ileal resection
   - Bacterial overgrowth in the small bowel

   (Reference: Arias practical guide to high-risk pregnancy and delivery; Williams obstetrics 25th edition)

4. **c.** Ferric carboxymaltose

   The given scenario is suggestive of pica associated with moderate iron deficiency anemia. Since the anemia was diagnosed late in pregnancy, the most appropriate treatment is parenteral iron therapy. Ferric carboxymaltose is a form of parenteral iron given as an intravenous (IV) infusion and in third trimester IV iron is preferred.

   (Reference: journal https://www.ncbi.nlm.nih.gov/pmc/article; Williams obstetrics 25th edition)

5. **b.** Avoided in chronic liver disease
   - Parenteral iron therapy for iron deficiency anemia in pregnancy is avoided if the patient has history of chronic liver disease.
   - Alternative to oral iron therapy for those who cannot tolerate oral iron

   Contraindications include:
   - Chronic liver disease
   - Active infection
   - First trimester of pregnancy
   - Anaphylactic reactions to oral iron therapy

   Sensitivity test prior to the infusion is not mandatory. Intravenous (IV) iron should be given with caution.

   (Reference: FOGSI – recommendation on management of iron deficiency anemia in pregnancy; Williams obstetrics 25th edition)

6. **c.** 7 g/dL

   Severe anemia is defined as hemoglobin (Hb) <7 g/dL. Anemia in pregnancy is said to occur when Hb level is <11 g/dL.

Hemoglobin values (g/dL)	World Health Organization (WHO) classification of anemia in pregnancy	Indian Council of Medical Research (ICMR) classification of anemia in pregnancy
>11	In the second trimester, hemoglobin (Hb) >10.5 g/dL is considered normal	Normal
10–10.9	Mild	Mild
7–9.9	Moderate	Moderate
<7	Severe	Severe
<4		Very severe

   (Reference: FOGSI – recommendation on management of iron deficiency anemia in pregnancy; Williams obstetrics 25th edition; Arias practical guide to high risk pregnancy and delivery)

7. **b.** 1,000 mg

   Maternal requirement of iron during a singleton gestation averages close to 1,000 mg.

   The average iron store in a nonpregnant female is around 300 mg and requirement of iron during pregnancy is 1,000 mg.

Iron requirement during pregnancy	
Fetus and placenta	300 mg
Expansion of maternal hemoglobin mass	500 mg
Losses through normal excretion routes	200 mg
Total	1,000 mg

(Reference: FOGSI – recommendation on management of iron deficiency anemia in pregnancy; Williams obstetrics 25th edition; Arias practical guide to high risk pregnancy and delivery)

8. **b.** Serum ferritin

Here, history suggestive of restless leg syndrome and hemoglobin (Hb) of 10.1 g/dL points to a diagnosis of iron deficiency anemia. Serum ferritin is the most sensitive indicator of iron deficiency.

Serum ferritin concentration <12 µg/L indicates complete depletion of iron stores and level <50 µg/L in early pregnancy is an indication for iron supplementation.

Restless leg syndrome causes unpleasant sensation in the legs along with an irresistible urge to move them.

(Reference: Williams obstetrics 25th edition. Arias practical guide to high-risk pregnancy and delivery)

9. **c.** Urinary tract infections

Sickle cell trait mostly is at a higher risk of developing urinary tract infections.

Sickle cell disease is associated with increased risk of:
- Miscarriages
- Fetal growth restrictions
- Preterm labor
- Venous thromboembolism
- Preeclampsia
- Placental abruptions

Sickle cell trait is a benign condition in which the affected person has only one abnormal hemoglobin (Hb) β gene allele, so do not have symptoms related to sickling; whereas, in sickle cell disease, the affected person has two abnormal Hb β gene alleles and hence severely symptomatic.

(Reference: Williams obstetrics 25th edition)

10. **a.** 5 mg

The amount of folic acid to be given to pregnant women suffering from sickle cell disease is 5 mg.

This is to reduce the risk of neutral tube defect and to compensate for the increased demand for folate during pregnancy.

(Reference: RCOG guidelines for management of iron deficiency anemia in pregnancy; Williams obstetrics 25th edition)

11. **b.** 2.4 × (target Hb – actual Hb) × body weight (kg) + 500 mg

The formula for calculating parenteral iron is:

Total dose in mg = 2.4 × (target Hb – actual Hb) × body weight (kg) + 500 mg

Iron preparation must be diluted with normal saline.

(Reference: journal http://www.ncbi.nlm.nih.gov/pmc/articles; Online Resource https://www.medicines.org.uk/emc/product/5911/smpc; Online Resource https://anemiamuktbharat.info/wp-content/uploads)

12. **d.** Folic acid deficiency

In the given clinical scenario, presence of microcytic hypochromic red blood cells (RBCs) indicates *iron deficiency anemia*, and hypersegmented neutrophils indicate anemia due to folic acid or vitamin B_{12} deficiency, called dimorphic anemia.

(Reference: FOGSI – recommendation on management of iron deficiency anemia in pregnancy; Williams obstetrics 25th edition; Arias practical guide to high-risk pregnancy and delivery)

13. **c.** Packed cell transfusion

The treatment of choice for severe anemia (<7 g/dL) in the third trimester is packed cell transfusion.

(Reference: FOGSI – recommendation on management of iron deficiency anemia in pregnancy. Williams obstetrics 25th edition; Arias practical guide to high-risk pregnancy and delivery)

14. **a.** Anemia associated with chronic disease

The second most common pathological cause of anemia during pregnancy is anemia associated with chronic disease.
- Chronic renal insufficiency
- Inflammatory bowel disease
- Connective tissue disorders
- Granulomatous infections
- Malignant neoplasms

And the first most common cause of anemia during pregnancy is iron deficiency anemia.

(Reference: Online Resource http://www.uptodate. com/contents/anemia- in-pregnancy; Williams obstetrics 25th edition)

15. **c.** Normocytic and normochromic
Hemodilution causes physiological anemia. The increase in plasma volume is far greater than the increase in red blood cell (RBC) mass.
Peripheral smear will be normocytic and normochromic.
(Reference: FOGSI - recommendation on management of iron deficiency anemia in pregnancy; Williams obstetrics 25th edition; Arias practical guide to high-risk pregnancy and delivery)

16. **a.** 32 weeks
32 weeks pregnancy-induced iron deficiency anemia, parenteral therapy is recommended as rise in hemoglobin (Hb) is 1 g/week.
(Reference: Williams obstetrics 25th edition; Arias practical guide to high-risk pregnancy and delivery)

17. **b.** 11.0 g%
According to standards laid by World Health Organization (WHO), anemia in pregnancy is defined as when hemoglobin is 11 g% or less or hematocrit is <33%
Also know
ICMR – Grades of Anemia in Pregnancy

Mild anemia	10–10.9 g%
Moderate anemia	7–9.9 g%
Severe anemia	6.9–4 g%
Very severe anemia	<4 g%

(Reference: Williams obstetrics 25th edition; Arias practical guide to high-risk pregnancy and delivery)

18. **b.** Serum ferritin
Serum ferritin is most sensitive test as it correlates best with iron stores and is the first test to become abnormal in case of iron deficiency.
(Reference: FOGSI - recommendation on management of iron deficiency anemia in pregnancy; Williams obstetrics 25th edition; Arias practical guide to high-risk pregnancy and delivery)

19. **d.** Combined iron and folic acid deficiency
Combined iron and folic acid deficiency
Anisocytosis is variation in size of red blood cells.
(Reference: Williams obstetrics 25th edition; Arias practical guide to high-risk pregnancy and delivery; Online Resource http://www.uptodate.com/contents/anemia- in-pregnancy)

20. **d.** Evans syndrome
Evans syndrome is an autoimmune disease in which individual antibodies attack their own red blood cell (RBC) and platelets, similar to autoimmune hemolytic anemia and idiopathic thrombocytopenic purpura and leads to formation of spherocytes.
Schistocytes are fragmented RBCs that are result of microangiopathic hemolysis.
Disseminated intravascular coagulation (DIC), thrombotic thrombocytopenic purpura (TTP), and HELLP syndrome all may presents with:
- Fever
- Anemia
- Thrombocytopenia
- Fragmented RBCs
- Normal total leukocyte count (TLC)

(Reference: Williams obstetrics 25th edition; Arias practical guide to high-risk pregnancy and delivery)

21. **c.** Routine iron therapy
In thalassemia, routine iron therapy should not be given as it leads to hemochromatosis, so given only in case of documented iron deficiency.
Moreover β-thalassemia major patient is iron overload, due to repeated transfusion, can lead to organ damage due to hemosiderosis.
(Reference: Williams obstetrics 25th edition; Arias practical guide to high-risk pregnancy and delivery)

22. **c.** 100 mg elemental iron + 500 µg of folic acid
To prevent nutritional anemia among mother and children, the government of India sponsored a National Nutritional Anaemia Prophylaxis Programme. The suggested prophylactic doses were initially 60 mg of elemental iron and 500 µg of folic acid for pregnant females. These tablets were distributed free of cost at all the primary health centers (PHCs). But survey done during the years 1985–1986 shows poor results and no impact was seen on the prevalence of anemia in pregnant female. So, the dosage of elemental iron was increased.
So presently, the tablets supplied contain 100 mg of elemental iron and 500 µg of folic acid.
(Reference: https://www.ncbi.nih.gov >pmc)

23. **b.** 3 weeks
Rise in hemoglobin with oral iron 0.7–1 g/week, which is seen after 3 weeks on initiation of oral therapy, and hemoglobin (Hb) level should increase by at least 0.3 g/dL/week, if the patient is responding to therapy.
(Reference: https://www.ncbi.nih.gov >pmc)

24. **b.** Duodenum
The absorption of most of the dietary iron occurs in the duodenum and proximal jejunum and depends heavily on the physical state of the iron atom.
(Reference: The obstetrics Hematology manual, Sue Pavord, Beverley Hunt. https://www.ncbi.nlm.nih.gov >pmc)

25. **d.** Antithrombin III and protein C—increase
As increase in plasma volume exceeds that of red blood cells (RBCs), which increases by 25%, leading to fall in hemoglobin (Hb) concentration and hematocrit (Hct) due to hemodilution. Pregnancy is hypercoagulable state due to increase in factor V, VII, VIII, X, XII, and vWF, but antithrombin III and protein C remains unchanged and protein S decreases.
(Reference: Arias practical guide to high-risk pregnancy and delivery)

26. **a.** 17 days
The sickle cells only live for about 10–20 days. The sickle-shaped cells do not pass easily through blood vessels. They clog or break apart which leads to decreased life of red cells. Also sickle cells may be destroyed by the spleen because of their shape and stiffness. Sickled cells get stuck in filter and die.
(Reference: https://www.ncbi.nlm.nih.gov > pmc; https://www.hopkinsmedicine.org/health/conditions-ans-diseases/sickle-cell-disease)

27. **b.** Greater iron absorption from gastrointestinal (GI) tract during pregnancy
Metabolism of any substance depends on amount of absorption and amount of excretion.
In case of iron, the increased demand is met by increasing the absorption in the GI tract.
Iron stores are greater in men than women as the loss is only epithelial cells (1 mg/dL) while in women there is increased loss of iron due to monthly loss during menses.
And iron requirements are increased more during the second trimester and near term due to active transport of iron to the fetus.
Ascorbic acid helps in increased iron absorption while phytates interfere with iron absorption from the GI tract.
(Reference: Williams obstetrics 25th edition; Arias practical guide to high-risk pregnancy and delivery)

28. **d.** No contraceptives are used.
Many clinicians do not recommend because of adverse vascular and thrombotic effects. Haddad and Coworkers found no higher complication with their use in women with sickle cell syndrome. The Centers for Disease Control and Prevention categorizes combined oral contraceptives (COCs), intrauterine devices (IUDs), implants and progestin-only contraception as having no risk or as having advantages that generally outweigh theoretical or proven risks.
(Reference: Williams obstetrics 25th edition; Arias practical guide to high-risk pregnancy and delivery)

29. **e.** Preimplantation testing is not possible.
All above mentioned points are true and pattern of inheritance of both α- and β-thalassemia are autosomal recessive and antenatal diagnosis is possible and advised. Preimplantation testing is also possible in couples undergoing in vitro fertilization (IVF).
(Reference: Williams obstetrics 25th edition; Arias practical guide to high-risk pregnancy and delivery)

30. **1.** All are true
All these conditions feature accelerated erythrocyte destruction.
Aberrant antibodies causes Autoimmune hemolysis., Can be primary syndrome or secondary due to lymphoma, leukemia, chronic inflammatory disease.
Cold agglutinin disease may be induced by infectious etiologies such as Mycoplasma pneumonia or Epstein Barr virus.
(Reference: Williams obstetrics 25th edition)

Chapter 28

Rh Isoimmunization

Soniya Dhiman

QUESTIONS

1. Consider the following statements regarding the risk of Rh isoimmunization:
   1. The overall risk of Rh immunization after the first Rh-positive pregnancy is 13.2%
   2. The risk of Rh isoimmunization after the first Rh-positive pregnancy with an ABO-incompatible blood group is 16%
   3. The risk of Rh isoimmunization with only postpartum anti-D will reduce from 12–13 to 1–2%
   4. The risk of Rh isoimmunization with both antenatal and postpartum anti-D will reduce from 2 to 0.1%

   Which of the following is the correct answer?
   a. 1, 3, and 4
   b. 1, 2, and 3
   c. 1, 2, and 4
   d. 1, 2, 3, and 4

2. A primigravida presented to outpatient department (OPD) at 28 weeks period of gestation (POG) with a USG report showing hydrops in the fetus. In investigating the cause of the hydropic baby, the patient's blood group was B-negative and her husband's blood group was O-positive. All other causes of hydrops have been ruled out. Which of the following explains the development of hydrops in this fetus?
   a. Mirror syndrome
   b. Grandmother theory
   c. Kohlberg's theory
   d. Spearman's two-factor theory

3. As a sensitizing event for a Rh-negative woman, consider the following etiologies:
   1. Threatened miscarriage
   2. Ectopic pregnancy
   3. Evacuation of molar pregnancy
   4. Intrauterine fetal death

   Which of the following option is correct?
   a. Only 1, 2, and 3 are correct
   b. Only 2, 3, and 4 are correct
   c. Only 1, 3, and 4 are correct
   d. 1, 2, 3, and 4 are correct

4. For quantification of fetomaternal hemorrhage, which of the following test is not used?
   a. Kleihauer–Betke test
   b. Acid elution test
   c. Rosette test
   d. Middle cerebral artery-peak systolic velocity (MCA-PSV)

5. A 26-year-old primigravida presented to the antenatal clinic for a routine antenatal visit at 16 weeks of POG. Her blood group was A-negative and her husband's blood group was O-positive. She advised for an indirect Coombs test (ICT) titer which came out negative. Consider the following statements regarding her management:
   1. Follow her up with ICT titer at 4 weeks intervals, provide an injection of anti-D immunoglobulin (IG), 300 µg at 28 weeks
   2. ABO and Rh typing of newborn need to be done.
   3. If the blood group of the newborn is negative, provide an injection of anti-D IG, 300 µg within 72 hours of delivery.
   4. If the blood group of the newborn is positive, no need to provide an injection of anti-D IG, 300 µg within 72 hours of delivery.

   Select the correct answer among the given options:
   a. 1, 2, and 3
   b. 2 and 3
   c. 1 and 2
   d. 1, 2, 3, and 4

6. A 28-year-old primigravida with Rh-negative nonisoimmunized pregnant woman presented to the labor room with labor pains. She progressed well. Junior resident was prepared to conduct the delivery. The senior resident has given the following instructions to the junior:
   1. No attempt to be done for manual removal of the placenta.
   2. During cord clamping, keep cord as long as possible -15 cm for exchange transfusion
   3. For any postpartum hemorrhage (PPH), you can use oxytocin, ergometrine, and carboprost.
   4. After delivery of the baby, send cord blood for blood group, direct Coombs test (DCT), bilirubin, hematocrit, hemoglobin, and reticulocyte count
   Select the correct answer among the given options:
   a. 1, 2, and 3 are correct
   b. 1, 2, and 4 are correct
   c. 2, 3, and 4 are correct
   d. 1, 2, 3, and 4 are correct

7. A primigravida with Rh-negative nonisoimmunized female presented at 32 weeks POG with antepartum hemorrhage. She was diagnosed with placenta previa and had recurrent episodes of hemorrhages. Which of the following is correct regarding her management for the prevention of Rh isoimmunization?
   a. If she received injection anti-D at 28 weeks, no need to repeat the dose of anti-D
   b. Consider the next dose of injection anti-D in the postpartum period with 72 hours of delivery
   c. Maternal antibody titer needs to be repeated every 3 weeks if negative repeat dose is to be given
   d. Maternal antibody titer needs to be repeated every 3 weeks if positive repeat dose is to be given

8. Which of the following is not correct regarding critical titer in case of Rh Alloimmunized pregnancy?
   a. A critical titer is that titer associated with a significant risk for severe erythroblastosis fetalis and hydrops
   b. In most centers this is between 1:8 and 1:32
   c. If the initial antibody titer is 1:8 or less, the patient may be monitored with titer assessment every 4 weeks.
   d. None of the above

9. Consider the following statements regarding fetal hemoglobin and fetal anemia:
   1. Fetal anemia is diagnosed when fetal hemoglobin level is more than 2 standard deviation below the mean for gestational age (GA)
   2. Normally, there is a linear fall of fetal hemoglobin value with GA
   3. Normally, there is a linear rise of fetal hemoglobin value with GA
   4. Normally, there is no change of fetal hemoglobin value with GA
   Identify the correct answer from the following options:
   a. 1 and 2   b. 1 and 3
   c. 1 and 4   d. Only 1

10. Consider the following statements regarding the following picture given below:

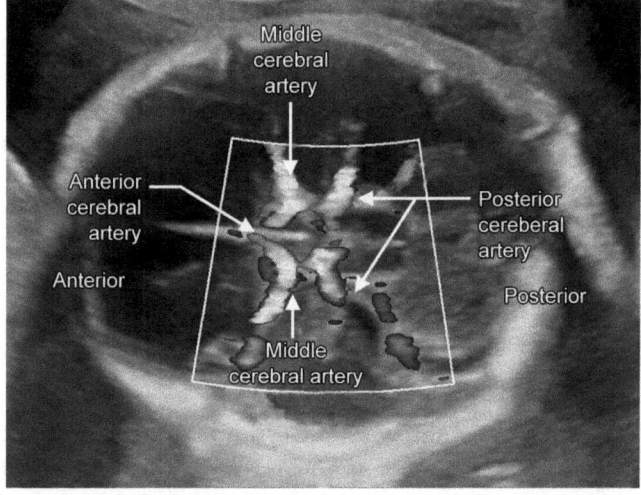

   A. MCA Doppler velocimetry is a noninvasive method of assessment of fetal anemia
   B. Other vessels are not used because a larger insonating angle is required
   C. In Rh-isoimmunized women, monitoring should begin at 18–20 weeks POG
   D. The threshold value of 1.5 multiples of median (MoM) suggests a fetus with moderate or severe anemia
   Select the correct answer from the given options:
   a. A, B, and C are correct
   b. B, C, and D are correct
   c. A, C, and D are correct
   d. A, B, C, and D are correct

11. Which of the following is correct regarding the amniotic fluid spectral analysis in Rh-isoimmunized antenatal women?
    a. It is more accurate than MCA velocimetry
    b. It is a direct test for fetal anemia
    c. Represented as change in absorbance at 450 nm—ΔOD450
    d. Queenan chart—valid from 27 to 42 weeks

12. The prevalence of red cell alloimmunization in pregnancy is:
    a. 1%
    b. 2%
    c. 0.1%
    d. 0.2%

13. Identify the incorrect statement regarding ABO blood group incompatibility:
    a. It is the most common cause of hemolytic disease of newborn
    b. ABO incompatibility is often seen in first born neonate
    c. Fetal surveillance and early delivery are not indicated in pregnancies with prior ABO incompatibility
    d. Neonates are not evaluated for hyperbilirubinemia as they do not need any treatment with phototherapy or transfusion

14. Which of the following is a correct statement regarding D-alloimmunized pregnancy?
    a. If alloimmunization is detected, irrespective of the value, the titer has to be repeated every 4 weeks
    b. If alloimmunization is detected and the titer is below the critical value, the titer has to be repeated every 4 weeks
    c. If alloimmunization is detected and the titer has reached a critical value, the titer has to be repeated every 4 weeks
    d. If a prior pregnancy was complicated by alloimmunization, the risk to this pregnancy will depend on the antibody titer

15. Management of alloimmunized pregnancy consist of:
    a. Maternal antibody titer surveillance at 4 weeks interval, provided the titer is below the critical level
    b. If maternal antibody titer reached the critical titer, than monitoring for fetal anemia by serial measurement of fetal middle cerebral artery velocimetry need to be done
    c. None of the above
    d. Both of the above

16. The characteristics of blood used for intrauterine transfusion include:
    1. Type O
    2. D negative
    3. Cytomegalovirus negative
    4. Irradiated
    5. Leukodepleted
    Select the correct option among the following:
    a. Only 1 and 2 are correct
    b. Only 1, 2, and 4 are correct
    c. Only 1, 2, and 5 are correct
    d. 1, 2, 3, 4, and 5 are correct

17. Which of the following is not an indication of fetal blood transfusion in a Rh-isoimmunized pregnancy?
    a. Fetal hematocrit less than 30%
    b. Fetal hydrops is there
    c. Middle cerebral artery, peak systolic velocity (MCA-PSV) is <1.5 MoM
    d. Middle cerebral artery, peak systolic velocity (MCA-PSV) is >1.5 MoM

18. One 300-μg dose of anti-D IG will neutralize how much amount of fetal blood?
    a. 15 mL of fetal red cells
    b. 30 mL of fetal whole blood
    c. Both of the above
    d. None of the above

19. A G3P2L1 at POG of 35^{+5} weeks Rh-isoimmunized woman presented to labor room with chief complaint of decreased fetal movement. On nonstress test (NST) testing, her NST trace showed sinusoidal heart rate pattern. What should be the best management for her?
    a. Repeat NST after 4 hours
    b. Provide her with injection of anti-D IG 300 μg
    c. Consider her delivery on urgent basis
    d. Proceed for complete biophysical profile after 4 hours

20. Which of the following sentence is not correct regarding hydrops fetalis?
    a. Hydrops is diagnosed by identifying two or more fetal effusions—pleural, pericardial, or ascites
    b. Sonographically measured skin thickness of >7 mm constitutes edema or anasarca
    c. Placentomegaly is defines as placental thickness ≥6 cm in third trimester

d. Placentomegaly is defines as placental thickness ≥4 cm in second trimester

21. Consider the following statements regarding hydrops:
    1. When fetal hydrops was found in association with red cell alloimmunization, it is termed nonimmune hydrops
    2. Transplacental passage of maternal antibodies destroy fetal red blood cells and causes anemia in immune hydrops
    3. At least 90% cases of hydrops are immune
    4. There is marrow erythroid hyperplasia and extramedullary hematopoiesis in the spleen and liver in immune hydrops

    Select the correct answer among the following options:
    a. 1 and 4 are correct
    b. 2 and 4 are correct
    c. 1 and 3 are correct
    d. 2 and 3 are correct

22. Which of the following is the most common chromosomal anomaly associated with non-immune hydrops when it presents before 24 weeks of gestation?
    a. 45,X: Turner syndrome
    b. Down syndrome: Trisomy 21
    c. Edward syndrome: Trisomy 18
    d. Patau syndrome: Trisomy 13

23. Which of the following is the most common infectious etiology of nonimmune hydrops?
    a. Parvovirus B19
    b. Syphilis
    c. Cytomegalovirus
    d. Toxoplasmosis

24. Which of the following statement is not correct regarding Mirror syndrome?
    a. This condition is also called triple edema
    b. It can be considered as a form of severe preeclampsia
    c. There is development of fetal hydrops along with development of maternal edema
    d. The etiology of fetal hydrops is related to the development of mirror syndrome

25. Which of the following statement regarding Kell alloimmunization is not correct?
    a. It develops more rapidly and may be more severe than with sensitization to D
    b. Kell immunization causes severe anemia even with less antibody titers
    c. Nearly 90% Kell sensitization results from transfusion
    d. An antibody titer of ≥1:16 can be used to target intensive clinical monitoring

26. Which of the following statement is not correct regarding fetal D genotyping using cell-free DNA (cfDNA)?
    a. It is a noninvasive test
    b. *First potential indication:* In isoimmunized condition, to know about fetus Rh status and thus can prevent fetal anemia surveillance
    c. *Second potential indication:* In cases without isoimmuniaztion, anti-D globulin may be withheld if fetus is Rh-negative
    d. ACOG (2019) recommended routine cfDNA in Rh-negative pregnancies

27. Which of the following statement is not correct regarding anti-D IG?
    a. Half-life is 24 days
    b. Provide protection for 12 weeks
    c. Both antenatal and postnatal anti-D reduces sensitization to 2%
    d. Postnatally anti-D given within 72 hours but can be given up to 28 days

28. Consider the following statements:
    1. Antenatal women with ICT positive titer
    2. Father is Rh-negative
    3. If fetal cfDNA test shows, fetus is Rh-negative.
    4. Antenatal women with ICT negative titer

    Which of the above is not an indication for providing anti-D prophylaxis to antenatal women who is Rh-negative?
    a. 1 and 3
    b. 2 and 4
    c. 1, 2, and 4
    d. 1, 2, and 3

29. Consider the following causes for failure of anti-D prophylaxis:
    1. Inadequate dose
    2. Patient already immunized but antibody titer too low for laboratory recognition
    3. Missed prophylactic antenatal dose
    4. Omission of Kell blood group typing

    Select the correct statement among the following options:
    a. 1, 2, and 3 are correct
    b. 2, 3, and 4 are correct

c. 1, 3, and 4 are correct
d. 1, 2, 3, and 4 are correct

30. **Which of the following is not a treatment option for Rh-isoimmunized pregnancy?**
    a. Intrauterine transfusions
    b. Intravenous immunoglobulins (IVIGs) therapy
    c. Anti-D IGs
    d. Plasmapheresis

ANSWERS

1. **a.** 1, 3, and 4
   Risk of Rh isoimmunization after first Rh-positive pregnancy
   - Without anti-D immune globulin prophylaxis, a D-negative woman delivered of a D-positive, ABO-compatible newborn has a 16-percent likelihood of developing alloimmunization.
   - If there is ABO incompatibility, the D alloimmunization risk decreases to 2 percent because erythrocyte destruction of incompatible cells limits sensitization.
   - Routine postpartum administration of anti-D immune globulin to at-risk pregnancies within 72 hours of delivery lowers the alloimmunization rate by 90 percent: from 12-13% to 1-2%
   - Additionally, provision of anti-D immune globulin at 28 weeks' gestation reduce the third-trimester alloimmunization rate from approximately 2 percent to 0.1 percent
   - Overall risk of immunization: 13.2%

   [References: Fetal disorders. In: Cunningham FG, Leveno KJ, Dashe JS, Hoffman BL, Spong CY, Casey BM (Eds). Williams Obstetrics, 26th edition. New York: McGraw Hill; 2022. pp. 354, 356; Bowman J. Rh-immunoglobulin: Rh prophylaxis. Best Pract Res Clin Haematol. 2006;19(1):27-34]

2. **b.** The Grandmother Theory/Effect
   In virtually all pregnancies, small amounts of maternal blood enter the fetal circulation. Polymerase chain reaction (PCR) has identified maternal D-positive DNA in peripheral blood from preterm and full-term D-negative newborns (Lazar, 2006). Thus, a D-negative female fetus exposed to maternal D-positive red cells might develop sensitization and later produce anti-D antibodies before or during pregnancy. This mechanism is called the grandmother effect because the fetus in the current pregnancy is jeopardized by maternal antibodies that were initially provoked by his or her grandmother's erythrocytes.

   [Reference: Fetal disorders. In: Cunningham FG, Leveno KJ, Dashe JS, Hoffman BL, Spong CY, Casey BM (Eds). Williams Obstetrics, 26th edition. New York: McGraw Hill; 2022. p. 354]

3. **d.** 1, 2, 3, and 4 are correct
   Causes of Feto-maternal Hemorrhage associated with Red Cell Antigen Alloimmunization or Sensitizing events for a Rh-Negative Mother

   Pregnancy Loss
   - Abortion, spontaneous or elective
   - Ectopic pregnancy
   - Fetal death (any trimester)

   Procedures
   - Amniocentesis
   - Chorionic villus sampling
   - Fetal blood sampling
   - Molar pregnancy evacuation

   Other
   - Antepartum bleeding, including threatened abortion
   - Delivery, vaginal or cesarean
   - External cephalic version
   - Placental abruption
   - Trauma to the abdomen during pregnancy

   [Reference: Fetal disorders. In: Cunningham FG, Leveno KJ, Dashe JS, Hoffman BL, Spong CY, Casey BM (Eds). Williams Obstetrics, 26th edition. New York: McGraw Hill; 2022. p. 354]

4. **d.** Middle cerebral artery-peak systolic velocity (MCA-PSV)
   In the setting of Rh incompatibility, or any time a large fetomaternal hemorrhage is suspected regardless of antigen status, a Kleihauer-Betke test or acid elution test, flow cytometry test and Rosette tests are used.

   [Reference: Fetal disorders. In: Cunningham FG, Leveno KJ, Dashe JS, Hoffman BL, Spong CY, Casey BM (Eds). Williams Obstetrics, 26th edition. New York: McGraw Hill; 2022. p. 354]

5. c. 1 and 2

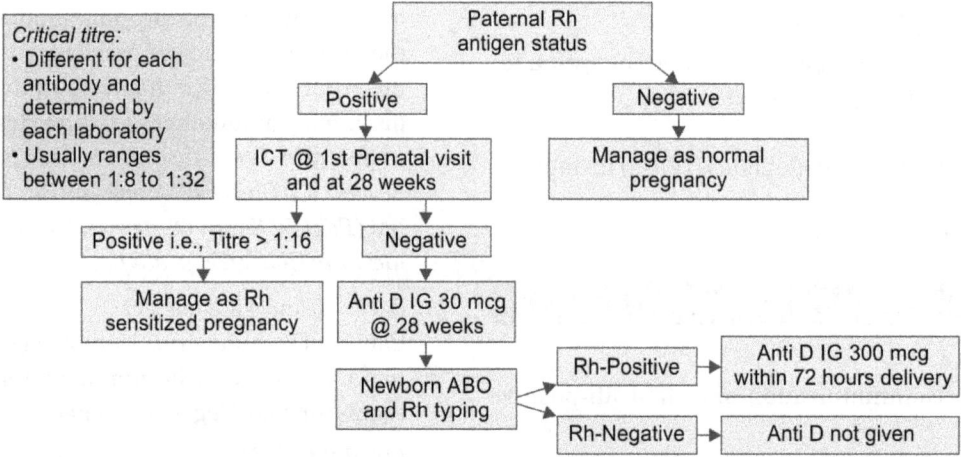

Anti-D and anti-c levels should be measured every 4 weeks up to 28 weeks of gestation and then every 2 weeks until delivery.
[References: 1. James D, Steer P, Weiner CP, Gonik B, Crowther CA, Robson SC (Eds). High Risk Pregnancy: Management Options, 5th edition. USA: Elsevier Saunders; 2018.
2. (RCOG GTG 65)]

6. b. 1, 2, and 4 are correct

Intrapartum measures to reduce the risk of Rh-immunization:
- No stripping of the membrane is to be done.
- No fundal pushing in 1st or 2nd stage of labor to be done.
- No uterine massage or uterine grasp and squeeze in 3rd stage of labor to be done.
- No attempt for Manual removal of placenta to be made.
- Placenta to be delivered spontaneously using control cord traction without squeezing the uterus
- Cord kept as long as possible -15 cm for exchange transfusion.
- For any PPH, oxytocin is used instead of ergometrine.
- Protect the vaginal and perineal wounds and lacerations from exposure to fetal blood spill from the cord
- *Cord Blood:* Blood group, DCT, Bilirubin, HCT, Hb, and Reticulocyte count need to be sent.

[Reference: James D, Steer P, Weiner CP, Gonik B, Crowther CA, Robson SC (Eds). High Risk Pregnancy: Management Options, 5th edition. USA: Elsevier Saunders; 2018]

7. c. Maternal antibody titer needs to be repeated every 3 weeks if negative repeat dose is to be given.

Anti-D immune globulin is recommended for Rh-D-negative women who experience antenatal hemorrhage after 20 weeks of gestation. Management of the patient with persistent or intermittent antenatal bleeding is complex. The most conservative approach may be to assess the volume of fetal–maternal hemorrhage with a quantitative test (such as the Kleihauer–Betke test). The appropriate amount of Rh D immune globulin then can be administered to cover the estimated volume of fetal–maternal hemorrhage. In cases of chronic or episodic bleeding this approach may need to be repeated. An intuitive but unproven strategy is to monitor the Rh D-negative patient with continuing antenatal hemorrhage with serial indirect Coombs testing for anti-D approximately every 3 weeks. If the result is positive, indicating the persistence of anti-D immune globulin, then theoretically no additional treatment with anti-D immune globulin is necessary. If the Coombs test result is negative, excessive fetal–maternal hemorrhage may have occurred, and a Kleihauer–Betke test should be performed in order to determine the amount of additional anti-D immune globulin necessary. Finally, it has been proposed in this clinical situation to use cell-free DNA testing to ascertain the fetal Rh D status and, thus, avoid repeated administration of doses of anti-D immune globulin with an Rh D-negative fetus.

(Reference: ACOG Practice Bulletin, Prevention of Rh D Alloimmunization August 2017)

8. **d.** None of the above

   A critical titer is a titer associated with a significant risk for severe erythroblastosis fetalis and hydrops. In most centers this is between 1:8 and 1:32. If the initial antibody titer is 1:8 or less, the patient may be monitored with titer assessment every 4 weeks.

   [Reference: (ACOG Practice Bulletin, Management of Alloimmunization during Pregnancy, Number 192, March 2018)]

9. **b.** 1 and 3

   Fetal anemia is diagnosed when the hemoglobin value is more than 2 SD below the mean for that gestational age. Normally, there is a linear rise in hemoglobin value with gestational age.

   [Reference: Abbasi N, Johnson JA, Ryan G. Fetal anemia. Ultrasound Obstet Gynecol. 2017;50(2):145-153. doi: 10.1002/uog.17555. PMID: 28782230]

10. **d.** A, B, C, and D are correct

    Methods of assessment of fetal anemia:

    1. *Non-Invasive method:*
       - Middle cerebral artery (MCA) doppler velocimetry
       - Ultrasound examination
    2. *Invasive method:*
       - *Indirect:* Amniotic fluid spectral analysis
       - *Direct:* fetal blood studies using a sample obtained by fetal blood sampling

    Recent advances in Doppler technology have led to the development of noninvasive methods to assess the degree of fetal anemia. Doppler was used to measure the peak systolic velocity in the fetal middle cerebral artery in 111 fetuses at risk for fetal anemia secondary to red cell alloimmunization. Moderate or severe anemia was predicted by values of peak systolic velocity in the fetal middle cerebral artery above 1.5 times the median for gestational age with a sensitivity of 100% and a false-positive rate of 12%. Correct technique is a critical factor when determining peak systolic velocity in the fetal middle cerebral artery with Doppler ultrasonography.

    [References: Cunningham FG, Leveno KJ, Bloom SL, Dashe JS, Hoffman BL, Casey BM, Spong CY (Eds). Williams Obstetrics, 25th edition. New York: McGraw Hill; 2018.

    ACOG Practice Bulletin, Management of Alloimmunization during Pregnancy, Number 192, March 2018]

11. **c.** Represented as change in absorbance at 450 nm—ΔOD450

    Amniotic fluid spectral analysis: The fetus with hemolytic anemia frequently has an elevated serum bilirubin. By the middle of the second trimester, the amniotic fluid bilirubin is also elevated. It is an indirect method where amniotic fluid bilirubin concentration measurement by spectrophotometer. Wiliam Liley has first standardized an approach that remains essentially unchanged since first reported in 1961. Amniotic fluid was obtained by ultrasound-guided amniocentesis. Change in absorbance at 450nm named as ΔOD450 is noted and plotted on a graph on the y-axis, against the period of gestation at x-axis. These are termed as Liley's graph. The graph is divided into three zones. Liley's chart is valid from 27 to 42 weeks. Another chart is made by Queenan, can be used as early as 14 weeks. MCA velocimetry is a more accurate and non-invasive method for assessment of fetal anemia.

    (Reference: James, High-Risk Pregnancy, chapter 13 fetal hemolytic disease page 217)

12. **a.** 1%

    The prevalence of red cell alloimmunization in pregnancy approximates 1 percent.

    [Reference: Fetal disorders. In: Cunningham FG, Leveno KJ, Dashe JS, Hoffman BL, Spong CY, Casey BM (Eds). Williams Obstetrics, 26th edition. New York: McGraw Hill; 2022. p. 353]

13. **d.** Neonates are not evaluated for hyperbilirubinemia as they do not need any treatment with phototherapy or transfusion.

    Incompatibility for the major blood group antigens A and B is the most common cause of hemolytic disease in newborns, but it does not cause appreciable hemolysis in the fetus. This is because most anti-A and anti-B antibodies are IgM types and do not cross the placenta. The condition differs from CDE incompatibility in several respects. First, ABO incompatibility is often seen in firstborn neonates, unlike sensitization to other blood group antigens. This is because most group O women have developed anti-A and anti-B isoagglutinin before pregnancy from exposure to bacteria displaying similar antigens. Additionally, ABO alloimmunization rarely becomes more severe in successive pregnancies. Fetal surveillance and early delivery are not indicated

in pregnancies with prior ABO incompatibility. Postnatally, however, neonates are evaluated for hyperbilirubinemia, which may require treatment with phototherapy or occasionally transfusion.
[Reference: Fetal disorders. In: Cunningham FG, Leveno KJ, Dashe JS, Hoffman BL, Spong CY, Casey BM (Eds). Williams Obstetrics, 26th edition. New York: McGraw Hill; 2022. p. 355]

14. **b.** If alloimmunization is detected and the titer is below the critical value, the titer has to be repeated every 4 weeks.
If alloimmunization is detected and the titer is below the critical value, the titer is generally repeated every 4 weeks for the duration of the pregnancy (American College of Obstetricians and Gynecologists, 2019a). In any pregnancy in which the antibody titer has reached a critical value, there is no benefit to repeating the titer. The pregnancy is at risk even if the titer drops, and further evaluation is required. Similarly, if a prior pregnancy was complicated by alloimmunization, the pregnancy is considered at risk regardless of titer.
[Reference: Fetal disorders. In: Cunningham FG, Leveno KJ, Dashe JS, Hoffman BL, Spong CY, Casey BM (Eds). Williams Obstetrics, 26th edition. New York: McGraw Hill; 2022. p. 355]

15. **d.** both of the above
Management of the alloimmunized pregnancy typically consists of maternal antibody titer surveillance followed by ultrasound monitoring of the fetal MCA peak systolic velocity if a critical antibody titer is reached.
[Reference: Fetal disorders. In: Cunningham FG, Leveno KJ, Dashe JS, Hoffman BL, Spong CY, Casey BM (Eds). Williams Obstetrics, 26th edition. New York: McGraw Hill; 2022. p. 355]

16. **d.** 1, 2, 3, 4, and 5 are correct
Fetal blood transfusion is generally recommended only if the fetal hematocrit is <30 percent (Society for Maternal-Fetal Medicine, 2015a). The red cells transfused are type O, D-negative, cytomegalovirus-negative, packed to a hematocrit of approximately 80 percent to prevent volume overload, irradiated to prevent fetal graft-versus-host reaction, and leukocyte poor.
[Reference: Fetal disorders. In: Cunningham FG, Leveno KJ, Dashe JS, Hoffman BL, Spong CY, Casey BM (Eds). Williams Obstetrics, 26th edition. New York: McGraw Hill; 2022. p. 356]

17. **c.** MCA-PSV is <1.5 MoM.
Fetal Blood Transfusion: If the MCA peak systolic velocity exceeds 1.5 MoM or if hydrops develops and anemia is the leading etiology, fetal blood sampling and intrauterine transfusion should be considered.
Fetal transfusion is typically performed before 34 to 35 weeks gestation (Society for Maternal-Fetal Medicine, 2015a). Transfusion is generally recommended only if the fetal hematocrit is <30 percent (Society for Maternal-Fetal Medicine, 2015a).
[Reference: Fetal disorders. In: Cunningham FG, Leveno KJ, Dashe JS, Hoffman BL, Spong CY, Casey BM (Eds). Williams Obstetrics, 26th edition. New York: McGraw Hill; 2022. p. 356]

18. **c.** Both of the above
The standard intramuscular dose of anti-D immune globulin—300 µg or 1500 IU—will protect the average-sized mother from a fetal hemorrhage of up to 30 mL of fetal whole blood or 15 mL of fetal red cells.
[Reference: Fetal disorders. In: Cunningham FG, Leveno KJ, Dashe JS, Hoffman BL, Spong CY, Casey BM (Eds). Williams Obstetrics, 26th edition. New York: McGraw Hill; 2022. p. 356]

19. **c.** Consider her delivery on urgent basis
With significant feto-maternal hemorrhage, the most common presenting complaint is decreased fetal movement. A sinusoidal fetal heart rate pattern is infrequently seen but warrants immediate evaluation. Sonography may demonstrate elevated MCA peak systolic velocity, and indeed this is reported to be the most accurate predictor. Hydrops is an ominous finding. If the MCA peak systolic velocity is elevated or hydrops is identified, urgent fetal transfusion or delivery should be considered depending on the period of gestation.
[Reference: Fetal disorders. In: Cunningham FG, Leveno KJ, Dashe JS, Hoffman BL, Spong CY, Casey BM (Eds). Williams Obstetrics, 26th edition. New York: McGraw Hill; 2022. p. 358]

20. **b.** Sonographically measured skin thickness of >7 mm constitutes edema or anasarca
Hydrops is diagnosed by identifying two or more fetal effusions—pleural, pericardial, or ascites—or one effusion plus anasarca. Sonographically measured

skin thickness of >5 mm constitutes edema or anasarca. Placentomegaly is defined as placental thickness ≥4 cm in the second trimester or ≥6 cm in the third trimester (Society for Maternal–Fetal Medicine, 2015b). As hydrops progresses in severity, anasarca is an invariable feature and is usually accompanied by placentomegaly and hydramnios.
[Reference: Fetal disorders. In: Cunningham FG, Leveno KJ, Dashe JS, Hoffman BL, Spong CY, Casey BM (Eds). Williams Obstetrics, 26th edition. New York: McGraw Hill; 2022. p. 358]

21. **b.** 2 and 4 are correct
If fetal hydrops is found in association with red cell alloimmunization, it is termed immune, otherwise, it is nonimmune. In immune hydrops, there is transplacental passage of maternal antibodies that destroy fetal red cells. The resultant anemia stimulates marrow erythroid hyperplasia and extramedullary hematopoiesis in the spleen and liver. The incidence of immune hydrops has decreased dramatically with the advent of anti-D immune globulin and with use of MCA Doppler to aid anemia detection. At least 90 percent of cases of hydrops are nonimmune.
[Reference: Fetal disorders. In: Cunningham FG, Leveno KJ, Dashe JS, Hoffman BL, Spong CY, Casey BM (Eds). Williams Obstetrics, 26th edition. New York: McGraw Hill; 2022. p. 360]

22. **a.** 45,X: Turner syndrome
When nonimmune hydrops presents before 24 weeks' gestation, the most frequent aneuploidy is 45,X—Turner syndrome, and in such cases, the survival rate is <5 percent.
[Reference: Fetal disorders. In: Cunningham FG, Leveno KJ, Dashe JS, Hoffman BL, Spong CY, Casey BM (Eds). Williams Obstetrics, 26th edition. New York: McGraw Hill; 2022. p. 362]

23. **a.** Parvovirus B19
Categories and Etiologies of Nonimmune Hydrops Fetalis:

A. Cardiovascular
Structural defects: Ebstein anomaly, tetralogy of Fallot with absent pulmonary valve, hypoplastic left or right heart, premature closure of ductus arteriosus, arteriovenous malformation (vein of Galen aneurysm) Cardiomyopathies

B. Tachyarrhythmias
Bradycardia, as may occur in heterotaxy syndrome with endocardial cushion defect or with anti-Ro/La antibodies

C. Chromosomal
Turner syndrome (45,X), triploidy, trisomies 21, 18, and 13

D. Hematological
- Hemoglobinopathies, such as α4-thalassemia
- Erythrocyte enzyme and membrane disorders
- Erythrocyte aplasia/dyserythropoiesis
- Decreased erythrocyte production (myeloproliferative disorders)
- Fetomaternal hemorrhage

E. Lymphatic abnormalities
Cystic hygroma, systemic lymphangiectasis, pulmonary lymphangiectasis

F. Infections
Parvovirus B19, syphilis, cytomegalovirus, toxoplasmosis, rubella, enterovirus, varicella, herpes simplex, coxsackievirus, listeriosis, leptospirosis, Chagas disease, Lyme disease

G. Syndromic
Arthrogryposis multiplex congenita, lethal multiple pterygium, congenital lymphedema, myotonic dystrophy type I, Neu-Laxova, Noonan, and Pena-Shokeir syndromes

H. Thoracic Abnormalities
- Cystic adenomatoid malformation
- Pulmonary sequestration
- Diaphragmatic hernia
- Hydro/chylothorax
- Congenital high airway obstruction sequence (CHAOS)
- Mediastinal tumors
- Skeletal dysplasia with very small thorax

I. Gastrointestinal
Meconium peritonitis, gastrointestinal tract obstruction

J. Kidney and Urinary Tract
- Kidney malformations
- Bladder outlet obstructions
- Congenital (Finnish) nephrosis, Bartter syndrome, mesoblastic nephroma

K. Placental, Twin, and Cord Abnormalities
Placental chorioangioma, twin-twin transfusion syndrome, twin reversed arterial

Perfusion sequence, twin anemia polycythemia sequence, cord vessel thrombosis

L. Other Rare Disorders
Inborn errors of metabolism: Gaucher disease, galactosialidosis, GM1 gangliosidosis, sialidosis, mucopolysaccharidoses, mucolipidoses
Tumors: sacrococcygeal teratoma, hemangioendothelioma with Kasabach-Merritt syndrome

M. Idiopathic
Among the infectious etiology, the most common is Parvovirus B19.
[Reference: Fetal disorders. In: Cunningham FG, Leveno KJ, Dashe JS, Hoffman BL, Spong CY, Casey BM (Eds). Williams Obstetrics, 26th edition. New York: McGraw Hill; 2022. p. 360]

24. **d.** The etiology of fetal hydrops is related to the development of mirror syndrome.
The association between fetal hydrops and the development of maternal edema, in which the mother mirrors the fetus, is attributed to Ballantyne. He called the condition triple edema because the fetus, mother, and placenta all became edematous. Mirror syndrome has been reported to complicate at least 20 percent of hydrops cases. The etiology of the hydrops is not related to development of mirror syndrome.
[Reference: Fetal disorders. In: Cunningham FG, Leveno KJ, Dashe JS, Hoffman BL, Spong CY, Casey BM (Eds). Williams Obstetrics, 26th edition. New York: McGraw Hill; 2022. p. 364]

25. **d.** An antibody titer of ≥1:16 can be used to target intensive clinical monitoring.
Kell Alloimmunization:
- Transfusion history is important, as nearly 90 percent of Kell sensitization cases result from transfusion with Kell-positive blood.
- Kell sensitization may develop more rapidly and may be more severe than with sensitization to D and other blood group antigens.
- This is because Kell antibodies attach to erythrocyte precursors in the fetal bone marrow and thereby impair the normal hemopoietic response to anemia. With fewer erythrocytes produced, there is less hemolysis, and thus severe anemia may not be predicted by the maternal Kell antibody titer.
- Slootweg and colleagues (2018) reviewed 93 pregnancies with Kell alloimmunization in which the fetus was confirmed to be Kell-positive. They found that a titer of 1:4 had 100 percent sensitivity, 27 percent specificity, and 60 percent positive predictive value for transfusion requirement in the fetal or neonatal period.
- Given the potential for severe anemia, the American College of Obstetricians and Gynecologists (2019a) has recommended that antibody titers not be used to monitor Kell-sensitized pregnancies.

[References: Slootweg YM, Lindenburg IT, Koelewijn JM, Van Kamp IL, Oepkes D, De Haas M. Predicting anti-Kell-mediated hemolytic disease of the fetus and newborn: diagnostic accuracy of laboratory management. Am J Obstet Gynecol. 2018;219(4):393. e8.
Fetal disorders. In: Cunningham FG, Leveno KJ, Dashe JS, Hoffman BL, Spong CY, Casey BM (Eds). Williams Obstetrics, 26th edition. New York: McGraw Hill; 2022. p. 354]

26. **d.** ACOG (2019) recommended routine cfDNA in Rh-negative pregnancies
Noninvasive fetal D genotyping has been performed using cell-free DNA (cfDNA) from maternal plasma. The reported sensitivity exceeds 99 percent, the specificity exceeds 95 percent, and positive or negative predictive values are similarly very high. Two potential indications for cfDNA use in D-negative pregnant women are: (1) in the setting of D alloimmunization, testing can identify fetuses who are also D-negative and do not require anemia surveillance, and (2) in women without D alloimmunization, anti-D immune globulin might be withheld if the fetus is D negative. In the case of the latter, the American College of Obstetricians and Gynecologists (2019b) does not recommend routine cfDNA screening in D-negative pregnancies until it has been demonstrated to be cost-effective.
[Reference: Fetal disorders. In: Cunningham FG, Leveno KJ, Dashe JS, Hoffman BL, Spong CY, Casey BM (Eds). Williams Obstetrics, 26th edition. New York: McGraw Hill; 2022. p. 364]

27. **c.** Both antenatal and postnatal anti-D reduces sensitization to 2%
- Depending on the preparation, the half-life of anti-D immune globulin ranges from 16 to 24 days, and a standard 300-μg dose provides 12 weeks of protection against exposure to up to 30 mL of blood, of 15 mL of erythrocytes

- Routine postpartum administration of anti-D immune globulin to at-risk pregnancies within 72 hours of delivery lowers the alloimmunization rate by 90 percent. Additionally, provision of anti-D immune globulin at 28 weeks gestation reduces the third-trimester alloimmunization rate from approximately 2 percent to 0.1 percent
- Following delivery, anti-D immune globulin should be given within 72 hours. Administration of immune globulin is recommended only after the newborn is confirmed to be D positive (American College of Obstetricians and Gynecologists, 2019b).
- If immune globulin is inadvertently not administered following delivery, it should be given as soon as the omission is recognized, because there may be some protection up to 28 days postpartum
- Anti-D immune globulin may produce a weakly positive—1:1 to 1:4—indirect Coombs titer in the mother. This is harmless and should not be confused with development of alloimmunization.

[Reference: Fetal disorders. In: Cunningham FG, Leveno KJ, Dashe JS, Hoffman BL, Spong CY, Casey BM (Eds). Williams Obstetrics, 26th edition. New York: McGraw Hill; 2022. p. 364]

28. **d.** 1, 2, and 3

Reasons for failure of prophylaxis:
a. Dose too small
b. Dose too late > 72 hours
c. Patient already immunized but antibody titre too low for laboratory recognition
d. Defective immunoglobulin given
e. Inadequate dosing of anti-D
f. Missed prophylactic antenatal dose
g. Unrecognized Fetomaternal hemorrhage
h. Omission of Kell blood group typing

(Reference: ACOG Practice Bulletin, Prevention of Rh D Alloimmunization August 2017)

29. **d.** 1, 2, 3, and 4 are correct

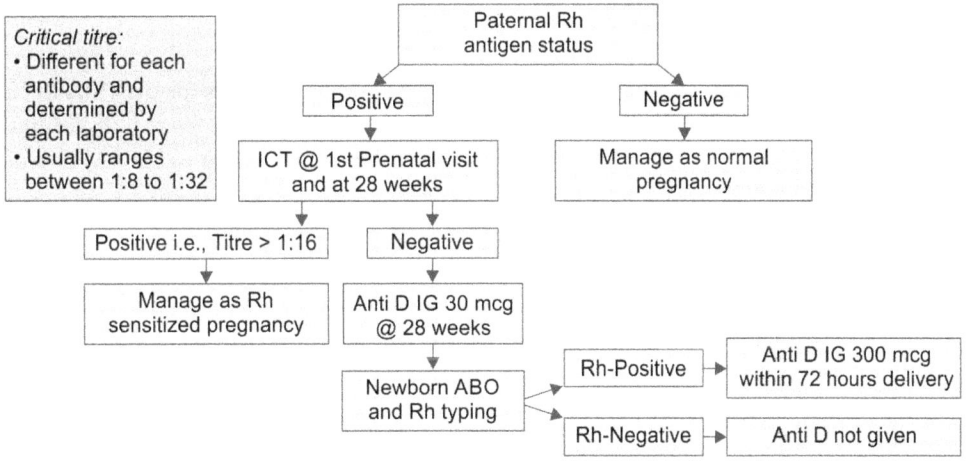

[Reference: James D, Steer P, Weiner CP, Gonik B, Crowther CA, Robson SC (Eds). High Risk Pregnancy: Management Options, 5th edition. USA: Elsevier Saunders; 2018]

30. **c.** Anti-D IGs

Treatment options for Rh Alloimmunized pregnancy:
1. **Intra uterine transfusion (IUT)**
   a. Intravascular transfusion
      - Placental Cord insertion (PCI)
      - Trans amniotic free loop
      - Intrahepatic
   b. Intraperitoneal transfusion
2. **Others**
   - Intravenous immunoglobulin,
   - Plasmapheresis

Anti-D immune globulin is indicated only in Rh-negative women who are not previously sensitized to D.

[Reference: Fetal disorders. In: Cunningham FG, Leveno KJ, Dashe JS, Hoffman BL, Spong CY, Casey BM (Eds). Williams Obstetrics, 26th edition. New York: McGraw Hill; 2022]

Chapter 29: Liver Dysfunction in Pregnancy

Shashi Lata Maheshwari (Kabra), Shakun Tyagi

QUESTIONS

Hepatic Disorders

1. Liver diseases specific to pregnancy are all, *except*:
   a. Hyperemesis gravidarum
   b. Intrahepatic cholestasis
   c. HELLP syndrome
   d. Autoimmune hepatitis

2. The usual level of bilirubin (in mg%) in intrahepatic cholestasis of pregnancy (ICP) is:
   a. 1–5
   b. 2–8
   c. 1–4
   d. 1–2

3. All are causes of acute liver failure in pregnancy, *except*:
   a. Acute fatty liver of pregnancy (AFLP)
   b. Fulminant viral hepatitis
   c. Autoimmune hepatitis
   d. Hyperemesis gravidarum

4. All features are common in pregnancy, *except*:
   a. Serum alkaline phosphatase levels
   b. Palmar erythema
   c. Spider angiomas
   d. Pruritus

5. Other names for intrahepatic cholestasis of pregnancy are all, *except*:
   a. Recurrent jaundice of pregnancy
   b. Cholestatic hepatitis
   c. Icterus gravidarum
   d. Gestational pruritus

6. All are true about the characteristics of pruritus in intrahepatic cholestasis, *except*:
   a. Generalized pruritus
   b. Shows predilection for the palms and soles
   c. Usually develops in late pregnancy
   d. Increases in the morning

7. The following are helpful in the diagnosis of ICP, *except*:
   a. Elevated total serum bile acid
   b. Elevated transaminase levels
   c. Pruritus
   d. Significant scratch marks

8. The risk of developing ICP in patients already suffering from hepatitis C is higher by how many times?
   a. 10
   b. 30
   c. 20
   d. 5

9. All are treatments for pruritus in ICP, *except*:
   a. Antihistamines
   b. Topical emollients
   c. Ursodeoxycholic acid
   d. Cholestyramine

10. Dose of ursodeoxycholic acid in ICP is:
    a. 5–10 mg/kg of weight
    b. 10–15 mg/kg of weight
    c. 20–30 mg/kg of weight
    d. 15–25 mg/kg of weight

11. The following are the actions of ursodeoxycholic acid in ICP, *except*:
    a. Decreases pruritus
    b. Decreases the incidence of stillbirth
    c. Decreases fetal distress
    d. Causes biochemical improvement

12. All are treatments for ICP, *except*:
    a. Ursodeoxycholic acid
    b. Cholestyramine
    c. Therapeutic plasma exchange
    d. Rifampin

13. Following comorbidities increase the risk of stillbirth in ICP, *except*:
    a. Gestational diabetes
    b. Preeclampsia
    c. Anemia in pregnancy
    d. Multifetal pregnancy

14. Following are the terminologies, which can be used for pregnant women with itching of normal skin, *except*?
    a. Mild ICP
    b. Moderate ICP
    c. Severe ICP
    d. Very severe ICP

15. The upper limit of normal bile acid concentrations in pregnancy is in (µmol/L):
    a. 18
    b. 10
    c. 14
    d. 20

16. What is the most common cause of acute liver failure during pregnancy?
    a. Intrahepatic cholestasis of pregnancy
    b. Acute fatty liver of pregnancy
    c. Autoimmune hepatitis
    d. Viral hepatitis

17. All are suggested as etiopathogenesis of acute fatty liver, *except*:
    a. Recessively inherited mitochondrial abnormalities of fatty acid oxidation
    b. G1528C and E474Q missense mutations of the gene on chromosome 2 that codes for long-chain 3-hydroxyacyl-CoA dehydrogenase (LCHAD) (Liu, 2017a)
    c. Autosomal dominant inheritance
    d. Mutations for medium-chain acyl-CoA dehydrogenase (MCAD) and for carnitine palmitoyl-transferase 1 (CPT1) deficiency

18. The most common time period for the appearance of acute fatty liver of pregnancy is:
    a. Third trimester
    b. Second trimester
    c. Late mid-trimester
    d. First trimester

19. The incidence of acute fatty liver of pregnancy in multiple pregnancies_____. Please choose the correct answer.
    a. Increases
    b. Decreases
    c. Remains same as in singleton pregnancy
    d. Decreases in dizygotic twins and increases in monozygotic twins

20. Pregnant woman with acute fatty liver of pregnancy can have all, *except*:
    a. Preeclampsia
    b. Hyperglycemia
    c. Epigastric pain
    d. Nausea/vomiting

21. In Swansea criteria for AFLP diagnosis, all clinical features are included, *except*:
    a. Abdominal pain
    b. Encephalopathy
    c. Polydipsia
    d. Polyphagia

22. The histologic pathognomonic of AFLP is:
    a. Perihepatic necrosis
    b. Zonal coagulative necrosis
    c. Massive or submassive steatosis
    d. Microvesicular steatosis

23. Cause of hemolysis in AFLP is:
    a. Effect of liver injury
    b. Effect of kidney injury
    c. Effect of endothelial injury
    d. Effect of hypercholesterolemia

24. All can be observed in blood and peripheral blood smear tests in acute fatty liver of pregnancy, *except*:
    a. Leukocytosis
    b. Burr cells
    c. Nucleated red cells
    d. Echinocytosis

25. Transient diabetes insipidus can be seen in:
    a. Intrahepatic cholestasis of pregnancy
    b. Acute fatty liver of pregnancy
    c. Autoimmune hepatitis
    d. Pancreatitis

26. Causes of maternal death in acute fatty liver of pregnancy are all, *except*:
    a. Liver failure
    b. Aspiration
    c. Renal failure
    d. Splenic rupture

27. Regarding hepatitis, all are RNA viruses, *except*:
    a. Hepatitis virus A
    b. Hepatitis virus B
    c. Hepatitis virus C
    d. Hepatitis virus D

28. All are true about Wilson's disease, *except*:
    a. Caused by copper overload
    b. Autosomal recessive mutations are responsible
    c. The disease can manifest with cardiomyopathy
    d. There is no endocrine abnormality

29. All pregnancy complications may occur in Wilson's disease, *except*:
    a. Infertility
    b. Spontaneous abortions
    c. Birth defects
    d. Liver disease

30. A Kayser–Fleischer ring surrounding the iris is highly specific of which disease?
    a. Nonalcoholic fatty liver disease
    b. Acute fatty liver of pregnancy
    c. Wilson's disease
    d. Autoimmune hepatitis

Biliary and Pancreatic Disease in Pregnancy

31. Alkaline phosphatase levels in pregnancy:
    a. Does not change
    b. Reduces
    c. Can increase up to three times the normal
    d. May increase or fall in pregnancy

32. **Following symptomatic cholelithiasis in pregnant patients should be operated in case of the following situations:**
    a. Immediately in case of any symptomatic cholelithiasis
    b. After 48 hours of detecting cholelithiasis
    c. Second trimester in case of multiple stones <1 cm
    d. Single large stone >2 cm

33. **Complication of cholecystitis in the third trimester of pregnancy is:**
    a. Preeclampsia
    b. Anemia
    c. Postdated pregnancy
    d. Preterm labor

34. **Recurrent severe pancreatitis in pregnancy:**
    a. Can result in stillbirth and preterm delivery
    b. Can result in jaundice
    c. Mimic preeclampsia
    d. Always requires urgent delivery of the baby

35. **Women with intrahepatic cholestasis of pregnancy (IHCP) are more prone to cholelithiasis:**
    a. False statement
    b. True due to increased hemolysis in IHCP
    c. True due to structural pathology in the biliary system
    d. True due to the abnormality of bile acid metabolism

36. **Delivery in case of pancreatitis:**
    a. Should be performed immediately
    b. Should be performed by cesarean section preferably
    c. Should be performed if no improvement of clinical or laboratory parameters near-term gestation
    d. Increases the chances of jaundice

37. **Laparoscopic cholecystectomy can be safely performed in pregnancy:**
    a. In the first trimester
    b. In midsecond trimester
    c. In the third trimester
    d. In all trimesters

38. **Normal lipase levels in pregnancy are:**
    a. Same as nonpregnant level
    b. More than nonpregnant level
    c. Less than nonpregnant level
    d. May be more or lower than nonpregnant level

39. **Normal amylase levels in pregnancy are:**
    a. Same as nonpregnant level
    b. More than nonpregnant level
    c. Less than nonpregnant level
    d. May be more or lower than nonpregnant level

40. **Acute pancreatitis is diagnosed in pregnancy based on:**
    a. Only amylase and lipase levels
    b. Pain and amylase and lipase levels
    c. Pain, fever, leukocytosis, and amylase lipase levels
    d. Pain, fever, leukocytosis, hyperglycemia, and amylase lipase levels

41. **Endoscopic retrograde cholangiopancreatography (ERCP) in pregnancy is:**
    a. Absolutely contraindicated
    b. May be performed with minimum radiation exposure if lifesaving
    c. Can always be replaced with magnetic resonance cholangiopancreatography (MRCP)
    d. Does not result in pancreatitis

42. **The most important association of pancreatitis in pregnancy is:**
    a. Alcohol
    b. Cholelithiasis
    c. Trauma
    d. Thrombosis

43. **Second trimester onward gallbladder size in pregnancy:**
    a. Reduces to half
    b. Remains same
    c. Double the nonpregnant size
    d. May increase or decrease

44. **Ascending cholangitis is suspected in case of biliary obstruction by the presence of the following symptoms:**
    a. Jaundice, abdominal pain, and fever
    b. Jaundice, itching, clay-colored stools
    c. Jaundice, itching, coagulopathy
    d. Jaundice, fever, and itching

ANSWERS

1. **d.** Autoimmune hepatitis
Liver diseases complicating pregnancy are placed into three general categories. The first includes those specific to pregnancy and resolve either spontaneously or following delivery. Hyperemesis gravidarum, intrahepatic cholestasis, acute fatty liver, and HELLP syndrome—which is characterized by hemolysis, elevated liver enzyme levels, and low platelet counts, are examples. The second category involves acute hepatic disorders that are coincidental to pregnancy, such as acute viral hepatitis. Last are chronic liver diseases that predate pregnancy, such

as chronic viral or autoimmune hepatitis, cirrhosis, or esophageal varices.
[Reference: Cunningham FG, Leveno KJ, Dashe JS, Hoffman BL, Spong CY, Casey BM (Eds). Williams Obstetrics, 26th edition. New York: McGraw Hill; 2022. p. 2675]

2. **a.** 1–5
Serum bilirubin value in intrahepatic cholestasis of pregnancy is usually between 1 and 5 mg%.
   1–5 mg% is seen in hyperemesis gravidarum.
   Acute fatty liver of pregnancy shows serum bilirubin 2–8 mg%
   HELLP syndrome usually has 1–2 mg% of bilirubin.
[Reference: Cunningham FG, Leveno KJ, Dashe JS, Hoffman BL, Spong CY, Casey BM (Eds). Williams Obstetrics, 26th edition. New York: McGraw Hill; 2022. p. 2677]

3. **d.** Hyperemesis gravidarum
Hyperemesis gravidarum is not associated with liver failure.
   Liver failure is uncommon during pregnancy. Of the various causes, drug-induced liver injury (DILI) is probably the most frequent nonpregnancy-related etiology. Acetaminophen toxicity is the most prevalent cause in the United States. Other sources of liver failure include acute fatty liver of pregnancy, fulminant viral hepatitis, environmental toxins, autoimmune hepatitis, shock liver, and alternative medicines. In a highly selective study of 70 referred women with hepatic encephalopathy, half were caused by AFLP, and half were associated with HELLP syndrome.
[Reference: Cunningham FG, Leveno KJ, Dashe JS, Hoffman BL, Spong CY, Casey BM (Eds). Williams Obstetrics, 26th edition. New York: McGraw Hill; 2022. p. 2678]

4. **d.** Pruritus
Pruritus is seen in specific diseases like intrahepatic cholestasis of pregnancy. Several normal pregnancy-induced physiological changes induce appreciable liver-related clinical and laboratory manifestations. Abnormalities such as increased serum alkaline phosphatase levels, palmar erythema, and spider angiomas are common during normal pregnancy.
[Reference: Cunningham FG, Leveno KJ, Dashe JS, Hoffman BL, Spong CY, Casey BM (Eds). Williams Obstetrics, 26th edition. New York: McGraw Hill; 2022. p. 2677]

5. **d.** Gestational pruritus
Gestational pruritus is a symptom, not an alternative name for intrahepatic cholestasis of pregnancy.
   All remaining names are alternative names of ICP.
[Reference: Cunningham FG, Leveno KJ, Dashe JS, Hoffman BL, Spong CY, Casey BM (Eds). Williams Obstetrics, 26th edition. New York: McGraw Hill; 2022. p. 2679]

6. **d.** Increases in the morning
Generalized pruritus that shows a predilection for the palms and soles usually develops in late pregnancy or occasionally earlier.
[Reference: Cunningham FG, Leveno KJ, Dashe JS, Hoffman BL, Spong CY, Casey BM (Eds). Williams Obstetrics, 26th edition. New York: McGraw Hill; 2022. p. 2680]

7. **d.** Significant scratch marks
Scratch marks are not significant in intrahepatic cholestasis of pregnancy. Serum transaminase and bile acid levels are measured in women with suspected ICP. As a threshold for comparison, total serum bile acid levels typically remain <10 μmol/L throughout normal pregnancy. Elevated total serum bile acid or transaminase levels plus pruritus support an ICP diagnosis. Biochemical tests may be abnormal at presentation or may follow initial pruritus after several weeks. Moreover, a rise in transaminase levels may precede an increase in serum bile acid levels.
   Approximately 10% of women have concurrent jaundice.
[Reference: Cunningham FG, Leveno KJ, Dashe JS, Hoffman BL, Spong CY, Casey BM (Eds). Williams Obstetrics, 26th edition. New York: McGraw Hill; 2022. p. 2680]

8. **c.** 20
Underlying chronic hepatitis C is associated with a significantly greater risk of developing intrahepatic cholestasis of pregnancy, which may be as much as 20-fold higher.
[Reference: Cunningham FG, Leveno KJ, Dashe JS, Hoffman BL, Spong CY, Casey BM (Eds). Williams Obstetrics, 26th edition. New York: McGraw Hill; 2022. p. 2680]

9. **d.** Cholestyramine
Pruritus may be troublesome and is thought to result from elevated serum bile salt concentrations. Antihistamines and topical emollients usually provide some relief. Cholestyramine is reported to be

effective, but this compound also lowers absorption of fat-soluble vitamins. This may lead to vitamin K deficiency and fetal coagulopathy. Subsequent fetal intracranial hemorrhage and stillbirth have been reported.
[Reference: Cunningham FG, Leveno KJ, Dashe JS, Hoffman BL, Spong CY, Casey BM (Eds). Williams Obstetrics, 26th edition. New York: McGraw Hill; 2022. p. 2680]

10. **b.** 10–15 mg/kg of weight
Currently, the most popular treatment is ursodeoxycholic acid, which relieves pruritus and reduces serum levels of bile salts and liver enzymes. It is available as 300 mg capsules. Oral dosing is 10–15 mg/kg maternal body weight daily, which is divided into two or three doses.
[Reference: Cunningham FG, Leveno KJ, Dashe JS, Hoffman BL, Spong CY, Casey BM (Eds). Williams Obstetrics, 26th edition. New York: McGraw Hill; 2022. p. 2680]

11. **d.** Causes biochemical improvement
Pruritus typically improves after 2–3 weeks of ursodeoxycholic acid therapy. Such treatment has also been reported to lower risks for stillbirth and fetal distress.
[Reference: Cunningham FG, Leveno KJ, Dashe JS, Hoffman BL, Spong CY, Casey BM (Eds). Williams Obstetrics, 26th edition. New York: McGraw Hill; 2022. p. 2681]

12. **b.** Cholestyramine
Pruritus typically improves after 2–3 weeks of ursodeoxycholic acid therapy. Such treatment has also been reported to lower risks for stillbirth and fetal distress. Other described treatments include therapeutic plasma exchange and rifampin. A randomized trial comparing ursodeoxycholic acid and rifampin is underway.
[Reference: Cunningham FG, Leveno KJ, Dashe JS, Hoffman BL, Spong CY, Casey BM (Eds). Williams Obstetrics, 26th edition. New York: McGraw Hill; 2022. p. 2681]

13. **c.** Anemia in pregnancy
The presence of risk factors or comorbidities (such as gestational diabetes and/or preeclampsia and/or multifetal pregnancy) appears to increase the risk of stillbirth and may influence decision-making around timing of planned birth (Grade D).
[Reference: Girling J, Knight CL, Chappell L; Royal College of Obstetricians and Gynaecologists. Intrahepatic cholestasis of pregnancy: Green-top Guideline No. 43 June 2022. BJOG. 2022;129(13):e95-e114]

14. **d.** Very severe ICP
Very severe intrahepatic cholestasis of pregnancy is not used in any terminology of ICP.

Diagnosis	Clinical features
Gestational pruritus	Itching and peak bile acid concentrations <19 µmol/L*
Mild ICP	Itching and raised peak bile acid concentrations 19–39 µmol/L
Moderate ICP	Itching and raised peak bile acid concentrations 40–99 µmol/L
Severe ICP	Itching and raised peak bile acid concentrations ≥100 µmol/L

*The upper limit of normal bile acid concentrations in pregnancy is 18 µmol/L.
Note: Peak bile acid concentrations refer to the highest bile acid concentration recorded during a woman's pregnancy. Thus, a woman's diagnosis may progress in pregnancy severity during pregnancy.
(ICP: intrahepatic cholestasis of pregnancy)

[Reference: Girling J, Knight CL, Chappell L; Royal College of Obstetricians and Gynaecologists. Intrahepatic cholestasis of pregnancy: Green-top Guideline No. 43 June 2022. BJOG. 2022;129(13): e95-e114]

15. **a.** 18

Diagnosis	Clinical features
Gestational pruritus	Itching and peak bile acid concentrations <19 µmol/L*
Mild ICP	Itching and raised peak bile acid concentrations 19–39 µmol/L
Moderate ICP	Itching and raised peak bile acid concentrations 40–99 µmol/L
Severe ICP	Itching and raised peak bile acid concentrations ≥100 µmol/L

*The upper limit of normal bile acid concentrations in pregnancy is 18 µmol/L.
Note: Peak bile acid concentrations refer to the highest bile acid concentration recorded during a woman's pregnancy. Thus, a woman's diagnosis may progress in pregnancy severity during pregnancy.
(ICP: intrahepatic cholestasis of pregnancy)

[Reference: Girling J, Knight CL, Chappell L; Royal College of Obstetricians and Gynaecologists. Intrahepatic cholestasis of pregnancy: Green-top Guideline No. 43 June 2022. BJOG. 2022;129(13): e95-e114]

16. **b.** Acute fatty liver of pregnancy
The most frequent cause of acute liver failure during pregnancy is acute fatty liver also called acute fatty metamorphosis or acute yellow atrophy. It is characterized by accumulation of microvesicular fat that literally "crowds out" normal hepatocytic function. Grossly, the liver is small, soft, yellow, and greasy. In its worst form, the incidence approximates 1 case per 10,000 births. Acute fatty liver of pregnancy recurring in subsequent pregnancy is rare.
(Reference: Williams Obstetrics. 26th edition, Page 2657-58)

17. **c.** Autosomal dominant inheritance
Although the underlying cause remains unclear, many cases of acute fatty liver of pregnancy are associated with recessively inherited mitochondrial abnormalities of fatty acid oxidation. Several mutations for the mitochondrial trifunctional protein enzyme complex that catalyzes the last oxidative steps in the pathway are implicated. The most common are the G1528C and E474Q missense mutations of the gene on chromosome 2 that codes for long-chain 3-hydroxyacyl-CoA dehydrogenase (LCHAD) (Liu, 2017a). Mutations for medium-chain acyl-CoA dehydrogenase (MCAD) and for carnitine palmitoyltransferase 1 (CPT1) deficiency are others. These are similar to mutations in children with Reye-like syndromes.
[Reference: Cunningham FG, Leveno KJ, Dashe JS, Hoffman BL, Spong CY, Casey BM (Eds). Williams Obstetrics, 26th edition. New York: McGraw Hill; 2022. p. 2683]

18. **a.** This is the most common observation.
[Reference: Cunningham FG, Leveno KJ, Dashe JS, Hoffman BL, Spong CY, Casey BM (Eds). Williams Obstetrics, 26th edition. New York: McGraw Hill; 2022. p. 2684]

19. **a.** Increases
Women with a multifetal gestation account for 20% of cases (Vigil-De Gracia, 2011), which are more than the incidence of acute fatty liver of pregnancy in singleton pregnancy.
[Reference: Cunningham FG, Leveno KJ, Dashe JS, Hoffman BL, Spong CY, Casey BM (Eds). Williams Obstetrics, 26th edition. New York: McGraw Hill; 2022. p. 2684]

20. **b.** Hyperglycemia
These patients have hypoglycemia.
Nausea/vomiting is one of the most common symptoms of acute fatty liver of pregnancy.
Half of affected women have hypertension, proteinuria, and edema, alone or in combination. Notably, these signs also suggest preeclampsia.
[Reference: Cunningham FG, Leveno KJ, Dashe JS, Hoffman BL, Spong CY, Casey BM (Eds). Williams Obstetrics, 26th edition. New York: McGraw Hill; 2022. p. 2684]

21. **d.** Polyphagia

Clinical features
Vomiting
Abdominal pain
Encephalopathy
Polydipsia/polyuria
Laboratory features
Bilirubin >0.8 mg/dL
Glucose <72 mg/dL
WBC >11,000/µL
AST or ALT >42 U/L
AKI or Cr >1.7 mg/dL
Ammonia >47 µmol/L
Coagulopathy or PT >14 s
Urea >340 µmol/L
Ultrasound features
Ascites or echogenic liver
Histologic features
Microvesicular steatosis

Note: The presence of six or more features without another explanation for them supports a diagnosis of AFLP.
(AFLP: acute fatty liver of pregnancy; AKI: acute kidney injury; ALT: alanine transaminase; AST: aspartate transaminase; Cr: creatinine; PT: protime; WBC: white blood cell count)

[Reference: Cunningham FG, Leveno KJ, Dashe JS, Hoffman BL, Spong CY, Casey BM (Eds). Williams Obstetrics, 26th edition. New York: McGraw Hill; 2022. p. 2686]

22. **d.** Microvesicular steatosis

Clinical features
Vomiting
Abdominal pain
Encephalopathy
Polydipsia/polyuria
Laboratory features
Bilirubin >0.8 mg/dL
Glucose <72 mg/dL
WBC >11,000/µL
AST or ALT >42 U/L
AKI or Cr >1.7 mg/dL
Ammonia >47 µmol/L
Coagulopathy or PT >14 s
Urea >340 µmol/L
Ultrasound features
Ascites or echogenic liver
Histologic features
Microvesicular steatosis
Note: The presence of six or more features without another explanation for them supports a diagnosis of AFLP. (AFLP: acute fatty liver of pregnancy; AKI: acute kidney injury; ALT: alanine transaminase; AST: aspartate transaminase; Cr: creatinine; PT: protime; WBC: white blood cell count)

[Reference: Cunningham FG, Leveno KJ, Dashe JS, Hoffman BL, Spong CY, Casey BM (Eds). Williams Obstetrics, 26th edition. New York: McGraw Hill; 2022. p. 2686]

23. **d.** Effect of hypercholesterolemia
Hemolysis can be severe and is thought to stem from effects of hypocholesterolemia on erythrocyte membranes.
[Reference: Cunningham FG, Leveno KJ, Dashe JS, Hoffman BL, Spong CY, Casey BM (Eds). Williams Obstetrics, 26th edition. New York: McGraw Hill; 2022. p. 2686]

24. **b.** Burr cells
Laboratory evidence includes leukocytosis, nucleated red cells, mild to moderate thrombocytopenia, and increased serum levels of lactic acid dehydrogenase (LDH) or decreased haptoglobin levels. The peripheral blood smear demonstrates echinocytosis. Burr cells are not seen in acute fatty liver of pregnancy.
[Reference: Cunningham FG, Leveno KJ, Dashe JS, Hoffman BL, Spong CY, Casey BM (Eds). Williams Obstetrics, 26th edition. New York: McGraw Hill; 2022. p. 2686]

25. **b.** Acute fatty liver of pregnancy
Hepatic function usually returns to normal within a week postpartum, but in the interim, intensive medical support may be required. Two associated conditions can be seen during this time. Perhaps a fourth of women have evidence of transient diabetes insipidus. This presumably stems from elevated vasopressinase concentrations caused by diminished hepatic production of its inactivating enzyme. Second, acute pancreatitis develops in approximately 20%.
[Reference: Cunningham FG, Leveno KJ, Dashe JS, Hoffman BL, Spong CY, Casey BM (Eds). Williams Obstetrics, 26th edition. New York: McGraw Hill; 2022. p. 2688]

26. **d.** Splenic rupture
Maternal deaths are caused by liver failure, sepsis, hemorrhage, aspiration, renal failure, pancreatitis, and gastrointestinal bleeding. Splenic rupture does not happen in acute fatty liver of pregnancy.
[Reference: Cunningham FG, Leveno KJ, Dashe JS, Hoffman BL, Spong CY, Casey BM (Eds). Williams Obstetrics, 26th edition. New York: McGraw Hill; 2022. p. 2688]

27. **b.** Hepatitis virus B
Hepatitis B virus is double-stranded DNA virus and is transmitted by exposure to blood or other body fluids from infected individuals. Hepatitis A virus (HAV) is an RNA picornavirus and is transmitted by the fecal–oral route and usually by contaminated food or water ingestion. Hepatitis C infection stems from a single-stranded RNA virus. Transmission is via blood and other body fluids, although sexual transmission is inefficient. Hepatitis D is a defective RNA virus that is a hybrid particle with a hepatitis B surface antigen (HBsAg) coat and a delta core. The hepatitis D virus (HDV) must coinfect with hepatitis B virus (HBV) either simultaneously or secondarily, and transmission is similar to HBV.
[Reference: Cunningham FG, Leveno KJ, Dashe JS, Hoffman BL, Spong CY, Casey BM (Eds). Williams Obstetrics, 26th edition. New York: McGraw Hill; 2022. p. 2693]

28. **d.** There is no endocrine abnormality.
Wilson's disease can manifest with endocrine abnormality.

It is caused by copper overload leading to chronic hepatitis and cirrhosis. Autosomal recessive mutations of the *ATP7B* gene underlie this disorder. This gene codes for the P-type ATPase involved in copper transport to ceruloplasmin and bile. This systemic condition can also manifest with cardiomyopathy, renal disease, neuropsychiatric symptoms, and certain endocrine abnormalities.
[Reference: Cunningham FG, Leveno KJ, Dashe JS, Hoffman BL, Spong CY, Casey BM (Eds). Williams Obstetrics, 26th edition. New York: McGraw Hill; 2022. p. 2700]

29. **c.** Birth defects
Birth defects were not increased with chelation treatment. With Wilson's disease, infertility may be present, but pregnancy outcomes among affected women are influenced by disease severity. In one multicenter study of 282 pregnancies, the miscarriage rate was 26%, and 6% of the women had worsening liver disease.
[Reference: Cunningham FG, Leveno KJ, Dashe JS, Hoffman BL, Spong CY, Casey BM (Eds). Williams Obstetrics, 26th edition. New York: McGraw Hill; 2022. p. 2701]

30. **c.** Wilson's disease
A Kayser–Fleischer ring surrounding the iris is highly specific of Wilson's disease, but a suspected diagnosis generally requires subsequent genetic analysis confirmation.
[Reference: Cunningham FG, Leveno KJ, Dashe JS, Hoffman BL, Spong CY, Casey BM (Eds). Williams Obstetrics, 26th edition. New York: McGraw Hill; 2022. p. 2701]

31. **c.** Can increase up to three times the normal
Serum alkaline phosphate levels may increase up to three times in pregnancy due to the contribution from placental alkaline phosphatase.
[Reference: Appendix 1: Serum and blood constituents. In: Cunningham FG, Leveno KJ, Dashe JS, Hoffman BL, Spong CY, Casey BM (Eds). Williams Obstetrics, 26th edition. New York: McGraw Hill; 2022. p. 3196]

32. **a.** Immediately in case of any symptomatic cholelithiasis
In acute cases, medical therapy consists of intravenous fluids, antibiotics, analgesics, and in some instances, nasogastric suction. Surgical therapy follows, and laparoscopic cholecystectomy is the preferred route for most.
Symptomatic cholelithiasis is common in pregnancy. Othman and colleagues (2012) showed that gravidas managed conservatively had greater pain, more recurrent emergency department visits, more hospitalizations, and higher cesarean delivery rate. Dhupar and associates (2010) reported more complications with conservative management of gallbladder disease compared with laparoscopic cholecystectomy in pregnancy. These included multiple admissions, prolonged total parenteral nutrition (TPN), and unplanned labor induction for worsening gallbladder symptoms. Therefore, operative and endoscopic interventions are increasingly favored over conservative measures.
[Reference: Cunningham FG, Leveno KJ, Dashe JS, Hoffman BL, Spong CY, Casey BM (Eds). Williams Obstetrics, 26th edition. New York: McGraw Hill; 2022. p. 2708]

33. **d.** Preterm labor
If cholecystitis occurs later in pregnancy, preterm labor is more likely.
[Reference: Cunningham FG, Leveno KJ, Dashe JS, Hoffman BL, Spong CY, Casey BM (Eds). Williams Obstetrics, 26th edition. New York: McGraw Hill; 2022. p. 2707]

34. **a.** Can result in stillbirth and preterm delivery
The increasing severity of pancreatitis is associated with adverse maternal and fetal outcomes. In one review of 101 pancreatitis cases, Eddy and coworkers (2008) found a 30% preterm delivery rate, and 11% were delivered before 35 weeks' gestation. There were also 4% stillbirths. There were two pancreatitis-related maternal deaths. Importantly, almost a third of women had recurrent pancreatitis during pregnancy. In another study of 342 pregnancies complicated by pancreatitis, preterm delivery and fetal mortality rates were comparable to the data from Eddy.
[Reference: Cunningham FG, Leveno KJ, Dashe JS, Hoffman BL, Spong CY, Casey BM (Eds). Williams Obstetrics, 26th edition. New York: McGraw Hill; 2022. p. 2712]

35. **d.** True due to the abnormality of bile acid metabolism
Liver biopsy shows mild cholestasis with bile plugs in the hepatocytes and canaliculi of the centrilobular regions in intrahepatic cholestasis of pregnancy (IHCP).

[Reference: Cunningham FG, Leveno KJ, Dashe JS, Hoffman BL, Spong CY, Casey BM (Eds). Williams Obstetrics, 26th edition. New York: McGraw Hill; 2022. p. 2679]

36. **c.** Should be performed if no improvement of clinical or laboratory parameters near-term gestation

    Increasing severity of pancreatitis is associated with adverse maternal and fetal outcomes. In one review of 101 pancreatitis cases, Eddy and coworkers (2008) found a 30% preterm delivery rate, and 11% were delivered before 35 weeks' gestation. There were also 4% stillbirths.
    [Reference: Cunningham FG, Leveno KJ, Dashe JS, Hoffman BL, Spong CY, Casey BM (Eds). Williams Obstetrics, 26th edition. New York: McGraw Hill; 2022. p. 2712]

37. **d.** In all trimesters

    When first used, 26–28 weeks became the upper gestational age limit recommended. However, as experience has accrued, many now describe laparoscopic surgery performed in the third trimester. In one report, a third of gravidas undergoing laparoscopic cholecystectomy or appendectomy were >26 weeks' gestation. No serious adverse sequelae are linked to these procedures, and laparoscopy can safely be performed in all trimesters.
    [Reference: Cunningham FG, Leveno KJ, Dashe JS, Hoffman BL, Spong CY, Casey BM (Eds). Williams Obstetrics, 26th edition. New York: McGraw Hill; 2022. p. 2260]

38. **b.** More than nonpregnant level

    The normal level of Lipase in non-pregnant adults is 0–160 U/L but it is lower during pregnancy. First trimester 0–104 U/L; Second trimester 0–140; Third Trimester 5–148.
    [Reference: Appendix 1: Serum and blood constituents. In: Cunningham FG, Leveno KJ, Dashe JS, Hoffman BL, Spong CY, Casey BM (Eds). Williams Obstetrics, 26th edition. New York: McGraw Hill; 2022. p. 3196]

39. **a.** Same as nonpregnant level

    Normal Amylase level in non-pregnant adults is 20–96 U/L. Although there is a slight fall in the second trimester (16–73 U/L) the level in pregnancy (First trimester: 24–83 U/L and third trimester (15–81U/L) are essentially similar to the non-pregnant level.
    [Reference: Appendix 1: Serum and blood constituents. In: Cunningham FG, Leveno KJ, Dashe JS, Hoffman BL, Spong CY, Casey BM (Eds). Williams Obstetrics, 26th edition. New York: McGraw Hill; 2022. p. 3196]

40. **a.** Only amylase and lipase levels

    Serum lipase levels are preferred for diagnosis; however, serum amylase levels can also be used.
    [Reference: Cunningham FG, Leveno KJ, Dashe JS, Hoffman BL, Spong CY, Casey BM (Eds). Williams Obstetrics, 26th edition. New York: McGraw Hill; 2022. p. 2710]

41. **b.** May be performed with minimum radiation exposure if lifesaving

    Symptomatic biliary duct gallstones during pregnancy can be retrieved by endoscopic retrograde cholangiopancreatography (ERCP). The procedure is performed if common duct obstruction is suspected or proven. ERCP can be modified in many cases so that radiation exposure from fluoroscopy is avoided. If standard fluoroscopy is used, a lead apron shield is placed between the radiation source and the fetus.
    [Reference: Cunningham FG, Leveno KJ, Dashe JS, Hoffman BL, Spong CY, Casey BM (Eds). Williams Obstetrics, 26th edition. New York: McGraw Hill; 2022. p. 2710]

42. **b.** Cholelithiasis

    In nonpregnant patients, alcohol and cholelithiasis are equally associated with pancreatitis but in pregnancy cholelithiasis is almost always the predisposing condition.
    [Reference: Cunningham FG, Leveno KJ, Dashe JS, Hoffman BL, Spong CY, Casey BM (Eds). Williams Obstetrics, 26th edition. New York: McGraw Hill; 2022. p. 2711]

43. **c.** Double the nonpregnant size

    After the first trimester, the gallbladder fasting volume and the residual volume after postprandial emptying are doubled.
    [Reference: Cunningham FG, Leveno KJ, Dashe JS, Hoffman BL, Spong CY, Casey BM (Eds). Williams Obstetrics, 26th edition. New York: McGraw Hill; 2022. p. 2708]

44. **a.** Jaundice, abdominal pain, and fever

    Nearly 70% of affected patients of ascending cholangitis develop Charcot triad—jaundice, abdominal pain, and fever.
    [Reference: Cunningham FG, Leveno KJ, Dashe JS, Hoffman BL, Spong CY, Casey BM (Eds). Williams Obstetrics, 26th edition. New York: McGraw Hill; 2022. p. 2710]

Chapter 30: Renal Disorders in Pregnancy

Kavita Mandrelle Bhatti

QUESTIONS

1. All the following renal changes occur during normal pregnancy, *except:*
   a. Dilatation of the renal calyces and pelvis
   b. Increase in renal plasma flow by 80%
   c. Increase in glomerular filtration rate by 65%
   d. Fall in serum concentrations of creatinine and urea

2. All the following complications in pregnancy can cause renal failure, *except:*
   a. Septic abortion
   b. Accidental hemorrhage
   c. Uncomplicated heart disease
   d. Eclampsia

3. A 24-year-old G2P1 comes for her first prenatal visit at 13 weeks of gestation. The urine culture showed > 10,000 *Escherichia coli* bacteria/mL of urine. The woman does not have any symptoms. Which of the following is the best course of action for this patient?
   a. Observation; no treatment required
   b. Initiate antibiotic therapy empirically
   c. Initiate antibiotic therapy based on the sensitivity
   d. Initiate treatment when the patient develops symptoms

4. Asymptomatic bacteriuria in pregnancy may be associated with an increased risk of the following, *except:*
   a. Maternal anemia   b. Hypertension
   c. Low birth weight   d. Renal failure

5. Acute renal failure may be encountered in the following complications of pregnancy, *except:*
   a. Eclampsia
   b. Gestational diabetes mellitus
   c. Severe postpartum hemorrhage
   d. Septic abortion

6. Nephrotic syndrome is characterized by the following, *except:*
   a. Proteinuria   b. Hypoalbuminemia
   c. Hyperlipidemia   d. Bacteriuria

7. The most common organism that causes asymptomatic bacteriuria is:
   a. *E. coli*   b. *Pseudomonas*
   c. *Proteus*   d. *Klebsiella*

8. Ideal time to screen a pregnant woman for asymptomatic bacteriuria:
   a. First trimester   b. Second trimester
   c. Early third trimester   d. Late third trimester

9. Gold standard to detect bacteriuria in pregnancy:
   a. Urine microscopy   b. Nitrite test
   c. Leukocyte esterase test   d. Urine culture test

10. Frequent Screening for asymptomatic bacteriuria is recommended for following, *except:*
    a. Previous history of asymptomatic bacteriuria
    b. Pre-existing renal disease
    c. Preeclampsia
    d. Renal Calculi

11. Risk of persistence of infection after treatment with antibiotics in a case of asymptomatic bacteriuria is:
    a. 20%   b. 30%
    c. 40%   d. 50%

12. Which statement is wrong for asymptomatic bacteriuria:
    a. Undiagnosed and untreated asymptomatic bacteriuria can progress to acute cystitis
    b. Acute cystitis can occur in 10% cases of untreated asymptomatic bacteriuria
    c. Cystitis presents with dysuria, urgency, fever, and hematuria
    d. Cystitis can progress to pyelonephritis

13. Acute pyelonephritis is a more common occurrence in:
    a. First trimester
    b. Second trimester
    c. Early third trimester
    d. Late third trimester

14. The most common organism which can cause pyelonephritis is:
    a. *Proteus*
    b. *Klebsiella*
    c. *E. coli*
    d. *Pseudomonas*

15. The mainstay of diagnosis of acute pyelonephritis is:
    a. Imaging
    b. Urine examination
    c. Blood culture
    d. Hemogram

16. Management of acute pyelonephritis includes the following, *except*:
    a. Intravenous hydration
    b. Antimicrobial therapy
    c. Hospitalization
    d. Induction of labor

17. Complications of pyelonephritis include all, *except*:
    a. Miscarriage
    b. Preterm labor
    c. Intrauterine fetal demise
    d. Preeclampsia

18. Nephrotic syndrome is characterized by the presence of proteinuria in excess of:
    a. 1 g per day
    b. 2 g per day
    c. 3 g per day
    d. 4 g per day

19. Acute pyelonephritis is more common:
    a. Left side renal involvement
    b. Right side renal involvement
    c. Bilateral involvement
    d. Both side involvement is equal affected

20. Acute renal failure is characterized by:
    a. Decrease in GFR
    b. Rise in creatinine levels
    c. Reduced urine output
    d. All of the above

21. The common form of renal failure in pregnancy is:
    a. Tubular necrosis
    b. Cortical necrosis
    c. Both tubular and cortical necrosis
    d. None of the above

22. Pathological changes are irreversible with poor prognosis in:
    a. Tubular necrosis
    b. Cortical necrosis
    c. Both tubular and cortical necrosis
    d. None of the above

23. Acute pyelonephritis in pregnancy is seen in:
    a. 2% of patients
    b. 10% of patients
    c. 12% of patients
    d. 20% of patients

24. The duration of treatment in acute pyelonephritis during pregnancy should be at least:
    a. 3 days
    b. 5 days
    c. 7 days
    d. 10 days

25. Women who have had renal transplant should ideally be advised to avoid pregnancy for:
    a. 1–2 years
    b. 3–4 years
    c. 5–6 years
    d. 7–8 years

26. An important sign of acutely impaired renal function is:
    a. Polyuria
    b. Oliguria
    c. Increased frequency
    d. Urgency

27. Acute renal failure is characterized by all, *except*:
    a. Increase in the GFR
    b. Rise in creatinine levels
    c. Reduced urine output
    d. None of the above

28. Hematuria in pregnancy can be caused by following, *except*:
    a. Severe pyelonephritis
    b. Rupture of bladder viscosities
    c. Lower segment cesarean scar rupture
    d. Ovarian cyst torsion

29. The term asymptomatic bacteriuria is used when the bacterial count of same species in midstream urine on two occasions without symptoms is more than:
    a. 10^2/mL
    b. 10^3/mL
    c. 10^4/mL
    d. 10^5/mL

30. A 28-year-old primigravida attends the casualty at 34 weeks of gestation with high fever associated with chills and severe pain in the flanks. In her past history, she was diagnosed with asymptomatic bacteriuria at 14 weeks of gestation and was treated. Her temperature is 102°F, pulse is 100 bpm, tongue is dry and BP is 100/70 mm Hg. There is costovertebral tenderness. The uterus corresponds to 34 weeks of gestation, is well-relaxed, and the FH is good. What is the most likely diagnosis?
    a. Appendicitis
    b. Pyelonephritis
    c. Ovarian cyst
    d. Colitis

ANSWERS

1. b.	2. c.	3. c.	4. d.	5. b.	6. d.	7. a.
8. a.	9. d.	10. c.	11. b.	12. b.	13. b.	14. c.
15. b.	16. d.	17. d.	18. c.	19. b.	20. d.	21. a.
22. b.	23. a.	24. d.	25. a.	26. b.	27. a.	28. d.
29. d.	30. b.					

Chapter 31: Thrombocytopenia in Pregnancy

Harshada Thakur, Rani Daruwale

QUESTIONS

1. **Platelet count for diagnosis of thrombocytopenia in pregnancy should be less than:**
   a. 100,000/μL
   b. 150,000/μL
   c. 125,000/μL
   d. 80,000/μL

2. **Causes of gestational thrombocytopenia are all, except:**
   a. Increase in blood volume
   b. Increase in platelet activation
   c. Decreased platelet synthesis
   d. Increased platelet clearance

3. **All of the following investigations should be done in a pregnant woman with thrombocytopenia, except:**
   a. Thyroid function test
   b. Viral markers
   c. Serology for dengue, malaria, and leptospirosis
   d. Platelet function test

4. **Clinical feature of primary immune thrombocytopenia is:**
   a. Normal spleen and lymph nodes
   b. Normal PT/INR and aPTT
   c. Severe thrombocytopenia which requires transfusion
   d. Normal peripheral smear and bone marrow biopsy

5. **Indication of treatment in a case of gestational thrombocytopenia is the following, except:**
   a. Platelet count below 20,000/μL
   b. Features of spontaneous bleeding
   c. Thrombocytopenia prior to any surgical procedure
   d. Thrombocytopenia in third trimester of pregnancy

6. **Options for medical treatment of primary immune thrombocytopenia are all, except:**
   a. Anti-D in Rh-negative women
   b. Intravenous immunoglobulin
   c. Immunosuppressants
   d. Corticosteroids

7. **Which of the following is a false statement with respect to prednisone administration in thrombocytopenia in pregnancy?**
   a. Response is seen within 7 days treatment
   b. Prolonged treatment causes gestational diabetes
   c. High dose steroids for longer duration can lead to fetal adrenal suppression
   d. It does not have any effect on fetal thrombocytopenia

8. **Regarding splenectomy in immune thrombocytopenic purpura in pregnancy, all are true, except:**
   a. Contraindicated in pregnancy
   b. Best done in second trimester
   c. Simultaneous cesarean section maybe needed in late pregnancy for better exposure
   d. Can be done by open or laparoscopic approach

9. **False statement among the following is:**
   a. Neonatal thrombocytopenia is not proportionate to maternal platelet count
   b. Platelet count should be >75,000/μL if an epidural block is planned
   c. Vaginal delivery has higher risk of neonatal intracranial hemorrhage in thrombocytopenia patients
   d. Cord blood platelet count should be done in all neonates born to mothers with thrombocytopenia

10. **All of the above can cause thrombocytopenia in pregnancy, except:**
    a. Acute fatty liver of pregnancy
    b. Prolonged heparin therapy
    c. Intrahepatic cholestasis of pregnancy
    d. Thrombotic thrombocytopenia purpura/hemolytic-uremic syndrome

CHAPTER 31: Thrombocytopenia in Pregnancy

11. **Most common reason for thrombocytopenias in pregnancy:**
    a. HELLP syndrome
    b. Disseminated intravascular coagulopathy
    c. Gestational thrombocytopenia
    d. Immune thrombocytopenic purpura

12. **Incidence of gestational thrombocytopenia:**
    a. 10%   b. 25%
    c. 50%   d. 75%

13. **Following are the features of gestational thrombocytopenia, *except*:**
    a. No past history of thrombocytopenia outside pregnancy
    b. Not associated with fetal thrombocytopenia
    c. Associated with maternal bleeding
    d. Occurs in mid second/third trimester of pregnancy

14. **A 27-year-old woman presents at 18 weeks of pregnancy with epistaxis, bleeding gums, and pancytopenia. She is found to have a prolonged activated partial thromboplastin time, prothrombin time, and very low fibrinogen. Which of the following statement is true?**
    a. The most likely diagnosis in this woman is Hodgkin's lymphoma
    b. This presentation is considered a hematological emergency and the woman will require urgent treatment with fresh frozen plasma, platelet transfusion, and cryoprecipitate
    c. ABVD chemotherapy (doxorubicin, bleomycin, vinblastine, dacarbazine) is the treatment of choice
    d. The most likely diagnosis is acute promyelocytic leukemia

15. **National Institute for Health and Care Excellence (NICE) guidelines for thrombocytopenia in pregnancy:**
    a. Platelet count between 20 and 30 × 10^9/L in a nonbleeding patient is safe for most pregnancy and a platelet count ≥50 × 10^9/L is preferred for delivery
    b. Platelet count between 40 and 50 × 10^9/L in a nonbleeding patient is safe for most pregnancy and a platelet count ≥100 × 10^9/L is preferred for delivery
    c. Platelet count between 20 and 30 × 10^9/L in a nonbleeding patient is safe for most pregnancy and a platelet count ≥150 × 10^9/L is preferred for delivery
    d. Platelet count between 40 and 50 × 10^9/L in a nonbleeding patient is safe for most pregnancy and a platelet count ≥75 × 10^9/L is preferred for delivery

16. **First-line treatment for ITP in pregnancy:**
    a. Platelet transfusion
    b. Corticosteroids and IVIG
    c. Rituximab
    d. All of the above

17. **Hematological changes in normal pregnancy include following, *except*:**
    a. Increased plasma volume
    b. Decreased platelet count
    c. Increase in RBC count
    d. Increased platelet count

18. **Fetal complications in gestational thrombocytopenia:**
    a. Prematurity
    b. Fetal thrombocytopenia
    c. Fetal hydrops
    d. None of the above

19. **What are the diagnostic criteria for HELLP syndrome as per Tennessee classification?**
    a. Hemolysis with increased LDH (>600 U/L), AST (≥70 U/L), and platelets <100 × 10^9/L
    b. Hemolysis with increased LDH (>500 U/L), AST (≥150 U/L), and platelets <150 × 10^9/L
    c. Hemolysis with increased LDH (>600 U/L), AST (≥100 U/L), and platelets <40 × 10^9/L
    d. None of the above

20. **The following statements are true about inherited bleeding disorders:**
    a. Von Willebrand disease (VWD) is the most common inherited bleeding disorder
    b. VWD is an X-linked genetic disorder
    c. The most common type of VWD is of the severe form
    d. Carriers of hemophilia may have low factor levels

21. **Thrombocytopenia is defined as platelet count:**
    a. <150 × 10^9/L   b. <100 × 10^9/L
    c. <50 × 10^9/L   d. <75 × 10^9/L

22. **A single unit of single donor platelet will raise patient's platelet by:**
    a. 10,000–30,000/μL   b. 30,000–60,000/μL
    c. 5,000–8,000/μL   d. 50,000–80,000/μL

23. **State true or false:**
    Blood grouping is a criterion for platelet transfusion.
    a. True
    b. False

24. **State true or false:**
    One unit of random donor platelet raises more platelets than one unit of single donor platelet.
    a. True
    b. False

25. A single unit of random donor platelet will raise patient's platelet by:
    a. 10,000–30,000/µL
    b. 30,000–60,000/µL
    c. 5,000–10,000/µL
    d. 50,000–80,000/µL

26. Single unit of single donor platelet contains a plasma volume of:
    a. 100–200 mL
    b. 200–300 mL
    c. 300–400 mL
    d. 40–70 mL

27. Single unit of random donor platelet contains a plasma volume of:
    a. 100–200 mL
    b. 200–300 mL
    c. 300–400 mL
    d. 40–70 mL

28. In a pregnant patient, first trimester tests were all normal. Now third trimester all tests are normal except low platelets, likely diagnosis is:
    a. Immune thrombocytopenic purpura
    b. Gestational thrombocytopenia
    c. Thrombotic thrombocytopenic purpura
    d. Both b and c

29. A 35-year-old woman is evaluated for worsening thrombocytopenia; she is at her 36 weeks of gestation. Medical history is significant for ITP, previous platelet counts during pregnancy were 80,000–100,000/µl. Her only medication is a prenatal vitamin.
    On examination, T—98.6°F, BP—165/110 mm Hg, pulse—95 beats/min, respiratory rate—15 breaths/min. Abdominal examination reveals mild right upper quadrant discomfort on palpation. Reflexes are normal, and no clonus is observed. She has lower extremity edema to level of the knees bilaterally.

    Laboratory studies:
    - Hb—10.5 g/dL
    - Platelet count—21,000/µL
    - SGOT—480 U/L
    - SGPT—600 U/L
    - Creatinine—1.2 mg/dL
    - Urinalysis—3 + Proteins

    Which of the following is the most appropriate management of this patient's thrombocytopenia?
    a. Platelet transfusion and emergent delivery
    b. Intravenous immune globulin only
    c. Plasma exchange and IV IgG
    d. Prednisone and plasma exchange

30. Recovery of gestational thrombocytopenia is seen after how many hours of delivery?
    a. After 72 hours
    b. Within 72 hours
    c. 48–96 hours
    d. 4–5 days

ANSWERS

1. **b.** 150,000/µL
   (Reference: Page no 1086, Chapter 56, Hematological disorders, Williams Obstetrics, 25th edition)

2. **c.** Decreased platelet synthesis
   (Reference: Page no 262, Chapter 13, Other Medical disorders, Ian Donald's Practical Obstetrics Problems, 7th edition)
   Gestational thrombocytopenia occurs due to increase in blood volume, increase in platelet activation, and increased platelet clearance. Platelet synthesis is not affected.

3. **d.** Platelet function test
   (Reference: Page no 263, Chapter 13, Other Medical Disorders, Ian Donald's Practical Obstetrics Problems, 7th edition)
   Platelet function tests usually do not have any significant role in the management of the patient. Thyroid function test should be done to rule out associated autoimmune disease whereas viral markers and serology for dengue, malaria, and leptospirosis help in diagnosing the cause of thrombocytopenia.

4. **a.** Normal spleen and lymph node
   Immune thrombocytopenia presents with changes in bone marrow and peripheral smear. The coagulation profile is also affected. Severity may vary. But splenomegaly and lymphadenopathy are uncommon in primary immune thrombocytopenia.
   (Reference: Chapter 56, Hematological disorders; Williams Obstetrics, 25th edition)

5. **d.** Thrombocytopenia in third trimester of pregnancy
   (Reference: Page no 263, Chapter 13, Other Medical Disorders, Ian Donald's Practical Obstetrics Problems, 7th edition)

Indication of transfusion is not dependent upon the gestational age. Severity of thrombocytopenia, symptoms of bleeding, and any planned surgical procedure in the patient require transfusion.

6. **c.** Immunosuppressants
    (Reference: Page no 263, Chapter 13, Other Medical Disorders, Ian Donald's Practical Obstetrics Problems, 7th edition)
    Immunosuppressants are contraindicated in pregnancy due to teratogenic effects.

7. **c.** High doses of steroids for longer duration can lead to fetal adrenal suppression.
    (Reference: Page no 263, Chapter 13, Other Medical Disorders, Ian Donald's Practical Obstetrics Problems, 7th edition)
    90% of prednisolone is metabolized in the placenta thus there is no serious side effect on fetus and nor does it help in treatment of fetal thrombocytopenia.

8. **a.** Contraindicated in pregnancy
    (Reference: Page no 1087, Chapter 56, Hematological Disorders, Williams Obstetrics, 25th edition)
    Splenectomy can be done in patients with no response to corticosteroids and intravenous immunoglobulin. It is best to perform the surgery in second trimester and can be with open or laparoscopic approach. Cesarean section may be needed for termination and better exposure during surgery in late pregnancy.

9. **c.** Vaginal delivery has higher risk of neonatal intracranial hemorrhage in TCP patients.
    (Reference: Page no 264, Chapter 13, Other Medical Disorders, Ian Donald's Practical Obstetrics Problems, 7th edition)
    The risk of intracranial hemorrhage in the fetus is similar irrespective of the mode of delivery whether vaginal or cesarean.

10. **c.** Intrahepatic cholestasis of pregnancy
    (Reference: Page no 262, Chapter 13, Other Medical Disorders, Ian Donald's Practical Obstetrics Problems, 7th edition)
    Intrahepatic cholestasis does not have any effect on platelet counts of the patients.

11. **c.** Gestational thrombocytopenia
    (Reference: Page no 1086, Chapter 56, Hematological Disorders, Williams Obstetrics, 25th edition)

12. **d.** 75%
    (Reference: Page no 1086, Chapter 56, Hematological Disorders, Williams Obstetrics, 25th edition)

13. **c.** Associated with maternal bleeding
    (Reference: Chapter 56, Hematological disorders, Williams Obstetrics, 25th edition)
    Gestational thrombocytopenia is not associated with maternal bleeding.

14. **b.** This presentation is considered a hematological emergency and the woman will require urgent treatment with fresh frozen plasma, platelet transfusion, and cryoprecipitate.
    (Reference: Salyer SW. Essential Emergency Medicine Chapter 11—Hematologic Emergencies, 2007, Pages 555-74).

15. **a.** Platelet count between 20 and 30×10^9/L in a nonbleeding patient is safe for most pregnancy and a platelet count $\geq 50 \times 10^9$/L is preferred for delivery.
    (Reference: NICE Guidelines - 2019)

16. **b.** Corticosteroids and IVIG
    (Reference: Chapter 56, Hematological disorders, Williams Obstetrics, 25th edition, NICE Guidelines)

17. **a.** Increased platelet count
    (Reference: Chapter 56, Hematological disorders, Williams Obstetrics, 25th edition)

18. **d.** None of the above
    (Reference: Chapter 13, Other Medical Disorders, Ian Donald's Practical Obstetrics Problems, 7th edition; Chapter 56, Hematological disorders, Williams Obstetrics, 25th edition)

19. **a.** Hemolysis with increased LDH (>600 U/L), AST ($\geq$70 U/L), and platelets <100×10^9/L
    (Reference: NICE Guidelines - 2019)

20. **d.** Carriers of hemophilia may have low factor levels.
    (Reference: Salyer SW. Essential Emergency Medicine, Chapter 11—Hematologic Emergencies, 2007, pages 555-74)

21. **a.** 150×10^9/L
    (Reference: Page no 1086, Chapter 56, Hematological disorders, Williams Obstetrics, 25th edition)

22. **b.** 30,000–60,000/μL
    (Reference: Salyer SW. Essential Emergency Medicine, Chapter 11—Hematologic Emergencies, 2007, pages 555-74)

23. **b.** False
    (Reference: Dunbar NM. Does ABO and RhD matching matter for platelet transfusion? Hematology Am Soc Hematol Educ Program. 2020;2020(1):512-17)

24. **b.** False
(Reference: Salyer SW. Essential Emergency Medicine, Chapter 11—Hematologic Emergencies, 2007, pp. 555-74)

25. **c.** 5,000–10,000/μL
(Reference: Salyer SW. Essential Emergency Medicine, Chapter 11—Hematologic Emergencies, 2007, pp. 555-74)

26. **b.** 200–300 mL
(Reference: Salyer SW. Essential Emergency Medicine, Chapter 11—Hematologic Emergencies, 2007, pp. 555-74)

27. **d.** 40–70 mL
(Reference: Kahn S, Chegondi M, Nellis ME, Karam O. Overview of Plasma and Platelet Transfusions in Critically Ill Children. Front Pediatr. 2020;8:601659)

28. **b.** Gestational thrombocytopenia
(Reference: Page no 1086, Chapter 56, Hematological disorders, Williams Obstetrics, 25th edition)

29. **a.** Platelet transfusion and emergent delivery
(Reference: Slayer SW, Essential Emergency Medicine; Chapter 11-Hematologic Emergencies. MKSAP QUIZ: Worsening thrombocytopenia, Hematology and Oncology section)

The most appropriate management for this patient's thrombocytopenia is immediate delivery of the fetus, because she has HELLP (hemolysis, elevated liver enzymes, and low platelets) syndrome. Although she has a history of immune thrombocytopenic purpura (ITP), and her platelet counts have been low throughout the pregnancy, her markedly decreased platelet count is worrisome and could indicate development of another condition. Worsening anemia, right upper quadrant pain, hypertension, proteinuria, and elevated liver enzymes are more consistent with a microangiopathy of pregnancy [HELLP syndrome, pre-eclampsia, thrombotic thrombocytopenic purpura (TTP)] rather than worsening ITP. Her clinical picture is more consistent with preeclampsia (new-onset hypertension at >20 weeks' gestation) with proteinuria or the HELLP syndrome. The relationship between preeclampsia and HELLP syndrome is unclear; HELLP syndrome occurs in 10–20% of women with preeclampsia but occasionally in some patients without hypertension or proteinuria. The primary treatment for both conditions, particularly in advanced pregnancy, is urgent delivery. Platelet counts tend to recover quickly after delivery; persistent thrombocytopenia several days after delivery should raise concern for another diagnosis, such as thrombotic thrombocytopenic purpura–hemolytic uremic syndrome (TTP-HUS).

Administering intravenous immune globulin is not indicated as a treatment for thrombocytopenia associated with preeclampsia and HELLP syndrome.

Plasma exchange can be undertaken if TTP is present earlier in the pregnancy before delivery is a viable option, but would not be a preferred treatment strategy in a patient in whom delivery is appropriate. Plasma exchange would be indicated if thrombocytopenia persisted after delivery and TTP-HUS were diagnosed.

Glucocorticoids such as prednisone are not indicated for microangiopathy of pregnancy. Additionally, if used as a treatment for ITP, prednisone typically takes 48–72 hours for effectiveness. Therefore, treatment with prednisone would not be appropriate in this patient.

Key point: Immediate delivery of the fetus is the best management approach for pregnant women experiencing thrombotic microangiopathy of pregnancy.

30. **a.** After 72 hours
(Reference: Chapter 56, Hematological disorders, Williams Obstetrics, 25th edition)

Chapter 32: Viral Infections in Pregnancy

Sreelatha S, Veena M Vernekar

QUESTIONS

1. Which of the following vaccinations is contraindicated in pregnancy?
   a. Influenza
   b. Hepatitis B
   c. MMR
   d. Tetanus diphtheria pertussis

2. Which of the following is true?
   a. Herpes simplex is RNA virus
   b. Parvovirus causes fetal hydrops
   c. Toxoplasmosis is a viral infection
   d. Vertical transmission of cytomegalovirus (CMV) occurs in 70%

3. Which of the following is a nonteratogenic pathogen in pregnancy?
   a. CMV
   b. Rubella
   c. Toxoplasmosis
   d. Herpes simplex

4. Which of the following is true?
   a. Pregnancy hastens the progression of HIV to AIDS
   b. The incidence of preeclampsia is decreased by ART
   c. Cesarean section is mandatory in all HIV-affected patients
   d. Stillbirth and intrauterine growth restriction (IUGR) is more common in HIV-affected individuals

5. Mode of transmission of measles:
   a. Through aerosols
   b. Fecal–oral
   c. Sexually
   d. Close contact

6. Highest maternal mortality is seen in which of the following types of viral hepatitis infection?
   a. Hepatitis A
   b. Hepatitis B
   c. Hepatitis C
   d. Hepatitis E

7. Which of the following marker indicated the infectivity of hepatitis infection?
   a. Anti-HBc
   b. HBeAg
   c. HBcAg
   d. Anti-HBs

8. Hepatitis A is best diagnosed by?
   a. IgM antibodies in serum
   b. Culture from blood
   c. Isolation from stool
   d. Isolation from sputum

9. Which of the following marker indicated the recent hepatitis infection during window period?
   a. HBsAg
   b. IgM anti-HBc
   c. Anti-HBs
   d. None

10. Hepatitis C virus belongs to which group?
    a. Picornavirus
    b. Herpes
    c. Flavivirus
    d. Hepadnavirus

11. Which of the following hepatitis infection is prevented by vaccines?
    a. Hepatitis A
    b. Hepatitis B
    c. Hepatitis C
    d. Both A and B

12. The greatest risk of transmission of rubella is up to how many days after the onset of rash?
    a. 7
    b. 10
    c. 12
    d. 18

13. All of the following about congenital rubella are true, *except*:
    a. It is diagnosed when the infant has IgM antibodies at birth
    b. It is diagnosed when IgG antibodies persists for > 6 months
    c. Most common congenital defects are deafness, cardiac defect, and cataract
    d. Infection after 16 weeks of gestation results in major congenital defects

14. What is the latent phase between time of HIV infection and developing AIDS in adults?
    a. 2-4 weeks b. 3-6 months
    c. 1-5 years d. 5-10 years

15. How does HIV damages immune system?
    a. Destroys CD4 lymphocytes
    b. Lowers antibody level
    c. Reduces CD8 lymphocytes
    d. Interferes with function of polymorphs

16. What is the risk of vertical transmission of HIV without ART prophylaxis?
    a. <10% b. 10-30%
    c. 30-50% d. >50%

17. Which of the following procedures increases the risk of HIV transmission during pregnancy?
    a. Amniocentesis
    b. Per vaginal examination
    c. Abdominal palpation
    d. Cytology

18. Neural tube defect is an adverse effect of which of the following drug?
    a. AZT (zidovudine) b. TDF (tenofovir)
    c. FTC (emtricitabine) d. DTG (dolutegravir)

19. In retroviral positive pregnant women, when should the membranes:
    a. Ruptured as soon as possible to initiate labor
    b. Ruptured when 4 cm dilated
    c. Ruptured when fully dilated
    d. Not to be artificially ruptured unless clinically indicated

20. Zika virus is transmitted by:
    a. Mosquito bite b. Contaminated water
    c. Sexual contact d. Blood transfusion

21. The outermost covering of HIV virus is:
    a. Lipid bilayer b. Matrix protein
    c. Capsid protein d. Nuclear membranes

22. Which of the following hepatitis virus is not an RNA virus?
    a. Hepatitis A b. Hepatitis B
    c. Hepatitis C d. Hepatitis E

23. Which of the following does not establish a diagnosis of congenital CMV infection in a neonate?
    a. Urine culture of CMV
    b. IgG CMV antibodies in blood
    c. Intranuclear inclusion bodies in hepatocytes
    d. CMV viral DNA in blood by PCR

24. A neonate with jaundice, petechiae, microcephalus, and hepatosplenomegaly is most likely infected with which of the following?
    a. Neonatal herpes infection
    b. Chlamydial infection
    c. Neonatal CMV infection
    d. Gonococcal infection

25. Neonatal varicella occurs when mother is infected:
    a. 4-5 days before to 2 days after delivery
    b. 10 days before to 1 week after delivery
    c. In early pregnancy
    d. Mid trimester

26. Hepatitis A virus is transmitted by:
    a. Fecal-oral b. Sexual
    c. Blood transfusion d. Aerosol

27. Cotrimoxazole should be started if CD4 count is:
    a. ≤250 cells/mm^3 b. ≤500 cells/mm^3
    c. ≤750 cells/mm^3 d. ≤1,000 cells/mm^3

28. The gold standard test for H1N1:
    a. RT PCR of throat swab b. IgM antibody in blood
    c. Sputum culture d. Rapid molecular assay

29. What is the incubation period of chickenpox?
    a. 1-2 days b. 3-5 days
    c. 10-14 days d. 21-28 days

30. Which HIV exposed infants should have NVP at birth?
    a. All HIV exposed infants
    b. Only if mother did not receive ARV treatment
    c. Only if maternal ARV treatment started in last month of pregnancy
    d. Only if mother received ARV treatment from 14 weeks

ANSWERS

1. **c.** Live-attenuated virus in a vaccine can cross the placental barrier to cause fetal infection; hence, measles-mumps-rubella vaccine which is a live attenuated vaccine is contraindicated in pregnancy.

2. **b.** Parvovirus B$_{19}$ infection causes severe fetal anemia leading to high-output cardiac failure (nonimmune fetal hydrops).

3. **d.** In utero congenital herpes simplex virus (HSV) transmission is rare, accounting for only 5% of all neonatal herpes infections.

4. **d.** Intrauterine growth restriction (IUGR) and stillbirth are common in HIV-affected pregnant women.

5. **a.** Measles is transmitted from person to person through aerosolized droplets from an infected person. No known animal reservoir or a carrier state has been documented for measles.

6. **d.** Hepatitis E usually progresses to fulminant hepatitis and has a mortality rate of 5-25%.

7. **b.** Hepatitis B virus serological markers:
   - HBsAg is hepatitis B surface antigen; anti-HBs is hepatitis B surface antibody
   - HBcAg is hepatitis B core antigen; anti-HBc hepatitis B core antibody
   - HBeAg hepatitis B envelope antigen; anti-HBe hepatitis B envelope antibody

   HBsAg is positive in early phase of acute infections and persists in chronic infection as well.

   HBeAg depicts the high viral load and high infectivity.

8. **a.** Hepatitis A causes mild to severe liver infection. It is transmitted by ingestion of contaminated water and food.

   But specific diagnosis is made by detecting HAV IgM antibodies in blood.

9. **b.** Antibodies in hepatitis B infection

   Anti-HBs—is a neutralizing antibody, appears after the infection is cleared, it indicates immunity from acute infection or vaccination

   Anti HBc-IgM: Appears following recent infection

   IgG: Marker of current or past exposure

   Anti-HBe—indicates host immune response to HBeAg, reduced infectivity

10. **c.** Hepatitis C virus is a small, enveloped, positive single-stranded RNA virus. It belongs to the Flaviviridae family, genus *Hepacivirus.*

11. **d.** Currently safe and effective vaccines are available to prevent both hepatitis B and hepatitis A infections.

12. **a.** A person with rubella may spread the disease to others up to 1 week before the rash appears, and remain contagious up to 7 days after the onset of rash.

13. **d.** Congenital rubella syndrome (CRS) is a condition that occurs when the mother is infected with the rubella virus and is transmitted to the fetus, most severe damage occurs when the mother is infected early in pregnancy, especially in the first trimester.

14. **d.** About 4-6 weeks after acute infection, a stage with no signs and symptoms called clinical latent period occurs which lasts for up to 5-10 years then progresses to an end-stage disease—AIDS

15. **a.** HIV attaches and penetrates host T cells through $CD4^+$ lymphocytes and destroys them.

16. **b.** In the absence of intervention or ART prophylaxis, the rate of mother to child transmission during pregnancy, delivery, or breastfeeding ranges from 10-30%.

17. **a.** Amniocentesis being an invasive procedure increases the risk of HIV transmission to the fetus.

    Other intrapartum risk factors are—prolonged rupture of membranes, episiotomy, vaginal lacerations, invasive fetal monitoring, and instrumental delivery.

18. **d.** In a recent study, a small increased risk of neural tube defects was found in children born to mothers with HIV who were on Dolutegravir compared to other antiretroviral drugs.

19. **d.** Artificial rupture of membranes should be avoided in people with HIV RNA ≥50 copies/mL, unless there is a clear obstetric indication.

20. **a.** Zika virus is primarily transmitted by an infected mosquito bite mainly Aedes aegypti and Aedes albopictus.

21. **a.** The HIV is composed of a capsid core which has the genetic material that is covered by a protein envelope and lipid bilayer. There is an outer gp120 docking glycoprotein which is attached to transmembrane gp41 glycoprotein. The genome has two helices of RNA molecules. Enzymes—reverse transcriptase, integrate, and protease are present.

22. **b.** Hepatitis B virus is a partially double-stranded DNA virus that belongs to Hepadnaviridae family of viruses.

23. **b.** Maternal IgG antibodies can pass into the fetal circulation. Hence, it is not possible to establish a diagnosis of congenital CMV infection just by demonstrating the presence of IgG antibodies. IgG avidity is often needed to determine the timing of primary infection. Viral culture and polymerase chain reaction using urine, saliva, and blood can be done.

24. **c.** Babies with congenital CMV infection can have signs at birth such as rashes, jaundice, microcephaly, hepatosplenomegaly, seizures, and retinitis.

25. **a.** If the mother develops varicella rash between day 4 and 5 antepartum to day 2 postpartum, generalized neonatal varicella can occur in the newborn.

26. **a.** Hepatitis A is transmitted primarily by fecal-oral route when an infected person in just food and water that has been contaminated with the faces of an infected person.

27. **a.** Cotrimoxazole is a fixed dose combination of sulfamethoxazole and trimethoprim. Prophylactic therapy with it is recommended in advanced HIV disease or WHO stage 3 or 4 and/or with $CD4^+$ count of <250 cells/mm^3.

28. **a.** Real-time polymerase chain reaction is considered as the gold standard for diagnosis of influenza viruses.

29. **c.** Incubation period of chickenpox is 10-14 days.

30. **a.** Nevirapine (NVP) often is used as part of newborn antiretroviral regimens to prevent perinatal transmission of HIV.

    ARV medications should begin as soon as possible, preferably within 6-12 hours of delivery.

Chapter 33: Malaria and Dengue in Pregnancy

Sunita Samal

MALARIA IN PREGNANCY

QUESTIONS

1. **Which of the antimalarial drug is safest in pregnancy?**
   a. Chloramphenicol
   b. Quinine
   c. Chloroquine
   d. Primaquine

2. **The WHO recommends the following interventions for malaria in pregnancy in areas of moderate-to-high transmission, *except*:**
   a. Use of insecticide-treated nets (ITNs)
   b. Intermittent preventive treatment (IPT) with sulfadoxine–pyrimethamine (SP)
   c. Indoor residual spraying (IRS)
   d. Early diagnosis and prompt treatment for those infected with malaria

3. **The WHO recommends that pregnant women in areas of moderate-to-high malaria transmission take IPT with SP:**
   a. At the beginning of pregnancy
   b. At least two times during pregnancy, after quickening
   c. At each scheduled antenatal care visit, starting the first dose as early as possible during the second trimester of gestation
   d. Only given to primigravida

4. **WHO has recommended the intermittent preventive treatment in pregnancy (IPTp) strategy, which is integral to antenatal care service. Choose the correct dose.**
   a. Single dose of three tablets of single-pill combination (SPC) of sulfadoxine–pyrimethamine (SP)
   b. Single dose of two tablets of single-pill combination (SPC) of sulfadoxine–pyrimethamine (SP)
   c. Double dose of two tablets of single-pill combination (SPC) of sulfadoxine–pyrimethamine (SP)
   d. Double dose of three tablets of single-pill combination (SPC) of sulfadoxine–pyrimethamine (SP)

5. **Sulfadoxine-pyrimethamine (SP) should not be taken by pregnant women who:**
   a. Take folic acid
   b. HIV positive and taking cotrimoxazole
   c. Take iron tablet
   d. Sleep under a insecticide net (ITN)

6. **All are components of malaria prevention in pregnancy, *except*:**
   a. Awareness of risk
   b. Bite prevention
   c. Chemoprophylaxis
   d. Avoidance of travel to Southeast Asian countries

7. **What is uncomplicated malaria in pregnancy?**
   a. Less than 2% parasitized red blood cells in a woman with no signs of severity and no complicating features
   b. Less than 1% parasitized red blood cells in a woman with no signs of severity and no complicating features
   c. Less than 3% parasitized red blood cells in a woman with no signs of severity and no complicating features
   d. Less than 4% parasitized red blood cells in a woman with no signs of severity and no complicating features

8. **Which drug is recommended for chemoprophylaxis for pregnant or breastfeeding women?**
   a. Mefloquine
   b. Chloroquine
   c. Primaquine
   d. Quinine

9. **Congenital malaria results from all, *except*:**
   a. The passage of parasites or infected red blood cells from the mother to the newborn while in utero
   b. The passage of parasites or infected red blood cells from the mother to the newborn during delivery
   c. By the bite of the female anopheline mosquito
   d. By the bite of the female aedes mosquito

10. **The most suitable test to diagnose malaria in pregnancy:**
    a. Microscopic examination of thick and thin blood films for parasites
    b. Rapid diagnostic tests which detect specific parasite antigen or enzyme
    c. PCR test for malaria
    d. Complete blood count

11. **The treatment of choice for severe falciparum malaria in pregnancy:**
    a. Primaquine
    b. Intravenous artesunate
    c. Intravenous quinine
    d. Intravenous clindamycin

12. **Common obstetric problems with acute symptomatic malaria are all, *except*:**
    a. Preterm labor
    b. Intrauterine growth restriction (IUGR)
    c. Fetal distress
    d. Preeclampsia

13. **Which of the following is true regarding women planning pregnancy and travelling to malaria endemic destination:**
    a. Chloroquine and proguanil can be used as chemoprophylaxis
    b. Women should be advised not to travel or to choose an alternative destination
    c. Prophylaxis is 100% effective
    d. Women should not be advised to delay either the pregnancy or the travel plan

14. **All are features of complicated or severe malaria in pregnancy, *except*:**
    a. Nausea and vomiting   b. Pulmonary edema
    c. Severe anemia   d. Multiple convulsions

15. **Non-falciparum malaria (*P. vivax*, *P. ovale*, and *P. malariae*) can be best treated with:**
    a. Oral chloroquine (base) 600 mg followed by 300 mg 68 hours later. Then 300 mg on day 2 and again on day 3
    b. Oral quinine 600 mg 8 hourly and oral clindamycin 450 mg 8 hourly for 7 days
    c. Artesunate IV 2.4 mg/kg at 0, 12, and 24 hours, then daily thereafter
    d. Primaquine oral 45–60 mg once a week for 8 weeks

ANSWERS

1. **c.** Safe in pregnancy, works against the asexual form of malarial parasite within RBC

2. **c.** WHO recommends a three-pronged approach to the prevention and management of malaria in pregnancy: Insecticide-treated nets (ITNs); Intermittent preventive treatment; Effective case management of malarial illness.
   (Reference: WHO guideline for malaria, 2022)

3. **c.** WHO has observed a slowing of efforts to scale-up IPTp for malaria with SP in a number of countries in Africa. Based on a recent WHO evidence review, WHO updated its policy recommendation for IPTp with SP. WHO recommends a schedule of four antenatal care visits. In areas of moderate-to-high malaria transmission, IPTp with SP is recommended for all pregnant women at each scheduled antenatal care visit, starting the first dose as early as possible during the 2nd trimester of gestation. In malaria-endemic areas, IPTp is now recommended for all pregnant women, regardless of the number of pregnancies. Previously, it was recommended only during a woman's first and second pregnancies.
   (Reference: WHO guideline for malaria, 2022)

4. **a.** The IPTp-SP is implemented in pregnant women starting as early as possible in the second trimester, with SP administered at monthly intervals up to the time of delivery. IPTp-SP should be administered under directly observed therapy (DOT) along with folic acid dose reduction (400 µg daily), usually with iron for prevention of maternal anemia. IPTp-SP should ideally be administered as DOT with three tablets of SP (each tablet containing 500 mg/25 mg SP), for the total required dosage of 1500 mg/75 mg SP.
   (Reference: WHO guideline for malaria, 2022)

5. **b.** Because cotrimoxazole and SP have similar properties (both contain sulfamides), there is concern about possible severe adverse reactions to sulfa drugs in HIV patients on daily cotrimoxazole.

WHO, therefore recommends that person on daily cotrimoxazole should not be given SP.
(Reference: WHO guideline for malaria, 2022)

6. **d.** The "ABCD" of malaria prevention is a useful formula to remember the components of malaria prevention:
   - Awareness of risk
   - Bite prevention
   - Chemoprophylaxis
   - Diagnosis and treatment which must be prompt
   (Reference: RCOG 54a, 2010)

7. **a.** Uncomplicated malaria in the UK is defined as fewer than 2% parasitized red blood cells in a woman with no signs of severity and no complicating features.
   (Reference: RCOG 54b, April 2010)

8. **a.** Mefloquine (5 mg/kg once a week) is the recommended drug of choice for prophylaxis in the second and third trimesters for chloroquine-resistant areas. With very few areas in the world free from chloroquine resistance, mefloquine is essentially the only drug considered safe for prophylaxis in pregnant travelers.
   (Reference: RCOG 54a, 2010)

9. **c.** Congenital malaria in the very young infant or newborn results from the passage of parasites or infected red blood cells from the mother to the newborn while in utero or during delivery and not by the bite of the female anopheline mosquito.
   (Reference: RCOG 54b, 2010)

10. **a.** Microscopy and rapid diagnostic tests are the standard tools available. The diagnosis of malaria in pregnancy, as in nonpregnant patients, relies on microscopic examination (the current gold standard) of thick and thin blood films for parasites or the use of rapid diagnostic tests which detect specific parasite antigen or enzyme. Rapid diagnostic tests are less sensitive than malaria blood film.
    (Reference: RCOG 54b, 2010)

11. **b.** *(Reference: RCOG, 2010)*

12. **d.** *(Reference: RCOG, 2010)*

13. **b.** Women planning pregnancy and travelling to a destination where there is a risk of contracting malaria should be advised there may be harmful consequences for the pregnancy. Prophylaxis is not 100% effective and malaria is associated with increased risk of miscarriage. Women should be advised not to travel or to choose an alternative destination. If it not possible to delay either the pregnancy or the travel plan, advice from a specialist with current experience of malaria should be sought. Chloroquine and proguanil are not efficacious in chloroquine-resistant areas and cannot be recommended because of this. There are very few chloroquine-sensitive areas remaining.
    (Reference: RCOG 54a, 2010)

14. **a.** *(Reference: RCOG 54b, 2010)*

15. **a.** *(Reference: RCOG 54b, 2010)*

DENGUE IN PREGNANCY

QUESTIONS

1. **Causative organism of dengue fever:**
   a. Togavirus
   b. Flavivirus
   c. Paramyxoma virus
   d. Varicella

2. **Major mode of transmission in dengue fever:**
   a. Bite of male culex mosquito
   b. Bite of female sandfly
   c. Bite of female aedes aegypti mosquito
   d. Bite of female anopheles mosquito

3. **Classical dengue fever is known as:**
   a. Black fever
   b. Break bone fever
   c. Saddle back fever
   d. Both b and c

4. **A patient presented with fever (104°F), chills, severe headache, and pain around the eyeballs, muscle, and severe bone pain. He also gave history of mosquito bite. On examination, there was maculopapular rash and lymph nodes were enlarged. Clinicians were suspecting some viral disease. Laboratory investigations showed positive IgM antibodies to the causative organism. What is the most likely diagnosis?**
   a. Chickenpox
   b. Dengue
   c. Malaria
   d. Measles

5. **Which of the following is true regarding secondary dengue infection or dengue hemorrhagic fever (DHF)?**
   a. A different serotype of dengue virus is responsible for DHF than the serotype in the primary infection
   b. Anopheles mosquito is involved in the transmission of DHF
   c. Cause of secondary infection is independent of the primary infection
   d. DHF is caused by same serotype of dengue virus as in the primary infection

6. **What is the main mechanism of pathogenesis in the dengue hemorrhagic fever?**
   a. Antibody-dependent immune enhancement and cross-reactivity of T cells
   b. Complement inactivation
   c. Depletion of clotting factors
   d. Release of excessive amount of exotoxins

7. **All are true regarding NS1 dengue antigen, *except*:**
   a. A glycoprotein produced by all flaviviruses and is essential for replication and viability of the virus
   b. Present in high concentrations in the sera of the dengue virus-infected patients during the early clinical phase of the disease
   c. Commercial kits for the detection of NS1 antigens are useful to differentiate between the serotypes
   d. Can be detected in both patients with primary and secondary dengue infections for up to 6 days after the onset of fever

8. **Primigravida at 34 weeks of pregnancy presented with dengue hemorrhagic fever. Which is not appropriate regarding the management of this patient?**
   a. Intense fluid resuscitation
   b. Immediate induction of labor
   c. Vitals monitoring (BP/P/Pulse pressure, capillary refill) hourly
   d. Catheterize to know precise urine output hourly

9. **Which of the following features differentiates dengue shock syndrome from septic shock?**
   a. High hematocrit
   b. Marked thrombocytopenia
   c. A low erythrocyte sedimentation rate (ESR) (<10 mm in 1st hour)
   d. Leukopenia

10. **Which is true regarding diagnostic test for dengue?**
    a. Immunological tests are the methods of choice for diagnosis up to 6 days of onset of illness
    b. Virus isolation and viral nucleic acid or antigen detection can be used to diagnose infection up to 6 days of onset of illness
    c. RT-PCR test detects dengue NS antigen
    d. MAC-ELISA detects IgG antibody

11. **Management of antenatal woman with dengue fever without warning signs are all, *except*:**
    a. Paracetamol can be given for control of fever
    b. Aspirin can be continued if she is taking earlier
    c. Oral intake of fluid at least up to 2.5 L/day
    d. Daily complete blood count (CBC) monitoring

12. **All are warning signs of dengue fever, *except*:**
    a. Persistent vomiting and severe abdominal pain
    b. Increasing liver size and a tender liver
    c. Progressive fall in WBC, platelets fall, rise in HCT (PCV)
    d. Progressive rise in WBC, platelets fall, rise in HCT (PCV)

13. **Diagnosis of dengue hemorrhagic fever includes all, *except*:**
    a. Fever with hemorrhagic manifestation
    b. Thrombocytopenia
    c. Evidence of plasma leakage
    d. Features of shock

14. **All are maternal complications due to dengue in pregnancy, *except*:**
    a. Acute pulmonary edema
    b. Preeclampsia
    c. Postpartum hemorrhage
    d. GDM

15. **Which is true regarding infection to fetus in dengue affected pregnancy:**
    a. Dengue is detected by IgM or viruses in the placental, cord, or peripheral blood of the newborn
    b. The rate of transmission is higher in the second trimester
    c. Dengue can cause birth defects
    d. Hepatomegaly and thrombocytopenia are more common features in newborn

ANSWERS

1. **b.**
2. **c.**
3. **d.**
4. **b.**
5. **a.** Dengue hemorrhagic fever is strongly associated with secondary, so-called heterotypic infections (two sequential infections caused by different serotypes) (*Reference: WHO, 2011*)
6. **a.** Various cytokines with permeability enhancing effect have been implicated in the pathogenesis of DHF. However, the relative importance of these cytokines in DHF is still unknown. Studies have

shown that the pattern of cytokine response may be related to the pattern of cross-recognition of dengue-specific T-cells. Cross-reactive T-cells appear to be functionally deficit in their cytolytic activity but express enhanced cytokine production including TNF-α, IFN-γ, and chemokines.
(Reference: WHO, 2011)

7. **c.** The NS1 gene product is a glycoprotein produced by all flaviviruses and is essential for replication and viability of the virus. The protein is secreted by mammalian cells but not by insect cells. NS1 antigen appears as early as Day 1 after the onset of the fever and declines to undetectable levels by 5-6 days. Hence, tests based on this antigen can be used for early diagnosis, can be detected in both patients with primary and secondary dengue infections for up to 6 days after the onset of illness. Commercial kits for the detection of NS1 antigens are now available; however, these kits do not differentiate between the serotypes.
(Reference: WHO, 2011)

8. **b.** *(Reference: FOGSI, 2014)*

9. **c.** In cases with shock, a high hematocrit and marked thrombocytopenia support the diagnosis of DSS. A low ESR (<10 mm in 1st hour) during shock differentiates DSS from septic shock.
(Reference: WHO, 2011)

10. **b.** During the early stages of the disease (up to 6 days of onset of illness), virus isolation, viral nucleic acid, or antigen detection can be used to diagnose infection. At the end of the acute phase of infection, immunological tests are the methods of choice for diagnosis. RT-PCR assays have been reported for detecting dengue virus. MAC-ELISA is based on detecting the dengue-specific IgM antibodies in the test serum by capturing them out of solution using anti-human IgM.
(Reference: WHO, 2011)

11. **b.** *(Reference: FOGSI, 2014)*

12. **d.** Warning signs of plasma leak persistent vomiting and severe abdominal pain increasingly lethargic but usually remain mentally alert. Increasing liver size and a tender liver progressive fall in WBC, platelets fall rise in HCT (PCV).
(Reference: FOGSI, 2014)

13. **d.**

14. **d.** Lack of evidence to suggest dengue increases the risk of developing GDM.
(Reference: Chong V, Tan JZL, Jayanthi V, Arasoo T. Dengue in Pregnancy: A Southeast Asian Perspective, 2023)

15. **a.** *Vertical transmission:* Although vertical transmission of dengue can happen, it is rare, especially if mothers are asymptomatic. However, a study involving 54 participants in French Guiana reported vertical transmission in about 18.5–22.7%. Dengue is detected by IgM or viruses in the placental, cord, or peripheral blood of the newborn. The rate of transmission is higher in the third trimester. Perinatally, dengue is transmitted through the placenta. New evidence suggests that the virus may also be transmitted by breast milk. Clinical presentations of the vertical transmission of dengue in neonates can range from mild (fever) to severe (DHF, DSS, death), where symptoms of fever and rash are most common, followed by hepatomegaly, thrombocytopenia, and DHF.
(Reference: Chong V, Tan JZL, Jayanthi V, Arasoo T. Dengue in Pregnancy: A Southeast Asian Perspective, 2023)

Chapter 34: Antepartum Hemorrhage

Sebanti Goswami

QUESTIONS

1. **Swiss cheese placenta is seen in which condition?**
   a. Gestational diabetes mellitus
   b. Hypertensive disorder in pregnancy
   c. Placenta accreta
   d. Abruptio placenta

2. **Triple P procedure includes all, *except*:**
   a. Subtotal hysterectomy
   b. Delivery of the fetus above the upper border of the placenta
   c. Pelvic devascularization
   d. Placental nonseparation with myometrial excision

3. **Sher and Statland classification is used in which condition?**
   a. Postpartum hemorrhage (PPH)
   b. Acute fatty liver of pregnancy
   c. Twin to twin transfusion syndrome
   d. Abruptio placentae

4. **How many % of placenta previa at 20 weeks remain so at term?**
   a. 42%
   b. 56%
   c. 40%
   d. 32%

5. **Hemostasis at the placental site depends upon:**
   a. Blood coagulability
   b. Myometrial contractions
   c. Placental size
   d. Blood volume of the mother

6. **Placenta previa is less likely to migrate in:**
   a. Previous cesarean pregnancy
   b. Breech presentation
   c. Transverse lie
   d. Bicornuate uterus

7. **Which one is true?**
   a. USG is the most sensitive tool for diagnosis of placental abruption
   b. Incidence of coagulopathy is 80% in case of placental abruption
   c. Retroplacental clot is hypoechogenic compared to the placenta
   d. There is some evidence suggestive of the genetic influence in pathogenesis of placental abruption

8. **Which one is true about placenta previa?**
   a. It is associated with an increase in the incidence of intrauterine growth restriction
   b. If anterior is best treated by classical cesarean section
   c. Becomes symptomatic in labor for the first time in about 1/6th of cases
   d. It is more common in teenage pregnancy

9. **Subchorionic hematoma has an overall miscarriage rate of what %?**
   a. 10%
   b. 27%
   c. 39%
   d. 50%

10. **What is the meaning of the word previa?**
    a. In front of
    b. Over and above
    c. Going before
    d. Going below

11. **What is the cervical length below which a placenta previa is more associated with hemorrhage, uterine activity, and preterm birth?**
    a. <50 mm
    b. < 30 mm
    c. <40 mm
    d. <20 mm

12. **A low-lying placenta lies within how much cm wide perimeter around the os?**
    a. 2.5 cm
    b. 3 cm
    c. 2 cm
    d. 5 cm

13. **What is the incidence of vasa previa?**
    a. 0.1–0.5 per 10,000 pregnancies
    b. 7–8 per 10,000 pregnancies
    c. 0.6–0.8 per 10,000 pregnancies
    d. 2–6 per 10,000 pregnancies

14. **Which is true about vasa previa type 2?**
    a. Vessels are a part of velamentous cord insertion
    b. Involved vessels span between portions of a bilobed or succenturiate placenta
    c. Involved vessels extend to the introitus
    d. None of the above

15. **What is the most common cause of unexplained antepartum hemorrhage?**
    a. Low-lying placenta
    b. Abruptio placenta
    c. Rupture of marginal sinus
    d. Scar dehiscence

16. **What is the full form of FASTER trial?**
    a. First and second trimester evaluation of rate
    b. First and second trimester evaluation of risk
    c. First and second trimester examination of risk
    d. First and secure test of early risks

17. **All of the following increase the risk of placenta previa, *except*:**
    a. Uterine leiomyoma
    b. Cigarette smoking
    c. Younger age of the mother
    d. Assisted reproduction techniques

18. **A TVS in placenta previa:**
    a. Is absolutely contraindicated
    b. Is safe when there is no active bleeding
    c. Is safe even if there is bleeding
    d. Does not give accurate results

19. **What is the recommended time of delivery in a morbidly adherent placenta?**
    a. 37 completed weeks
    b. 34–35 completed weeks
    c. 39 weeks
    d. 38 weeks

20. **What is the name of the first episode of bleeding in placenta previa?**
    a. The first bleed
    b. The warning bleed
    c. The primary bleed
    d. Sentinel bleed

21. **Couvelaire uterus is also known as:**
    a. Abruptio placentae
    b. Placental abruptioplexy
    c. Uteroplacental apoplexy
    d. Abruptio apoplexy

22. **What is the full form of CAOS in antepartum hemorrhage?**
    a. Chronic abruption oligohydramnios syndrome
    b. Chronic abruption oligohydramnios sequence
    c. Chronic antepartum oligohydramnios system
    d. Complete antepartum oligohydramnios syndrome

23. **What is the most common high-risk factor for placental abruption?**
    a. Preeclampsia   b. Chorioamnionitis
    c. Multiparity   d. Prior abruption

24. **All of the following are risk factors for placental abruption, *except*:**
    a. Single umbilical artery
    b. Multifetal gestations
    c. Oligohydramnios
    d. Cigarette smoking

25. **In one-third of the women with abruption severe enough to kill the fetus, the fibrinogen level will be:**
    a. <50 mg/dL   b. <115 mg/dL
    c. <150 mg/dL   d. <100 mg/dL

26. **Consumptive coagulopathy is more likely with:**
    a. Revealed abruption
    b. Placenta previa
    c. Concealed abruption
    d. Partially revealed abruption

27. **How does smoking cause placental abruption?**
    a. By teratogenesis
    b. By increasing intrauterine pressure
    c. By causing necrosis at the edge of the placenta
    d. By increasing fragility of amniotic membrane

28. **What is the maternal mortality rate in placental abruption?**
    a. 2.5%   b. 3%
    c. 1%   d. 0.5%

29. **The indication of tocolytics in abruption is:**
    a. All cases
    b. Very preterm who need transfer to a hospital to provide neonatal intensive care
    c. PPROM cases
    d. In severe hypertension

30. **Which placental abnormality is specifically associated with placental abruption?**
    a. Circumvallate placenta
    b. Placenta spuria
    c. Placenta succenturiata
    d. Battledore placenta

ANSWERS

1. c.
2. **a.** It is a conservative surgical alternative to peripartum hysterectomy for morbidly adherent placenta.
3. d.
4. c.
5. b.
6. a.
7. **d.** (*Reference: JAMES High Risk Pregnancy*)
8. c.
9. a.
10. c.
11. b.
12. c.
13. d.
14. b.
15. c.
16. b.
17. c.
18. c.
19. b.
20. d.
21. c.
22. b.
23. d.
24. c.
25. c.
26. **c.** As intrauterine pressure is higher. Forces more thromboplastin into large veins draining the implantation site
27. **c.** (*Reference: James High-risk Pregnancy*)
28. **c.** (*Reference: James High-risk Pregnancy*)
29. b.
30. **a.** (*Reference: James High-risk Pregnancy*)

Note: All the questions and answers have been made from Williams Textbook.

Few have been framed from High-Risk Pregnancy of James and mentioned with the answer.

Chapter 35: Gynecological Problems in Pregnancy

Hemant Damle

QUESTIONS

1. Which is the most common cancer diagnosed during pregnancy?
   a. Lymphoma
   b. Breast cancer
   c. Thyroid cancer
   d. Cervical cancer

2. A 32-year-old primigravida diagnosed with cervical cancer. She is preparing to start chemotherapy and radiation. Which of the following fertility sparing options is not recommended?
   a. Cryopreservation
   b. Surgical transposition of the ovaries
   c. Gonadotropin-releasing hormone agonist
   d. All of the above can be recommended

3. The Pap smear at 9 weeks of gestation shows a low-grade squamous intraepithelial lesion. You perform a colposcopy, which is consistent with a cervical intraepithelial neoplasia 2 lesion. What is the chance of lesion regression upon revaluation in the postpartum period?
   a. 40–50%
   b. 50–60%
   c. 60–70%
   d. 70–80%

4. Which of the following is not a significant risk of cervical conization performed during pregnancy?
   a. Residual neoplasia
   b. Membrane rupture
   c. Bleeding requiring transfusion
   d. All are significant risks

5. A 23-year-old primigravida with 28 weeks of gestation is diagnosed with stage IA1 cervical cancer. What is correct regarding her management?
   a. Vaginal delivery is contraindicated.
   b. Early delivery at 34 weeks is recommended.
   c. Definitive therapy is reserved until 12 weeks postpartum.
   d. None of the above

6. Which of the following hormones can stimulate growth of leiomyomas?
   a. Estrogen
   b. Progesterone
   c. Both of these
   d. Neither stimulates leiomyoma growth

7. Which of the following pregnancy complications is not increased in the presence of uterine leiomyomas?
   a. Preterm labor
   b. Oligohydramnios
   c. Placental abruption
   d. Postpartum hemorrhage

8. What pregnancy-specific condition is associated with abnormally elevated cancer antigen 125 levels?
   a. Placenta previa
   b. Placental abruption
   c. Severe preeclampsia
   d. All of the above

9. A 20-year-old primigravida at 18 weeks gestation has an asymptomatic 10-cm complex adnexal mass with thick septa and solid components on a routine prenatal ultrasound. What management is recommended?
   a. Expectant management
   b. Magnetic resonance imaging
   c. Immediate laparoscopic removal
   d. Emergent exploratory laparotomy

10. What is the most common type of ovarian cancer in pregnancy?
    a. Epithelial tumor
    b. Germ cell tumor
    c. Sex cord-stromal tumor
    d. Low-malignant-potential tumor

11. What is the most common cause of cervical erosion in pregnancy?
    a. Premalignant lesions
    b. Cancer cervix
    c. Oral contraceptives
    d. Physiological

12. Most common extraplacental cause of antepartum hemorrhage in pregnancy:
    a. Cancer cervix
    b. Varicose veins
    c. Cervical polyp
    d. Local trauma

13. Diagnosis for congenital malformation of the uterus can be made by:
    a. Hysterosalpingography/hysteroscopy/laparoscopy
    b. Fundal notching on abdominal palpation
    c. During manual removal of placenta or C section
    d. All of the above

14. Most common obstetric adverse effect due to uterine malformation:
    a. Recurrent mid-trimester abortion
    b. Malposition
    c. Preterm labor
    d. Abnormal uterine action

15. Which category of unicornuate uterus poses the greatest risk for ectopic pregnancy?
    a. Agenesis of one horn
    b. Communicating noncavitary rudimentary horn
    c. Noncommunicating cavitary rudimentary horn
    d. Noncommunicating noncavitary rudimentary horn

16. Which of the following is not a cause of torsion of uterus in pregnancy?
    a. Leiomyoma
    b. Bicornuate uterus
    c. Adnexal pathology
    d. Retroverted uterus

17. What is the treatment of choice in a case of torsion in pregnancy?
    a. Exploratory laparotomy and detorsion
    b. Wait and watch
    c. Vaginal delivery
    d. Expectant management

18. Which of the following is not a pitfall in the diagnosis of cancer cervix in pregnancy?
    a. Indurated feel of malignancy is not evident
    b. Extension to parametrium is not well defined
    c. Benign lesions may bleed on touch
    d. Patient is noncooperative

19. Which of the following is not an effect of cancer cervix in pregnancy?
    a. Hyperemesis gravidarum
    b. Secondary cervical dystocia
    c. Sepsis
    d. Increased incidence of cesarean section

20. Which type of route of delivery is preferred in a case of advanced cancer cervix?
    a. Vaginal delivery
    b. Instrumental delivery
    c. Classical cesarean section
    d. Lower segment cesarean section

21. Which type of degeneration of leiomyoma is common during pregnancy?
    a. Hyaline
    b. Calcific
    c. Red
    d. Myxoid

22. What is the treatment of red degeneration of leiomyoma?
    a. Delivery
    b. Induction of labor
    c. NSAIDs and supportive management
    d. Termination of labor

23. What is the proposed treatment of a leiomyoma in pregnancy?
    a. Myomectomy
    b. Hysterectomy
    c. Cesarean section in all cases
    d. Assessment at term to formulate mode of delivery

24. Which of the following is not a characteristic of luteoma of pregnancy?
    a. Virilization of female fetus
    b. Elevation of Sr. testosterone
    c. Recurrence in subsequent pregnancies
    d. Occurs due to stimulating effects of pregnancy hormones in ovarian stroma

25. Following are true about hyperreactio-luteinalis, *except*:
    a. Maternal virilization
    b. USG "spoke wheel appearance"
    c. Increased levels of HCG
    d. Risk of recurrence is rare

26. Hingorani sign is present in which of the following conditions in pregnancy?
    a. Leiomyoma
    b. Retroverted gravid uterus
    c. Ovarian tumor
    d. Prolapse tumor

CHAPTER 35: Gynecological Problems in Pregnancy

27. Which of the following tumor markers is unaffected in pregnancy?
    a. Ca-125
    b. AMH
    c. Inhibin B
    d. LDH

28. Causes of incarceration of a retroverted gravid uterus may be due to all of these, *except*:
    a. Pelvic tumors
    b. Prolapse uterus
    c. Projected sacral promontory
    d. Uterine adhesions

29. Treatment if prolapsed uterus in pregnancy does not include:
    a. Manual correction
    b. Hodge Smith's pessary
    c. Hysterectomy
    d. Vaginal packing

30. Which of the following can be done during labor in a prolapsed uterus?
    a. Duhrssen's incisions
    b. Cesarean section
    c. Instrumental delivery
    d. All of the above

ANSWERS

1. **b.** *(Reference: Williams Obstetrics, 25th edition)*
2. **c.** *(Reference: Williams Obstetrics, 25th edition)*
3. **c.** *(Reference: Williams Obstetrics, 25th edition)*
4. **d.** *(Reference: Williams Obstetrics, 25th edition)*
5. **d.** *(Reference: Williams Obstetrics, 25th edition)*
6. **c.** *(Reference: Williams Obstetrics, 25th edition)*
7. **b.** *(Reference: Williams Obstetrics, 25th edition)*
8. **c.** *(Reference: Williams Obstetrics, 25th edition)*
9. **c.** *(Reference: Williams Obstetrics, 25th edition)*
10. **b.** *(Reference: Williams Obstetrics, 25th edition)*
11. **d.** *(Reference: Dutta Obstetrics, 9th edition)*
12. **c.** *(Reference: Dutta Obstetrics, 9th edition)*
13. **d.** *(Reference: Dutta Obstetrics, 9th edition)*
14. **a.** *(Reference: Dutta Obstetrics, 9th edition)*
15. **c.** *(Reference: Williams Obstetrics, 25th edition)*
16. **d.** *(Reference: Dutta Obstetrics, 9th edition)*
17. **a.** *(Reference: Dutta Obstetrics, 9th edition)*
18. **d.** *(Reference: Dutta Obstetrics, 9th edition)*
19. **a.** *(Reference: Dutta Obstetrics, 9th edition)*
20. **c.** *(Reference: Dutta Obstetrics, 9th edition)*
21. **c.** *(Reference: Dutta Obstetrics, 9th edition)*
22. **c.** *(Reference: Dutta Obstetrics, 9th edition)*
23. **d.** *(Reference: Dutta Obstetrics, 9th edition)*
24. **c.** *(Reference: Williams Obstetrics, 25th edition)*
25. **d.** *(Reference: Williams Obstetrics, 25th edition)*
26. **c.** *(Reference: DC Dutta Obstetrics, 9th edition)*
27. **a.** *(Reference: Ian Donald's Practical Obstetric Problems, 8th edition)*
28. **b.** *(Reference: Dc Dutta Obstetrics, 9th edition)*
29. **c.** *(Reference: DC Dutta Obstetrics, 9th edition)*
30. **d.** *(Reference: DC Dutta Obstetrics, 9th edition)*

Chapter 36

Preterm Labor

Shikha Seth

QUESTIONS

1. The risk of preterm delivery is increased if the cervical length is less than:
   a. 2.5 cm
   b. 3.0 cm
   c. 3.5 cm
   d. 4.0 cm

2. A 30-year-old lady, G2P1L0, comes for routine ANC check-up with normal TIFFA scan report at 19 weeks gestation with a history of pre-term labor at 32 weeks in her first pregnancy and currently receiving micronized progesterone suppositories (100 mg) daily PV on the prescription of her gynecologist. Sonogram demonstrates a cervical length of 18 mm. Which of the following is the most appropriate next step in the management of this patient?
   a. Place patient on bed rest
   b. Substitute 17-hydroxyprogesterone caproate for the micronized progesterone suppositories
   c. Perform a reduction amniocentesis
   d. Perform a cerclage
   e. Perform a D and C to empty the uterus

3. Choose the correct statement regarding chorioamnionitis:
   a. It causes all cases of preterm labor
   b. It always follows preterm rupture of the membranes
   c. It may cause and complicate preterm rupture of the membranes
   d. It only occurs in patients with vaginitis

4. A 27-year-old G2P1 twin gestation at 28 weeks presents with abdominal pain and an irritable uterus. She reports vaginal discharge with slight bleeding with stools in the morning, but no gush of fluid. She is feeling the fetal movements as usual. No gastrointestinal or urinary symptoms are noted. Her vitals are normal with PR—96 bpm afebrile, and BP of 130–80 mm Hg. On external fetal monitoring, uterine contractions every 2–4 minutes were notified by staff. Her gravid uterus is 32 weeks size and non-tender. You will advise all of the following assessments, *except*:
   a. Sterile digital exam
   b. Intravenous hydration
   c. Bedside ultrasound
   d. Urinalysis and urine culture
   e. Rectovaginal swab for Group B Streptococcus

5. A bedside transabdominal sonography was done which showed both fetuses are in the cephalic presentation and rules out the presence of a placenta previa. A sterile speculum examination was performed, and vaginal swab was obtained. The fern and nitrazine tests were negative. A subsequent digital examination indicates that the cervix is half-effaced soft and mid-positioned. All of the following are appropriate next steps to manage this patient, *except*:
   a. Prep the patient for an emergent cesarean
   b. Administer tocolytics
   c. Administer betamethasone
   d. Obtain a neonatal consultation

6. Nifedipine should not be used in a patient with:
   a. Asthma
   b. Preterm rupture of the membranes
   c. Multiple pregnancy
   d. Hypertension

7. The strength of using fetal fibronectin as a screening test for preterm labor is in its:
   a. Positive predictive value
   b. Specificity
   c. Negative predictive value
   d. Sensitivity

8. **Indomethacin may be more dangerous to the fetus if given at or beyond:**
   a. 28 weeks
   b. 32 weeks
   c. 34 weeks
   d. 36 weeks

9. **It is recommended that pregnancy be allowed to continue in the presence of preterm rupture of the membranes (unless there are contraindications) until the duration of pregnancy reaches:**
   a. 40 weeks
   b. 37 weeks
   c. 34 weeks
   d. 32 weeks

10. **In regard to etiological factors in spontaneous preterm labor, all are correct, except:**
    a. Delivery before 34 weeks occurs in 40% of twins
    b. Spontaneous preterm labor is common in the presence of fetal compromise
    c. Uterine abnormalities such as fibroids or Mullerian abnormalities are risk factors
    d. Cervical surgery and recurrent terminations of pregnancy predispose it

11. **Statement in regard to investigations and management in diagnosed preterm labor is correct:**
    a. Fetal fibronectin in cervical mucus as a test for **onset of** preterm labor which has high negative predictive value
    b. Raised WBC count indicates chorioamnionitis
    c. Steroids should be given from 24 until 32 weeks to reduce perinatal mortality by promoting pulmonary maturity
    d. Tocolysis may allow steroid administration or *in utero* transfer to a unit with neonatal intensive care facilities
    e. Oral antibiotics are given

12. **Tocolytic drugs are all, except:**
    a. Atosiban
    b. Anticholinergics
    c. Ca channel blockers
    d. B agonists
    e. Prostaglandin synthesis inhibitors

13. **Identify the incorrect statement regarding PPROM.**
    a. PPROM occurs in one-third of established preterm labor cases
    b. Infection of the placenta (chorioamnionitis) or cord (funisitis) is uncommon
    c. Preterm delivery follows within 48 hours in 50% of cases of PPROM
    d. If there is evidence of chorioamnionitis, the delivery may be delayed 48 hours to give antibiotics and steroid cover
    e. Absence of liquor in the second trimester can result in pulmonary hypoplasia and postural deformities

14. **Tocolytic drug that inhibits uterine contractility but can cause pulmonary edema as a side effect:**
    a. Ritodrine
    b. Nifedipine
    c. Indomethacin
    d. Atosiban
    e. Magnesium sulfate

15. **Maximum daily dose of nifedipine for the tocolysis purpose recommended to avoid side effects is:**
    a. 40 mg
    b. 60 mg
    c. 100 mg
    d. 120 mg

16. **Preterm labor is associated with all, except:**
    a. Esophageal atresia
    b. Asymptomatic bacteriuria
    c. Premature rupture of membranes
    d. Fibronectin in cervicovaginal discharge in the first trimester

17. **The most important factors in regard to a baby's survival chances and long-term damage due to preterm birth are:**
    a. Birth weight and mother's health
    b. Birth weight and mother's age
    c. Weeks of gestation and birth weight
    d. Weeks of gestation and delivery method

18. **Identify the wrong statement in regard to subcategories of preterm birth, based on gestational age:**
    a. Extremely preterm (less than 28 weeks)
    b. Very preterm (28 to less than 32 weeks)
    c. Moderate preterm (32-36 weeks)
    d. Late preterm (34-36 weeks)

19. **Maternal factors which are associated with preterm labor are all, except:**
    a. Black race
    b. Adolescent pregnancy
    c. Low socioeconomic strata
    d. High BMI

20. **Cervicovaginal swab is collected in suspected preterm labor cases for diagnosing the associated common infections, except:**
    a. Chlamydia
    b. Gonorrhea
    c. Candida
    d. B-Streptococcus

21. **For GBS antibiotic prophylaxis, identify the incorrect statement.**
    a. GBS antibiotic prophylaxis be given to all preterm labor cases in developing countries
    b. Prophylaxis with I/V Penicillin G is recommended
    c. GBS antibiotic prophylaxis be given to selected preterm labor cases with rectovaginal swab positivity, maternal fever, and prolonged PPROM
    d. GBS antibiotic prophylaxis reduces the incidence of early onset sepsis by 85–90%
    e. 2 g ampicillin IV as an initial bolus followed by 1 g IV every 4 hours until delivery is an alternative commonly available option for GBS prophylaxis

22. **Find the incorrect statement in regard to steroid dosage for preterm labor.**
    a. A repeat dose of corticosteroid may be given in extreme preterm labor cases if the earlier dose is received 2 weeks before and still the patient having chance of preterm labor
    b. Repeat doses of corticosteroids be avoided in moderate preterm labor cases
    c. Prophylactic corticosteroid dose is responsible for the glucose intolerance which persists for 48 hours
    d. Prophylactic corticosteroid dose can be responsible for the raised WBC count and the abnormalities in fetal heart rate, particularly variability and tachycardia suggesting fetal distress

23. **Find the incorrect statement in regard to magnesium neuroprotection in preterm labor:**
    a. Optimal regimen for neuroprotection is loading dose 4 g over 20–30 min followed by 1 g/h infusion for maintenance
    b. Regimen once started it must be continued till delivery
    c. $MgSO_4$ be stopped if delivery does not take place in 24 hours of start of regimen
    d. $MgSO_4$ is effective if started before 4 hours of delivery of baby
    e. $MgSO_4$ be started in cases of established preterm labor when birth is planned or expected within 24 hours

24. **Find the incorrect statement regarding preterm birth management:**
    a. Cerebral palsy was reduced (RR—0.68) when $MgSO_4$ was administered before 34 weeks
    b. Delayed umbilical cord clamping at least 30 seconds is recommended with preterm birth
    c. Steroid prophylaxis is for women with an imminent preterm birth delivery based on the woman's symptoms or an accurate predictive test
    d. Vaginal progesterone has a similar preventive effect as that of oral progesterone therapy in high-risk cases of PTL
    e. Preterm birth is one of the leading causes of under-five mortality

25. **Which statement is incorrect in regard to preterm labor?**
    a. Vaginal microbiota can evaluate the risk of preterm labor
    b. 5–18% is the prevalence of preterm birth worldwide
    c. Limiting the number of vaginal examinations after PPROM can reduce chorioamnionitis
    d. Subclinical or histological chorioamnionitis based on a semiquantitative assessment of inflammatory cells in the membranes, and umbilical cord after birth does not affect the fetus
    e. Fetal inflammatory response syndrome (FIRS) is diagnosed when fetal plasma interleukin-6 is >11 pg/mL

26. **Find the incorrect statement related to chorioamnionitis:**
    a. Gibbs criteria are related to subclinical chorioamnionitis
    b. Fever along with two of the clinical signs like maternal and fetal tachycardia, leukocytosis >15,000, uterine tenderness, and foul-smelling liquor are diagnostic of chorioamnionitis
    c. Clinical chorioamnionitis criteria are not sensitive for the prediction of intra-amniotic infection in pregnant women with preterm labor or PPROM
    d. Biomarkers IGFBP-1 or PAMG-1 are recommended in vaginal fluid as it has high sensitivity and specificity

27. **Criteria for tocolytic therapy in PTL are:**
    a. All threatened preterm labor cases
    b. Women having three uterine contractions per hour with cervical changes
    c. Sonographic findings of cervical length <25 mm, effacement 50%, and dilatation >20 mm
    d. Fulfilling Gibbs clinical criteria

28. **Statements regarding methods of predicting preterm birth are correct, *except*:**
    a. HUAM—home uterine activity monitoring
    b. Salivary estriol

c. Cervico-vaginal fluid fetal fibronectin
d. Transvaginal sonographic cervical length with full bladder

29. **All statements regarding cerclage are true,** *except:*
    a. Ultrasound-indicated cerclage be given to those with cervical shortening <25 mm
    b. Emergency cerclage means premature cervical dilatation with exposed fetal membranes in the vagina
    c. History of one spontaneous second-trimester loss or preterm birth may be offered serial sonographic surveillance
    d. In women with abdominal cerclage requires birth by C-section and cerclage is removed during the surgical delivery
    e. There is a limited role of cervical length assessment postcerclage and therefore not recommended

30. **Sonographic cervical changes responsible for predicting preterm labor are all,** *except:*
    a. Cervical length of <25 mm any time after 24 weeks
    b. Funneling or protrusion of amniotic sac beyond the internal os
    c. Uterocervical angle (UCA) of >105°
    d. Amniotic sludge or debris concentrated near the internal os or dispersed in the amniotic cavity

ANSWERS

1. **a.** 2.5 cm. Cervical length of <2.5 cm (as per transvaginal USG) is an important predictor of preterm labor.

2. **d.** Perform a cerclage. In patients with a prior history of preterm labor, cervical length can be monitored by transvaginal ultrasound screening. This patient's ultrasound examination demonstrates a shortened cervix.

3. **c.** Chorioamnionitis is there in 10–15% of cases of prolonged PROM and does not always associate with the rupture of membranes.

4. **a.** Sterile digital examination. Since this patient has multiple gestations along with bleeding, cramping, and increased vaginal discharge, PTL must be ruled out. Dehydration can be a cause of premature contractions and uterine irritability, so IVF would be appropriate here A U/A with C and S would be appropriate because UTIs can cause uterine contractions. A GBS infection can also be associated with PTL, so you should obtain a culture for this as well. An SVE should *not* be performed until placenta previa has been ruled out by ultrasound since the patient reported a history of vaginal bleeding.

5. **a.** Prepare the patient for an emergent cesarean. The patient is in preterm labor because she has a dilated and effaced cervix in the presence of regular uterine contractions. Therefore, treatment is aimed at delaying delivery to allow continued fetal growth and maturity. The administration of tocolytic therapy to treat preterm contractions is indicated. In addition, from 24 to 34 weeks, management also includes the administration of steroids such as betamethasone to promote fetal lung maturity. Respiratory distress syndrome (RDS) is a sequela of preterm neonates and occurs less often in infants given betamethasone in utero. If delivery seems likely, intravenous antibiotics are administered to prevent possible neonatal sepsis. If the patient's contractions subside and if there is no evidence of infection, then the antibiotics can be discontinued. It is advantageous to obtain a neonatology consult on any patient who appears to be in preterm labor so the parents know what to expect if they give birth to preterm infants. There is no need to prepare for a cesarean section in this patient. Attempts are made to stop the labor first. If the patient continues to progress, then vaginal delivery is preferred since the twins do not have a malpresentation.

6. **d.** Hypertension. Nifedipine is an antihypertensive agent and may interfere with or have a synergistic effect with other antihypertensives they may be taking to control the BP. Normotensive women have good adaptation and their BP does not fall much with antihypertensive agents.

7. **c.** Negative predictive value. fFN has a high negative predictive value, which means if it is negative, there is a very small chance a patient will deliver in the next 7–10 days. However, if it is positive, it does not tell you that the patient will deliver prematurely. So use it to rule out preterm labor.

8. **b.** 32 weeks indomethacin

9. **c.** 34 weeks

10. **a.** Delivery before 34 weeks occurs in 40% of twins delivery before 34 weeks occurs in approximately 15–20% cases of twin gestation. Fetal compromise, either from infection, preeclampsia, or IUGR, is

associated with spontaneous preterm labor, possibly as a survival mechanism.

11. **d.** Fetal fibronectin is a sensitive test. A negative result means preterm delivery is unlikely, but it has a high false-positive rate so not routinely advised and never in clinically diagnosed cases. Steroid treatment may cause the WBC to rise. Steroids are traditionally given between 24 and 34 weeks. Tocolysis delays rather than stop preterm labor and should be used only for 24-48 hours for in utero transfer of the baby to the tertiary care center and buys some time for steroid to work. Antibiotics, intravenously, are given once the diagnosis of preterm labor is confirmed.

12. **b.** Anticholinergics. Indomethacin is a prostaglandin synthesis inhibitor that is used as a tocolytic. B_2 agonists—ritodrine, CCB—nifedipine, and $MgSO_4$ are the proven tocolytic agents.

13. **d.** Steroids in case of established infection may turn harmful for the mother. Because of the risks of infection, delivery, usually induction of labor, is offered in established chorioamnionitis.

14. **a.** Ritodrine. It is a beta-2 adrenergic receptor agonist—a class of medication used for smooth muscle relaxation. Since ritodrine has a bulky N-substituent, it has high β2-selectivity. Most side effects of beta-2 agonists result from their concurrent beta-1 activity, and include increase in heart rate, rise in systolic pressure, decrease in diastolic pressure, chest pain secondary to MI, and arrhythmia. Beta-agonists may also cause fluid retention secondary to a decrease in water clearance, which when added to the tachycardia and increased myocardial work may result in cardiac failure.

15. **b.** 60 mg. A total dose above 60 mg appears to be associated with a threefold to fourfold increase in adverse events such as headache and hypotension.

16. **d.**

17. **c.** Weeks of gestation and birth weight. The strongest predictors of survival were birth weight [OR 1.0; 95% confidence intervals (CI): 1.0-1.01] and gestational age (OR = 1.1, 95% CI: 1.05-1.17)

18. **c.** WHO has defined the subcategories to define the outcome of babies and accordingly plan the management of preterm. Extremely preterm (less than 28 weeks), very preterm (28 to less than 32 weeks), moderate preterm (32 to 34 weeks), late preterm (34 to 36 weeks)

19. **d.**

20. **c.**

21. **a.**

22. **c.** Prophylactic corticosteroid dose is responsible for the glucose intolerance which persists for 5-7 days so blood sugar screening be done before giving steroid prophylaxis, and in diabetics, proper monitoring is required during steroid coverage and dose of insulin may need to be titrated (ACOG).

23. **b.**

24. **d.** Improved neonatal hematologic indices and reduced hospital mortality with delayed cord clamping. Vaginal progesterone has proven to be more efficacious then oral form in preventing the PTL

25. **d.**

26. **a.** Gibbs criteria are for clinical chorioamnionitis.

27. **c.** Six uterine contractions per hour with cervical changes are the criteria for tocolytics clinically.

28. **d.** The transvaginal sonographic cervical length should be measured with an empty bladder.

29. **d.** Women with abdominal cerclage requires birth by C-section and the abdominal suture may be left in place following birth for future pregnancies.

30. **d.** Uterocervical angle (UCA) of >105° poses a high risk for preterm delivery. It is not considered as effective solo criterion of prediction.

Chapter 37

Preterm Premature Rupture of Membranes

Geetha Balsarkar, Sunil Tambvekar

QUESTIONS

1. Which of the following is the most common complication associated with preterm rupture of membranes (PROM)?
   a. Chorioamnionitis
   b. Postpartum hemorrhage
   c. Preeclampsia
   d. Gestational diabetes

2. What is the primary goal of managing preterm rupture of membranes before 34 weeks of gestation?
   a. Prolonging pregnancy to achieve near term delivery
   b. Immediate induction of labor
   c. Administering tocolytic therapy
   d. Administering corticosteroids for fetal lung maturity

3. A multigravida presents with preterm premature rupture of membranes.
   According to RCOG (Royal College of Obstetrician and Gynaecologists) guidelines, which of the following antibiotics is preferred for her?
   a. Ampicillin
   b. Amoxicillin
   c. Erythromycin
   d. Azithromycin

4. Which of the following is a risk factor for preterm rupture of membranes?
   a. Multifetal gestation
   b. Maternal age over 35
   c. Prepregnancy obesity
   d. Previous full-term pregnancy

5. What is the role of corticosteroids in the management of preterm rupture of membranes?
   a. They help prevent chorioamnionitis
   b. They promote uterine contractions
   c. They enhance fetal lung maturity
   d. They reduce maternal blood pressure

6. Which of the following is an important consideration in the management of preterm rupture of membranes at term (37 weeks or later)?
   a. Expectant management for up to 24-72 hours
   b. Immediate induction of labor
   c. Administration of tocolytic therapy
   d. Intravenous antibiotics for 7 days

7. In cases of preterm rupture of membranes, which intervention is aimed at reducing the risk of neonatal sepsis?
   a. Administration of corticosteroids
   b. Early initiation of antibiotics
   c. Immediate induction of labor
   d. Administration of tocolytic therapy

8. Which of the following is a potential fetal complication associated with preterm rupture of membranes?
   a. Intraventricular hemorrhage
   b. Neonatal jaundice
   c. Hypoglycemia
   d. Respiratory distress syndrome

9. Which of the following is a potential complication of expectant management in cases of preterm rupture of membranes?
   a. Chorioamnionitis
   b. Neonatal hypoglycemia
   c. Maternal hypertension
   d. Fetal macrosomia

10. What is the primary goal of tocolytic therapy in cases of preterm rupture of membranes?
    a. Enhancing fetal lung maturity
    b. Reducing uterine contractions
    c. Preventing chorioamnionitis
    d. Inducing labor

11. Which of the following factors is associated with an increased risk of recurrent preterm rupture of membranes?
    a. Recurrent vaginal infections
    b. Smoking during pregnancy
    c. Primigravidity
    d. Normal body mass index (BMI)

12. What is the recommended initial antibiotic regimen for intrapartum prophylaxis in cases of preterm rupture of membranes?
    a. Ampicillin and erythromycin
    b. Ceftriaxone and vancomycin
    c. Clindamycin and gentamicin
    d. Doxycycline and azithromycin

13. What is the role of fetal fibronectin testing in cases of preterm rupture of membranes?
    a. It helps predict the risk of preterm birth
    b. It measures fetal lung maturity
    c. It assesses amniotic fluid volume
    d. It evaluates fetal heart rate patterns

14. What is the primary risk associated with expectant management in cases of preterm rupture of membranes?
    a. Prolonged hospitalization
    b. Maternal infection
    c. Fetal malpresentation
    d. Placental abruption

15. Which of the following is a potential complication of corticosteroid administration in cases of preterm rupture of membranes?
    a. Maternal hypertension
    b. Maternal hyperglycemia
    c. Fetal bradycardia
    d. Fetal hypoglycemia

16. In cases of preterm rupture of membranes, what is the significance of a positive nitrazine test result versus a ferning test result?
    a. Positive nitrazine indicates rupture of membranes; ferning indicates presence of fetal fibronectin
    b. Positive nitrazine indicates cervical mucus alkalinity; ferning indicates presence of amniotic fluid
    c. Positive nitrazine indicates presence of fetal fibronectin; ferning indicates rupture of membranes
    d. Positive nitrazine indicates presence of amniotic fluid; ferning indicates cervical mucus alkalinity

17. What are the potential long-term neurodevelopmental outcomes for infants born following preterm rupture of membranes? How might these outcomes be influenced by various clinical factors?
    a. Potential for cognitive deficits, cerebral palsy, and sensory impairments; influenced by gestational age at delivery and exposure to repeated courses of antenatal corticosteroids
    b. Potential for autism spectrum disorders, attention deficit hyperactivity disorder (ADHD), and intellectual giftedness; influenced by maternal age and parity
    c. Potential for emotional dysregulation, learning disabilities, and motor coordination deficits; influenced by neonatal Apgar scores and birth weight
    d. Potential for language delays, visual impairments, and fine motor difficulties; influenced by maternal pre-pregnancy BMI and smoking status

18. What is the significance of a positive ferning test in cases of preterm rupture of membranes and how does it differ from a positive nitrazine test?
    a. Positive ferning indicates the presence of amniotic fluid, while positive nitrazine indicates cervical mucus alkalinity
    b. Positive ferning indicates rupture of membranes, while positive nitrazine indicates the presence of fetal fibronectin
    c. Positive ferning indicates the presence of fetal fibronectin, while positive nitrazine indicates cervical mucus alkalinity
    d. Positive ferning indicates cervical mucus alkalinity, while positive nitrazine indicates the presence of amniotic fluid

19. In cases of preterm rupture of membranes complicated by maternal fever, what are the potential etiologies of the fever and how should they be managed?
    a. Maternal fever is most commonly due to chorioamnionitis; intrapartum antibiotics and expeditious delivery are indicated
    b. Maternal fever is usually benign and does not require intervention; symptomatic management with antipyretics is sufficient

c. Maternal fever is indicative of fetal distress; immediate cesarean delivery is warranted to prevent further complications

d. Maternal fever is a sign of urinary tract infection; prophylactic antibiotics should be administered during labor

20. A 32-year-old G3P2 pregnant woman presents at 28 weeks gestation with complaints of a sudden gush of clear fluid from her vagina. She has been experiencing regular contractions for the past 3 hours. On examination, there is evidence of pooling of amniotic fluid, the cervix is 3 cm dilated and 50% effaced. Fetal heart rate tracing shows early decelerations. What is the most appropriate next step in management?
    a. Administer corticosteroids for fetal lung maturity
    b. Administer tocolytic therapy to delay labor
    c. Perform a cesarean section for fetal distress
    d. Administer intravenous antibiotics and prepare for immediate delivery

21. A 35-year-old G5P4 pregnant woman presents at 24 weeks gestation with complaints of fever, abdominal pain, and a foul-smelling vaginal discharge. She reports that she experienced a gush of clear fluid from her vagina 4 days ago. On examination, there is evidence of cervical dilation and effacement, and there is tenderness over the lower abdomen. Fetal heart rate tracing shows late decelerations. What is the most appropriate next step in management?
    a. Administer intravenous antibiotics and perform an immediate cesarean section
    b. Administer corticosteroids for fetal lung maturity and prepare for immediate delivery
    c. Perform an amniocentesis to assess for infection
    d. Administer tocolytic therapy to delay labor

22. A 28-year-old G1P0 pregnant woman presents at 29 weeks gestation with complaints of a continuous trickle of clear fluid from her vagina for the past 12 hours. She has no contractions, abdominal pain, or vaginal bleeding. On examination, a nitrazine paper test is positive for amniotic fluid, and there is minimal cervical dilation. Fetal heart rate tracing shows a reassuring pattern. What is the most appropriate next step in management?
    a. Admit the patient for expectant management with close fetal monitoring
    b. Administer tocolytic therapy to delay labor
    c. Administer corticosteroids for fetal lung maturity
    d. Perform an immediate cesarean section

23. A 34-year-old pregnant woman presents at 31 weeks gestation with preterm rupture of membranes and is found to have a positive ferning test. What does the positive ferning test indicate, and how might it influence the management plan for this patient?
    a. Positive ferning indicates cervical mucus alkalinity; no impact on management plan
    b. Positive ferning indicates the presence of amniotic fluid; supports the diagnosis of PROM
    c. Positive ferning indicates rupture of membranes; suggests chorioamnionitis
    d. Positive ferning indicates bacterial vaginosis; requires immediate antibiotics

24. A 26-year-old pregnant woman presents at 29 weeks gestation with preterm rupture of membranes and is found to have a Bishop score of 8. How might the Bishop score influence the management plan for this patient, and what are the potential implications of this finding?
    a. Bishop score suggests unfavorable cervix; consider expectant management
    b. Bishop score indicates favorable cervix for induction; consider labor induction
    c. Bishop score is not relevant in cases of PROM; continue with expectant management
    d. Bishop score indicates high risk of chorioamnionitis; expedite delivery

25. A 31-year-old pregnant woman presents at 30 weeks gestation with preterm rupture of membranes and is found to have a positive nitrazine test, but a negative ferning test. What might this combination of test results indicate, and how should it influence the management plan?
    a. Positive nitrazine indicates rupture of membranes; continue with expectant management
    b. Positive nitrazine indicates cervical mucus alkalinity; consider further assessment
    c. Positive nitrazine indicates presence of amniotic fluid; prepare for immediate delivery
    d. Positive nitrazine indicates bacterial vaginosis; administer antibiotics

26. A sample of the vaginal fluid from the posterior fornix of a patient gave a positive nitrazine paper test. Which of the following conditions does not give a false positive result?
    a. Abruptio placenta
    b. Recent sexual intercourse

c. Bacterial vaginosis
d. Oligohydramnios

27. A 28-year-old primigravida presents with premature rupture of membranes at 27 weeks and 5 days with onset of uterine activity which drug you would prefer as a choice for tocolysis?
    a. Capsule Isoxsuprine
    b. Tablet form Isoxsuprine
    c. Capsule Nifedipine
    d. Injection Atosiban

ANSWERS

1. **a.** Chorioamnionitis
   (Reference: Dashe JS, Bloom SL, Spong CY, Hoffman BL. Williams Obstetrics, 26th edition. New York: McGraw-Hill Education; 2022)

2. **a.** Prolonging pregnancy to achieve near term delivery
   (Reference: American College of Obstetricians and Gynecologists. Prelabor rupture of membranes. ACOG Practice Bulletin No. 217. Obstet Gynecol. 2020;135:e80-97)

3. **c.** Erythromycin
   According to RCOG guidelines, erythromycin is the preferred antibiotic in the case of PPROM (preterm premature rupture of membranes).
   Spontaneous rupture of membranes before the onset of labor between 28 and 37 weeks is called preterm premature rupture of membranes.
   If PPROM occurs between 28 and 34 weeks, prophylactic antibiotics and corticosteroids are given to the patient.
   (Reference: RCOG green top guidelines, No. 73)

4. **a.** Multifetal gestation
   (Reference: Dashe JS, Bloom SL, Spong CY, Hoffman BL. Williams Obstetrics, 26th edition. New York: McGraw-Hill Education; 2022)

5. **c.** They enhance fetal lung maturity
   (Reference: American College of Obstetricians and Gynecologists. Prelabor rupture of membranes. ACOG Practice Bulletin No. 217. Obstet Gynecol. 2020;135:e80-97)

6. **a.** Expectant management for up to 24–72 hours
   (Reference: American College of Obstetricians and Gynecologists. Prelabor rupture of membranes. ACOG Practice Bulletin No. 217. Obstet Gynecol. 2020;135:e80-97)

7. **b.** Early initiation of antibiotics
   (References: Dashe JS, Bloom SL, Spong CY, Hoffman BL. Williams Obstetrics, 26th Edition. New York: McGraw-Hill Education; 2022)

8. **d.** Respiratory distress syndrome
   (Reference: Dashe JS, Bloom SL, Spong CY, Hoffman BL. Williams Obstetrics, 26th Edition. New York: McGraw-Hill Education; 2022)

9. **a.** Chorioamnionitis
   (References: American College of Obstetricians and Gynecologists. Prelabor rupture of membranes. ACOG Practice Bulletin No. 217. Obstet Gynecol. 2020;135:e80-97)

10. **b.** Reducing uterine contractions
    (Reference: American College of Obstetricians and Gynecologists. Prelabor rupture of membranes. ACOG Practice Bulletin No. 217. Obstet Gynecol. 2020;135:e80-97)

11. **a.** Recurrent vaginal infections

12. **a.** Ampicillin and erythromycin
    (Reference: American College of Obstetricians and Gynecologists. Prelabor rupture of membranes. ACOG Practice Bulletin No. 217. Obstet Gynecol. 2020;135:e80-97)

13. **a.** It helps predict the risk of preterm birth.
    (Reference: American College of Obstetricians and Gynecologists. Prelabor rupture of membranes. ACOG Practice Bulletin No. 217. Obstet Gynecol. 2020;135:e80-97)

14. **b.** Maternal infection
    (Reference: American College of Obstetricians and Gynecologists. Prelabor rupture of membranes. ACOG Practice Bulletin No. 217. Obstet Gynecol. 2020;135:e80-97)

15. **b.** Maternal hyperglycemia
    (Reference: American College of Obstetricians and Gynecologists. Prelabor rupture of membranes. ACOG Practice Bulletin No. 217. Obstet Gynecol. 2020;135:e80-97)

16. **b.** Positive nitrazine indicates cervical mucus alkalinity; ferning indicates presence of amniotic fluid.
    (Reference: Cunningham. Williams Obstetrics, 26th edition. New York: McGraw-Hill Education; 2022)

17. **a.** Potential for cognitive deficits, cerebral palsy, and sensory impairments; influenced by gestational age at delivery and exposure to repeated courses of antenatal corticosteroids.
[Reference: Mercer BM, Goldenberg RL. Evidence-Based Management of Preterm Prelabor Rupture of Membranes. Semin Perinatol. 2018;42(1):19-24]

18. **a.** Increased risk of recurrent PROM; closer surveillance for signs of preterm labor in subsequent pregnancies

19. **a.** Maternal fever is most commonly due to chorioamnionitis; intrapartum antibiotics and expeditious delivery are indicated.

20. **d.** Administer intravenous antibiotics and prepare for immediate delivery

21. **a.** Administer intravenous antibiotics and perform an immediate cesarean section

22. **c.** Administer corticosteroids for fetal lung maturity

23. **b.** Positive ferning indicates the presence of amniotic fluid; supports the diagnosis of PROM.

24. **b.** Bishop score indicates favorable cervix for induction; consider labor induction.

25. **b.** Positive nitrazine indicates cervical mucus alkalinity; consider further assessment.
(Reference: Dashe JS, Bloom SL, Spong CY, Hoffman BL. Williams Obstetrics, 26th edition. New York: McGraw-Hill Education; 2022)

26. **d.** Oligohydramnios
Oligohydramnios shows a false negative nitrazine paper test.

Nitrazine paper test detects the pH of the secretions from the vaginal pool. It turns blue at pH >6. Amniotic fluid is slightly alkaline with a pH of 7.1–7.3 and vaginal secretions have a pH of 4.5–6.0.

False-positive nitrazine test can be seen in contamination of the discharge with blood, semen, and bacterial infections. False-negative nitrazine test can be seen in the case of scanty amniotic fluid.
(Reference: Dashe JS, Bloom SL, Spong CY, Hoffman BL. Williams Obstetrics, 26th edition. New York: McGraw-Hill Education; 2022)

27. **d.** Injection Atosiban

Chapter 38

Postmaturity

Arnav Pai, Rishma Dhillon Pai

QUESTIONS

1. **What is meant by full term?**
   a. 38 0/7 weeks through 41 weeks
   b. 37 0/7 weeks through 42 weeks
   c. 39 0/7 weeks through 40 6/7 weeks
   d. 38 0/7 weeks through 40 6/7 weeks

2. **The most common cause of prolonged pregnancy:**
   a. Ethnic and race related
   b. Miscalculated gestational age
   c. Genetic
   d. Nutritional status

3. **A patient has a history of previous post-term delivery at 44 weeks. What will be the risk of recurrence of post-term pregnancy in this patient and what is the general rate of recurrence of post-term pregnancy?**
   a. 30%, 15%
   b. 20%, 15%
   c. 40%, 10%
   d. 15%, 5%

4. **What is the stillbirth rate at 42 weeks of gestation?**
   a. 3.18/1,000
   b. 2/1,000
   c. 6/1,000
   d. 11/1,000

5. **What is fetal dysmaturity syndrome?**
   a. Fetal hypoxia in post-term pregnancies
   b. Small for gestational age fetus
   c. Chronic intrauterine malnutrition and meconium staining
   d. Fetal metabolic disturbances

6. **Common metabolic dysfunction seen in post-term fetus:**
   a. Hyperlipidemia
   b. Normal glucose levels
   c. Hyperglycemia
   d. Hypoglycemia

7. **Why is fetal hypoxia more common in post-term pregnancies?**
   a. Placental dysfunction
   b. Anemia
   c. Meconium-stained liquor
   d. Larger size of the fetus

8. **Which enzyme deficiency can lead to post-term pregnancy?**
   a. Acid phosphatase
   b. Alkaline phosphatase
   c. Placental sulfatase
   d. Transferase

9. **How does anencephaly cause postmaturity?**
   a. Malpresentation
   b. Disrupts pituitary axis
   c. Polyhydramnios
   d. Hampers placental sulfatase

10. **What does SWEPIS study state?**
    a. Induction should not be offered prior to 41 weeks
    b. Higher perinatal mortality in induced group
    c. Expectant treatment group has worst results
    d. No significant differences in either group

11. **ARRIVE trial says to induce labor at what weeks of gestation?**
    a. 38 weeks
    b. 39 weeks
    c. 40 weeks
    d. 41 weeks

12. **Which of the following is true about postmaturity?**
    a. Modified BPP monitoring can be done
    b. Completed BPP monitoring must be done
    c. Once weekly NST
    d. AFI is preferred over SDP for amniotic fluid

13. **Which of the following is true in meconium-stained amniotic fluid?**
    a. Pharyngeal aspiration not recommended
    b. Pharyngeal aspiration should be done
    c. Pharyngeal aspiration can be done in vigorous baby
    d. Tracheal aspiration recommended

14. A patient with 42 weeks gestation is in labor and has a cervical dilatation of 3 cm, cervical length of 2 cm, soft cervix, central cervix, and station-2. What is the Bishop score?
    a. 6
    b. 7
    c. 8
    d. 9

15. WHO 2018 guidelines recommend induction of labor at what weeks of gestation?
    a. 39 weeks
    b. 40 weeks
    c. 41 weeks
    d. 42 weeks

16. All of the following are true, *except:*
    a. Foley's catheter induction is recommended
    b. Sublingual misoprostol is recommended
    c. Prostaglandins are fist line for cervical ripening
    d. Oxytocin can be used in previous cesarean patients

17. Incidence of fetal dysmaturity syndrome in postmaturity cases:
    a. 5%
    b. 10%
    c. 15%
    d. 20%

18. Color of meconium in postmaturity is:
    a. Straw color
    b. Deep yellow
    c. Golden
    d. Saffron

19. False about onset of labor:
    a. Progesterone levels decrease
    b. Estrogen levels decrease
    c. Cortisol levels rise
    d. Prostaglandins rise

20. Correct estimation of gestational age is important to avoid postmaturity error. At 11–13.6 weeks, the CRL is estimated to be:
    a. 40–90 mm
    b. 45–84 mm
    c. 46–94 mm
    d. 48–88 mm

21. All can occur in post-term fetus, *except:*
    a. Polycythemia
    b. Hypoglycemia
    c. Persistent pulmonary hypotension
    d. Neurodevelopmental problems

22. All commonly occur in post-term delivery, *except:*
    a. Increased instrumentation
    b. Pelvic floor trauma
    c. Meconium-stained liquor
    d. Precipitate labor

23. Which of the following is false?
    a. In the first trimester, CRL is the best measurement to determine gestational age
    b. Dating ultrasound can lead to reduction in pregnancies considered post-term by 70%
    c. Previous history of postmaturity is a risk factor
    d. Paternal genes do not play role in postmaturity

24. What is the term commonly used to describe the condition when a postmature fetus develops thick, peeling, and cracked skin due to prolonged exposure to the amniotic fluid?
    a. Erythroblastosis fetalis
    b. Fetal hydrops
    c. Meconium aspiration syndrome
    d. Postmature desquamation

25. Postmature infants are at a higher risk for hypoglycemia because:
    a. They have a decreased insulin production
    b. Their liver is less efficient at storing glycogen
    c. They have excessive fat stores
    d. Their pancreas is more active

26. Which of the following is a potential complication of postmaturity for the mother?
    a. Gestational diabetes
    b. Preeclampsia
    c. Ectopic pregnancy
    d. Placenta accreta

27. In postmature pregnancies, what is the primary concern regarding the umbilical cord?
    a. The risk of cord compression and decreased oxygen supply to the fetus
    b. The risk of a nuchal cord
    c. The risk of an umbilical hernia in the fetus
    d. The risk of a true knot in the umbilical cord

28. Postmature infants are more likely to experience difficulties with thermoregulation because:
    a. They have a thicker subcutaneous fat layer
    b. They have an underdeveloped hypothalamus
    c. They have lower metabolic rates
    d. They have less brown fat

29. In postmature pregnancies, the fetus may be at risk for which of the following complications due to the aging of the placenta?
    a. Polyhydramnios
    b. Fetal hydrops
    c. Meconium aspiration syndrome
    d. Placental abruption

30. What is the typical method used for estimating gestational age and determining postmaturity?
    a. Measuring fundal height
    b. Counting fetal movements
    c. Ultrasound dating
    d. Evaluating maternal weight gain

ANSWERS

1. **c.**
    - Early term is 37 0/7 weeks through 38 6/7 weeks
    - Full term is 39 0/7 weeks through 40 6/7 weeks
    - Late term is 41 0/7 weeks through 41 6/7 weeks
    - Post-term beyond 42 weeks

2. **b.** Most common cause of prolonged pregnancy is error in gestational age calculation. No relation has been found between post-term and age, parity or nutritional status.

3. **a.** In a patient with previous history of 44 weeks delivery the rate of post-term recurrence can go up to 30%. General rate of post-term recurrence is 15%.

4. **a.** As per meta-analysis, the stillbirth rate at 42 weeks is 3.18/1000. At 43 weeks, the rate is 11.5/1,000.

5. **c.** Fetal dysmaturity syndrome is characterized by chronic fetal malnutrition with decreased subcutaneous fat and vernix and meconium staining of amniotic fluid, skin, and placenta. It is seen in post-term pregnancy.

6. **d.** Hypoglycemia is commonly seen in post-term fetus.

7. **a.** In post-term pregnancy, there is placental dysfunction due to microinfarcts and calcifications thereby reducing blood flow to the fetus resulting in fetal hypoxia and eventual meconium passage.

8. **c.** Placental sulfatase deficiency can lead to postmaturity.

9. **b.** In anencephaly, there is no skull vault and pituitary therefore there is hampered pituitary axis leading to reduced cortisol level for onset of labor.

10. **c.** In SWEPIS study, it showed that expectant management in 42 weeks gestation had greater perinatal mortality rates and induction of labor should be offered no later than 41 weeks.

11. **b.** ARRIVE trial states that induction of labor at 39 weeks showed lesser complications as opposed to expectant management until 41 weeks.

12. **a.** Modified BPP which contains NST with amniotic fluid evaluation is preferred over completed BPP. Amniotic fluid measurement should be done by SDP and NST must be done twice weekly.

13. **a.** Pharyngeal aspiration is not recommended. If the baby is nonvigorous and has aspirated thick meconium then aspiration must be done.

14. **c.**

Bishop score = (total)		Date of Bishop score:.........		
Score	0	1	2	3
Dilation	Closed	1–2	3–4	5
Length	>4	3–4	1–2	0
Consistency	Firm	Medium	Soft	—
Position	Posterior	Midline	Anterior	—
Head—station	–3	–2	–1,0	4-1,+2

15. **c.** WHO 2018 recommends induction of labor at 41 completed weeks.

16. **b.** Sublingual misoprostol is not recommended as it is associated with higher rates of hyperstimulation and hence oral misoprostol is preferred. Also, prostaglandins are not recommended in previous cesarean patients.

17. **d.** The incidence is 20%.

18. **d.** Color of amniotic fluid in postmaturity is saffron.

19. **b.** Cortisol rise leads to preferential production of estradiol which rises, drop in progesterone and rise in prostaglandins in labor.

20. **b.** 11–13.6 weeks corresponds to CRL of 45–84 mm.

21. **c.** There is persistent pulmonary hypertension that occurs.

22. **d.** Not seen commonly precipitate labor.

23. **d.** Paternal genes do play a role in post-term risk as per studies.

24. **d.** Postmature desquamation which occurs in postmaturity.

25. **b.** The liver less efficiently stores glycogen which leads to hypoglycemia.

26. **b.** Rates of preeclampsia are increased as per certain studies.

27. **a.** The reason for hypoxia could be placental insufficiency or umbilical cord compression due to macrosomia or oligohydramnios.

28. **d.** Less fat stores hence lesser brown fat leading to reduced energy and heat production.

29. **c.** Hypoxia leads to autonomic nervous system stimulation and passage of meconium.

30. **c.** USG dating is the preferred method.

Chapter 39

Intrauterine Fetal Demise

Vaidehi Thakur, Mandakini Megh, Deep Kamal

QUESTIONS

1. **The most common complication of intrauterine fetal demise (IUFD):**
   a. Choriocarcinoma
   b. Disseminated intravascular coagulopathy
   c. Transfusion syndrome
   d. Retinopathy and nephropathy

2. **The following is not true for intrauterine fetal demise**
   a. Half of world's stillbirths are linked to intrapartum complication
   b. Intrapartum fetal demises could likely be averted with increased access to skilled healthcare
   c. The risk of stillbirth is greater in women with prior unexplained stillbirth
   d. Prior preterm birth <34 weeks does not increase the risk of a subsequent stillbirth

3. **Correlation between gestational age and IUFD, one of the following is not true:**
   a. Stillbirth risk is increased by early and late-term gestational age
   b. Induction of labor at 40 weeks will not change the incidence of cesarean delivery
   c. Neonatal and maternal adverse outcomes, must be considered while considering the induction of labor
   d. Induction of labor might be considered at 41 weeks and is recommended after 42 weeks of gestation

4. **Possible causes of stillbirth are:**
   a. Genetic abnormalities
   b. Rupture uterus
   c. Abruptio placentae
   d. All of the above

5. **In intrahepatic cholestasis of pregnancy, what is not true?**
   a. Higher stillbirth risk is seen with severe OC (bile acids >100 µmol/L)
   b. Serum bile acids should be tested fasting
   c. Bile acid concentration should be monitored weekly
   d. Ursodeoxycholic acid does not reduce the risk of stillbirth

6. **The most accurate method for diagnosis of IUFD:**
   a. No fetal movements by the mother
   b. Recurrent bleeding per vagina
   c. FHS not heard on Auscultation
   d. Ultrasound suggestive of absent cardiac activity

7. **Which sign appears earliest in IUFD?**
   a. Roberts sign
   b. Spalding sign
   c. Crowding of ribs
   d. Hyperflexion of spine

8. **Following routine investigations are required to detect the cause of IUFD immediately:**
   a. Amniocentesis if delivery is not imminent
   b. CBC and glucose
   c. Viral markers
   d. Thrombophilia testing

9. **The following is not true with diabetes and intrauterine fetal demise:**
   a. Poor diabetic control determined in pregnancy is associated with increased incidence of stillbirth
   b. If birth weight is <10th percentile, risk for stillbirth is elevated
   c. If birth weight is over 95th percentile, the risk of stillbirth is twofold
   d. Highest rate for stillbirth is between 32 and 34 weeks in type 1 and 2 diabetes mellitus

10. **The most common cause of IUFD is:**
    a. True knots in the cord
    b. Unexplained
    c. Infections
    d. Placental abruption

11. **The incidence of intrauterine fetal demise is:**
    a. More in non-Hispanic black women of United States
    b. More in white women of European countries
    c. Not related with race
    d. More in Asian black women

12. **All of the following are signs of IUFD, except:**
    a. Spalding's sign
    b. Hegar's sign
    c. Robert's sign
    d. Halo sign

13. **The following is true for maternal and paternal age and IUFD:**
    a. The risk of stillbirth is not related to advanced maternal age
    b. Maternal age over 35 has an increased risk for stillbirth, which is accentuated by nulliparity
    c. Stillbirth is not related with lethal chromosomal abnormalities
    d. Paternal age is not related with incidence of stillbirth

14. **In cases of IUFD, what is true?**
    a. Cause can be identified in most cases
    b. Immediate delivery is indicated
    c. More common with good antenatal care
    d. Careful examination of the newborn is important

15. **Spalding's sign appears in IUFD:**
    a. 12–24 hours after demise
    b. 24–48 hours after demise
    c. 48 hours to 7 days after demise
    d. More than 7 days of demise

16. **Which is incorrect regarding the options for suppression of lactation in IUFD?**
    a. Nonpharmacological measures cause excessive discomfort
    b. Dopamine agonists are well tolerated by majority of women
    c. Cabergoline is superior to bromocriptine
    d. Dopamine agonists can be given to women with hypertension or pre-eclampsia

17. **What is incorrect with IUFD?**
    a. Detection of congenital defects antenatally will decrease the incidence of stillbirth
    b. The risk of stillbirth with persistent polyhydramnios is more than resolved polyhydramnios
    c. The risk of stillbirth in polyhydramnios decreases with gestational age
    d. Alcohol consumption increases the risk of stillbirth

18. **One of the following options is incorrect while examination is done postdelivery in IUFD:**
    a. Photography of placenta and cord
    b. Culture of placenta with aerobic and anaerobic culture swabs
    c. Written consent for autopsy
    d. Skin biopsy of macerated skin

19. **What is Robert's sign seen in IUFD?**
    a. Hyperflexion of spines
    b. Crowding of rib shadows
    c. Appearance of gas shadows in heart and great blood vessels
    d. Hyperextension of neck

20. **Following is the recommendation for management of future delivery after unexplained stillbirth:**
    a. Recommend birth at a specialist maternity unit
    b. Previous IUFD related to a known nonrecurrent cause merits individual assessment for place of birth
    c. Maternal request for scheduled birth should consider gestational age of the previous IUFD, previous intrapartum history, and safety of induction of labor
    d. All of the above

21. **What is wrong in the management of IUFD?**
    a. Standard doses of synthetic oxytocin are used for delivery with favorable cervix
    b. Misoprostol can be given with unfavorable cervix with no hysterotomy scar
    c. Large fetuses can be delivered vaginally
    d. Trial of labor is contraindicated in women with unfavorable cervix and a prior history of a cesarean section

22. **What is not true for induction of labor in IUFD for a woman with an unscarred uterus?**
    a. A combination of mifepristone and misoprostol for induction of labor is safe and effective
    b. Misoprostol can be used in preference to prostaglandin E2 because of equivalent safety and efficacy
    c. Vaginal misoprostol is as effective as oral therapy but associated with fewer adverse effects
    d. Women with poor Bishop's score should not be given trial of labor and delivered immediately in view of risk of DIC

23. **What is incorrect in the management of IUFD?**
    a. ARM should be done in early labor
    b. Antibiotics covering anaerobic cover should be given
    c. Active management of third stage of labor is done
    d. DIC is rare before 3-4 weeks after the IUFD

24. **Chromosomal study in cases of IUFD, what is incorrect?**
    a. Chromosome testing for aneuploidy should be offered for all stillbirths to seek a cause
    b. Chromosomal microarray testing is now the preferred test
    c. Patient consent is necessary for amniocentesis and chorionic villus sampling
    d. Consent is necessary to save placental tissue or amniotic fluid containing amniocyte

25. **What is incorrect in induction of labor in scarred uterus in IUFD?**
    a. Trial of labor is contraindicated in midline incision scarred uterus
    b. Pharmacological induction of labor can be given in previous lower segment cesarean section
    c. Mifepristone can be used alone to increase the chance of labor significantly within 72 hours
    d. Repeat cesarean section is indicated in all the cases of previous scarred uterus

26. **Following is not true of Babygram done to investigate the cause of IUFD:**
    a. Babygram is a lateral and anterior–posterior X-ray of the whole fetus
    b. It uncovers skeletal dysplasia, costovertebral malformations, ectopic calcifications, and gas collections suggestive of infection
    c. This study may confirm or suggest a cause of stillbirth in 80% of cases
    d. All of the above

27. **The following is incorrect about autopsy of stillbirth:**
    a. Autopsy may identify the cause for stillbirth in 46% of cases
    b. Performance of an autopsy requires written consent
    c. If someone with this expertise is not locally available, the fetus and/or placenta can be transferred to another center for evaluation.
    d. Autopsy cannot evaluate cardiac malformations in stillbirths

28. **What is not true of smoking and IUFD?**
    a. Quitting by the beginning of the second trimester reduces the risk of stillbirth
    b. Active smoking is associated with increased incidence for having one or more stillbirths
    c. Passive smoking increases the incidence of smoking
    d. There is no association of stillbirth and smoking

29. **Antiphospholipid antibody syndrome and IUFD—what is not true?**
    a. Stillbirth risk is lowest when the lupus anticoagulant is negative
    b. Family history of thromboembolism increases the risk for stillbirth
    c. With diagnosis of pregnancy, warfarin must be stopped, and low molecular weight heparin started
    d. Low molecular weight heparin should be given till the end of first trimester

30. **Infections and IUFD, what is incorrect?**
    a. Infection accounts for 2% of stillbirths at term
    b. Human immunodeficiency virus increases the risk of stillbirth
    c. *Escherichia coli* is the most common bacterial infection responsible for stillbirth
    d. Serologic screening for toxoplasmosis, chlamydia, rubella, or herpes is indicated in all cases of IUFD

ANSWERS

1. **b.** Most common complication of IUFD is DIC—22.5%, followed by sepsis (10%), ARF (3.7%), and maternal mortality (1.2%).

2. **d.** Half of the world's stillbirths are linked to intrapartum complications; most of these deaths could likely be averted with increased access to skilled healthcare. Prior preterm birth less than 34 weeks increases the risk of a subsequent stillbirth three times. Compared to a woman with a prior stillbirth, the risk of stillbirth is even greater for women who have delivered a viable, growth-restricted fetus before 32 weeks gestational age.

3. **b.** Stillbirth risk is increased by early and late-term gestational age. Induction of labor after 40 weeks may decrease the risk of stillbirth and cesarean delivery. Induction of labor is recommended after 42 weeks and might be considered after 41 weeks of gestation.

4. **d.** *Placental and umbilical cord factors:* Fetomaternal hemorrhage, placental abruption, placental insufficiency, premature rupture of membranes, and umbilical cord accident (compression, twisting, knotting, etc.)

    Fetal risk factors: Infection, hereditary or genetic abnormalities, multiple fetuses, fetal growth restriction

    Maternal risk factors: Advanced maternal age (35 years or older), diabetes that is poorly controlled, ABO incompatibility, preeclampsia or eclampsia, postdatism, rupture uterus, use of alcohol, drugs, or tobacco during pregnancy

5. **b.** A higher stillbirth risk is only noted in severe OC defined by bile acids at or above 100 µmol/L. Medical induction after 37 weeks, in this group, is still advised. The majority of women with OC will have bile acids <100 µmol/L and can be reassured that their risk for stillbirth is not elevated. Bile acid concentration can change quickly in late pregnancy and, therefore, should be measured weekly. Although bile acids may be elevated after eating compared to fasting, median levels are similar, and therefore testing may be performed either fasting or postprandially. Whether the treatment of OC with ursodeoxycholic acid reduces the risk of stillbirth warrants future study.

6. **d.** Absence of fetal cardiac activity by real-time ultrasound is diagnostic for IUFD.

7. **a.** Robert's sign occurs within 12 hours. It is appearance of gas shadows in heart and great blood vessels.

8. **d.** All patients should be offered amniocentesis if delivery is not imminent, even if a prior cell-free DNA screening was unremarkable. All patients require CBC, glucose, as well as type and screen for HIV and syphilis. These helps screen for maternal hemoglobinopathy, infection, poor glycemic control, or undiagnosed diabetes and red cell alloimmunization. Most maternal and fetal thrombophilias are not associated with stillbirth, and routine testing for thrombophilias is not recommended. Screening may be considered if there is a history of growth restriction or a personal or family history of blood clots. Testing for thrombophilia includes: Factor V Leiden, prothrombin mutation, antithrombin III, MTHFR, protein C, and S. Of these factors, only protein S levels are affected by the pregnancy, and therefore protein S should only be tested 3 months after the delivery.

9. **d.** Third of the stillbirths associated with diabetes occur at term. The highest rate for stillbirth is in the 38th week for type 1 diabetes and in the 39th week for type 2 diabetes.

10. **b.** The cause of IUFD remains unexplained in majority of cases. Many stillbirths are due to placental complications.

11. **a.** Non-Hispanic, black women in US have a higher rate of stillbirth (11 per 1,000 births) compared to other racial groups. This group also has a higher incidence of diabetes, hypertension, premature membrane rupture, and abruption may account for the higher rate of stillbirth.

12. **b.** Hegar's sign is nonspecific indication of pregnancy characterized by compressibility and softening of cervical isthmus.

13. **b.** The risk of stillbirth is augmented by advanced maternal age due to an increased risk for aneuploidy and medical complications of pregnancy. Even after controlling for these risk factors, maternal age over 35 has an increased risk for stillbirth, which is accentuated by nulliparity. Stillbirth may be caused by lethal chromosomal abnormalities, which are more prevalent when the maternal age is greater than 35. 13% of stillbirths have an abnormal karyotype. A paternal age over 40 also increases the risk of stillbirth.

14. **d.** Cause of IUFD mostly remains undetected, in most cases and incidence decreases with good antenatal care.

15. **d.** Spalding's sign is irregular overlapping of cranial bones due to liquefaction of brain matter. It generally appears after 7 days of IUFD.

16. **d.** Dopamine agonists should not be given to women with hypertension or preeclampsia as it causes intracranial hemorrhage.

17. **c.** Compared with pregnancies unaffected by polyhydramnios, the risk of stillbirth for women with polyhydramnios increases with gestational age, with the lowest risk at 26 weeks gestation, seven times increased relative risk at 37 weeks, and 11 times increased relative risk at 40 weeks. The risk persists even after excluding confounding variables and sharply increases at term.

18. **d.** Avoid skin biopsy for cytogenetic testing if there is any maceration as this tissue will not yield a result.
19. **c.** Robert's sign is appearance of gas shadows in heart and great blood vessels. It appears 12 hours after stillbirth. It is difficult to interpret.
20. **d.** Recommend birth at a specialist maternity unit. Previous IUFD related to a known nonrecurrent cause merits individual assessment for place of birth. Maternal request for scheduled birth should consider gestational age of the previous IUFD, previous intrapartum history, and safety of induction of labor.
21. **d.** Women with third-trimester fetal demise and an unfavorable cervix, and a prior history of a cesarean section should use a mechanical method of cervical ripening followed by oxytocin for induction. Misoprostol may be considered as an option only after rigorous informed consent. The lowest dose of 25–50 µg vaginally should be used, and the dose should not be doubled to reduce the risk of uterine rupture
22. **d.** Trial of labor should be given in all the cases of IUFD with unscarred uterus.
23. **a.** ARM is contraindicated in early labor as it can lead to ascending infection.
24. **d.** No consent is required to save placental tissue or amniotic fluid containing amniocyte.
25. **d.** Trial of labor can be given under proper supervision.
26. **c.** This study may confirm or suggest a cause of stillbirth in 16% of cases.
27. **d.** Cardiac malformations are not readily detected on postmortem imaging, and hence an autopsy is invaluable to evaluate for them.
28. **d.** Women exposed to second-hand smoke for greater than 10 years in childhood or 20 years in adulthood at home or 10 years at adult work have an increased risk for having one or more stillbirths.
29. **d.** A personal or family history of thromboembolism appears to have an increased risk for stillbirth. LMWH should be given throughout the pregnancy.
30. **d.** Infection is unlikely the cause of stillbirth unless it results in significant autopsy or placental findings. Serologic screening for toxoplasmosis, chlamydia, rubella, or herpes is usually not indicated when these infections are not detected on placental or autopsy examination.

Chapter 40: Malpresentation, Malposition, and Cephalopelvic Disproportion

Surekha Tayade

QUESTIONS

1. A 36-year-old pregnant woman at 41 weeks of gestation is in active labor, and the obstetrician suspects a malpresentation due to an atypical fetal heart rate pattern. Upon examination, the baby is found to have its head flexed, but the head is presenting upward. The fetal heart rate tracing shows a late deceleration pattern. What is the most likely fetal presentation, and what are the potential implications for the baby's well-being?
   a. Occiput posterior presentation; risk of shoulder dystocia and umbilical cord prolapse
   b. Occiput anterior presentation; increased risk of uterine rupture and cephalopelvic disproportion (CPD)
   c. Brow presentation; increased risk of fetal head entrapment and prolonged labor
   d. Face presentation; risk of fetal head hyperextension and compromised oxygenation

2. A 32-year-old pregnant woman at 35 weeks of gestation is diagnosed with a compound presentation during an ultrasound examination. Upon palpation, the obstetrician confirms that the baby's head is presenting downward, but one of the arms is alongside the head. What is the most appropriate management plan for delivery?
   a. Proceed with a trial of vaginal delivery with close fetal monitoring
   b. Attempt external cephalic version (ECV) to correct the malpresentation
   c. Prepare for an emergency cesarean section due to the increased risk of cord prolapse
   d. Administer tocolytic drugs to prevent preterm labor and facilitate cephalic presentation

3. A 37-year-old pregnant woman at 40 weeks of gestation with a breech presentation is contemplating her delivery options. She wants to avoid a cesarean section if possible. What information should the healthcare provider provide to facilitate an informed decision-making process?
   a. The risks and benefits of vaginal breech delivery, including the potential for complications and success rates
   b. The indications and procedure for ECV to attempt to convert the baby to a cephalic presentation
   c. The advantages and disadvantages of planned cesarean section, including the recovery period and potential long-term consequences
   d. The possibility of using forceps or vacuum extraction during vaginal breech delivery to reduce the need for a cesarean section

4. A 30-year-old pregnant woman at 38 weeks of gestation presents to the labor ward in active labor. On examination, the obstetrician finds that the baby is in a shoulder presentation. The baby's head is not engaged, and the fetal heart rate tracing shows a sinusoidal pattern. What is the most appropriate management for this situation?
   a. Attempt an ECV to convert the baby to a cephalic presentation
   b. Proceed with a trial of vaginal delivery with close fetal monitoring and possible vacuum extraction if the head descends
   c. Prepare for an emergency cesarean section due to the risk of cord prolapse and fetal distress
   d. Administer tocolytic drugs to delay labor and allow for the baby's head to engage in the pelvis

5. A 34-year-old pregnant woman at 36 weeks of gestation is diagnosed with a transverse lie during an ultrasound examination. The woman has a history of two previous cesarean sections. She is adamant about attempting a vaginal birth this time. What is the most appropriate approach for managing this malpresentation in the context of her previous cesarean deliveries?
   a. Offer a trial of ECV to convert the baby to a cephalic presentation
   b. Plan for an elective cesarean section to avoid the risk of uterine rupture
   c. Attempt a vaginal breech delivery with careful monitoring of fetal position and progress
   d. Induce labor and proceed with a trial of vaginal delivery, considering her previous obstetric history

6. A 29-year-old pregnant woman at 38 weeks of gestation is in active labor, and her baby is diagnosed with a shoulder presentation. The obstetrician attempts to perform Rubin's maneuver to resolve the malpresentation, but it is unsuccessful. What is the next appropriate step in managing this situation?
   a. Proceed with a trial of ECV to convert the baby to a cephalic presentation
   b. Prepare for an emergency cesarean section due to the risk of cord prolapse and fetal distress
   c. Attempt the Woods' screw maneuver to rotate the baby to a more favorable position
   d. Administer tocolytic drugs to delay labor and allow for the baby's head to engage in the pelvis

7. A 33-year-old pregnant woman at 36 weeks of gestation is diagnosed with a transverse lie during a routine ultrasound examination. The obstetrician discusses the management options with the patient, including ECV. The patient asks about the success rate and potential complications of ECV. Which of the following statements is the most accurate regarding ECV?
   a. ECV is successful in approximately 80% of cases and carries a low risk of fetal distress
   b. ECV has a success rate of around 50%, and the most common complication is maternal discomfort
   c. ECV is successful in about 30% of the cases, and the main risk is the potential for umbilical cord compression
   d. ECV has a success rate of over 90% and is associated with a low risk of maternal discomfort

8. A 34-year-old pregnant woman at 39 weeks of gestation is admitted to the labor ward with a breech presentation. She is considering the option of vaginal breech delivery after counseling on the risks and benefits. What factors should be taken into consideration when deciding the appropriateness of vaginal breech delivery?
   a. Estimated fetal weight, parity, placental location, and the obstetrician's experience in managing breech deliveries
   b. Maternal age, fetal gender, gestational age, and previous birth experience
   c. Rupture of membranes, maternal body mass index (BMI), and the position of the baby's feet
   d. Presence of fetal anomalies, maternal occupation, and family history of breech presentation

9. A 36-year-old pregnant woman at 40 weeks of gestation with a breech presentation is considering the option of vaginal breech delivery to avoid a cesarean section. The obstetrician discusses the risks and benefits of vaginal breech delivery with the patient, and the patient remains uncertain about her decision. What additional information could be provided to facilitate the decision-making process?
   a. A simulation of the labor process and potential maneuvers used during vaginal breech delivery
   b. The experience and success rates of other patients who have attempted vaginal breech delivery
   c. A list of alternative birthing positions that might be considered to optimize the chances of successful vaginal breech delivery
   d. A description of the potential long-term effects of cesarean section and its implications for future pregnancies

10. A 31-year-old pregnant woman at 37 weeks of gestation presents to the labor ward in active labor. The obstetrician finds that the baby is in a frank breech presentation. The woman expresses her preference for a vaginal delivery and asks about the techniques used during vaginal breech delivery. Which technique is recommended to facilitate the delivery of the aftercoming head during vaginal breech delivery?
    a. Mauriceau–Smellie–Veit maneuver
    b. Rubin maneuver
    c. Lovset maneuver
    d. Zavanelli maneuver

11. **Scenario:** A 32-year-old pregnant woman at 39 weeks of gestation presents to the labor ward in active labor. On examination, the obstetrician finds that the baby's head is in a transverse position, and the baby's head is not engaging into the pelvis. The woman is experiencing intense contractions. Fetal heart rate monitoring shows decelerations. What is the most appropriate management for this situation?
    a. Proceed with a trial of vaginal delivery and assist with forceps if necessary
    b. Prepare for an emergency cesarean section due to the risk of cord prolapse and fetal distress
    c. Administer tocolytic drugs to delay labor and attempt ECV
    d. Attempt the Woods' screw maneuver to rotate the baby's head to a more favorable position

12. A 29-year-old pregnant woman at 35 weeks of gestation presents for a routine check-up. The obstetrician palpates the baby's back on the left side of the mother's abdomen, and the small parts (hands and feet) are felt on the right side. The woman has a history of a previous cesarean section. What type of malposition is most likely present, and what factors should be considered for the management?
    a. Left occiput transverse (LOT) presentation; consider ECV after 37 weeks of gestation
    b. Right occiput anterior (ROA) presentation; proceed with a trial of vaginal delivery
    c. Left sacroanterior (LSA) presentation; plan for an elective cesarean section
    d. Right sacrotransverse (RST) presentation; attempt manual rotation during the labor

13. A 31-year-old pregnant woman at 37 weeks of gestation presents for a routine check-up. The obstetrician palpates the baby's back on the right side of the mother's abdomen, and the small parts (hands and feet) are felt on the left side. What type of malposition is most likely present, and what are the potential implications for labor and delivery?
    a. LOA presentation; increased risk of persistent occiput posterior position during labor
    b. RSA presentation; increased risk of prolonged labor and fetal malposition
    c. LOT presentation; potential for spontaneous rotation into the occiput anterior position during labor
    d. RST presentation; potential for spontaneous rotation into the occiput posterior position during labor

14. A 34-year-old pregnant woman at 38 weeks of gestation presents in labor. The obstetrician performs a vaginal examination and finds that the baby's head is in a transverse position, and the head is not engaging into the pelvis. This is the woman's first pregnancy. The patient desires a vaginal delivery and asks about the potential risks of continuing with labor. What is the most appropriate response?
    a. Continuing with labor may result in a higher likelihood of uterine rupture, given the transverse lie position
    b. The baby's head is not engaging into the pelvis, and there is a risk of cord prolapse if labor continues
    c. Transverse lie in the first pregnancy is associated with an increased risk of fetal distress and shoulder dystocia
    d. In transverse lie positions, vaginal delivery is usually not feasible, and a cesarean section may be necessary

15. A 30-year-old pregnant woman at 37 weeks of gestation with a previous cesarean section presents in labor. The obstetrician performs a vaginal examination and finds that the baby's head is in a transverse position, and the head is not engaging into the pelvis. The patient expresses her desire for a trial of vaginal delivery after a previous cesarean section. What information should be provided to the patient regarding the risks and benefits of continuing with a trial of labor?
    a. The risk of uterine rupture and the potential for emergent cesarean section during labor
    b. The risk of shoulder dystocia and potential for prolonged labor
    c. The risk of cord prolapse and the likelihood of successful vaginal birth
    d. The risk of infection and potential for neonatal respiratory distress

16. A 32-year-old pregnant woman at 36 weeks of gestation presents for a routine check-up. The obstetrician performs an ultrasound to assess the fetal presentation. The ultrasound shows that the baby's head is presenting downward, but the baby's face is looking upward. What type of malpresentation is this, and what potential complications may arise during delivery?
    a. Brow presentation; increased risk of fetal head entrapment and prolonged labor

b. Face presentation; risk of fetal head hyperextension and compromised oxygenation
c. Occiput transverse presentation; risk of shoulder dystocia and uterine rupture
d. Compound presentation; potential for umbilical cord prolapse and cord compression

17. A 28-year-old pregnant woman at 41 weeks of gestation is in labor. The obstetrician observes an arrest of labor despite strong uterine contractions, and the baby's head fails to descend despite adequate maternal effort. What is the most likely cause of this situation?
    a. Macrosomia (large fetal size)
    b. Breech presentation
    c. Cord prolapse
    d. Premature rupture of membranes

18. A 30-year-old pregnant woman at 39 weeks of gestation presents to the labor ward in active labor. The obstetrician observes a persistent occiput posterior position during labor. Despite repositioning the mother and trying different birthing positions, the baby's head remains in the posterior position. What is the most appropriate management for this situation?
    a. Administer tocolytic drugs to delay labor and allow the baby's head to rotate
    b. Proceed with a trial of vacuum extraction to assist in delivering the baby
    c. Prepare for an emergency cesarean section due to the risk of CPD
    d. Attempt an ECV to convert the baby to a cephalic presentation

19. A 35-year-old pregnant woman at 40 weeks of gestation is in labor. The obstetrician observes a prolonged second stage of labor with the baby's head not descending despite good maternal pushing efforts. The fetal heart rate remains reassuring. What could be the reason for the prolonged second stage of labor?
    a. Malpresentation of the baby's head
    b. Maternal exhaustion and fatigue
    c. CPD
    d. Uterine atony

20. A 29-year-old pregnant woman at 37 weeks of gestation is in labor. The obstetrician observes a lack of progress in the dilation of the cervix despite regular contractions. On pelvic examination, the baby's head is high and not engaged in the pelvis. The woman is a first-time mother. What could be the possible cause of this lack of cervical dilation progress?
    a. Uterine atony
    b. Breech presentation
    c. CPD
    d. Occiput posterior position

21. A 32-year-old pregnant woman at 40 weeks of gestation is in labor. The obstetrician observes a slow progress of labor despite regular contractions. The woman has a history of pelvic surgery for a pelvic fracture sustained during a previous accident. What could be the reason for the slow progress of labor in this case?
    a. Fetal macrosomia
    b. Breech presentation
    c. Maternal pelvic deformity due to pelvic surgery
    d. Premature rupture of membranes

22. A 36-year-old pregnant woman at 42 weeks of gestation is in labor. The obstetrician observes a high fetal station and a persistent occiput posterior position during labor. The woman is experiencing intense back pain. What could be the reason for the persistent occiput posterior position, and what interventions can be considered to aid the delivery process?
    a. Fetal macrosomia; consider induction of labor to facilitate the delivery
    b. Pelvic outlet obstruction; attempt manual rotation of the baby's head during labor
    c. CPD; prepare for an emergency cesarean section
    d. Occiput transverse position; consider vacuum extraction to assist the delivery

23. A 33-year-old pregnant woman at 38 weeks of gestation is admitted to the labor ward with prolonged and difficult labor. The obstetrician observes a persistent occiput posterior position and a lack of progress in the descent of the baby's head through the birth canal. The fetal heart rate is concerning, and the baby's head is not molding well. What intervention may be considered in this situation to expedite delivery and improve fetal well-being?
    a. Induction of labor using oxytocin to strengthen contractions
    b. Vacuum extraction to assist in the delivery of the baby's head
    c. ECV to convert the baby to a cephalic presentation
    d. Epidural anesthesia to alleviate pain and allow the mother to rest

24. A 34-year-old pregnant woman at 39 weeks of gestation presents in labor. The obstetrician observes a prolonged second stage of labor with inadequate descent of the baby's head despite the strong maternal effort and regular contractions. The woman has a history of pelvic inflammatory disease (PID). What could be the possible reason for the prolonged second stage of labor in this case?
   a. Uterine atony
   b. Fetal macrosomia
   c. Pelvic outlet obstruction due to PID
   d. Premature rupture of membranes

ANSWERS

1. **c.** Brow presentation; increased risk of fetal head entrapment and prolonged labor.

   In a brow presentation, the baby's head is partially extended, causing the fetal skull to present in an intermediate position between flexion and extension. This can lead to fetal head entrapment and prolonged labor, putting the baby at risk of hypoxia and cephalopelvic disproportion (CPD). The presence of a late deceleration pattern in the fetal heart rate tracing further indicates fetal compromise.

2. **c.** Prepare for an emergency cesarean section due to the increased risk of cord prolapse.

   In a compound presentation, where one or more extremities (e.g., arm or hand) are present alongside the baby's head, there is an increased risk of cord prolapse. Cord prolapse can lead to cord compression and compromise the baby's oxygen supply, making an emergency cesarean section the most appropriate and timely management option.

3. **a.** The risks and benefits of vaginal breech delivery, including the potential for complications and success rates.

   Informed decision-making involves providing the patient with a comprehensive understanding of the risks and benefits associated with each delivery option. As the patient is considering vaginal breech delivery, she should be informed about the potential complications and success rates of such a delivery, considering her specific circumstances and individual factors.

4. **c.** Prepare for an emergency cesarean section due to the risk of cord prolapse and fetal distress.

   In a shoulder presentation, the baby is positioned transversely in the uterus, and the presence of a sinusoidal fetal heart rate pattern indicates severe fetal distress. There is an increased risk of cord prolapse and umbilical cord compression, making an emergency cesarean section the most appropriate and expedited management option to ensure the baby's safety.

5. **b.** Plan for an elective cesarean section to avoid the risk of uterine rupture.

   Given the woman's history of two previous cesarean sections, attempting a vaginal birth with a transverse lie carries an increased risk of uterine rupture and complications. An elective cesarean section is the safest approach to avoid potential obstetric emergencies and ensure the well-being of both the mother and the baby.

6. **b.** Prepare for an emergency cesarean section due to the risk of cord prolapse and fetal distress.

   The failure of the Rubin maneuver indicates that the shoulder presentation is likely fixed, making vaginal delivery impossible. An emergency cesarean section is the most appropriate and timely management option to ensure the baby's safety.

7. **a.** ECV is successful in approximately 80% of the cases and carries a low risk of fetal distress.

   External cephalic version is a procedure where the healthcare provider attempts to manually convert the baby to a cephalic presentation by external manipulation. It has a success rate of around 80%, making it an effective method in many cases. The most common complication is transient fetal heart rate changes during the procedure, but it generally carries a low risk of fetal distress.

8. **a.** Estimated fetal weight, parity, placental location, and the obstetrician's experience in managing breech deliveries.

   When considering vaginal breech delivery, various factors need to be taken into account to ensure the safety of both the baby and the mother. These factors include estimated fetal weight, parity (previous pregnancies and deliveries), placental location, and the experience and skills of the healthcare provider in managing breech deliveries. The decision-making process should be individualized based on these factors to optimize the chances of a successful and safe delivery.

9. **a.** A simulation of the labor process and potential maneuvers used during vaginal breech delivery.

Providing a simulation of the labor process and potential maneuvers during vaginal breech delivery can help the patient visualize the birthing process and understand the procedures involved. This visual representation may provide the patient with a better understanding of the potential challenges and benefits of vaginal breech delivery, aiding her decision-making process.

10. **a.** Mauriceau-Smellie-Veit maneuver.
The Mauriceau-Smellie-Veit maneuver is a technique used during vaginal breech delivery to facilitate the delivery of the aftercoming head. It involves applying gentle upward pressure on the baby's maxillary bones to help deliver the head, followed by a controlled downward flexion of the baby's head to complete the delivery process. The Rubin maneuver (option b) is used to rotate the baby's shoulder during delivery, while the Lovset maneuver (option c) is used to flex the baby's head for delivery in a face presentation. The Zavanelli maneuver (option d) involves returning the fetal head to the uterus and proceeding with an emergency cesarean section.

11. **b.** Prepare for an emergency cesarean section due to the risk of cord prolapse and fetal distress.

In this scenario, the baby's head is in a transverse position, and the head is not engaging into the pelvis. This is a malposition that poses a risk of cord prolapse and umbilical cord compression, leading to fetal distress. An emergency cesarean section is the most appropriate management to ensure the baby's safety.

12. **c.** LSA presentation; plan for an elective cesarean section

In this scenario, the baby's back is on the left side of the mother's abdomen, and the small parts (hands and feet) are felt on the right side. This indicates a LSA presentation, which is a malposition. Given the woman's history of a previous cesarean section, planning for an elective cesarean section is the most appropriate management to reduce the risk of uterine rupture during labor.

13. **d.** RST presentation; potential for spontaneous rotation into the occiput posterior position during labor.

In this scenario, the baby's back is on the right side of the mother's abdomen, and the small parts (hands and feet) are felt on the left side. This indicates a RST presentation, which is a malposition; however, it is important to note that RST presentation allows the baby's head to freely rotate during labor, which may result in spontaneous rotation into the occiput posterior (OP) position. The OP position is associated with a longer and more difficult labor and an increased risk of back pain for the mother. Obstetric interventions and positioning changes may be necessary to facilitate labor progress and optimize delivery outcomes.

14. **d.** In transverse lie positions, vaginal delivery is usually not feasible, and a cesarean section may be necessary.

In this scenario, the baby's head is in a transverse position, and it is not engaging into the pelvis. Transverse lie is an abnormal presentation that is incompatible with vaginal delivery. Attempting vaginal delivery in this case would carry a significant risk of uterine rupture and cord prolapse. A cesarean section is the most appropriate management to ensure the baby's safety.

15. **a.** The risk of uterine rupture and the potential for emergent cesarean section during labor.

In this scenario, the baby's head is in a transverse position, and the head is not engaging into the pelvis. Given the woman's history of a previous cesarean section, attempting a trial of vaginal delivery in the presence of a malpresentation carries an increased risk of uterine rupture, which can be life-threatening for both the mother and the baby. The patient should be informed about this serious complication and the likelihood of emergent cesarean section during labor to make an informed decision about her preferred mode of delivery.

16. **b.** Face presentation; risk of fetal head hyperextension and compromised oxygenation.

In a face presentation, the baby's head is presenting downward, but the face is looking upward, making it an abnormal malpresentation. During delivery, there is a risk of fetal head hyperextension, which can impede the baby's descent and compromise oxygenation. Assistance with maneuvers such as the Lovset maneuver may be required to flex the baby's head for a safer delivery.

17. **a.** Macrosomia (large fetal size).
Cephalopelvic disproportion occurs when there is inadequate space in the mother's pelvis to accommodate the size of the baby's head. Macrosomia, which

refers to a baby with a birth weight significantly above average, is a common cause of CPD. The large size of the baby's head can prevent it from descending through the birth canal, leading to an arrest of labor.

18. **c.** Prepare for an emergency cesarean section due to the risk of CPD.

    In this scenario, the baby's head is persistently in the occiput posterior position, which is associated with a higher risk of CPD. Attempting a vaginal delivery in this situation could lead to prolonged labor, fetal distress, and an increased risk of instrumental delivery or potential trauma to the baby. An emergency cesarean section is the most appropriate management to ensure a safe delivery for both the mother and the baby.

19. **c.** CPD.
    Cephalopelvic disproportion occurs when the baby's head is too large or the maternal pelvis is too small, making it difficult for the baby's head to pass through the birth canal. In this scenario, the prolonged second stage of labor with the baby's head not descending despite good maternal pushing efforts suggests the possibility of CPD. This situation may require further evaluation, and if CPD is confirmed, the most appropriate management may involve assisting the delivery through vacuum extraction or cesarean section.

20. **c.** CPD
    In this scenario, the lack of progress in cervical dilation and the high position of the baby's head suggest the possibility of CPD. Cephalopelvic disproportion occurs when the baby's head is too large or the maternal pelvis is too small, leading to inadequate space for the baby to descend through the birth canal. In a first-time mother, the pelvis may be less flexible, increasing the risk of CPD.

21. **c.** Maternal pelvic deformity due to pelvic surgery.
    In this scenario, the woman's history of pelvic surgery for a pelvic fracture indicates the possibility of a pelvic deformity. Pelvic deformities resulting from previous trauma or surgery can lead to inadequate pelvic space for the baby to descend during labor, causing slow progress or arrest of labor. Cephalopelvic disproportion is a common issue in such cases, leading to the need for alternative delivery methods, such as cesarean section.

22. **b.** Pelvic outlet obstruction; attempt manual rotation of the baby's head during labor.

    In this scenario, the persistent occiput posterior position, coupled with intense back pain, suggests the possibility of pelvic outlet obstruction. Pelvic outlet obstruction can prevent the baby's head from descending through the birth canal and lead to a prolonged and difficult labor. Attempting manual rotation of the baby's head during labor (e.g., using the Rubin maneuver) can help change the position of the baby's head and aid in the delivery process. If the rotation is successful, a vaginal delivery may still be possible.

23. **b.** Vacuum extraction to assist in the delivery of the baby's head.

    In this scenario, the persistent occiput posterior position, lack of progress in descent, and concerning fetal heart rate suggest the possibility of CPD, making the vaginal delivery challenging. Vacuum extraction is a surgical technique that involves using a vacuum cup to apply traction to the baby's head, aiding its descent through the birth canal. This intervention may expedite the delivery and reduce the risk of fetal distress in this situation.

24. **c.** Pelvic outlet obstruction due to PID.
    In this scenario, the woman's history of PID suggests the possibility of pelvic scarring and adhesions, leading to a pelvic outlet obstruction. Pelvic outlet obstruction can prevent the baby's head from descending through the birth canal, resulting in a prolonged second stage of labor. Cephalopelvic disproportion is a common issue in such cases, and alternative delivery methods such as vacuum extraction or cesarean section may be necessary.

Chapter 41: Abnormal Uterine Action Section Malpresentations

Mugdha L Jungari

QUESTIONS

1. The most common cause of _____ disorder is inadequate or abnormal uterine contraction.
   a. Protraction
   b. Retraction
   c. Contraction
   d. Atony

2. The most common type of abnormal uterine action
   a. Cervical dystocia
   b. Atony
   c. Uterine inertia
   d. All of the above

3. What is another name for Bandl's ring?
   a. Constriction ring
   b. Schroeder's ring
   c. Retraction ring
   d. Cervical dystocia

4. Which is a false statement about the constriction ring?
   a. Schroeder's ring is another name
   b. Injudicious oxytocin use may cause it
   c. Palpable per abdominal
   d. Better maternal prognosis

5. Hematuria in a patient in labor is diagnostic of which of the following?
   a. Impending scar rupture
   b. Urethral injury
   c. Obstructed labor
   d. Cystitis

6. What is the most common cause of breech presentation?
   a. Prematurity
   b. Hydrocephalus
   c. Placenta previa
   d. Polyhydramnios

7. Which is not linked with breech presentation at normal full-term pregnancy
   a. Placenta accreta
   b. Fetal malformation
   c. Uterine anomaly
   d. Corneal implantation

8. Zavanelli maneuver is performed in which of the following?
   a. Deep transverse arrest
   b. Face presentation
   c. Retained placenta
   d. Shoulder dystocia

9. What is the best approach to deliver arms in breech?
   a. Lovset's method
   b. Smellie-Veit maneuver
   c. Pinard's maneuver
   d. Wood's maneuver

10. Which of the following is not a cause of breech presentation?
    a. Hydrocephalus
    b. Oligohydramnios
    c. Pelvic contracture
    d. Placenta previa

11. The aftercoming head of the breech is delivered by which of the following?
    a. Maricelli technique
    b. Burns–Marshal method
    c. Lovset's method
    d. Manual rotation and extraction with Piper forceps

12. What is the treatment of choice for a 38-week primiparous woman in early labor with transverse presentation?
    a. Wait for the cervix to dilate
    b. Internal podalic version
    c. Cesarean section (CS)
    d. Forceps

13. Which is the most common breech presentation?
    a. Frank breech
    b. Complete breech
    c. Footling
    d. Knee

14. The prevailing reason for the occipitoposterior position of the fetal head during childbirth is commonly attributed to.
    a. Maternal obesity
    b. Deflexion of the fetal head
    c. Multiparity
    d. Android pelvis

15. When in labor, you diagnose occipitoposterior presentation of the fetal head. What is the most effective approach to managing this?
    a. Emergency CS
    b. Wait and watch for the progress of labor
    c. Early rupture of membrane
    d. Start oxytocin drip

16. In the second stage of labor, if the anterior fontanelle and the supraorbital ridge is felt on per vaginal (PV) examination, then what is the presentation?
    a. Brow presentation
    b. Deflexed head
    c. Flexed head
    d. Face presentation

17. Cord prolapse happens less often in which of the following?
    a. Frank breech
    b. Footling presentation
    c. Transverse lie
    d. Brow presentation

18. What is the most common form of fetal traumatic injury sustained during breech delivery?
    a. Rupture of the liver
    b. Rupture of the spleen
    c. Intra-adrenal hemorrhage
    d. Intracranial hemorrhage

19. When a baby is in a direct occipitoposterior position, the biggest issue that often occurs is which of the following?
    a. Intracranial injury
    b. Cephalhematoma
    c. Paraurethral tears
    d. Complete perineal tears

20. Deep transverse arrest is a condition that is not found in all cases except for which of the following?
    a. Android pelvis
    b. Epidural analgesia
    c. Transverse lie
    d. Uterine inertia

21. What is the presentation in a transverse lie?
    a. Vertex
    b. Breech
    c. Brow
    d. Shoulder

22. What would be the best management for 30-year-old primipara in labor with a transverse lie?
    a. Internal cephalic version CS
    b. Emergency CS
    c. Wait and watch
    d. External cephalic version

23. Which of the following is not a complication of shoulder presentation?
    a. Fetal death
    b. Uterine rupture
    c. Obstructed labor
    d. Shoulder dystocia

24. The usual placental position in the case of an unstable lie of the fetus is?
    a. Corneal
    b. Lateral wall
    c. Fundus
    d. Segment

25. What is not related to the face presentation?
    a. The most common position is LMA
    b. Engaging diameter is submentobregmatic
    c. The diameter distending the vulval outlet is mentovertical
    d. During molding, there is the elongation of the occipitofrontal diameter

26. In which fetal presentation vaginal delivery can be expected?
    a. Face presentation when the chin lies directly to the sacrum
    b. Brow presentation
    c. Shoulder presentation
    d. Face presentation when the chin lies under the symphysis pubis

27. Which method is not useful in shoulder dystocia?
    a. McRobert's maneuver
    b. Hegar's maneuver
    c. Zavanelli maneuver
    d. Wood's maneuver

28. Which of the following may not be a complication of shoulder dystocia?
    a. Sternomastoid swelling
    b. Erb's palsy
    c. Klumpke's paralysis
    d. None of the above

29. In McRobert's maneuver, which of the following nerves is commonly involved?
    a. Common peroneal nerve
    b. Obturator nerve
    c. Lumbosacral trunk
    d. The lateral cutaneous nerve of the thigh

30. What may be the cause of fetal death in breech delivery?
    a. Intracranial hemorrhage
    b. Aspiration
    c. Atlantoaxial dislocation
    d. Asphyxia

31. If A 28-year-old primigravida was admitted with an undiagnosed breech and opted to try for a vaginal delivery after counseling disproportion is unlikely to happen? What is the best indication that a cephalopelvic is likely to happen?
    a. A clinically adequate pelvis.
    b. An estimated fetal weight that is <3,800 g
    c. A frank breech presentation
    d. Good progress to full dilatation
    e. Simultaneous easy passage of the fetal thighs and trunk through the pelvis

32. A 20-year-old primigravida with 32 weeks gestation age, presents to the hospital with rupture of membranes and labor pains for one hour. A 5-day-old scan showed flexed breech with mild oligohydramnios, with an estimated baby weight of 2,050 g. She is having regular contractions, and the cervix is 5 cm dilated, fully effaced with breech presentation at 0 stations. On examination in OT, the breech was delivered with a fetal head inside with a tight cervix. What is the best way to help ensure a safe delivery in this scenario?
    a. Injection of terbutaline
    b. Emergency CS and use lower segment incision
    c. Emergency section and use vertical midline uterine incision
    d. Lateral cervical incisions
    e. Deliver head by Burns–Marshall technique

33. You are asked to review a 26-year-old primigravid woman in spontaneous labor with a continuing bradycardia. Examination findings are: Vertex 0/5 palpable per abdomen; cervix 10 cm dilated; cephalic presentation at zero station; anterior fontanelle palpable with orbital ridges and nasal bridge felt anteriorly. What is the most appropriate management?
    a. Category 1 emergency CS
    b. Commence pushing
    c. Fetal blood sample
    d. Forceps delivery
    e. Ventouse delivery in the room

34. A 24-year-old primigravida goes into spontaneous labor at 39 + 6 weeks of gestation following an uncomplicated pregnancy. She progresses to 8 cm dilatation but fails to dilate any further. You have examined and found that the baby is in the deflexed occipitoposterior position. What will be the diameter of the presenting part in this baby?
    a. Mentovertical
    b. Occipitofrontal
    c. Submentobregmatic
    d. Suboccipitobregmatic
    e. Suboccipitofrontal

35. You have been called to see a 30-year-old woman with immune thrombocytopenic purpura (ITP) who has been fully dilated for over 3 hours and pushing for the last one of these. You examine and find that the baby is in an occipitoposterior position and at the level of the ischial spines (station zero). What would be the next step in the management of this patient?
    a. Emergency CS
    b. Kielland's forceps delivery
    c. Manual rotation and forceps
    d. Neville–Barnes forceps delivery
    e. Ventouse delivery

36. A 25-year-old woman presents in labor at 39 weeks gestation in her second pregnancy. She had an emergency CS in her first pregnancy following a failed forceps delivery, 11 months ago. She now complains of constant abdominal pain, worsening over the last hour. There are unprovoked prolonged decelerations on the cardiotocograph (CTG) and the baseline has risen from 140 to 160 BPM. Her cervix is 8 cm dilated, with irregular contractions. What is your management plan?
    a. Category 1 CS
    b. Instrumental delivery in the delivery room
    c. Perform fetal blood sampling (FBS)
    d. Start oxytocin infusion and commence active pushing when contractions re-established
    e. Trial of instrumental delivery in operating theater

37. A 23-year-old primigravida whose pregnancy was complicated by gestational diabetes went into spontaneous labor at 40 weeks of gestation. She started pushing but had shoulder dystocia after the delivery of the head of the baby. What factor is likely to increase the risk of brachial plexus injury (BPI) in the baby?
    a. The weight of the baby
    b. The time it takes to deal with the dystocia
    c. Whether it is an anterior or posterior shoulder impacted
    d. The gestational age of delivery

38. A 36-year-old woman in her first pregnancy has been referred to see you at 39 weeks gestation. She is upset about finding out that her baby is in a breech presentation. What is the incidence of spontaneous version from breech to cephalic presentation in nulliparous women after 36 weeks?
    a. 2%
    b. 4%
    c. 6%
    d. 8%
    e. 10%

39. A 34-year-old primigravid woman presents in labor, having been pushing for 75 minutes. You are asked to review whether she is suitable for an operative vaginal delivery. Which of the following is correct?
    a. Epidural with oxytocin in the second stage of labor increases the incidence of nonrotational forceps delivery in primiparous women
    b. Fetal alloimmune thrombocytopenia is a relative contraindication to operative vaginal delivery
    c. Instrumental delivery is contraindicated if any part of the fetal head is palpable abdominally
    d. Maternal body mass index (BMI) over 30 is not associated with a higher rate of failed instrumental delivery until BMI is above 40
    e. Ventouse delivery is safe beyond 35 weeks of gestation

40. A 26-year-old primigravida is undergoing a trial of vaginal breech delivery. The breech is frank with an estimated birth weight of 3,100 g. She progressed at a normal rate, but the cervix has remained at 7 cm for the past 3 hours. The fetal heart rate is normal. What would be the next plan for her?
    a. Augment with Oxytocin and manage as for a cephalic presentation
    b. Augment with oxytocinon for 2 hours and then reassess
    c. Proceed to a caesarean section
    d. Re-examine in 2 hours and if no progress, perform a CS
    e. Re-examine in 3–4 hours and if no progress, perform a CS

41. At what gestational age should an external cephalic version be attempted on a primigravida who is diagnosed with a breech presentation at 35 weeks of gestation?
    a. At 35 weeks
    b. At 36 weeks
    c. At 37 weeks
    d. At 38 weeks
    e. At 39 weeks

42. A 26-year-old nulliparous woman was admitted in labor at 4 cm dilation. The pregnancy was uncomplicated. After 4 hours, she had dilated to 5 cm. A decision was therefore taken to perform an artificial rupture of membrane (ARM). 2 hours later, the cervix was still 5 cm dilated.
    a. Emergency CS-category III: Fetal
    b. Emergency CS-category III: Maternal epidural and commence Syntocinon
    c. Fetal blood sampling to assess the degree of urgency for delivery
    d. Neville–Barnes forceps delivery

43. A primigravida has been diagnosed as having slow progress in labor at 4 cm dilation (a VE demonstrated no change in the cervix after 4 hours). She was admitted 4 hours ago, having started contracting at home 2 hours after rupturing her membranes. An epidural has been sited and Syntocinon has been commenced.
    a. Re-examine in 1 hour
    b. Re-examine in 4 hours
    c. Rotational ventouse
    d. Start pushing

44. A 30-year-old primigravida went into spontaneous labor at 41 weeks and was diagnosed with failure to progress at 5 cm dilatation. Syntocinon was commenced, and 4 hours later, she is now 6 cm dilated. The fetal heart rate is normal and the presenting part is at the level of the spines.
    a. ARM and Syntocinon
    b. Re-examine in 1 hour
    c. Emergency CS-category I: Fetal
    d. Emergency CS-category I: Maternal
    e. Emergency CS-category II: Fetal

45. You have been called to see a primipara in labor at 38 weeks of gestation who is fully dilated (contractions are described as good) with CTG that has a normal baseline of 145 BPM, a baseline variability of 5–10 BPM and variable decelerations of >60 BPM, lasting >60 seconds and present in over 50% of the contractions. You examine her, and the head is found to be two-fifths palpable per abdomen and at the level of the spines vaginally with no caput but but molding present. What will be the best next step of management?
    a. Reassess in 30 minutes
    b. Category I LSCS
    c. Fetal scalp blood sampling
    d. Ventouse delivery

46. You are reviewing a multiparous woman in labor at term on account of an abnormal CTG She is fully dilated, and the vertex is at 0–1 in the occipitoposterior position. The CTG shows a baseline of 180 BPM, with late decelerations that have persisted over the last 30 minutes.
    a. ARM and oxytocin (Syntocinon)
    b. Emergency CS-category I: Fetal
    c. Emergency CS-category I: Maternal
    d. Emergency CS-category II: Fetal

47. You have been called to the room because a primigravida in the late first stage has had a prolonged deceleration for the past 5 minutes. The baseline has dropped from 138 to 95 BPM and has not recovered yet.
    a. Perform a FBS to measure pH or lactate
    b. Repeat FBS in 30 minutes
    c. Repeat FBS in 1 hour
    d. Stop Syntocinon and administer subcutaneous terbutaline 0.25 mg stat

48. A 31-year-old primigravida in spontaneous labor was subjected to CTG because of fetal heart rate abnormality on intermittent auscultation. The CTG has had a baseline of 185 BPM for the past 50 minutes with no other nonreassuring features. Maternal temperature was checked and was found to be normal. She was also moved to the left lateral position, was given fluids, and encouraged to mobilize, but the tachycardia has persisted. There are no accelerations and no decelerations.
    a. Offer oral fluids and paracetamol and encourage to mobilize or adopt a left lateral position
    b. Auscultation for at least 1 minute after contraction and then every 15 minutes
    c. Palpate and measure maternal pulse
    d. Perform an FBS to measure pH or lactate

49. A 30-year-old woman who is being induced because of preeclampsia is now 7 cm dilated. She has an epidural, which is working well. The CTG has been showing variable decelerations (a drop-in heart rate of over 60 BPM lasting for >60 seconds and for >50% of contractions) over the last 30 minutes. You decide to perform a FBS, and the lactate level has been reported to be 4.4 mmol/L (or pH-7.22).
    a. Repeat FBS in 30 minutes
    b. Repeat FBS in 1 hour
    c. Stop Syntocinon and administer subcutaneous terbutaline 0.25 mg stat
    d. Turn to lateral position and encourage to mobilize

50. A 30-year-old primigravida whose pregnancy is uncomplicated went into spontaneous labor last night. She progressed to full dilatation and after 2 hours in the passive second stage was encouraged to start pushing. She has now been pushing for 1.5 hours and the vertex which is in the occipitotransverse position is at 0 + 1.
    a. Syntocinon and re-examine in 2 hours
    b. Emergency CS category III: Fetal
    c. Emergency CS category III: Maternal
    d. Syntocinon and re-examine in 4 hours

ANSWERS

1. **a.** Protraction
2. **c.** Uterine inertia
3. **c.** Retraction ring
4. **c.** Palpable per abdominal
5. **c.** Obstructed labor
6. **a.** Prematurity
7. **a.** Placenta accreta
8. **d.** Shoulder dystocia
9. **a.** Lovset's method
10. **b.** Oligohydramnios
11. **d.** Manual rotation and extraction with Piper forceps
12. **c.** Cesarean section (CS)
13. **a.** Frank breech
14. **d.** Android pelvis.
15. **b.** Wait and watch for the progress of labor.
16. **a.** Brow presentation
17. **a.** Frank breech
18. **d.** Intracranial hemorrhage.
19. **a.** Intracranial injury
20. **c.** Transverse lie
21. **d.** Shoulder
22. **b.** Emergency
23. **d.** Shoulder dystocia
24. **d.** Segment
25. **c.** The diameter distending the vulval outlet is mentovertical.
26. **a.** Face presentation when the chin lies directly to the sacrum.

27. **b.** Hegar's maneuver.
28. **a.** Sternomastoid swelling.
29. **d.** The lateral cutaneous nerve of the thigh.
30. **d.** Asphyxia
31. **b.** An estimated fetal weight that is <3,800 g.
32. **d.** Lateral cervical incisions.
33. **a.** Category 1 emergency CS.
34. **b.** Occipitofrontal
35. **a.** Emergency CS
36. **a.** Category 1 CS
37. **a.** The weight of the baby.
38. **a.** 2%
39. **c.** Instrumental delivery is contraindicated if any part of the fetal head is palpable abdominally.
40. **b.** Augment with oxytocinon for 2 hours and then reassess.
41. **c.** At 37 weeks
42. **c.** Fetal blood sampling to assess the degree of urgency for delivery.
43. **a.** Re-examine in 1 hour.
44. **a.** ARM and Syntocinon.
45. **d.** Ventouse delivery
46. **b.** Emergency CS-category II: Fetal
47. **d.** Stop syntocinon and administer subcutaneous terbutaline 0.25 mg stat
48. **d.** Perform an FBS to measure pH or lactate.
49. **c.** Stop Syntocinon and administer subcutaneous terbutaline 0.25 mg stat.
50. **a.** Syntocinon and re-examine in 2 hours.

Chapter 42: Breech

Shrutika Thakkar

QUESTIONS

1. What is the engagement diameter in the breech presentation?
   a. Biparietal
   b. Bitrochanteric
   c. Ischiopubic
   d. Bimastoid

2. All the following are prerequisites of vaginal breech delivery, *except*?
   a. Frank breech
   b. Adequate pelvis
   c. Extended head
   d. Gestational age of 36–42 weeks

3. The most appropriate forceps for an aftercoming head of breech is?
   a. Monroe's forceps
   b. Piper's forceps
   c. Wrigley's forceps
   d. Sampson's forceps

4. The incidence of breech presentation in singleton-term pregnancies is?
   a. 3.5%
   b. 10%
   c. 8.5%
   d. 15%

5. External cephalic version (ECV) for breech presentation is to be done at all gestational ages, *except*?
   a. 28 weeks
   b. 32 weeks
   c. 34 weeks
   d. 37 weeks

6. The contraindications for the ECV for breech are all, *except*?
   a. Complete breech
   b. Contracted pelvis
   c. Uterine scar
   d. Ruptured membranes

7. Mauriceau-Smellie-Veit method of delivery of aftercoming head of breech means?
   a. Jaw traction and shoulder extraction
   b. Hyperextension of fetus
   c. Jaw flexion and shoulder traction
   d. Hands off and leave the fetus hanging

8. The method of bringing down the leg in breech delivery is called?
   a. Burns-Marshall method
   b. Piper's method
   c. Pinard's method
   d. Mauriceau method

9. All of the following are associated with breech presentation at normal full-term pregnancy, *except*:
   a. Placenta accreta
   b. Fetal malformation
   c. Uterine anomaly
   d. Cornual implantation of the placenta

10. Best method to deliver shoulders in breech is which one of the following?
    a. Lovset's method
    b. Smellie-Veit
    c. Pinard
    d. Any of the above

11. The most common cause of breech presentation is which one of the following?
    a. Prematurity
    b. Hydrocephalus
    c. Placenta previa
    d. Polyhydramnios

12. Which of the following is the most common breech presentation?
    a. Footling breech
    b. Complicated breech
    c. Complete breech
    d. Frank breech

13. Which is the bone that is perforated during decapitation of an aftercoming head of breech?
    a. Parietal
    b. Occiput
    c. Frontal
    d. Temporal

14. All of the following methods are meant to deliver the aftercoming head of breech, *except*:
    a. Lovset's method
    b. Mauriceau-Smellie-Veit
    c. Burns-Marshal method
    d. Piper's forceps

15. During an assisted breech delivery:
    a. Pinard's maneuver can be used to deliver legs in the extended position
    b. Mauriceau-Smellie-Veit's maneuver is used to deliver extended arms
    c. Forceps should not be applied to the fetal head
    d. Epidural analgesia is mandatory

16. The Zatuchni-Andros scoring system is used for:
    a. Predicting the outcome of occipitoposterior position
    b. Prediction of labor
    c. Fetal well-being
    d. Selecting cases of breech presentation for vaginal delivery

17. Depending on the attitude of the fetus the types of breech are classified as all, *except*:
    a. Frank breech
    b. Complete breech
    c. Footling
    d. Aftercoming breech

18. All of the following are true about Frank breech, *except*:
    a. It is also called "Pike"
    b. Hips are flexed and knees are extended
    c. Both the hips and knees are flexed
    d. Its more common in primigravidae

19. The most common type of breech presentation in primigravidae is:
    a. Frank breech
    b. Complete breech
    c. Footling
    d. Flexed breech

20. The maximum score in the Z-A prognostic scoring system for vaginal birth with presentation is which one of the following?
    a. 10
    b. 11
    c. 15
    d. 13

21. The Newman scoring system for the ECV involves all the following parameters, *except*:
    a. Parity
    b. Gestational age
    c. Cervical dilatation
    d. Estimated fetal weight

22. The scoring system for the ECV is called:
    a. Bishop's score
    b. Zatuchni score
    c. Newman-Peacock score
    d. Bishops score

23. The Zatuchni-Andros scoring system involves all the following parameters, *except*:
    a. Parity
    b. Gestational age
    c. Cervical dilatation
    d. Station

24. The Burns–Marshall method involves which of the following?
    a. Shoulder traction and malar flexion
    b. Traction on the arms
    c. Applying forceps to deliver the breech
    d. Hanging the fetus by its weight and then holding both feet and swinging the fetus onto the maternal abdomen to deliver the fetal head

25. Frank breech position of the fetus is:
    a. Hip flexed and knee extended
    b. Hip flexed and knee flexed
    c. One leg hip flexed and knee flexed
    d. Partial extension at hip and knee

26. These findings from the abdominal examination confirm the presentation:
    a. Hard and round ballotable mass on pelvic palpation
    b. Fetal size larger than period of gestation on fundal height
    c. A smooth, hard, and round ballotable mass felt on fundal palpation
    d. Fetal back on lateral palpation corresponds to the period of gestation

27. The type of breech presentation in which the hips of the fetus are flexed, and the knees are also flexed is called:
    a. Frank breech
    b. Complete breech
    c. Footling
    d. Extended breech

28. The most typical complication associated with footling breech is:
    a. Fetal hypoxia
    b. Obstructed labor
    c. Postpartum hemorrhage
    d. Cord prolapse

29. The absolute contraindications of the ECV are all, *except*:
    a. Placenta previa
    b. Bleeding per vaginum within last 7 days
    c. Multiple gestation
    d. Transverse lie

30. Which of the following is incorrect about the breech delivery mechanism?
    a. When the anterior hip is beneath the pubis symphysis the intertrochanteric diameter rotates around a 45° axis
    b. Anterior hip descends rapidly as compared to the posterior hip

c. If the posthip is beneath the symphysis pubis it has to go through 225° axis rotation

d. The axis of rotation is 45° degrees for the sacrum anterior or posterior position

ANSWERS

1. **b.** Bitrochanteric
   The engagement diameter in the breech presentation is the bitrochanteric diameter.

2. **c.** Extended head.

   The prerequisites of vaginal delivery of breech are:
   - Frank breech
   - Estimated fetal weight not >3.75 kg
   - *Gestational age*: 36–42 weeks
   - Flexed head
   - Adequate pelvis
   - Normal progress of labor by using the partogram
   - Uncomplicated pregnancy
   - Multiparas
   - An experienced obstetrician
   - In case of intrauterine fetal death

3. **b.** Piper's forceps.
   Piper's forceps is more suitable than the ordinary forceps as it has a perineal but not pelvic curve and has longer shanks. It is applied from the ventral aspect of the fetus.

4. **a.** 3.5%
   Only 3.5% of the term singleton deliveries are in breech presentation but about 25% of cases before 30 weeks of gestation are breech as most cases undergo spontaneous cephalic version up to term.

5. **a.** 28 weeks
   Most authors have recommended an external cephalon version after 32 weeks and up to 37 weeks only

   Version is not done earlier because:
   - Spontaneous version is liable to occur.
   - Return to breech presentation is liable to occur.
   - If labor occurs the fetus will have a lesser chance for survival.

   Version is difficult after 37th weeks due to:
   - Larger fetal size
   - Relatively less liquor
   - More irritability of the uterus

6. **a.** Complete breech:
   The contraindications for ECV are:
   - Contracted pelvis
   - Multiple pregnancy
   - Hydrocephalus
   - Antepartum hemorrhage
   - Uterine scar
   - Hypertension as the placenta is more susceptible to separation
   - Elderly primigravida
   - Ruptured membranes

7. **c.** Jaw flexion and shoulder traction.
   The Mauriceau-Smellie-Veit method is described as Jaw flexion and shoulder traction:
   - Two fingers of the left hand, (as originally described) or better on the malar eminences (the maxillae) to avoid dislocation of the jaw.
   - The index and ring finger of the right hand are placed on each shoulder while the middle finger is pressing against the occiput to promote flexion and act as a splint for the neck, preventing hyperextension and hence cervical spine injury.
   - Traction is commenced downward and backward till the nape of the fetus appears, and the body is lifted toward the mother's abdomen.

8. **c.** Pinard's method.
   Bringing down a leg is done by Pinard's method. It is done as follows:
   - Under general anesthesia.
   - Press it by two fingers in the popliteal fossa of the anterior leg to flex it then grasp the ankle and bring it down. This will prevent the anterior buttock from over-riding the symphysis pubis.
   - If the posterior leg was brought down first it must be rotated anteriorly with the trunk then bring the other leg which is now becomes posterior.

9. **a.** Placenta accreta.
   Most breech presentations seem to be chance occurrences. However, in up to 15% of cases, it may be due to fetal or uterine causes. The *risk factors* are listed below:

Uterine	Fetal
• Multiparity	• Prematurity
• Uterine malformations (e.g., septate uterus)	• Macrosomia
	• Polyhydramnios (raised amniotic fluid index)
• Fibroids	• Twin pregnancy (or higher order)
• Placenta previa	• Abnormality (e.g., anencephaly)

10. **a.** Lovset's method.
    The Lovset's maneuver to rotate the body and deliver the shoulders.

11. **a.** Prematurity
    Prematurity is the most common cause of breech presentation.

12. **b.** Complicated breech.
    If the after-coming head is to be perforated, make sure the occiput is the bone chosen, rather than the face or jaw. The perforator is now used to evacuate the cranial contents. This is done by agitating the perforator inside the cranium of the fetus.

13. **b.** Occiput
    If the aftercoming head is to be perforated, make sure the occiput is the bone chosen, rather than the face or jaw. The perforator is now used to evacuate the cranial contents. This is done by agitating the perforator inside the cranium of the fetus.

14. **a.** Lovset's method.
    The Lovset's maneuver is done to rotate the body and deliver the shoulders in a breech presentation.

15. **a.** Pinard's maneuver can be used to deliver legs in the extended position.
    Bringing down a leg is done by Pinard's method to deliver the legs in an extended position.

16. **d.** Selecting cases of breech presentation for vaginal delivery.
    The Zatuchni-Andros scoring system offers a means of predicting the outcome of breech delivery and selecting cases in which vaginal delivery may be preferable for both mother and infant.

17. **d.** Aftercoming breech.
    Depending on the attitude of the fetus, the breech presentation has been classified as:
    - Frank or extended breech presentation when the fetal hips are flexed and the knees extended.
    - Complete or flexed breech presentation when both the hips and the knees are flexed.
    - Footling or Incomplete breech presentation when one or both hips are extended.

18. **c.** Both the hips and knees are flexed.
    Frank or extended breech presentation when the fetal hips are flexed and the knees extended. It is also called "pike". This accounts for 50–70% of breech presentations and is commoner in primigravidae.

19. **a.** Frank breech.
    Frank or extended breech presentation when the fetal hips are flexed and the knees extended. This accounts for 50–70% of breech presentations and is commoner in primigravidae.

20. **b.** 11
    - The maximal score is 11
    - A score > 7 indicates a good prognosis for vaginal delivery.

21. **b.** Gestational age.
    The Newman-Peacock score includes five parameters before a planned ECV procedure—parity, estimated fetal weight, cervical dilation, placental location, and fetal station.

22. **c.** Newman-Peacock score.
    The Newman-Peacock score includes five parameters before a planned ECV procedure—parity, estimated fetal weight, cervical dilation, placental location, and fetal station

23. **d.** Station
    The Zatuchni-Andros score includes five parameters—(1) parity, (2) gestational age, (3) estimated fetal weight, (4) cervical dilation, and (5) previous breech.

24. **d.** Hanging the fetus by its weight and then holding both feet and swinging the fetus onto the maternal abdomen to deliver the fetal head.
    The Burns-Marshall method involves allowing the breech to "hang'" by its weight until the nape of the neck (or the 'hairline') is visible. This is followed by holding both feet and the swinging fetus onto the maternal abdomen to deliver the fetal head.

25. **a.** Hip flexed and knee extended.
    Frank or extended breech presentation when the fetal hips are flexed and the knees extended.

26. **c.** A smooth, hard, and round ballotable mass felt on fundal palpation.
    The findings to diagnose breech presentation on abdominal examination are as follows:
    - On abdominal palpation head feels as distinct hard spherical mass under the hypochondrium.
    - If the presenting part is irregular and not ballotable or if the fetal head is ballotable at the fundus.
    - Fetal heart heard higher in the abdomen.

27. **b.** Complete breech.
    The complete breech has the fetus sitting with flexion of both hips and both knees in a tuck position.

28. **d.** Cord prolapse.
    Incomplete or footling breech carries the highest risk of cord prolapse at 15–18%, while complete breech is lower at 4–6%, and frank breech is uncommon at 0.5%.

29. **d.** Transverse lie.
    The absolute contraindications of ECV are:
    - Placenta previa
    - Bleeding within last 7 days
    - Abnormal CTG
    - Major uterine anomaly
    - Ruptured membranes
    - Multiple gestations

30. **c.** If the posthip is beneath the symphysis pubis it has to go through a 225° axis rotation.
    Presentation engagement usually occurs in some form of oblique position, including four possibilities—left sacrum anterior, right sacrum anterior (LSA and RSA, respectively), and left sacrum posterior, right sacrum posterior (LSP and RSP, respectively). A 45° internal rotation occurs once the fetal pelvic pole is in contact with the lower strait. In the anterior varieties, there is a one-eight-of-a-circle backward rotation, whereas in the posterior varieties, an equal forward rotation occurs. This is the first of the classical rotations in breech delivery.

Chapter 43: Quiz on Occipitoposterior Position

Shashi R Goyal

QUESTIONS

1. What is the attitude of the fetal head in the occipitoposterior (OP) position?
   a. Fully flexed
   b. Fully extended
   c. Deflexed

2. What is the engaging diameter in OP?
   a. Suboccipitobregmatic
   b. Occipitofrontal
   c. Mentovertical

3. In which type of pelvis occipitoposterior position is common?
   a. Android
   b. Gynecoid
   c. Platypelloid

4. How much internal rotation is needed for the normal vaginal delivery?
   a. 45°
   b. 90°
   c. 135°

5. Deep transverse arrest cases (station zero) are delivered by which of the following options?
   a. Rotational forceps delivery
   b. Vacuum rotation and vaginal delivery
   c. Lower segment cesarean section (LSCS)

6. Which of the following options are the causes of Deep Transverse Arrest?
   a. Android pelvis
   b. Poor uterine contractions
   c. Both of the above causes

7. Obstetric forceps can be applied for which of the following?
   a. Breech presentation
   b. Face presentation
   c. Face to pubis position

8. Which of the following is the correct option for per abdominal examination findings in OP?
   a. Sinciput is lower than occiput
   b. Sinciput is at the same level as occiput
   c. Occiput is lower than sinciput

9. The location of Fetal Heart Sound in OP cases lies in which of the following options?
   a. Spinoumbilical line
   b. Midline
   c. Flanks

10. Timings of rupture of the membrane in OP are:
    a. Early
    b. Late
    c. Regular

11. On per vaginal (PV) examination which fontanelle is easily palpable?
    a. Anterior
    b. Posterior
    c. Lateral

12. What is reverse rotation? Choose the correct option.
    a. Occiput goes to the symphysis pubis
    b. Occiput goes on the lateral sides of the pelvis
    c. Occiput goes to sacrum

13. Direct occipitoposterior delivery occurs by which of the following movements?
    a. Extension
    b. Flexion
    c. Flexion followed by extension

14. Which pelvis is better for vaginal delivery in OP cases?
    a. Android
    b. Anthropoid
    c. Platypelloid

15. Occipitoposterior is more common in which gravida?
    a. Primigravida
    b. Multigravida
    c. Grand multigravida

16. Per vaginal examination findings in OP cases?
    a. Flat membrane
    b. Elongated membrane
    c. Well-applied fetal head

17. What percentage is the favorable outcome in OP?
    a. 10%   b. 50%
    c. 90%
18. Face-to-pubis delivery occurs in which of the following options?
    a. Face presentation
    b. After coming head of breech
    c. Occipitoposterior position
19. Obstetric forceps can be used for which of the following options?
    a. Face presentation   b. Face-to-pubis position
20. Direct Occipitoposterior is common in which type of the pelvis?
    a. Anthropoid pelvis   b. Platypelloid pelvis
    c. Android pelvis
21. Occipitoposterior in primigravida will lead to:
    a. Significant backache
    b. Prolonged first stage
    c. Prolonged second stage
    d. All of the above
22. Causes of unfavorable outcomes in OP cases:
    a. Week uterine contractions
    b. Big baby
    c. Early rupture of membrane
    d. Android pelvis
    e. All of the above
23. Which one is the abnormal position?
    a. Left occiput anterior (LOA)
    b. Right occiput anterior (ROA)
    c. Right occiput anterior (ROP)
24. The most common OP position is which one of the following?
    a. ROP   b. LOP
    c. Occipitosacral
25. Posterior fontanelle position in LOP is:
    a. Near right (RT) sacroiliac joint
    b. Near left (LT) sacroiliac joint
26. Engaging diameter in OP is which of the following options?
    a. Suboccipitofrontal   b. Occipitofrontal
    c. Anyone of the above
27. Occipitofrontal diameter measurement is:
    a. 11.5 cm   b. 10 cm
    c. 9 cm
28. Right oblique diameter starts from:
    a. RT sacroiliac joint   b. LT sacroiliac joint
29. Occipitoposterior can lead to:
    a. Increased postpartum hemorrhage (PPH)
    b. Increased perineal tears
    c. Prolonged labor
    d. All of the above complications
30. Floating head in primi is more common in which of the following options?
    a. ROA   b. LOA.
    c. ROP

ANSWERS

1. **c.** Deflexed
   Deflexed head. The posterior compartment of the pelvis is relatively larger and hence larger diameter of the deflexed head can be accommodated in the occipitoposterior (OP) position.
2. **b.** Occipitofrontal
   Occipitofrontal diameter is the engaging diameter.
3. **a.** Android
   Android pelvis is very narrow anteriorly, so the larger part occiput comes to the wider posterior compartment of the pelvis.
4. **c.** 135°
   About 135° of the internal rotation is needed for the occiput to come below the symphysis pubis because it is engaged in the posterior compartment of the pelvis.
5. **c.** Lower segment cesarean section (LSCS)
   Deep transverse arrest with station zero will be extremely high for forceps application. It will be traumatic.
6. **c.** Both of the above causes.
   Android pelvis and poor uterine contractions prevent further anterior rotation of the fetal head.
7. **c.** Face to pubis position.
   Obstetrical forceps can be applied for face-to-pubis delivery, as your forceps blades are on the side of the vertex only. Nose is behind symphysis pubis.
8. **b.** Sinciput is at the same level as the occiput.
   Occipitoposterior position will have a deflexed head with a military attitude, so sinciput and occiput will be at the same level.

9. **c.** Flanks
Flanks, Fetal Heart Sounds will be in the flanks because the back goes to the side and limbs come near the anterior abdominal wall.

10. **a.** Early rupture of the membrane occurs due to improper application of the head over the cervix. The membrane is elongated and ruptures early with uterine contractions.

11. **a.** Anterior
The anterior fontanelle is palpated easily, as is big and anterior. The posterior fontanelle is very posterior.

12. **c.** Occiput goes to sacrum
In reverse rotation, the occiput goes posterior as the sinciput touches the pelvic floor first and rotates anteriorly.

13. **c.** Flexion followed by extension
In reverse rotation, the occiput goes posterior as the sinciput touches the pelvic floor first and rotates anteriorly.

14. **b.** Anthropoid
Anthropoid pelvis has a long anteroposterior (AP) diameter, so the head can be accommodated in AP diameter and face-to-pubis delivery can take place.

15. **a.** Primigravida
It is more common in primigravida. The space is relatively more in multigravida.

16. **b.** Elongated membrane
Elongated membrane because the head is not well applied to the cervix.

17. **c.** 90%
Outcome is favorable in about 90% of cases with good uterine contractions and descent of the head anterior rotation takes place in cases without cast partial dentures (CPD).

18. **c.** Occipitoposterior position
Face to pubis delivery occurs in occipitoposterior cases when it becomes a direct sacral position and the AP diameter of the pelvis is adequate.

19. **b.** Face-to-pubis position
Forceps can be applied to both sides of the vertex, as the face is behind the symphysis pubis.

20. **a.** Anthropoid pelvis
Anthropoid pelvis has a large AP diameter, so it can accommodate a larger Occipitofrontal diameter of OP position.

21. **d.** All of the above due to posterior position & long Internal Rotation

22. **e.** All of the above factors lead to unfavorable outcomes

23. **c.** Anterior Position is normal. Right or Left doesn't matter

24. **a.** Right Occipitoposterior is most common amongst all

25. **b.** Left OP will be left Posterior compartment

26. **c.** Anyone of above depending upon degree of Deflection of head.

27. **a.** 11.5 cm

28. **a.** Oblique diameter is named with respective Sacro iliac Joint.

29. **d.** All of the above complications

30. **d.** All the factors have problems in Vaginal Deliver.

Chapter 44: Transverse Lie, Brow, and Face

Rajshree Dayanand Katke, Gayathri AK

QUESTIONS

1. What is the incidence of a transverse lie?
   a. One in 300 births
   b. One in 200 births
   c. One in 400 births
   d. One in 800 births

2. What is the percentage of transverse lies in twin pregnancy?
   a. 30%
   b. 50%
   c. 60%
   d. 40%

3. Which of the following are the common causes for transverse lies?
   a. Placenta previa
   b. Preterm fetus
   c. Abnormal uterine anatomy
   d. All of the above

4. Which of the following is presenting part of a transverse lie?
   a. Sacrum
   b. Brow
   c. Acromion and scapula
   d. Face

5. A 28-year-old female came to the labor ward and, on examination found to be a transverse lie, which of the following findings goes in favor for a transverse lie, *except*?
   a. The position is to be confirmed on vaginal examination by palpating supraorbital ridges and anterior fontanel
   b. Pelvic grip—the lower pole of the uterus is found empty
   c. On per vaginal (PV) examination the scapula and the clavicle are distinguished
   d. All of the above

6. When the long axis of the fetus lies perpendicularly to the maternal spine or uterine axis, it is called?
   a. Breech
   b. Transverse lie
   c. Face
   d. Brow

7. A multiparous woman came to the labor ward with hand prolapse. On examination her fetal heart sounds is absent. Which will be your line of management?
   a. Normal vaginal delivery
   b. Normal vaginal delivery with episiotomy
   c. Lower segment cesarean section
   d. Classical cesarean section

8. During a cesarean section, how to deliver a baby in a transverse lie?
   a. Delivery by breech extraction
   b. Delivery by vertex presentation
   c. Delivery by mentum
   d. None of the above

9. Which of the following is a complication of a transverse lie?
   a. Cord prolapse
   b. Hand prolapse
   c. Abruption
   d. None of the above

10. Which of the following is the most common uterine anomaly causing transverse lie?
    a. Unicornuate
    b. Bicornuate
    c. Arcuate
    d. None of the above

11. What is the incidence of brow presentation?
    a. One in 300 births
    b. One in 200 births
    c. One in 1000 births
    d. One in 800 births

12. Which pelvis favors brow presentation?
    a. Gynecoid
    b. Android
    c. Anthropoid
    d. Flat pelvis

13. Which of the following is true regarding brow presentation?
    a. The fetal head thus occupies a position midway between full flexion (occiput) and full extension (face)
    b. Presenting part of brow presentation is mentum
    c. Area between coronal suture behind and supraorbital ridge in front
    d. Both (a) and (c)

14. What is the engaging diameter in brow presentation?
    a. Submentobregmatic   b. Mentovertical
    c. Occipitofrontal   d. Suboccipitobregmatic

15. Denominator of brow presentation?
    a. Occiput   b. Sinciput
    c. Mentum   d. Sacrum

16. Mentovertical diameter how much it measures:
    a. 9.5 cm   b. 12 cm
    c. 13.5 cm   d. 14 cm

17. The given picture shows:

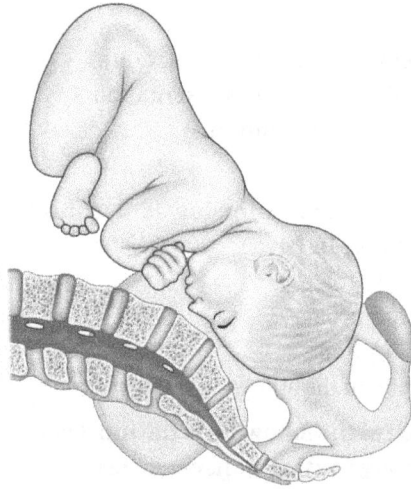

    a. Face presentation   b. Breech presentation
    c. Brow presentation   d. Transverse lie

18. Most appropriate mode of delivery in persistent brow presentation?
    a. Normal vaginal delivery
    b. Assisted breech delivery
    c. Cesarean section
    d. None of the above

19. What is the engaging diameter in face presentation?
    a. Submentobregmatic   b. Mentovertical
    c. Occipitofrontal   d. Suboccipitobregmatic

20. What is the incidence of the face presentation?
    a. One in 300 births
    b. One in 200 births
    c. One in 500 births
    d. One in 800 births

21. Which of the following point differentiate face presentation from breech presentation?
    a. The mouth and the malar eminence are not in a line, but in the breech, the anus and the ischial tuberosities are in one line
    b. Sucking effect of the mouth
    c. Hard alveolar margin
    d. All of the above

22. The denominator of face presentation is which of the following?
    a. Mentum   b. Sinciput
    c. Occiput   d. Sacrum

23. The neck is hyperextended so that the occiput is in contact with the fetal back, and the chin (mentum) is presenting part represent _____ presentation.
    a. Breech   b. Brow
    c. Cephalic   d. Face

24. Which of the following are the common causes for the face presentation?
    a. Neck swelling
    b. Flat pelvis
    c. Pelvic tumors
    d. All of the above

25. How is a fetus with face presentation delivered?
    a. The delivery of head by flexion
    b. The delivery of head by extension
    c. Internal rotation of chin
    d. None of the above

26. Which of the following is/are complications of face presentation?
    a. Cord prolapse
    b. Postpartum hemorrhage (PPH)
    c. Increased operative delivery
    d. All of the above

27. Trial of vaginal delivery is given in _____ position of face presentation.
    a. Mentoanterior
    b. Mentoposterior
    c. Elective cesarean section is the definitive management
    d. None of the above

28. **What are the complications while delivering the baby with face presentation?**
    a. Shoulder dystocia
    b. Injury to neck
    c. Injury to cervix and vagina
    d. All of the above

29. **The diagnostic feature of mentoposterior presentation is which of the following?**
    a. Groove between the head and back is not so prominent
    b. Back is felt to the front and better palpated only toward the podalic pole because of the extension of the spine
    c. Fetal heart sounds is distinctly audible anteriorly through the chest wall of the fetus toward the side of the limbs
    d. None of the above

30. **What are the fetal complications of face presentation?**
    a. Facial edema
    b. Injury to neonatal eyes
    c. Injury to lips
    d. All of the above

ANSWERS

1. **b.** One in 200 births
   The incidence is about one in 200 births. It is common in premature and macerated fetuses, and five times more common in multipara than primigravidae. Transverse lie in twin pregnancy is found in 40% of cases.

2. **d.** 40%
   Transverse lie in twin pregnancy is found in 40% of the cases.

3. **c.** Abnormal uterine anatomy
   The common causes include:
   - Abdominal wall relaxation from high parity
   - Preterm fetus
   - Placenta previa
   - Abnormal uterine anatomy
   - Hydramnios
   - Contracted maternal pelvis

4. **c.** Acromion and scapula
   During vaginal examination, in the early stages of labor, if the side of the thorax can be reached, the sequential parallel ribs are felt. With further dilation, the scapula and the clavicle are distinguished on opposite sides of the thorax. The position of the axilla indicates the side of the mother toward which the shoulder is directed.

5. **a.** The position is to be confirmed on vaginal examination by palpating supraorbital ridges and anterior fontanel.

   Palpation:
   - *Fundal height* is less than the period of amenorrhea.
   - *Fundal grip*—the fetal pole (breech or head) is not palpable.
   - Lateral grip—(1) soft, broad, and irregular breech is felt to one side of the midline, and the smooth, hard, and globular head is felt on the other side. The head is usually placed at a lower level on one iliac fossa and (2) the back is felt anteriorly across the long axis in the dorsoanterior or the irregular small parts are felt anteriorly in the dorsoposterior.
   - Pelvic grip—the lower pole of the uterus is found empty. This; however, is evident only during pregnancy but during labor, it may be occupied by the shoulder.

6. **b.** Transverse lie
   When the long axis of the fetus lies perpendicularly to the maternal spine or uterine axis, it is called a transverse lie.

7. **c.** Lower segment cesarean section
   Spontaneous delivery of a fully developed newborn is impossible with a persistent transverse lie. The active labor in a woman with a transverse lie typically requires cesarean delivery.

8. **a.** Delivery by breech extraction
   - Spontaneous delivery of a fully developed newborn is impossible with a persistent transverse lie. The active labor in a woman with a transverse lie typically requires cesarean delivery.
   - With a dorsoposterior or backup position, one or both feet can be grasped through a low transverse incision and delivered by breech extraction.

9. **b.** Hand prolapse
   Complication of transverse lie is hand prolapse.

10. **c.** Arcuate
    The arcuate uterus is the most common uterine anomaly in a transverse lie.

11. **c.** One in 1,000 births
    The incidence of brow is very rare, about one in 1,000 births.
12. **d.** Flat pelvis
    This happens especially in a flat pelvis where the biparietal diameter is held in the sacrocotyloid diameter.
13. **d.** Both (a) and (c)
    The fetal head thus occupies a position midway between full flexion (occiput) and full extension (face).
    The area between the coronal suture behind and the supraorbital ridge in front.
14. **b.** Mentovertical
    As the engaging diameter of the head is mentovertical (14 cm), there is no mechanism of labor in an average-sized baby with a normal pelvis.
15. **b.** Sinciput
    - *Denominator:* Arbitrary bony fixed point on the presenting part
    - *Brow:* Sinciput
    - *Vertex:* Occiput
    - *Face:* Mentum
    - *Breech:* Sacrum
    - *Shoulder:* Acromion
16. **d.** 14 cm
    As the engaging diameter of the head is mentovertical (14 cm), there is no mechanism of labor in an average-sized baby with a normal pelvis.
17. **c.** Brow presentation
    - The fetal head thus occupies a position midway between full flexion (occiput) and full extension (face).
    - The area between the coronal suture behind and the supraorbital ridge in front
18. **c.** Cesarean section
    The most appropriate mode of delivery in persistent brow presentation is a cesarean section.
19. **a.** Submentobregmatic
    As the engaging diameter of the head is submentobregmatic (9.5 cm)
20. **c.** One in 500 births
    Its frequency is about one in 500 births. Face presentation present during pregnancy (primary) is rare, while that developing after the onset of labor (secondary) is common. It occurs more frequently in multiparous women (70%).
21. **d.** All of the above
    - The mouth and the malar eminence are not in a line, but in the breech, the anus and the ischial tuberosities are in one line.
    - Sucking effect of the mouth
    - Hard alveolar margin
    - Absence of meconium staining on the examination finger
22. **a.** Mentum
    - *Denominator:* Arbitrary bony fixed point on the presenting part
    - *Brow:* Sinciput
    - *Vertex:* Occiput
    - *Face:* Mentum
    - *Breech:* Sacrum
    - *Shoulder:* Acromion
23. **d.** Face
    The neck is hyperextended so that the occiput is in contact with the fetal back, and the chin (mentum) is presented as part of representing face presentation.
24. **d.** All of the above
    - *Maternal*: (1) Multiparity with the pendulous abdomen, (2) lateral obliquity of the uterus especially, if it is directed to the side toward which the occiput lies, (3) contracted pelvis is associated in about 40% of cases, and (4) flat pelvis favors face presentation and pelvic tumors.
    - *Fetal*:
        - Congenital malformations:
            - The most common one is anencephaly.
            - Congenital goiter—prevalent in endemic areas
            - Dolichocephalic head with long anteroposterior diameter
            - Congenital
        - Twist of the cord several turns around the neck.
        - Increased tone of the extensor group of neck muscles.
25. **a.** The delivery of head by flexion
    In face presentation the head delivers by flexion
26. **d.** All of the above
    - Cord prolapse
    - Increased operative delivery
    - Cerebral congestion due to poor venous return from the head and neck and

- Neonatal infection due to bacterial contamination within the vagina

27. **a.** Mentoanterior

    Trial of vaginal delivery is given in the mentoanterior position of face presentation.

28. **d.** All of the above

    Complications while delivering the baby with facial presentation include:
    - Shoulder dystocia
    - Injury to the neck
    - Injury to cervix and vagina

29. **b.**
    - *Lateral grip*: The back is felt to the front and better palpated only toward the podalic pole because of the extension of the spine.
    - *Pelvic grip*:
        - Head seems big and is not engaged.
        - Cephalic prominence is to the side toward which the back lies.
        - Groove is so prominent.
    - *Auscultation*: FHS is not so distinct and is audible on the flank toward the side of the limbs.

30. **d.** All of the above

    Fetal complications of face presentation include:
    - Facial edema
    - Injury to neonatal eyes
    - Injury to lips

    (*Reference: Cunningham GF, Leveno KJ, Dashe JS, Hoffman BL, Spong CY, Casey BM. Williams Obstetrics, 26th edition. Noida: McGraw Hill Education (India) Private Limited; 2022*)

    (*Reference: Konar H. DC Dutta's Textbook of Obstetrics Including Perinatology & Contraception, 10th edition. New Delhi: Jaypee Brothers Medical Publishers (P) Ltd; 2022*)

Chapter 45

Medicolegal Aspects in Gynecology and Obstetrics

Kavita Tilwani, Vivek Tilwani

QUESTIONS

1. The upper age limit of a male for an intending couple for surrogacy is:
   a. 65 years
   b. 55 years
   c. 45 years
   d. 35 years

2. The highest age of gestation for medical termination of pregnancy without referral of the matter to the board is:
   a. 12 weeks
   b. 20 weeks
   c. 22 weeks
   d. 24 weeks

3. Which of the following is not a ground for termination of pregnancy under the Medical Termination of Pregnancy Act, 1971?
   a. Fetal anencephaly
   b. Pregnancy as a result of rape
   c. Pendency of divorce proceedings
   d. Failure of contraception

4. Failure to obtain an undertaking in "Form–F" under the Pre-Conception and Pre-Diagnostic Techniques (Regulation and Prevention of Misuse) Act, 1994 for the performance of obstetric ultrasonography constitutes an offense punishable with which one of the following?
   a. A fine only
   b. Imprisonment only
   c. Imprisonment with or without a fine
   d. No penalty

5. Proceedings for medical negligence against a doctor can be filed before which of the following?
   a. A Criminal Court
   b. A Consumer Disputes Redressal Commission
   c. A State Medical Council
   d. All of the above

6. An adult male accused of rape is brought by the police for medical examination but he is refusing to give consent for medical examination. Which of the following is the right course of action?
   a. Obtain consent by force and then examine him
   b. Refuse to examine him and send him back with the police
   c. Examine him against his consent with the use of reasonable force as may be necessary for the same
   d. Obtain blood, semen, and fingerprint samples without conducting a medical examination

7. For consent for surgery to be valid, which of the following criterion/criteria must be satisfied?
   a. Clarity of information
   b. Absence of coercion
   c. Mental stability
   d. All of the above

8. A 24-year-old married woman with a pregnancy of 13 weeks gestation wants to terminate her pregnancy on the grounds of failure of contraceptive without informing her husband of the same and without the consent of her husband. She also wants a tubal ligation to be performed at the same time. Which of the following would be the right course of action?
   a. Refuse to perform tubal ligation without the consent of the patient's husband
   b. Perform medical termination of pregnancy with tubal ligation without the consent of the patient's husband
   c. Inform the husband of the patient about the patient's desire to undergo a medical termination of pregnancy
   d. Inform the police

9. The lower age limit for a woman to act as an oocyte donor is:
   a. 18 years
   b. 21 years
   c. 23 years
   d. 35 years

10. **The upper age limit for a woman to act as an oocyte donor is:**
    a. 18 years b. 21 years
    c. 23 years d. 35 years

11. **The lower age limit for a male to act as a sperm donor is:**
    a. 18 years b. 21 years
    c. 33 years d. 55 years

12. **The upper age limit for a male to act as a sperm donor is:**
    a. 18 years b. 21 years
    c. 33 years d. 55 years

13. **Which of the following statements is true regarding the donation of oocytes by a woman in India?**
    a. A woman can donate her oocytes only once in a lifetime
    b. A woman who has donated her oocytes once can donate her oocytes again after 2 years
    c. A 42-year-old married woman can donate oocytes only if she does not want to conceive any further
    d. Oocyte donation is banned in India

14. **Which of the following statements is false for surrogacy in India?**
    a. A woman can act as a surrogate mother by providing her own gametes
    b. A woman cannot act as a surrogate mother more than once in her lifetime
    c. The age of a woman acting as a surrogate mother shall be between 25 and 35 years as on the date of implantation
    d. A child born through surrogacy is deemed to be a biological child of the intending couple

15. **A 25-year-old pregnant woman with a full-term pregnancy in labor was hit by a bus while crossing the road and has presented with hemorrhagic shock and altered sensorium. She is not accompanied by any relatives. She needs to undergo an emergency cesarean section. Which of the following is the course of action?**
    a. Proceed with medical treatment immediately
    b. Contact the relatives telephonically and wait for their arrival to obtain consent for surgery upon the patient
    c. Inform the police and wait for their arrival since a road traffic accident has occurred in the case
    d. Refuse treatment and send her to a government hospital

16. **A pregnant girl at the age of 18 years and 1 month has presented with 10 weeks of gestation. As per her history, she had consented to sexual intercourse with a 24-year-old man which led to the present pregnancy. The girl is demanding medical termination of pregnancy since she is unmarried. What is the right course of action?**
    a. Perform medical termination of pregnancy as demanded by the patient
    b. Intimation of the case to the police under Protection of Children from Sexual Offences (POCSO)
    c. Refer the patient for marital counseling and solemnization of marriage with the 24-year-old man
    d. Let the pregnancy continue till full term and register the woman for surrogacy so that her baby may be given to an intending couple

17. **Which of the following statements is true with respect to the medical examination of a survivor of rape and an accused of rape?**
    a. The consents of both a survivor of rape and an accused of rape are mandatory for their medical examination
    b. Both a survivor of rape and an accused of rape can be subjected to a medical examination without their consent
    c. Reasonable force can be used, if necessary, for subjecting a survivor of rape to a medical examination if she does not consent for her medical examination but an accused of rape cannot be subjected to medical examination without his consent
    d. Reasonable force can be used, if necessary, for subjecting an accused of rape to a medical examination if he does not consent for his medical examination but a survivor of rape cannot be subjected to a medical examination without her consent

18. **Which of the following statements is true for a case of medical termination of pregnancy in the case of a 24-year-old unmarried pregnant woman with 16 weeks of gestation detected with anencephaly?**
    a. Only the consent of the woman is sufficient
    b. The consent of the woman and the biological father of the fetus is necessary
    c. Medical termination of pregnancy cannot be performed for an unmarried woman under any circumstances

d. No consent is required for performing medical termination of pregnancy in case of proven anencephaly

19. **Which of the following statements are true for the performance of vasectomy in a 32-year-old married male?**
    a. Consent of the patient alone is sufficient
    b. Consent of the patient and his wife is necessary
    c. Consent of the wife alone is sufficient if the couple has more than three children
    d. No consent is required if the couple has >12 children

20. **Which of the following statements is true for the performance of tubal ligation in a 32-year-old married woman?**
    a. Consent of the patient alone is sufficient
    b. Consent of the patient and her husband is necessary
    c. Consent of the husband alone is sufficient if the couple has more than three children
    d. No consent is required if the couple has >12 children

21. **Which of the following statements is true for the registration of a case for offenses under the POCSO, 2013?**
    a. A case can be registered only if the survivor is a female
    b. A case can be registered if the survivor is a male or a female or a transgender below the age of 18 years
    c. A case cannot be registered if the sexual offense complained of had been committed with the consent of the survivor
    d. A case cannot be registered if the sexual offense complained of had been committed with the consent of the parents of the minor survivor

22. **Which of the following statements is true for the PCPNDT, 1994?**
    a. In India, sex selection and sex determination are totally banned
    b. In India, sex selection and sex determination are both permitted
    c. In India, sex selection is permitted but sex determination is banned
    d. In India, sex selection is banned but sex determination is permitted

23. **Which of the following statements is true about surrogacy in India?**
    a. It must necessarily be altruistic
    b. Payment of rental fees for utilization of "rent a womb" is exempted from taxation
    c. If the woman of the intending couple is unable to produce oocytes, the oocytes of the surrogate woman may be used for surrogacy
    d. A child born through surrogacy involving an oocyte donor is not entitled to inherit property of the intending couple

24. **Which of the following statements is true in vitro fertilization technology in India?**
    a. It is not permissible to be carried out using a sperm donor
    b. It is not permissible to be carried out using an ovum donor
    c. If the sperm count of the male is good, the unutilized part of the semen sample can be used for another couple
    d. The unutilized zygotes cannot be sold to other couples

25. **Which of the following are not included in maternal mortality?**
    a. Death during cesarean section
    b. Death after 40 days of parturition
    c. Death during medical termination of pregnancy
    d. Death after 45 days of normal delivery

26. **A pregnant woman has given birth to a child by normal delivery but out of wedlock. The lady does not want to keep the child because her husband is not aware of this pregnancy and delivery. Which of the following options are available to the woman under the law?**
    a. Abandon the child on the streets
    b. Refuse to accept the child from the hospital at the time of discharge
    c. The doctor who has conducted the delivery directly can directly give the child in adoption to a childless couple after obtaining the written consent of the biological mother of the baby
    d. None of the above

27. **Which of the following is true about adoptions in India?**
    a. The doctor who has conducted the delivery directly can directly give the child in adoption to a childless couple after obtaining the written consent of the biological mother of the baby

b. The doctor who has conducted the delivery directly can directly give the child in adoption to a childless couple after obtaining the written consent of the biological father of the baby

c. The doctor who has conducted the delivery directly can directly give the child in adoption to a childless couple after obtaining the written consent of the biological father and mother of the baby

d. None of the above

28. **Which of the following statements is not true about a case of rape?**
    a. The doctor to whom the rape survivor has presented should not give intimation of the case to the police if the rape survivor gives her written consent and/or instructions to that effect
    b. The doctor to whom the rape survivor has presented must necessarily give intimation of the case to the police even if the rape survivor does not want such intimation to be given
    c. Police intimation is not necessary if rape was committed >1 month ago
    d. Police intimation is not necessary if rape was committed >6 months ago

29. **Which of the following is the correct advice for contraception in the case of a woman who has undergone bilateral oophorectomy?**
    a. Tubal ligation
    b. Intrauterine contraceptive device
    c. Oral contraceptive pills
    d. None of the above

30. **Which of the following is true for the performance of a medical termination of pregnancy?**
    a. The place where the medical termination of pregnancy is to be performed must be recognized under the provisions of the Medical Termination of Pregnancy Act, of 1971
    b. The doctor who performs the medical termination of pregnancy must be recognized under the provisions of the Medical Termination of Pregnancy Act, 1971
    c. The indication for performing the medical termination of pregnancy must be as prescribed under the provisions of the Medical Termination of Pregnancy Act, 1971
    d. All of the above

ANSWERS

1. **b.** 55 years
   Under section 4 (iii)(c)(I), the male has to be between 26 and 55 years of age.

2. **d.** 24 weeks
   Under section 3 (2) (b) of the Medical Termination of Pregnancy Act, 1971 as amended vide the Medical Termination of Pregnancy (Amendment) Act, 2021, where the length of the pregnancy exceeds twenty weeks but does not exceed *24 weeks* the pregnancy can be terminated if not less than two registered medical practitioners are of the opinion formed in good faith in that regard.

3. **c.** Pendency of divorce proceedings
   Pendency of divorce proceedings is not a ground for termination of pregnancy under sections 3 and 5 of the Medical Termination of Pregnancy Act, 1971.

4. **c.** Imprisonment with or without a fine.

5. **d.** All of the above
   Under Regulation 2.4 of the Indian Medical Council (Professional Conduct, Etiquette and Ethics) Regulations, 2002, a provisionally or fully registered medical practitioner shall not willfully commit an act of negligence that may deprive his patient or patients from necessary medical care; thus, in addition to criminal cases as well as consumer protection cases, a complaint can also be filed before the State Medical Council.

6. **c.** Examine him against his consent with the use of reasonable force as may be necessary for the same.
   Under section 53 of the Code of Criminal Procedure, 1973.

7. **d.** All of the above
   Consent is not valid unless all of the above criteria are satisfied.

8. **a.** Refuse to perform tubal ligation without the consent of the patient's husband.
   Under Regulation 7.16 of the Indian Medical Council (Professional Conduct, Etiquette and Ethics) Regulations, 2002. "In an operation which may result in sterility the consent of both husband and wife is needed."

9. **c.** 23 years
   Under section 27 (2)(b) of the Assisted Reproductive Technology (Regulation) Act, 2021, the age of an oocyte donor must be between 23 and 35 years.

10. **d.** 35 years
    Under section 27 (2)(b) of the Assisted Reproductive Technology (Regulation) Act, 2021, the age of an oocyte donor must be between 23 and 35 years.

11. **b.** 21 years
    Under section 27 (2)(a) of the Assisted Reproductive Technology (Regulation) Act, 2021, the age of an oocyte donor must be between 21 and 55 years.

12. **d.** 55 years
    Under section 27 (2)(a) of the Assisted Reproductive Technology (Regulation) Act, 2021, the age of an oocyte donor must be between 21 and 55 years.

13. **a.** A woman can donate her oocytes only once in a lifetime.
    Under the Assisted Reproductive Technology (Regulation) Act, 2021, a woman can donate oocytes only once in her lifetime.

14. **a.** A woman can act as a surrogate mother by providing her own gametes.
    Under the Surrogacy (Regulation) Act, 2021, no woman shall act as a surrogate mother by providing her own gametes.

15. **a.** Proceed with medical treatment immediately.
    Immediate treatment is necessary in the face of a lifesaving emergency.

16. **b.** Intimation of the case to the police under POCSO.
    The patient was a minor at the time of sexual activity and hence it is a case of POCSO.

17. **d.** Reasonable force can be used, if necessary, for subjecting an accused of rape to a medical examination if he does not consent for his medical examination but a survivor of rape cannot be subjected to a medical examination without her consent.
    A survivor of rape cannot be forced for a medical examination.

18. **a.** Only the consent of the woman is sufficient.
    The consent of the woman alone is sufficient to perform a medical termination of pregnancy in such a case as per law.

19. **b.** Consent of the patient and his wife is necessary.
    Under Regulation 7.16 of the Indian Medical Council (Professional Conduct, Etiquette and Ethics) Regulations, 2002. "In an operation which may result in sterility the consent of both husband and wife is needed."

20. **b.** Consent of the patient and her husband are necessary.
    Under Regulation 7.16 of the Indian Medical Council (Professional Conduct, Etiquette and Ethics) Regulations, 2002. "In an operation which may result in sterility the consent of both husband and wife is needed."

21. **b.** A case can be registered if the survivor is a male a female or a transgender below the age of 18 years.
    Under the POCSO Act, a case can be registered if any child is subjected to a sexual offense.

22. **a.** In India, sex selection and sex determination are totally banned.
    Under the PCPNDT Act, 1994, sex selection and sex determination are totally banned in India.

23. **a.** It must necessarily be altruistic.
    Under the Surrogacy (Regulation) Act, 2021, only altruistic surrogacy is permitted in India.

24. **d.** The unutilized zygotes cannot be sold to other couples.
    Under the Assisted Reproductive Technology (Regulation) Act, 2021, the unutilized zygotes cannot be sold.

25. **d.** Death after 45 days of normal delivery.
    This is in according to the definition of the term "maternal mortality."

26. **d.** None of the above

27. **d.** None of the above
    According to the adoption laws in India, a doctor cannot give a child of a couple directly in adoption to any person.

28. **b.** The doctor to whom the rape survivor has presented must necessarily give intimation of the case to the police even if the rape survivor does not want such intimation to be given.
    This is necessary under the Indian Penal Code, of 1860.

29. **d.** None of the above

30. **d.** None of the above

Chapter 46

Cord Prolapse

Priya Vora, Nishita Shah

QUESTIONS

1. Cord prolapse is defined as the descent of the umbilical cord through the cervix:
   a. Occult
   b. Overt
   c. Either of the above
   d. None of the above

2. The overall incidence of cord prolapse is:
   a. 0.1–0.6%
   b. 0.8–1.2%
   c. 0.05–0.1%
   d. 1–2%

3. One of the following is not a high-risk factor for cord prolapse:
   a. Multiple pregnancies
   b. Nonvertex presentation
   c. Singleton term pregnancy
   d. Polyhydramnios

4. Diagnosis to the delivery interval with the adverse neonatal outcome:
   a. >3 minutes
   b. >5 minutes
   c. >10 minutes
   d. >7 minutes

5. Which of the following is a sign of cord prolapse—Fetal Heart Rate?
   a. Acceleration
   b. Decelerations
   c. Both of the above
   d. None of the above

6. When to consider for umbilical cord prolapse?
   a. Every vaginal examination in labor
   b. After artificial rupture of membranes (ARM)
   c. Decelerations after spontaneous rupture of membranes (ROM)
   d. All of the above

7. How to relieve pressure? Choose the correct option.
   a. Manually push the presenting part down
   b. Empty bladder
   c. Stop tocolysis
   d. Knee-chest position

8. Steps in management involve which of the following?
   a. Call for help—obstetrician
   b. Perioperative team—anesthetist
   c. Competent neonatal team
   d. All of the above

9. This type of presentation has the highest risk of cord prolapse:
   a. Footling breech
   b. Complete breech
   c. Frank breech
   d. Vertex

10. The frequency is highest in this type of presentation:
    a. Vertex
    b. Breech
    c. Transverse
    d. All of the above

11. Risk factor for cord prolapse includes which of the following?
    a. Term fetus
    b. Preterm fetus
    c. Post-term fetus
    d. All of the above

12. Polyhydramnios is an independent risk factor because:
    a. Increased risk of unstable lie
    b. Unengaged presenting part
    c. Fetal anomalies
    d. All of the above

13. The Cord abnormalities which are associated with:
    a. Cord length of approximately 55 cm
    b. Cord length < 35 cm
    c. Cord length > 70 cm
    d. Cord length < 20 cm

14. The mode of delivery is:
    a. Always vaginal
    b. Always cesarean
    c. Assess and assist birth by the quickest means
    d. Wait for labor

15. Choose the correct option for Tocolysis:
    a. Primary modality of treatment
    b. As an adjunct to mechanical methods
    c. When delivery is imminent
    d. Longer acting should be used

16. At threshold of viability
    a. Continue pregnancy
    b. Terminate pregnancy
    c. Expectant management only
    d. Counsel patient on both continuation and termination

17. Contraindications of immediate cesarean delivery
    a. Fetal demise
    b. Previable gestation
    c. Fetus with lethal anomalies
    d. All of the above

18. Regional anesthesia is preferred in the presence of:
    a. Fetal distress
    b. Normal fetal pattern
    c. Presence of fetal bradycardia
    d. None of the above

19. Which one of these is a pushing method to reduce cord compression?
    a. Retrograde bladder filling
    b. Knee-chest position
    c. Trendelenburg position
    d. Exaggerated Sim's position

20. The best method during transport is?
    a. Knee-chest position
    b. Trendelenburg position
    c. Wedging the maternal pelvis
    d. Supine position

21. Steps for clinical approach include all, except:
    a. Call for help
    b. Intrauterine resuscitation
    c. Fetal Heart Rate monitoring
    d. Maximum manipulation

22. Steps to prevent cord prolapse include all, except:
    a. Controlled ARM
    b. Gentle fundal pressure
    c. Disengaging fetal presenting part
    d. Early elective admission for patients with an abnormal lie

23. Perinatal mortality and morbidity:
    a. 91/1,000
    b. 81/1,000
    c. 71/1,000
    d. 61/1,000

24. Cord abnormalities that can be associated with a higher incidence of cord prolapse is:
    a. True knot
    b. False knot
    c. Single umbilical artery
    d. Both (a) and (c)

25. Procedures associated with an increased risk of cord prolapse are all, except:
    a. External cephalic version
    b. Internal podalic version
    c. Artificial rupture of membranes with engaged presenting part
    d. Large balloon catheter induction of labor

26. Cord prolapse leads to which of the following?
    a. Vasoconstriction and fetal hypoxia
    b. Vasodilatation and fetal hypoxia
    c. Vasoconstriction and fetal tachycardia
    d. Vasodilatation and fetal tachycardia

27. With transverse, oblique, or unstable lie, elective admission to hospital after ____ weeks of gestation should be discussed.
    a. 36
    b. 37
    c. 38
    d. 35

28. Vaginal birth can be attempted:
    a. At full dilatation
    b. Breech extraction under some circumstances
    c. After the internal podalic version for the second twin
    d. All of the above

29. Cardiotocographic (CTG) findings in the case of umbilical cord prolapse can be:
    a. Recurrent decelerations
    b. Prolonged deceleration
    c. Acute bradycardia
    d. All of the above

30. Bradycardia-to-delivery interval is:
    a. Significant correlation with cord arterial pH with fetal bradycardia
    b. Significant correlation between cord arterial pH with normal heart rate
    c. The risk of significant acidosis (pH < 7) was 80% when the bradycardia-to-delivery interval is <20 minutes
    d. All of the above

31. Marginal insertion of the placenta is when cord insertion is within ____ of the placental edge.
    a. 3-4 cm
    b. 1-2 cm
    c. 4-5 cm
    d. 6 cm

32. **Increased risk of fetal demise is seen with which of the following?**
    a. True knot
    b. False knot
    c. Both of the above
    d. None of the above

33. **Which of the following is associated with the cord prolapse?**
    a. Short cord
    b. Long cord
    c. Velamentous insertion
    d. Vasa previa

34. **Umbilical cord consists of which of the following?**
    a. Two arteries one vein
    b. Two veins one artery
    c. Two arteries two veins
    d. 1 artery one vein

35. **Which of the following is correct?**
    a. The umbilical artery carries oxygenated blood
    b. The umbilical artery carries deoxygenated blood
    c. The umbilical vein carries deoxygenated blood
    d. The umbilical vein carries waste products from the fetus to the placenta

ANSWERS

1. **c.** Either of the above.
   There are two forms of umbilical cord prolapse. The first, overt prolapse, occurs when the cord exits the cervix before the fetal presenting part; the second, occult prolapse, occurs when the cord exits the cervix with the fetal presenting part.
   [Reference: Boushra M, Stone A, Rathbun KM. Umbilical cord prolapse. In: StatPearls (Internet). Treasure Island (FL): StatPearls Publishing; 2023]

2. **a.** 0.1–0.6%
   Umbilical cord prolapse is an unpredictable obstetrical emergency with an incidence ranging from 1 to 6 per 1,000 pregnancies.
   [Reference: Wong L, Kwan AHW, Lau SL, Sin WTA, Leung TY. Umbilical cord prolapse: revisiting its definition and management. Am J Obstet Gynecol. 2021;225(4):357-66]

3. **c.** Singleton term pregnancy.
   Prolapsed amniotic bag, labor, and rupture of the membrane during the premature period, fetal abnormal presentation induced by multiple pregnancies, and polyhydramnios was a high-risk situation for umbilical cord prolapse.
   [Reference: Hasegawa J, Ikeda T, Sekizawa A, Ishiwata I, Kinoshita K; Japan Association of Obstetricians and Gynecologists, Tokyo, Japan. Obstetric risk factors for umbilical cord prolapse: a nationwide population-based study in Japan. Arch Gynecol Obstet. 2016;294(3):467-72]

4. **c.** >10 minutes.
   A diagnosis to delivery interval greater than ten minutes is independently associated with an adverse neonatal outcome.
   [Reference: Kaymak O, Iskender C, Ibanoglu M, Cavkaytar S, Uygur D, Danisman N. Retrospective evaluation of risk factors and perinatal outcome of umbilical cord prolapse during labor. Eur Rev Med Pharmacol Sci. 2015;19(13):2336-9]

5. **b.** Decelerations
   [Reference: Cleveland Clinic. Umbilical cord prolapse. (online) Available from https://my.clevelandclinic.org/health/diseases/12345-umbilical-cord-prolapse (Last accessed December, 2023)]

6. **d.** All of the above.
   [Reference: Cleveland Clinic. Umbilical Cord Prolapse (Green-top Guideline No. 50) (online). Available from https://www.rcog.org.uk/guidance/browse-all-guidance/green-top-guidelines/umbilical-cord-prolapse-green-top-guideline-no-50/#:~:text=Cord%20prolapse%20has%20been%20defined,with%20or%20without%20membrane%20rupture (Last accessed December, 2023)]

7. **d.** Knee-chest position.
   [Reference: Wong L, Kwan AHW, Lau SL, Sin WTA, Leung TY. Umbilical cord prolapse: revisiting its definition and management. Am J Obstet Gynecol. 2021;25(4):357-66]

8. **d.** All of the above.
   [Reference: Cleveland Clinic. Umbilical Cord Prolapse (Green-top Guideline No. 50) (online). Available from https://www.rcog.org.uk/guidance/browse-all-guidance/green-top-guidelines/umbilical-cord-prolapse-green-top-guideline-no-50/#:~:text=Cord%20prolapse%20has%20been%20defined,with%20or%20without%20membrane%20rupture (Last accessed December, 2023)]

9. **a.** Footling breech.
   [Reference: Barclay M. Umbilical cord prolapse and other cord accidents. In: Gynecology and Obstetrics, Sciarra JJ (Ed). Philadelphia: JB Lippincott; 1989. p. 1]

10. **c.** Transverse
[Reference: Barclay M. Umbilical cord prolapse and other cord accidents. In: Gynecology and Obstetrics, Sciarra JJ (Ed). Philadelphia: JB Lippincott; 1989. p. 1]

11. **b.** Preterm fetus.
[References: Koonings PP, Paul RH, Campbell K. Umbilical cord prolapse. A contemporary look. J Reprod Med. 1990;35(7):690-2.
Ylä-Outinen A, Heinonen PK, Tuimala R. Predisposing and risk factors of umbilical cord prolapse. Acta Obstet Gynecol Scand. 1985;64(7):567-70.
Murphy DJ, MacKenzie IZ. The mortality and morbidity associated with umbilical cord prolapse. Br J Obstet Gynaecol. 1995;102(10):826-30]

12. **d.** All of the above.
[Reference: Holbrook BD, Phelan ST. Umbilical cord prolapse. Obstet Gynecol Clin North Am. 2013;40(1):1-14]

13. **c.** Cord length > 70 cm.
[References: Rayburn WF, Beynen A, Brinkman DL. Umbilical cord length and intrapartum complications. Obstet Gynecol. 1981;57(4):450-2.
Krakowiak P, Smith EN, de Bruyn G, Lydon-Rochelle MT. Risk factors and outcomes associated with a short umbilical cord. Obstet Gynecol. 2004;103(1):119-27]
Linde LE, Rasmussen S, Kessler J, Ebbing C. Extreme umbilical cord lengths, cord knot, and entanglement: Risk factors and risk of adverse outcomes, a population-based study. PLoS One. 2018;13(3):e0194814]

14. **c.** Assess and assist birth by the quickest means.
[Reference: Cleveland Clinic. Umbilical Cord Prolapse (Green-top Guideline No. 50) (online). Available from https://www.rcog.org.uk/guidance/browse-all-guidance/green-top-guidelines/umbilical-cord-prolapse-green-top-guideline-no-50/#:~:text=Cord%20prolapse%20has%20been%20defined,with%20or%20without%20membrane%20rupture (Last accessed December, 2023)]

15. **b.** As an adjunct to mechanical methods.
[Reference: Wong L, Kwan AHW, Lau SL, Sin WTA, Leung TY. Umbilical cord prolapse: revisiting its definition and management. Am J Obstet Gynecol. 2021;225(4):357-66]

16. **d.** Counsel the patient on both continuation and termination.
[Reference: Cleveland Clinic. Umbilical Cord Prolapse (Green-top Guideline No. 50) (online). Available from https://www.rcog.org.uk/guidance/browse-all-guidance/green-top-guidelines/umbilical-cord-prolapse-green-top-guideline-no-50/#:~:text=Cord%20prolapse%20has%20been%20defined,with%20or%20without%20membrane%20rupture (Last accessed December, 2023)]

17. **d.** All of the above.
(Reference: Ahmed WAS, Hamdy MA. Optimal management of umbilical cord prolapse. Int J Womens Health. 2018;10:459-65)

18. **b.** Normal fetal pattern.
[Reference: Wong L, Kwan AHW, Lau SL, Sin WTA, Leung TY. Umbilical cord prolapse: revisiting its definition and management. Am J Obstet Gynecol. 2021;225(4):357-66]

19. **a.** Retrograde bladder filling.
[Reference: Kwan AHW, Chaemsaithong P, Wong L, Tse WT, Hui ASY, Poon LC, et al. Transperineal ultrasound assessment of fetal head elevation by maneuvers used for managing umbilical cord prolapse. Ultrasound Obstet Gynecol. 2021;58(4):603-8]

20. **c.** Wedging the maternal pelvis.
[Reference: Wong L, Kwan AHW, Lau SL, Sin WTA, Leung TY. Umbilical cord prolapse: revisiting its definition and management. Am J Obstet Gynecol. 2021;225(4):357-66]

21. **d.** Maximum manipulation.
[Reference: Cleveland Clinic. Umbilical Cord Prolapse (Green-top Guideline No. 50) (online). Available from https://www.rcog.org.uk/guidance/browse-all-guidance/green-top-guidelines/umbilical-cord-prolapse-green-top-guideline-no-50/#:~:text=Cord%20prolapse%20has%20been%20defined,with%20or%20without%20membrane%20rupture (Last accessed December, 2023)]

22. **c.** Disengaging fetal presenting part.
[Reference: Cleveland Clinic. Umbilical Cord Prolapse (Green-top Guideline No. 50) (online). Available from https://www.rcog.org.uk/guidance/browse-all-guidance/green-top-guidelines/umbilical-cord-prolapse-green-top-guideline-no-50/#:~:text=Cord%20prolapse%20has%20been%20defined,with%20or%20without%20membrane%20rupture (Last accessed December, 2023)]

23. **a.** 91/1,000
    [Reference: Murphy DJ, MacKenzie IZ. The mortality and morbidity associated with umbilical cord prolapse. Br J Obstet Gynaecol. 1995;102(10):826-30]

24. **d.** Both (a) and (c).
    [References: Hayes DJL, Warland J, Parast MM, Bendon RW, Hasegawa J, Banks J, et al. Umbilical cord characteristics and their association with adverse pregnancy outcomes: A systematic review and meta-analysis. PloS One. 2020;15(9):e0239630.
    Merz E, Pashaj S. True or false umbilical cord knot? Differentiation via 3D/4D color Doppler ultrasound. Ultraschall Med. 2018;39(2):127-8]

25. **c.** Artificial rupture of membranes with engaged presenting part.
    [Reference: Cleveland Clinic. Umbilical Cord Prolapse (Green-top Guideline No. 50) (online). Available from https://www.rcog.org.uk/guidance/browse-all-guidance/green-top-guidelines/umbilical-cord-prolapse-green-top-guideline-no-50/#:~:text=Cord%20prolapse%20has%20been%20defined,with%20or%20without%20membrane%20rupture (Last accessed December, 2023)]

26. **a.** Vasoconstriction and fetal hypoxia.
    [Reference: Boushra M, Stone A, Rathbun KM. Umbilical cord prolapse. In: StatPearls (Internet). Treasure Island (FL): StatPearls Publishing; 2023]

27. **b.** 37
    [Reference: Cleveland Clinic. Umbilical Cord Prolapse (Green-top Guideline No. 50) (online). Available from https://www.rcog.org.uk/guidance/browse-all-guidance/green-top-guidelines/umbilical-cord-prolapse-green-top-guideline-no-50/#:~:text=Cord%20prolapse%20has%20been%20defined,with%20or%20without%20membrane%20rupture (Last accessed December, 2023)]

28. **d.** All of the above.
    [Reference: Cleveland Clinic. Umbilical Cord Prolapse (Green-top Guideline No. 50) (online). Available from https://www.rcog.org.uk/guidance/browse-all-guidance/green-top-guidelines/umbilical-cord-prolapse-green-top-guideline-no-50/#:~:text=Cord%20prolapse%20has%20been%20defined,with%20or%20without%20membrane%20rupture (Last accessed December, 2023)]

29. **d.** All of the above.
    [Reference: Botezatu R, Gica N, Peltecu G, Panaitescu AM. Umbilical Cord Prolapse—Interesting CTG Traces. Diagnostics (Basel). 2022;12(11):2845]

30. **a.** Significant correlation between cord arterial pH with fetal bradycardia
    [Reference: Wong L, Tse WT, Lai CY, Hui ASY, Chaemsaithong P, Sahota DS, et al. Bradycardia-to-delivery interval and fetal outcomes in umbilical cord prolapse. Acta Obstet Gynecol Scand. 2021;100(1):170-7]

31. **b.** 1–2 cm
    [Reference: Wax JR, Pinette MG. Imaging the Placental Cord Insertion: Just Do It. J Ultrasound Med. 2020;39(4):811-5]

32. **a.** True knot.
    [Reference: Hayes DJL, Warland J, Parast MM, Bendon RW, Hasegawa J, Banks J, et al. Umbilical cord characteristics and their association with adverse pregnancy outcomes: A systematic review and meta-analysis. PloS One. 2020;15(9):e0239630]

33. **b.** Long cord.
    [References: Rayburn WF, Beynen A, Brinkman DL. Umbilical cord length and intrapartum complications. Obstet Gynecol. 1981;57(4):450-2.
    Linde LE, Rasmussen S, Kessler J, Ebbing C. Extreme umbilical cord lengths, cord knot, and entanglement: Risk factors and risk of adverse outcomes, a population-based study. PLoS One. 2018;13(3):e0194814]

34. **a.** Two arteries one vein.
    [Reference: Ramesh S, Hariprasath S, Anandan G, Solomon PJ, Vijayakumar V. Single umbilical artery. J Pharm Bioallied Sci. 2015;7(Suppl 1):S83-4]

35. **b.** The umbilical artery carries deoxygenated blood.
    [Reference: Ramesh S, Hariprasath S, Anandan G, Solomon PJ, Vijayakumar V. Single umbilical artery. J Pharm Bioallied Sci. 2015;7(Suppl 1):S83-4]

Chapter 47

Prolonged Labor, Obstructed Labor, and Dystocia

Suvarna Khadilkar, Rutuja Bodake

QUESTIONS

1. **Prolonged labor can be defined as:**
   a. When the first and second stage of labor combined is >6 hours
   b. When the first and second stage of labor combined is >18–20 hours
   c. When the first and second stage of labor combined is <2 hours
   d. When the first and second stages are about 10 hours

2. **A 37-week primigravida has mild pain in the abdomen for 20 hours and the cervix persistently 1 cm dilated but non-effaced. What would be the appropriate management?**
   a. Sedation and wait
   b. Augmentation with oxytocin
   c. Cesarean section
   d. Amniotomy

3. **A 28-year-old primigravida is brought to the room in the latent phase of labor. How long will you wait till you declare her latent phase to be prolonged?**
   a. 12 hours   b. 14 hours
   c. 18 hours   d. 20 hours

4. **A 26-year-old primigravida presents with pains. At 39 weeks of gestation, she was diagnosed with a prolonged phase of labor. Which of the following is false regarding this condition?**
   a. >14 hours in nullipara
   b. Oxytocin stimulation given
   c. Excessive sedation can prolong this phase
   d. Morphine is used in management

5. **Which among the following is false with respect to the active phase of labor?**
   a. The minimum rate of cervical dilatation is 1.2 cm/h in nullipara
   b. Arrest of dilatation is cessation of dilatation for >2 hours
   c. Arrest of descent is the cessation of descent for >1 hour
   d. Poor cervical dilatation causes prolonged active phase

6. **Post-term pregnancy refers to pregnancy continuing beyond:**
   a. 41 weeks of gestation   b. 42 weeks of gestation
   c. 44 weeks of gestation   d. 40 weeks of gestation

7. **Abdominal examination of a 28-year-old primigravida who is in the prolonged second stage of labor, reveals a retraction ring between the active upper segment and the distended lower segment. Which would best describe this ring?**
   a. Physiological retraction ring
   b. Pathological retraction ring
   c. Physiological contraction ring
   d. Pathological contraction ring

8. **Protracted descent in a nullipara is:**
   a. <1 cm/h   b. <1.2 cm/h
   c. 1.5 cm/h   d. <2 cm/h

9. **What is the most common cause of true cephalopelvic disproportion in India?**
   a. Malpresentation
   b. Rickets
   c. Trauma
   d. Occipitoposterior position

10. **You are monitoring uterine contractions in the term primigravida in labor. You find that the contractions are uncoordinated and the frequency is about 8 contractions every 10 minutes. Which of the following is incorrect regarding your finding?**
    a. Commonly associated with occipitoposterior
    b. It is common in multiparous labor

c. Oxytocin administration is beneficial
d. Management includes waiting and watching fetal heart, action if necessary

11. A young primigravida at 36 weeks of gestation came with complaints of decreased perception of fetal movements for the past 2 days. NST is nonreactive and on ultrasonography (USG) fetal cardiac activity is absent. What will be the best management for this patient?
    a. Forceps extraction
    b. Induce if she does not have a spontaneous expulsion
    c. Caesarean section
    d. Artificial rupture of membranes

12. A pregnant woman presents with obstructed labor and is grossly dehydrated. Investigations reveal fetal demise. What will be the management?
    a. Craniotomy
    b. Decapitation
    c. Cesarean section
    d. Forceps extraction

13. Abdominal examination of a 28-year-old primigravida, who is in second stage of labor, reveals retraction ring between the active upper segment and the distended lower segment. Which would best describe the ring?
    a. Physiological ring
    b. Pathological ring
    c. Physiological contraction ring
    d. Pathological contraction ring

14. A 32-year-old nulliparous woman at 38 weeks' gestation comes to the labor and delivery ward with regular painful contractions after a gush of fluid two hours ago. Her temperature is 98.6°F (37°C). She is found to have a gross rupture of membranes and to have a cervix that is 6 cm dilated. The fetus is in a breech position. The patient is then brought to the operating room for cesarean delivery. Which of the following represents the correct procedure for antibiotic administration?
    a. Administer intravenous antibiotics 30 minutes before the procedure
    b. Administer intravenous antibiotics after the cord is clamped
    c. Administer intravenous antibiotics immediately after the procedure
    d. Administer intravenous antibiotics for 24 hours after the procedure
    e. Administer oral antibiotics for 1 week following the procedure

15. A 21-year-old primigravida at 39 weeks' gestation comes to the labor ward with painful contractions every three minutes. Her prenatal course was unremarkable. Examination shows her cervix to be 3 cm dilated and 90% effaced. The fetal heart rate (FHR) tracing is in the 150 bpm and is reactive. About 5 hours later cervical examination reveals that the patient is 9 cm dilated and at −1 station. The FHR tracing shows moderate variable decelerations with each contraction and decreased variability. Fetal scalp sampling is performed that yields fetal scalp pHs of 7.04, 7.05, and 7.06. Which of the following is the most appropriate next step in management?
    a. Expectant management
    b. Episiotomy
    c. Forceps-assisted vaginal delivery
    d. Vacuum-assisted vaginal delivery
    e. Cesarean delivery

16. A 31-year-old, human immunodeficiency virus (HIV)-positive woman, gravida 3, para 2, at 32 weeks gestation comes to the physician for a prenatal visit. Her prenatal course is significant for the fact that she has taken zidovudine throughout the pregnancy. Otherwise, her prenatal course has been unremarkable. She has no history of mental illness. She states that she has been weighing the benefits and risks of cesarean delivery in preventing transmission of the virus to her baby. After much deliberation, she has decided that she does not want a cesarean delivery and would like to attempt a vaginal delivery. Which of the following is the most appropriate next step in management?
    a. Contact psychiatry to evaluate the patient
    b. Contact the hospital lawyers to get a court order for cesarean delivery
    c. Perform cesarean delivery at 38 weeks
    d. Perform cesarean delivery once the patient is in labor
    e. Respect the patient's decision and perform the vaginal delivery

17. Which of the following maneuvers is not used for the management of shoulder dystocia?
    a. McRoberts maneuver
    b. Suprapubic pressure
    c. Woods corkscrew maneuver
    d. Mauriceau-Smellie-Veit maneuver

18. Oligohydramnios is characteristically associated with which one of the following?
    a. Diabetes mellitus
    b. Rhesus iso-immunization
    c. Fetal renal agenesis
    d. Hemangioma of the placenta
    e. Fetal duodenal atresia

19. Dystocia is a characteristic feature of all of the following, *except* which one of the following?
    a. Mentoposterior position
    b. A breech presentation
    c. An android pelvis
    d. Mentoanterior position
    e. Cervical fibroid

20. All of the following cause labor dystocia, *except* which of the following?
    a. Hydrocephalus
    b. Occipitoanterior
    c. Face presentation
    d. Occipitoposterior
    e. Ovarian mass
    f. Shoulder dystocia

21. Effects of labor dystocia include all, *except* for which one of the following?
    a. Chorioamnionitis
    b. Uterine rupture
    c. Reassuring FHR trace
    d. Pelvic floor injury

22. A few hours into labor induction cardiotocograph (CTG) shows a late deceleration after episodes of frequent contraction. The most likely explanation of deceleration is which one of the following?
    a. Maternal position on the left lateral side
    b. Uterine hyperstimulation from cervical ripening agent
    c. Compression of the fetal head mediated by the vagus
    d. Umbilical cord compression

23. Management of shoulder dystocia includes the following, *except* which of the following?
    a. McRobert's maneuver: Sharply flex the maternal thigh
    b. Episiotomy if needed for more room
    c. Fundal pressure
    d. Woods screw maneuver
    e. Delivery of the posterior arm

24. Intrapartum computed tomography (CT) a finding of late deceleration is which of the following?
    a. Relied by maternal position on the left side
    b. Compression of fetal head mediated by the vagus
    c. Caused by umbilical cord compression
    d. Is not worrisome if nonrecurrent
    e. Is mostly due to placental insufficiency

25. What is Robin's maneuver to release shoulder dystocia?
    a. Rotation of posterior shoulder to deliver anterior shoulder
    b. Abduction of shoulders
    c. Flex of mother's knees and suprapubic pressure
    d. Rotation and extraction of anterior shoulder

26. Which of the following is the best definition for dystocia?
    a. Abnormal or difficult labor or childbirth
    b. Excessively long labor
    c. Breech presentation of the baby during labor
    d. Labor during which requires a C-section required

27. Progress in labor is determined by which of the following?
    a. Dilation and intensity of contraction
    b. Dilation and effacement
    c. Frequency of contraction and descent
    d. All of the above

28. Related to shoulder dystocia which of the following statements are true?
    a. The obstruction is at the pelvic outlet
    b. The incidence is about one in 200 deliveries
    c. It can be prevented in the majority of cases
    d. Maternal diabetes is a risk factor
    e. The most effective treatment is strong, sustained traction on the neck

29. Which of the following are complications of prolonged labor?
    a. Fetal hypoxia
    b. Intrauterine infection
    c. Chorioamnionitis
    d. All of the above

30. Related to progress in labor—problems and their treatment which of the following statements are true?
    i. The partogram aids identification of abnormal progress.
    ii. Cephalopelvic disproportion is the most common cause of slow progress in labor.
    iii. When hyperactive uterine contractions occur, tocolysis can be given.
    iv. In a multiparous woman, if descent is poor in the second stage, an oxytocin infusion should be started and pushing delayed by up to 2 hours.
    a. (i) and (ii) are correct
    b. (ii) and (iii) are correct
    c. (i) and (iii) are correct
    d. All are correct

31. Which of the following can cause shoulder dystocia?
    a. Diabetes
    b. Obesity [body mass index (BMI) >30 kg/m²]
    c. Prolonged first stage or second stage of labor
    d. Postmaturity
    e. All of the above

32. What must always be done in the event of shoulder dystocia?
    a. Lower the bed
    b. Call for help
    c. Apply suprapubic pressure
    d. Apply fundal pressure

33. A 28-year-old gravida 2, para 2 (G2P1) at 8 weeks of gestation presents for her first antenatal visit. The provider reviews her history and notes her prior pregnancy 24 months ago was complicated by well-controlled gestational diabetes mellitus and macrosomia. She underwent induction of labor at 39 weeks of gestation. Her delivery was complicated by a shoulder dystocia that was relieved after 56 seconds by the McRoberts maneuver and suprapubic pressure. She sustained a third-degree laceration during the delivery that was repaired, and she reports no current issues with fecal incontinence. Her infant weighed 4,400 g and did not sustain any injuries during delivery. A 2-hour glucose tolerance test was within normal limits at her postpartum exam. Her current BMI is 23 kg/m², and the pelvic exam is normal. What is the most appropriate recommendation regarding the mode of delivery in her current pregnancy?
    a. A trial of labor should be recommended
    b. Induction of labor scheduled at 37-39 weeks of gestation should be recommended
    c. A scheduled primary cesarean delivery at 39 weeks of gestation should be recommended
    d. Waiting to make a decision until later in the pregnancy should be recommended

ANSWERS

1. **b.** When the first and second stage of labor combined is >18-20 hours
   Labor is defined as prolonged when the total duration of the first and second stage is >18 hours
   Causes:
   - Fetal malposition and presentation
   - Cervical dystocia
   - Cephalic disproportion

2. **a.** Sedation and wait
   - The given clinical scenario is suggestive of either false labor pain or a prolonged latent phase.
   - The appropriate management is to sedate the patient and wait.
   - False labor can be differentiated from the latent phase of labor by therapeutic rest and also enema which will increase true labor pains and reduce false labor pains.
   - Augmentation with oxytocin is done only in those patients who even after therapeutic rest continue to be in prolonged latent phase.

3. **d.** 20 hours
   - The latent phase is said to be prolonged in a primigravida if it lasts for >20 hours
   - Friedman defined the prolonged latent phase as:
   - A nullipara who has not entered the active phase by 20 hours after the onset of the latent phase
   - A multipara who has not entered the active phase by 14 hours after the onset of the latent phase

4. **a.** >14 hours in nullipara
   The given clinical features suggest that the patient is in the latent phase of labor. The latent phase is said to be prolonged if it is:
   - >20 hours in nullipara
   - >14 hours in multipara

   Causes:
   - Excessive sedation/epidural analgesia
   - Poor cervical conditions (thick and uneffaced)
   - False labor (most common cause in multipara)
   - Friedman's curve is used in the diagnosis of prolonged labor. It is the sigmoid curve plotting the pattern of cervical dilatation during the latent and active phase of normal labor.

5. **d.** Poor cervical dilatation causes prolonged active phase
   - Poor cervical dilatation causes prolonged latent phase
   - The active phase of labor starts from ≥6 cm dilatation
   - An active phase arrest can be diagnosed for a patient when she is ≥6 cm dilatation with ruptured membranes with no cervical change despite 4 hours of adequate uterine contraction or 6 hours of inadequate contraction.

6. **b.** 42 weeks of gestation
   - The American College of Obstetricians and Gynecologists (ACOG) defines post-term pregnancy as a pregnancy continuing beyond 42 completed weeks of gestation
   - For clinical purposes, a pregnancy continuing beyond 2 weeks off EDD (>294 days) is called post-term pregnancy
   - Inaccurate LMP is the most common cause of misdiagnosis of post-term pregnancy.

7. **b.** Pathological retraction ring
   - Bandl's ring refers to the pathological retraction ring. It is formed in cases of obstructed labor.
   - The upper segment of the uterus contracts and retracts vigorously in an attempt to overcome the obstruction while the lower segment dilates.
   - With each contraction there is myometrial shortening so that the actively contracting upper segment becomes progressively thicker and shorter. The passive lower segment is progressively stretched and becomes thinner.
   - The junction between the two segments stands out prominently as a Pathological retraction ring.

8. **a.** <1 cm/h
   The protracted descent in labor in a nullipara is <1 cm/h.

9. **b.** Rickets
   The most common cause of true cephalic disproportion in India is rickets.

10. **c.** Oxytocin administration is beneficial
    The given clinical finding is suggestive of uterine tachycardia. Oxytocin administration is not beneficial here as it leads to hyperstimulation of the uterus.

11. **b.** Induce if she does not have a spontaneous expulsion.
    The given clinical picture is suggestive of intrauterine fetal death. The best management for such cases at 36 weeks is waiting for spontaneous expulsion. If expulsion does not take place, induction of labor may be done for the fear of disseminated intravascular coagulation (DIC).

12. **c.** Cesarean section
    The best management in the above case is the cesarean section.

13. **b.** Bandl's ring refers to the pathological ring. It is formed in cases of obstructed labor.

14. **b.** Administer intravenous antibiotics after the cord is clamped
    One of the major risk factors for developing postpartum endometritis is cesarean delivery. Therefore, prophylactic antibiotics are recommended in all cases of nonscheduled cesarean delivery (i.e., a cesarean delivery that is not anticipated). This patient is having a cesarean delivery because she is a nulliparous woman in labor with a fetus in the breech position.

15. **e.** Cesarean delivery
    Fetal scalp sampling (FSS) is a method of fetal assessment that is used during labor and delivery to obtain fetal blood for pH assessment. Normal labor and delivery are characterized by a lowering of the fetal pH as the labor progresses. However, most fetuses tolerate labor and delivery without a dangerous drop in pH (i.e., an acidosis that will result in organ damage).

16. **e.** Respect the patient's decision and perform the vaginal delivery
    Cesarean delivery has been shown to decrease the rate of transmission of the human immunodeficiency virus from an infected mother to her fetus. Some reports have shown that the transmission rate can be decreased to as low as 2% with the combination of antiretroviral medication and elective cesarean delivery prior to labor or rupture of membranes; however, although cesarean delivery benefits the infant by decreasing the risk of transmission, the risks of the surgery accrue to the mother.

17. **d.** Mauriceau-Smellie-Veit maneuver
    Mauriceau-Smellie-Veit maneuver is used in the management of after-coming head in case of breech delivery.

18. **c.** Fetal renal agenesis
    Fetal renal agenesis; the major contribution to amniotic fluid volume is urine hence absence of kidneys leads to oligohydramnios.

19. **d.** Mentoanterior position
    Mentoanterior face presentation can have a vaginal delivery.

20. **b.** Occipitoanterior

21. **c.** Reassuring fetal heart rate trace

22. **b.** Uterine hyperstimulation from cervical ripening agent

23. **c.** Fundal pressure
24. **e.** Is mostly due to placental insufficiency
25. **b.** Abduction of shoulders
    Option A—Woods screw
    Option C—McRoberts maneuver
    Option D—Zavanelli maneuver
26. **a.** Abnormal or difficult labor or childbirth
27. **d.** All of the above
28. **b.** The incidence is about one in 200 deliveries, **d.** Maternal diabetes is a risk factor, and **e.** Maternal diabetes is a risk factor, are true.

    The obstruction is at the pelvic inlet. Although, high birth weight is the most important risk factor, most affected babies weigh <4.5 kg. Maternal diabetes is an additional risk factor. Prevention is problematic because of the difficulties in determining fetal weight using ultrasound, and elective cesarean section for large babies of nondiabetic mothers is seldom advised. Excessive traction is pointless and will cause an Erb's palsy from tearing the brachial plexus. This may resolve or be permanent.

29. **d.** All of the above
    Dangers of prolonged labor are: (1) Fetal—hypoxia and intrauterine infection and (2) Maternal—Chorioamnionitis, increased operative delivery, and postpartum hemorrhage (PPH)

30. **c.** a and c correct
    A partogram is a graphic representation of labor progress and of key observations. Use of an appropriate partogram can influence obstetric management and prevent excessive delay and unnecessary intervention. Inefficient uterine action is the most common cause of slow progress in primiparous labor, therefore (b) is false. Oxytocin in a multiparous should only be used with great caution and after exclusion of malpresentation.

31. **e.** All of the above
    Risk factors for shoulder dystocia are: (1) Previous shoulder dystocia, (2) macrosomia (>4.5 kg), (3) diabetes, (4) obesity (BMI > 30 kg/m^2), (5) induced labor, (6) prolonged first stage or second stage of labor, (7) secondary arrest of labor, (8) postmaturity, (9) multiparity, (10) anencephaly, (11) midpelvic instrumental delivery (more following ventouse than forceps), and (12) fetal ascites.

32. **b.** Call for help
    As soon as shoulder dystocia is detected, the team should call for additional help immediately every time. In addition to calling for more experienced labor and delivery personnel, the neonatology and anesthesia teams should also be notified.

    It is helpful for neonatologists to be present once the infant is delivered to provide resuscitation if needed and evaluate the infant for birth trauma.

    There is no role for fundal pressure in shoulder dystocia because this action further impacts the shoulder against the pubic bone and makes the situation worse. The McRoberts maneuver should always be attempted first, according to professional guidelines. Suprapubic pressure is usually applied concurrently; however, because the McRoberts maneuver may relieve up to 40% of shoulder dystocias when used alone, suprapubic pressure may not always be necessary. Relieve up to 40% of shoulder dystocias when used alone, suprapubic pressure may not always be necessary.

33. **d.** Waiting to make a decision until later in the pregnancy should be recommended.

    In patients with a history of shoulder dystocia, mode-of-delivery decisions in future pregnancies should be individualized based on risk factors present in the prior and current pregnancies and take into account patient preference. This patient had gestational diabetes (GDM) and macrosomia in her last pregnancy, and her third-degree laceration was likely related to the macrosomia and shoulder dystocia; therefore, it would be prudent to wait until further into the pregnancy to see if she develops these risk factors again before deciding the mode of delivery. If, e.g., she does not develop GDM, and an estimated fetal weight near term is only 3,500 g, a trial of labor would likely be appropriate to consider. If; however, she develops GDM and macrosomia again, a cesarean delivery would probably be more prudent.

Chapter 48

Placenta Accreta Spectrum

Poonam Yadav

QUESTIONS

1. The incidence of the placenta accreta spectrum is on the rise in 1982 it was 1 in 2,510 pregnancies and the currently estimated incidence of the placenta accreta spectrum is 1 in_____ pregnancy.
   a. 100–250
   b. 250–400
   c. 400–700
   d. 700–1,000

2. In the setting of the placenta previa with one or more prior cesarean sections, the placenta accreta spectrum is dramatically increased. However, placenta previa alone contributes to placenta accreta spectrum (PAS) in women even without cesarean section in ____ pregnancies.
   a. 1%
   b. 2%
   c. 3%
   d. 5%

3. Various risk factors for PAS are all of the following, *except*:
   a. Grand multipara
   b. Scarred uterus
   c. Prior history of dilatation and curettage (D&C)
   d. Primi with myoma
   e. In vitro fertilization (IVF) pregnancy

4. Conservative management following placenta accreta is followed by recurrence of repeat placenta accreta in _____ of women.
   a. 10%
   b. 20%
   c. 30%
   d. 40%

5. Ultrasound is the cornerstone of the diagnosis of PAS. In the first trimester, one should be alert on which of the following findings?
   a. Abnormal placental appearance
   b. Abnormal uterine shape
   c. Abnormal vascularity of myometrium
   d. Current scar pregnancy
   e. All of the above

6. Magnetic resonance imaging (MRI) findings of PAS are given below, *except* for:
   a. Uterine bulging
   b. Heterogenous signal intensity within the placenta
   c. Echogenic intraplacental bands on T2 weighted imaging
   d. Invasion of the placenta in an adjacent structure

7. Magnetic resonance imaging is used in which of the following selected situations in PAS?
   a. Anterior placenta
   b. Posterior placenta
   c. Lateral placenta
   d. Low-lying placenta

8. Use of color flow Doppler facilitates the diagnosis of PAS. Which of the following signs are most strongly associated with PAS on color Doppler?
   a. Increased subplacental vascularity
   b. Gaps in myometrial blood flow
   c. Vessels bridging the placenta through the uterine margin
   d. Multiple lacunae and turbulent blood flow

9. For optimizing the fetomaternal outcome, the delivery is to be planned at what gestation in PAS?
   a. 34–35 weeks
   b. 35–36 weeks
   c. 36–37 weeks
   d. 37–38 weeks

10. Current clinical indication of the use of methotrexate in PAS are which of the following?
    a. Evidence are in favor of methotrexate in PAS
    b. Can be used in selected cases of PAS
    c. Not found effective and hence serious side effects
    d. None of the above

11. In case of focal placenta accreta triple P procedure includes the following, *except*:
    a. Placental location
    b. Perioperative ballooning of internal iliac arteries
    c. Perioperative clamping of aorta
    d. Peroperative excision of uterine muscles with adherent placenta and subsequent repair

12. A 35-year-old G3P2L2A0 at 39 weeks of gestation undergoes a cesarean section after delivery. Placenta tears during removal. A small fraction of the placenta cannot be removed from the uterus and the patient begins to bleed heavily. Her medical history is significant for two previous cesarean sections. Which of the following would most likely be found on histological examination of the uterus and placenta of the patient?
    a. Infarction, decidual necrosis, intervillous thrombus, and hemosiderosis
    b. Macrophages, neutrophils in both amnion and chorion
    c. Absence of decidual plate trophoblastic invasion into myometrium and trophoblastic inclusion
    d. Infiltrative pattern of intermediate trophoblast

13. Ultrasound (USG) features of the placenta accreta spectrum are all, *except* for:
    a. Loss of the normal hypoechoic retroplacental zone between the placenta and uterus
    b. Plancental vascular lacunae or lakes
    c. Distance between uterus serosa-bladder wall interface and the retroplacental vessels measures <10 mm
    d. Placenta bulging into the posterior bladder wall

14. The placenta that has placental villi extending into the myometrium but not reaching the serosa is called?
    a. Placenta accreta   b. Placenta increta
    c. Placenta membranacea   d. Placenta percreta

15. At what gestation period, placenta accreta spectrum can be screened on MRI?
    a. 12–18 weeks gestation   b. 20–22 weeks gestation
    c. 28–32 weeks gestation   d. 36–40 weeks gestation

16. All of the following are the features of the placenta accreta spectrum, *except* for?
    a. Abnormal vascularization of placental bed
    b. Loss of retroplacental hypointense line on T2
    c. Placenta/uterus bulge with intraplacental bands
    d. Three layers of myometrium adjacent to the myometrium

17. A 22-year-old women is noted to have marginal placenta on USG at 24 weeks. How do we manage the patient?
    a. Schedule cesarean section at 38 weeks
    b. Reassess placental position by USG at 33–34 weeks
    c. Reassess placental position digitally at 32–34 weeks
    d. Recovered termination of pregnancy

18. Which of the following women is most likely to have placenta previa?
    a. 19-year-old, G1P0, vertex presentation
    b. 24-year-old G2P1, cephalic presentation two-fifths prolapse
    c. 34-year-old G5P3A1 vertex presentation
    d. 36-year-old G3P2 previous two lower segment cesarean section (LSCS) transverse lie
    e. 28-year-old, G3P1 + 1 (abortion), head at 0 station

19. All of the following are risk factors of the placenta accreta, *except* for:
    a. Previous LSCS scar
    b. Previous curettage
    c. Previous myomectomy
    d. Previous placenta previa

20. A 24-year G2 with a previous cesarean section at 30 weeks with complaints of painless vaginal bleeding. The USG shows a low-lying placenta. The resident thinks it is a placenta accreta and orders which investigation?
    a. Color Doppler
    b. Computed tomography (CT) scan
    c. Computed tomography angiography
    d. Magnetic resonance imaging

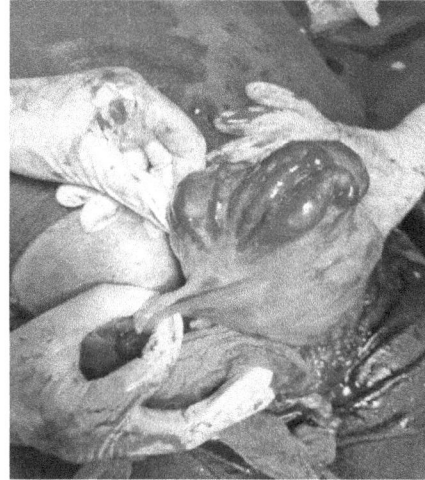

21. What will be the most likely clinical diagnosis of the intraoperative image of gravid uterus given below?
    a. Placenta accreta
    b. Arteriovenous malformation
    c. Placenta previa
    d. Abruptio placenta

ANSWERS

1. **b.** 250–400
2. **c.** 3%
3. **d.** Primi with myoma
4. **b.** 20%
5. **e.** All of the above
6. **c.** Echogenic intraplacental bands on T2 weighted imaging
7. **b.** Lateral placenta
8. **d.** Multiple lacunae and turbulent blood flow
9. **b.** 35–36 weeks
10. **c.** Not found effective and hence serious side effects.
11. **c.** Perioperative clamping of aorta.
12. **c.** Absence of decidual plate trophoblastic invasion into myometrium and trophoblastic inclusion.
13. **c.** Distance between uterus serosa-bladder wall interface and the retroplacental vessels measures <10 mm
14. **b.** Placenta increta
15. **c.** 28–32 weeks gestation
16. **d.** Three layers of myometrium adjacent to the myometrium
17. **b.** Reassess placental position by USG at 33–34 weeks
18. **d.** 36-year-old G3P2 previous two lower segment cesarean section (LSCS) transverse lie
19. **d.** Previous placenta previa
20. **a.** Color Doppler
21. **a.** Placenta accreta

Chapter 49: Gestational Diabetes Mellitus

Kiranmai Devineni, Kalpana Basany

QUESTIONS

1. **The proportion of gestational diabetes mellitus (GDM) affected women who have no risk factors?**
   a. 30–50%
   b. 5–10%
   c. 10–15%
   d. 60–70%

2. **The risk factor to evaluate the risk of GDM is which one of the following?**
   a. Body mass index (BMI) >30 kg/m^2
   b. Previous macrosomic baby ≥4.5 kg
   c. Previous GDM
   d. All of the above

3. **To determine the risk of GDM, which of the following tests listed below is utilized?**
   a. Fasting plasma glucose
   b. Glycated hemoglobin (HbA1c)
   c. Random blood glucose
   d. 75 g oral glucose tolerance test (GTT)

4. **What is the chance of type 2 diabetes in females with GDM after 5–10 years? Choose the correct option.**
   a. 20–30%
   b. 50–70%
   c. 5–10%
   d. <5%

5. **With one exception, all of the findings from the Metformin in Gestational Diabetes trial is?**
   a. No difference in perinatal outcomes in women treated with metformin or insulin
   b. Women preferred metformin to insulin treatment.
   c. Metformin-exposed offspring were smaller than insulin-exposed offspring
   d. Metformin with or without insulin is a safe treatment option for GDM

6. **Trials related to GDM are all the following, *except* for:**
   a. ACHOIS trial
   b. CHIPS trial
   c. HAPO study
   d. IGDPC project

7. **"Using insulin pumps during pregnancy" which of the following statement is correct?**
   a. Small but significant improvement in HbA1c levels
   b. Reduce the rate of hypoglycemic episodes
   c. Useful in women who suffer from recurrent hypoglycemia or the dawn phenomenon
   d. All are true

8. **Which of the following is not a drawback of using insulin pumps during pregnancy?**
   a. Greater education and clinical support needed
   b. Higher cost of pump and supplies
   c. Potential for diabetic ketoacidosis if pump malfunctions
   d. Avoidance of multiple daily injections

9. **Which statement is false about breastfeeding and GDM?**
   a. Oral antidiabetic drug (OAD) medications cause hypoglycemia in babies
   b. Breastfeeding helps in postpartum weight loss in the mother
   c. Helps in the reduction of childhood obesity
   d. Helps in the reduction of type 2 diabetes mellitus (T2DM)

10. **Which of the following is not true according to National Institute for Health and Clinical Excellence (NICE) recommendations on postnatal care for women with GDM?**
    a. Offer a fasting plasma glucose test 6–13 weeks after the birth
    b. Offer routinely a 75 g 2-hour oral glucose tolerance test (OGTT)

c. After 13 weeks, an HbA1c test is offered if a fasting plasma glucose test is not possible
d. Offer lifestyle advice

11. **Which statement is true among the following?**
    a. Breastfeeding should start as soon as possible after birth and then at frequent intervals
    b. Routinely start the babies on tube feeding
    c. Pre-feed capillary plasma glucose levels maintained at a minimum of 3.0 mmol/L
    d. Routinely start the babies on intravenous (IV) dextrose

12. **Which of the following is true based on the Diabetes Prevention Program Outcomes Study (DPPOS)?**
    a. Over 10 years, women with GDM assigned to placebo had a 48% higher risk of developing overt diabetes compared with women without a history of GDM
    b. In women with GDM, an "intensive lifestyle" reduced progression to diabetes compared with placebo by 35%
    c. In women with GDM, metformin reduced progression to diabetes compared with placebo by 40%
    d. All of the above

13. **Which of the following insulins are recommended and work well during pregnancy?**
    a. Regular insulin
    b. Neutral protamine Hagedorn (NPH)
    c. Lispro
    d. Detemir
    e. All of the above

14. **Which of the following is not a reason to use insulin as the first choice for women with GDM?**
    a. Fasting plasma glucose levels >110 mg/dL
    b. Pregnancy weight gain <7 kg
    c. 1-hour postprandial glucose >140 mg/dL
    d. Diagnosis of diabetes <20 weeks of gestation

15. **How much insulin is needed during pregnancy? Choose the correct option.**
    a. 0.7 units/kg/day in the first trimester
    b. 0.8 units/kg/day from week 18
    c. 0.9 units/kg/day from week 26
    d. 1.0 units/kg/day from week 36 until delivery
    e. All of the above

16. **What is low blood sugar in a newborn?**
    a. Blood glucose <25 mg/dL
    b. Blood glucose <35 mg/dL
    c. Blood glucose <45 mg/dL
    d. Blood glucose <50 mg/dL

17. **Which of the following is not a special measure for women with diabetes during childbirth?**
    a. Pregnant women (PW) with GDM on insulin require plasma glucose monitoring during labor by a glucometer
    b. The morning dose of Insulin is withheld on the day of induction/labor
    c. PW should be started on 1/2 hourly monitoring of plasma glucose
    d. IV infusion with normal saline (NS) to be started and regular insulin to be added according to blood glucose levels

18. **How much weight should obese women gain during pregnancy? Choose the correct option.**
    a. 5-9 kg
    b. 11.5-16 kg
    c. 12.5-18 kg
    d. 7-11.5 kg

19. **What are the glycemic targets for women with gestational diabetes? Choose the correct option.**
    a. Fasting glucose < 5.3 mmol/L (95 mg/dL)
    b. 1-hour postprandial glucose < 7.8 mmol/L (140 mg/dL)
    c. 2 hours postprandial glucose < 6.7 mmol/L (120 mg/dL)
    d. During labor and delivery 4-7 mmol/L (72-126 mg/dL)
    e. All of the above

20. **Choose the correct statement from the following:**
    a. Elective cesarean delivery is offered when the fetal weight is >4 kg
    b. Labor should be induced if the baby is large-for-gestational age (LGA) at 36-37 weeks
    c. In women with GDM and previous stillbirth, labor should be induced at 37 weeks if the fetal weight is >3,800 g
    d. In women with GDM and poor compliance, labor should be induced at 37 weeks if the fetal weight is >3,800 g

21. **How often fetal growth assessment be done? Choose the correct option.**
    a. 2-4 weeks from diagnosis until term
    b. 6 weeks from diagnosis until term
    c. Weekly once from diagnosis until term
    d. Biweekly once from diagnosis until term

22. **Choose the wrong statement from the following about the insulin vials.**
    a. Use an insulin vial within a month after opening it
    b. Keep insulin vials away from heat or sunlight, and below 25–30°C
    c. You do not need to refrigerate or keep insulin vials in a cool and dark place if you are using them
    d. You can freeze insulin vials

23. **Which of the following is false about metformin?**
    a. You can take up to 2,500 mg/day
    b. Taking it with food can reduce side effects
    c. It lowers blood sugar before and after meals
    d. It does not pass through the placenta

24. **What are the signs of diabetic ketoacidosis (DKA) in pregnancy?**
    a. High levels of ketones in blood or urine
    b. High blood sugar or diagnosed diabetes
    c. Low levels of bicarbonate and/or pH in blood
    d. All of the above

25. **A woman diagnosed with GDM is in preterm labor. Which of the following tocolytic is avoided?**
    a. Atosiban   b. Nifedipine
    c. Ritodrine   d. Magnesium sulfate

26. **What can precipitate DKA in pregnancy?**
    a. Hyperemesis gravidarum
    b. Steroid treatment
    c. Infections
    d. Beta sympathomimetic drugs
    e. All of the above

27. **A pregnant woman undergoes Diabetes in Pregnancy Study Group of India (DIPSI) at the first antenatal visit and is diagnosed with GDM. She is on medical nutrition therapy (MNT). After 2 weeks, her second-hour plasma glucose value is 156 mg/dL. What is the best management?**
    a. Continue MNT
    b. Start insulin
    c. Start metformin
    d. Repeat testing

28. **Criteria to consider referral to a nephrologist in pregnant woman with diabetes include the following, *except*:**
    a. Serum creatinine is 90 µmol/L or more
    b. Serum creatinine is 120 µmol/L or more
    c. The urinary albumin:creatinine ratio is >30 mg/mmol
    d. Total protein excretion exceeds 0.5 g/day

29. **Fetal origins of disease (programming and imprinting) include which of the following?**
    a. Diabetes   b. Obesity
    c. Hypertension   d. Metabolic syndrome
    e. All of the above

30. **Which of the following contraceptive methods are safe to use [UK Medical Eligibility Criteria for Contraceptive Use (UKMEC-1)] in women with GDM?**
    a. Progestogen-only pill (POP)
    b. Copper-bearing intrauterine device (Cu-IUD)
    c. Progestogen-only implant (IMP)
    d. Levonorgestrel-releasing intrauterine system (LNG-IUS)
    e. All of the above

ANSWERS

1. **a.** 30–50%
   Women with the following characteristics are at higher risk of developing gestational diabetes mellitus in pregnancy: Body mass index >30 kg/m^2, previous GDM, previous macrosomic baby, family history of diabetes, ethnicity with a high risk of diabetes, advanced maternal age (particularly 40 years), multiple pregnancies, polycystic ovary syndrome (PCOS), and subfertility or conception via assisted reproductive technologies. Additionally, women taking some classes of antipsychotic or steroid medications, and those with cystic fibrosis are at increased risk of developing GDM. Factors including low or high maternal birthweight, and increased early pregnancy weight gain have also been proposed as risk factors for developing GDM, but these have been less well studied. It is important to note that 30–50% of the cases of GDM occur in women without known risk factors.
   [Reference: Stewart-Field ZA. Gestational diabetes: screening, diagnosis, treatment and management. Obstet Gynaecol Reprod Med. 2023;33(7):185-9]

2. **d.** All of the above
   Assess the risk of gestational diabetes using risk factors in a healthy population. At the booking appointment, check for the following risk factors:
   - BMI above 30 kg/m^2, previous macrosomic baby weighing 4.5 kg or more
   - Previous gestational diabetes

- Family history of diabetes (first-degree relative with diabetes)
- An ethnicity with a high prevalence of diabetes. Offer women with any of these risk factors testing for gestational diabetes

[Reference: National Institute for Health and Care Excellence. Diabetes in pregnancy: management from preconception to the postnatal period. London: National Institute for Health and Care Excellence (NICE); 2020]

3. **d.** 75 g oral glucose tolerance test

Do not use fasting plasma glucose, random blood glucose, glycated hemoglobin (HbA1c), glucose challenge test, or urinalysis for glucose to assess the risk of developing gestational diabetes.

[Reference: National Institute for Health and Care Excellence. Diabetes in pregnancy: management from preconception to the postnatal period. London: National Institute for Health and Care Excellence (NICE); 2020]

4. **b.** 50–70%

Women who develop GDM in pregnancy face a far higher risk of developing type 2 diabetes, with a 50–70% chance in the following 5-10 years.

[Reference: Stewart-Field ZA. Gestational diabetes: screening, diagnosis, treatment and management. Obstet Gynaecol Reprod Med. 2023;33(7):185-9]

5. **c.** Metformin-exposed offspring were smaller than insulin-exposed offspring.

In women with gestational diabetes mellitus, metformin (alone or with supplemental insulin) is not associated with increased perinatal complications as compared with insulin. The women preferred metformin to insulin treatment.

[Reference: Rowan JA, Hague WM, Gao W, Battin MR, Moore MP; MiG Trial Investigators. Metformin versus Insulin for the Treatment of Gestational Diabetes. N Engl J Med. 2008;358(19):2003-15]

The landmark Metformin in Gestational Diabetes (MiG) trial was a randomized controlled trial of insulin versus metformin therapy (with or without supplemental insulin therapy) in women with gestational diabetes, conducted in Australia and New Zealand. It found that there was no difference in perinatal outcomes between women treated with insulin and those treated with metformin. In the 7-9 years follow-up of the offspring from this trial, children had similar total and abdominal fat percentage and metabolic markers regardless of whether their mothers had received metformin or insulin treatment.

[Reference: Stewart-Field ZA. Gestational diabetes: screening, diagnosis, treatment and management. Obstet Gynaecol Reprod Med. 2023;33(7):185-9]

6. **b.** CHIPS trial

Australian Carbohydrate Intolerance Study in Pregnant Women (ACHOIS) trial to assess whether the treatment of gestational diabetes would reduce perinatal complications and to assess the effects of treatment on maternal outcome, mood, and quality of life.

Control of Hypertension in Pregnancy Study (CHIPS) trial—interventions of "less tight" [target diastolic blood pressure (DBP) 100 mm Hg] versus "tight" control (target DBP 85 mm Hg).

[References: Crowther CA, Hiller JE, Moss JR, McPhee AJ, Jeffries WS, Robinson JS; et al. Effect of treatment of gestational diabetes mellitus on pregnancy outcomes. N Engl J Med. 2005;352(24):2477-86.

Stewart-Field ZA. Gestational diabetes: screening, diagnosis, treatment, and management. Obstet Gynaecol Reprod Med. 2023;33(7):185-9]

7. **d.** All are true

Outside of pregnancy, particularly in observational studies, pump therapy has been shown to allow a small but significant improvement in HbA1c levels, reduce the rate of hypoglycemic episodes, and improve quality of life. In addition, expert opinion indicates that pumps ameliorate care, particularly in individuals who have inadequately controlled diabetes, those who suffer from recurrent hypoglycemia or the "dawn phenomenon" (requiring an increased dose of insulin for a short time in the early morning), and those who need only a very small daily insulin requirement, which is difficult to administer using injections.

[Reference: White SL, Brackenridge A, Rajasingam D. Insulin pumps and pregnancy. Obstet Gynaecol. 2016;18(3):199-203]

8. **d.** Avoidance of multiple daily injections

Advantages of insulin pump therapy: Potential for improved glucose control preconception and during pregnancy, greater flexibility for exercise and meals, avoidance of multiple daily injections, catheter change only every 2–3 days, multiple programmable basal rates aid night time hypoglycemia and dawn phenomenon, and periods of nausea or vomiting.

Disadvantages: Greater education and clinical support needed, higher cost of pump and supplies, potential for diabetic ketoacidosis if pump malfunctions or is unwittingly removed, greater potential for difficulties if poor compliance, and higher risk for site infection.

[Reference: White SL, Brackenridge A, Rajasingam D. Insulin pumps and pregnancy. Obstet Gynaecol. 2016;18(3):199-203]

9. **a.** Oral antidiabetic drug medications cause hypoglycemia in babies

    Breastfeeding has been shown to be protective against the occurrence of infant and maternal complications including a reduction in childhood obesity, type 2 diabetes mellitus (T2DM), and even type 1 diabetes (T1D). Moreover, breastfeeding helps postpartum weight loss. Treatment with insulin or commonly used OADs, such as glyburide and metformin, is not a contraindication to breastfeeding as levels of OAD medications in breast milk are negligible and do not cause hypoglycemia in the baby

    [Reference: Hod M, Kapur A, Sacks DA, Hadar E, Agarwal M, Di Renzo GC, et al. The International Federation of Gynecology and Obstetrics (FIGO) Initiative on gestational diabetes mellitus: A pragmatic guide for diagnosis, management, and care. 2015;131(Suppl 3):S173-211]

10. **b.** Offer routinely a 75 g 2-hour oral glucose tolerance test

    For women who were diagnosed with gestational diabetes and whose blood glucose levels returned to normal after the birth:
    - Offer lifestyle advice (including weight control, diet, and exercise), offer a fasting plasma glucose test 6–13 weeks after the birth to exclude diabetes, after 13 weeks offer a fasting plasma glucose test if this has not been done earlier, or an HbA1c test if a fasting plasma glucose test is not possible
    - Do not routinely offer a 75 g 2-hour OGTT

    [Reference: National Institute for Health and Care Excellence. Diabetes in pregnancy: management from preconception to the postnatal period. London: National Institute for Health and Care Excellence (NICE); 2020]

11. **a.** Breastfeeding should start as soon as possible after birth and then at frequent intervals

    Women with diabetes should feed their babies: As soon as possible after birth (within 30 minutes) and then at frequent intervals (every 2–3 hours) until feeding maintains their prefeed capillary plasma glucose levels at a minimum of 2.0 mmol/L. Only use additional measures (such as tube feeding and intravenous dextrose) if—capillary plasma glucose values are below 2.0 mmol/L on two consecutive readings despite maximal support for feeding or there are abnormal clinical signs or the baby will not effectively feed orally. For babies with clinical signs of hypoglycemia, test blood glucose levels and provide intravenous dextrose as soon as possible.

    [Reference: National Institute for Health and Care Excellence. Diabetes in pregnancy: management from preconception to the postnatal period. London: National Institute for Health and Care Excellence (NICE); 2020]

12. **d.** All of the above

    Data from the Diabetes Prevention Program Outcomes Study have been published and show that the benefits of lifestyle intervention and metformin seen in the DPP study continue over a longer period. DPPOS is a long-term follow-up of the DPP participants to investigate whether the delay in the development of diabetes observed during DPP is sustained and to assess the long-term effects of the interventions on health. DPPOS followed participants from the DPP study for an additional 7 years, during which time the lifestyle and metformin groups were encouraged to continue those interventions, and all participants were offered group lifestyle classes. Over 10 years, women with a history of GDM assigned to a placebo had a 48% higher risk of developing overt diabetes compared with women without a history of GDM. In women with a history of GDM, "intensive lifestyle" and metformin reduced progression to diabetes compared with placebo by 35% and 40%, respectively. Among women without a history of GDM, an "intensive lifestyle" reduced the progression to diabetes by 30%, while metformin did not reduce the progression to diabetes.

    [Reference: Aroda VR, Christophi CA, Edelstein SL, Zhang P, Herman WH, Barrett-Connor E, et al. The effect of lifestyle intervention and metformin on preventing *or delaying diabetes among women with and without gestational diabetes: the diabetes prevention program outcomes study 10-year follow-up. J Clin Endocrinol Metab. 2015;100(4):1646-53]*

13. **e.** All of the above

    The following insulins may be considered safe and effective treatment during pregnancy—regular insulin, neutral protamine Hagedorn (NPH), lispro, aspart, and detemir.

    [Reference: Hod M, Kapur A, Sacks DA, Hadar E, Agarwal M, Di Renzo GC, et al. The International Federation of Gynecology and Obstetrics (FIGO) Initiative on gestational diabetes mellitus: A pragmatic guide for diagnosis, management, and care. 2015;131(Suppl 3):S173-211]

14. **b.** Pregnancy weight gain <7 kg

    Insulin should be considered as the first-line treatment in women with GDM who are at high risk of failing on OAD therapy, including some of the following factors:
    - Diagnosis of diabetes 30 weeks
    - Fasting plasma glucose levels >110 mg/dL
    - 1-hour postprandial glucose >140 mg/dL
    - Pregnancy weight gain >12 kg

    [Reference: Hod M, Kapur A, Sacks DA, Hadar E, Agarwal M, Di Renzo GC, et al. The International Federation of Gynecology and Obstetrics (FIGO) Initiative on gestational diabetes mellitus: A pragmatic guide for diagnosis, management, and care. 2015;131(Suppl 3):S173-211]

15. **e.** All of the above

    In women with diabetes, insulin requirements gradually increase throughout pregnancy: 0.7 units/kg/day in the first trimester, 0.8 units/kg/day from week 18, 0.9 units/kg/day from week 26, and 1.0 units/kg/day from week 36 until delivery. In some instances, lower doses may suffice.

    [Reference: Hod M, Kapur A, Sacks DA, Hadar E, Agarwal M, Di Renzo GC, et al. The International Federation of Gynecology and Obstetrics (FIGO) Initiative on gestational diabetes mellitus: A pragmatic guide for diagnosis, management, and care. 2015;131(Suppl 3):S173-211]

16. **c.** Blood glucose <45 mg/dL

    The operational definition cut off of plasma glucose by glucometer is 45 mg/dL. Any newborn with blood glucose <45 mg/dL should be considered as a "baby with hypoglycemia."

    [Reference: Maternal Health Division, Ministry of Health and Family Welfare, Government of India. (2014). National Guidelines for Diagnosis & Management of Gestational Diabetes Mellitus. [online] Available from: https://nhm.gov.in/images/pdf/programmes/maternal-health/guidelines/National_Guidelines_for_Diagnosis_&_Management_of_Gestational_Diabetes_Mellitus.pdf (Last accessed December, 2023)]

17. **c.** PW should be started on 1/2 hourly monitoring of plasma glucose

    Pregnant women with GDM on Insulin require plasma glucose monitoring during labor by a glucometer. The morning dose of Insulin is withheld on the day of induction/labor and the PW should be started on 2-hourly monitoring of plasma glucose. Intravenous infusion with normal saline (NS) is to be started and regular insulin is to be added according to blood glucose levels. Blood glucose level amount of insulin added in 500 mL NS rate of NS infusion 90–120 mg/dL, 0 100 mL/h (16 drops/min) 120–140 mg/dL, 4 U 100 mL/h (16 drops/min) 140–180 mg/dL, 6 U 100 mL/h (16 drops/min) > 180 mg/dL, 8 U 100 mL/h (16 drops/min).

    [Reference: Maternal Health Division, Ministry of Health and Family Welfare, Government of India. (2014). National Guidelines for Diagnosis & Management of Gestational Diabetes Mellitus. (online) Available from: https://nhm.gov.in/images/pdf/programmes/maternal-health/guidelines/National_Guidelines_for_Diagnosis_&_Management_of_Gestational_Diabetes_Mellitus.pdf (Last accessed December, 2023)]

18. **a.** 5–9 kg

    Weight gain targets for pregnancy are based on women's pre pregnancy BMI.

    Normal weight (18.5–24.9): 11.5–16 kg, underweight (<18.5): 12.5–18 kg, overweight (25–29.9): 7–11.5 kg), obese (include all classes namely grade I, II, and III), and ≥30: 5–9 kg.

    *[Reference: Maternal Health Division, Ministry of Health and Family Welfare, Government of India. (2014). National Guidelines for Diagnosis & Management of Gestational Diabetes Mellitus. (online) Available from: https://nhm.gov.in/images/pdf/programmes/maternal-health/guidelines/National_Guidelines_for_Diagnosis_&_Management_of_*

Gestational_Diabetes_Mellitus.pdf (Last accessed December, 2023)]

19. **e.** All of the above
Targets for glucose control during pregnancy: Fasting glucose <5.3 mmol/L (95 mg/dL) 1 hour, postprandial glucose <7.8 mmol/L (140 mg/dL), 2-hour postprandial glucose <6.7 mmol/L, (120 mg/dL), during labor and delivery 4–7 mmol/L (72–126 mg/dL).
[Reference: Hod M, Kapur A, Sacks DA, Hadar E, Agarwal M, Di Renzo GC, et al. The International Federation of Gynecology and Obstetrics (FIGO) Initiative on gestational diabetes mellitus: A pragmatic guide for diagnosis, management, and care.2015;131(Suppl 3): S173-211]

20. **a.** Elective cesarean delivery is offered when the fetal weight is >4 kg

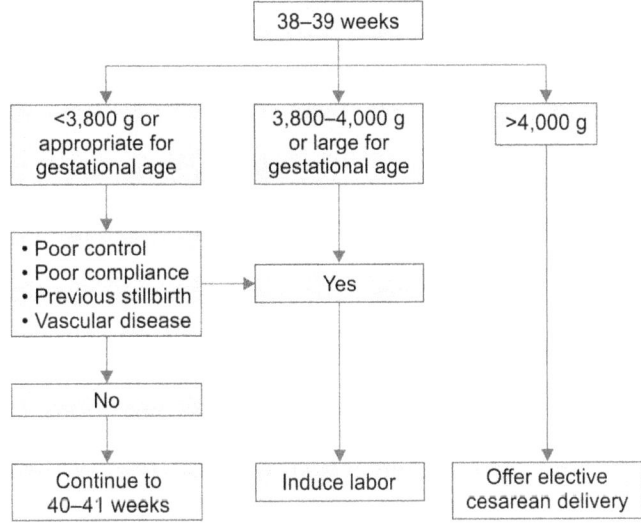

[Reference: Hod M, Kapur A, Sacks DA, Hadar E, Agarwal M, Di Renzo GC, et al. The International Federation of Gynecology and Obstetrics (FIGO) Initiative on gestational diabetes mellitus: A pragmatic guide for diagnosis, management, and care. 2015;131(Suppl 3): S173-211]

21. **a.** 2–4 weeks from diagnosis until term
Clinical and sonographic growth assessments every 2–4 weeks from diagnosis until term.
[Reference: Hod M, Kapur A, Sacks DA, Hadar E, Agarwal M, Di Renzo GC, et al. The International Federation of Gynecology and Obstetrics (FIGO) Initiative on gestational diabetes mellitus: A pragmatic guide for diagnosis, management, and care. 2015;131(Suppl 3):S173-211]

22. **d.** You can freeze insulin vials
[Reference: Maternal Health Division, Ministry of Health and Family Welfare, Government of India. (2014). National Guidelines for Diagnosis & Management of Gestational Diabetes Mellitus. (online) Available from https://nhm.gov.in/images/pdf/programmes/maternal-health/guidelines/National_Guidelines_for_Diagnosis_&_Management_of_Gestational_Diabetes_Mellitus.pdf (Last accessed December, 2023)]

23. **d.** It does not pass through the placenta
Metformin is an inexpensive, oral medication with a maximum dose of 2,500 mg daily and does not contribute to hypoglycemia. It should be titrated every 5–7 days in increments of 500 or 850 mg to a therapeutic dose of 2,000–2,500 mg. Although not required to be taken with food, metformin's side effects may be better tolerated when taken with food. Titration can occur more gradually if gastrointestinal (GI) side effects continue but switching agents should also be considered if GI intolerance persists. Metformin is the only oral medication used in pregnancy that can treat both fasting and postprandial hyperglycemia.
[Reference: Rickert M, Caughey AB, Valent AM. Medications for Managing Preexisting and Gestational Diabetes in Pregnancy. Obstet Gynecol Clin North Am. 2023;50(1):121-36]

24. **d.** All of the above
The Joint British Diabetes Societies Inpatient Care Group guidelines state the following diagnostic criteria for diabetic ketoacidosis in pregnancy (DKP): Blood ketone level ≥3.0 mmol/L (or) urine ketone level >2+, blood glucose level > 11.0 mmol/L or known diabetes mellitus, bicarbonate level <15.0 mmol/L and/or venous pH <7.3.
[Reference: Mohan M, Baagar KAM, Lindow S. Management of diabetic ketoacidosis in pregnancy. Obstet Gynaecol. 2017;19(1):55-62]

25. **c.** Ritodrine
If tocolysis is required, it is preferable to avoid betamimetics (they increase susceptibility for DKP) and use a different class of tocolytics. Tocolytics that are safer to use are the oxytocin receptor antagonist atosiban or a calcium channel blocker, e.g., nifedipine
[Reference: Mohan M, Baagar KAM, Lindow S. Management of diabetic ketoacidosis in pregnancy. Obstet Gynaecol. 2017;19(1):55-62]

26. e. All of the above

Diabetic ketoacidosis in pregnancy is more commonly observed along with T1D, but can also be observed with type II diabetes and gestational diabetes. It is likely to be precipitated by specific factors; such as protracted vomiting, hyperemesis gravidarum, starvation, infections, insulin noncompliance, medications precipitating DKP (e.g., β-sympathomimetic agents), steroid prophylaxis/steroid treatment, insulin pump failure (as pumps deliver rapid-acting insulin, interruption for a few hours completely deprives the patient of insulin), and conditions; such as diabetic gastroparesis.

[Reference: Mohan M, Baagar KAM, Lindow S. Management of diabetic ketoacidosis in pregnancy. Obstet Gynaecol. 2017;19(1):55-62]

27. b. Start insulin

If 2 hours postprandial plasma glucose (PPPG) ≥120 mg/dL medical management (insulin therapy) to be started as per guidelines.

[Reference: Maternal Health Division, Ministry of Health and Family Welfare, Government of India. (2014). National Guidelines for Diagnosis & Management of Gestational Diabetes Mellitus. (online) Available from: https://nhm.gov.in/images/pdf/programmes/maternal-health/guidelines/National_Guidelines_for_Diagnosis_&_Management_of_Gestational_Diabetes_Mellitus.pdf (Last accessed December, 2023)]

28. a. Serum creatinine is 90 μmol/L or more

Consider referring pregnant woman with diabetes to a nephrologist if: • their serum creatinine is 120 μmol/L or more or the urinary albumin:creatinine ratio is >30 mg/mmol or total protein excretion exceeds 0.5 g/day.

[Reference: National Institute for Health and Care Excellence. Diabetes in pregnancy: management from preconception to the postnatal period. London: National Institute for Health and Care Excellence (NICE); 2020]

29. e. All of the above

Early in the first trimester, intrauterine growth restriction and organ malformation, described by Freinkel as "fuel-mediated teratogenesis" may occur. During the second trimester, at the time of brain development and differentiation, behavioral, intellectual, or psychological damage may occur. During the third trimester, abnormal proliferation of fetal adipocytes and muscle cells, together with hyperplasia of pancreatic beta cells and neuroendocrine cells may be responsible for the development of obesity, hypertension, and T2DM mellitus later in life.

[Reference: Hod M, Kapur A, Sacks DA, Hadar E, Agarwal M, Di Renzo GC, et al. The International Federation of Gynecology and Obstetrics (FIGO) Initiative on gestational diabetes mellitus: A pragmatic guide for diagnosis, management, and care. 2015;131(Suppl 3): S173-211]

30. e. All of the above
- UK Medical Eligibility Criteria for Contraceptive Use (UKMEC) categorization for women with diabetes.
- Copper-bearing intrauterine device (Cu-IUD), levonorgestrel-releasing intrauterine system (LNG-IUS), implant, progestin-only pill (POP), and combined hormonal contraception (CHC) (UKMEC-1)

[Reference: Aiken C, Bolton H, Guerrero K, Mathur R (Eds). Obstet Gynaecol Reprod Med. 2022;32(1):20-7]

Chapter 50

Genital Tract Injuries

Rajeshwari Laxman Khyade

QUESTIONS

1. **Anterior perineum includes:**
   a. Clitoris
   b. Urethra
   c. Labia
   d. Anterior vaginal wall
   e. All of the above
   f. None of the above

2. **Posterior perineum includes:**
   a. Posterior vaginal wall
   b. Perineal and levator ani muscles
   c. The anal sphincter complex
   d. All of the above
   e. None of the above

3. **First-degree perineal tear includes:**
   a. Vagina and perineal skin only
   b. <50% external anal sphincter
   c. Cervical tear
   d. None of the above
   e. All of the above

4. **When both the external and internal anal sphincters are involved, _____ degree of perineal tear.**
   a. 3a
   b. 3b
   c. 3c
   d. Fourth degree
   e. Second degree

5. **Fourth-degree perineal tear includes:**
   a. Injury to external anal sphincter
   b. Injury to internal anal sphincter
   c. Injury to anorectal epithelium
   d. All of the above
   e. b and c only

6. **Which anesthesia is better for perineal tear repair?**
   a. Regional anesthesia
   b. General anesthesia
   c. Local anesthesia
   d. All of the above
   e. None of the above

7. **The torn anorectal epithelium is closed with:**
   a. 3-0 Dexon
   b. 3-0 Vicryl
   c. 3-0 Ethilon
   d. 3-0 Silk
   e. a and b

8. **Internal anal sphincter is sutured with:**
   a. 3-0 Vicryl
   b. 3-0 Dexon
   c. 3-0 PDS polydioxanone
   d. 3-0 Ethilon
   e. None of the above

9. **Two techniques for repair of the torn external sphincter muscle are:**
   a. End-to-end technique
   b. Overlapping technique
   c. Continuous interlocking
   d. a + b
   e. b + c

10. **Periurethral and periclitoral lacerations are common in:**
    a. Multipara
    b. Grand multipara
    c. Nullipara
    d. All of the above
    e. None of the above

11. **Vaginal lacerations commonly involve:**
    a. The lower two-thirds of posterior vaginal sulci
    b. In the anterior sulcus of vagina
    c. a + b
    d. None of the above

12. **Lacerations of the upper third of vagina are associated with:**
    a. Vacuum delivery
    b. Forceps rotation delivery
    c. Outlet forceps delivery
    d. None of the above

13. **Cervical lacerations are:**
    a. Rare
    b. Mostly do not bleed
    c. Requires no treatment
    d. All of the above
    e. None of the above

14. **Cervical laceration requires suturing if:**
    a. Tear is <2 cm, no bleeding
    b. Tear is >2 cm, no bleeding
    c. Tear is >2 cm and bleeding
    d. All of the above
    e. b + c

15. **Annular detachment of the cervix, which of the following are not true:**
    a. Normally seen
    b. Seen with prolonged late first and second stage
    c. Associated with scared cervix
    d. Requires no treatment if no bleeding
    e. It is doughnut-shaped

16. **Vulval hematomas are:**
    a. Painful and tender
    b. May extend to ischiorectal fossa
    c. Purple colored swelling in labia majora
    d. All of the above
    e. None of the above

17. **Paravaginal hematomas are:**
    a. Not visible externally
    b. Inability to void
    c. Associated with rectal tenesmus
    d. All of the above
    e. None of the above

18. **Broad ligament hematoma occur if vessel rupture**
    a. Above urogenital diaphragm
    b. Below urogenital diaphragm
    c. All of the above
    d. None of the above

19. **Which of the following is true about broad ligament hematoma?**
    a. May cause profound hypovolemic shock
    b. May extend to kidney
    c. USG or MRI is required for diagnosis
    d. All of the above
    e. None of the above

20. **Broad ligament hematomas are treated by:**
    a. Laparotomy
    b. Angiographic embolization
    c. Both a and b
    d. None of the above

21. **Principle for all hematomas, which of the following are not true:**
    a. Incision and evacuation
    b. Under regional or general anesthesia
    c. Tamponade
    d. Foleys catheterization
    e. Conservative management

22. **According to ACOG (2016), _____ % of women sustain some type of vaginal laceration at vaginal delivery.**
    a. 50%
    b. 60%
    c. 80%
    d. 70%

23. **In vulval hematoma, bleeding is from:**
    a. Obturator artery
    b. Pudendal artery
    c. Uterine artery descending branch
    d. None of the above

24. **Paravaginal hematoma bleeding is from:**
    a. Pudendal artery
    b. Uterine artery descending branch
    c. Obturator artery
    d. External iliac artery

25. **Bakri balloon can be used for**
    a. Vulval hematoma
    b. Paracervical hematoma
    c. Retroperitoneal hematoma
    d. All of the above

26. **Drawback of midline episiotomy:**
    a. Blood loss is more
    b. Extension to external anal sphincter
    c. Cuts the belly of the muscle
    d. All of the above

27. **Muscles cut during episiotomy:**
    a. Bulbocavernosus
    b. Transverse perineal
    c. Puborectalis
    d. All of the above
    e. None of the above

28. **The incidence of third and fourth-degree tears is:**
    a. 0.5–5%
    b. 0.1–10%
    c. 2–20%
    d. 5–15%

29. **Postpartum dissipation of external anal sphincter and internal anal sphincter is diagnosed by:**
    a. Ultrasound (USG) abdomen
    b. Endoanal ultrasound (USG)
    c. Magnetic resonance imaging (MRI) pelvis
    d. Computed tomography (CT) scan

CHAPTER 50: Genital Tract Injuries

30. Birth after fourth-degree perineal tear is by:
   a. Vaginal delivery
   b. Elective lower segment cesarean section (LSCS)
   c. Vacuum delivery
   d. Forceps delivery

ANSWERS

1. **d.** Anterior vaginal wall
   Anatomically the perineum is between the coccyx and pubic arch. The anterior perineum includes the clitoris, urethra, labia, and anterior vaginal wall.

2. **d.** All of the above
   Anatomically the perineum is between the coccyx and pubic arch. The posterior perineum includes the posterior vaginal wall, the perineal and levator ani muscles, and the anal sphincter

3. **a.** Vagina and perineal skin only
   Standard definition of perineal tear that can be correlated with the subsequent pelvic floor morbidity.
   - First-degree: Vaginal and perineal skin only
   - Second-degree: Separation of the skin and perineal muscle

4. **c.**
   Standard definition of perineal tear that can be correlated with subsequent pelvic floor morbidity.
   - First-degree: Vaginal and perineal skin only
   - Second-degree: Separation of the skin and perineal muscle
   - 3a: <50% external anal sphincter
   - 3b: >50% external anal sphincter
   - 3c: Both external and internal anal sphincter
   - 4: Injury to external anal sphincter, internal anal sphincter, and anal mucosa

5. **c.** Injury to anorectal epithelium
   Standard definition of perineal tear that can be correlated with subsequent pelvic floor morbidity.
   - First-degree: Vaginal and perineal skin only
   - Second-degree: Separation of the skin and perineal muscle
   - 3a: <50% external anal sphincter
   - 3b: >50% external anal sphincter
   - 3c: Both external and internal anal sphincter
   - 4: Injury to external anal sphincter, internal anal sphincter, and anal mucosa

6. **a.** Regional anesthesia
   It is optimal as this allows relaxation of the sphincter and better identification and approximation of the separated ends of muscle.

7. **e.** A and B
   - Better tensile strength
   - Less chances of dehiscence

8. **c.** 3-0 PDS polydioxanone
   This suture has longer half-life and greater tensile strength than Dexon and Vicryl

9. **d.** a + b
   These are the two accepted techniques for repair as they ensure accurate placement of suture:
   1. End-to-end—torn muscle ends are reapproximated with 2-3 figure-of-eight suture.
   2. Overlapping technique—the torn muscle ends are mobilized such that they can be overlapped by 1-1.5 cm

10. **c.** Nullipara
    Periurethral and periclitoral seen in nullipara when episiotomy is not given, pressure from delivering head is transferred to anterior perineum by the intact posterior perineum.

11. **a.** The lower two-thirds of posterior vaginal sulci
    - Vaginal lacerations are common and usually involve the lower two-thirds and the posterolateral vaginal sulcus, they also occur as extension of episiotomy.
    - Lacerations in anterior sulcus of the vagina are less frequent but are seen with narrow subpubic arch and elevation and the forceps application before occiput has descended completely below pubic symphysis.

12. **b.** Forceps rotation delivery
    Lacerations of the upper third of the vagina are rare and most often associated with for forceps rotation delivery. They produce eccentric laceration high in vaginal vault which can be difficult to expose.

13. **d.** All of the above
    The cervix can usually be inspected by applying ring or sponge forceps and traced and entire cervix is inspected if no bleeding and tear is small in size, requires no treatment.

14. **c.** Tear is >2 cm and bleeding
    Lacerations usually occur laterally and if they are <2 cm and not bleeding, do not require suture, if they are >2 cm and bleeding continuous locking sutures are taken.

15. **a.** Normally seen
    Annular detachment of the cervix is an extremely rare condition associated with cervical dystocia from rigid or scarred cervix causing annular detachment of the lower portion of cervix in its entirety such that a

doughnut-shaped portion of the cervix is detached in front of the fetal head.

16. **d.** All of the above
    Vulval hematomas have an obvious clinical presentation with an acutely painful, tender purple swelling in the area of labia majora, these may extend to the lower vagina into the ischiorectal fossa.

17. **d.** All of the above
    Paravaginal lacerations are not visible externally and usually present with pain, restlessness, inability to void and rectal tenesmus. A gentle one finger, vaginal examination will reveal the tender mass bulging into vagina.

18. **a.** Above urogenital diaphragm
    Broad ligament or retroperitoneal hematoma occurs when vessels rupture above the urogenital diaphragm. The bleeding extends into the supravaginal space between the leaves of broad ligament and retroperitoneally up to kidney.

19. **d.** All of the above
    Broad ligament hematoma when large and extensive, retroperitoneal may cause hypovolemic shock, may extend to kidney and diagnosis is normally by ultrasound and MRI. These type of hematomas may be associated with cervical laceration extending to lower uterine segment or with rupture of lower uterine segment.

20. **c.** Both a and b
    - Broad ligament hematoma and retroperitoneal hematoma may be self-limiting and may absorb when treated conservatively.
    - If the sign of progressive bleeding persists then laparotomy or if angiographic embolization facilities available can be done.

21. **e.** Conservative management
    Not all hematomas are treated conservatively. If the hematomas are large then they need intervention like incision and evacuation under regional or general anesthesia with Foleys catheterization.

22. **c.** 80%
    According to ACOG 2016, 80% of women sustain some laceration during vaginal delivery they may lie proximally or distally along the lower genital tract.

23. **b.** Pudendal artery
    Vulval hematoma may involve the vestibular bulb or branches of pudendal artery which are the inferior rectal, perineal, and clitoral arteries.

24. **b.** Uterine artery descending branch
    Paravaginal hematoma involves the descending branch of the uterine artery. Torn vessels may lie above the pelvic fascia cause superior levator hematomas, continuous bleeding may dissect retroperitoneal to form a mass palpable above the inguinal ligament in some case may ascend behind the ascending colon in hepatic flexure.

25. **c.** Retroperitoneal hematoma
    The use of Bakri balloon for a paracervical hematoma has been described (GIZZO 2013, CRONVALT 2013). USG-guided drainage of recurrent supralevator hematomas has also been reported.

26. **b.** Extension to external anal sphincter
    Advantages are blood loss is less, muscle belly is not cut; the two sides of the incised area are anatomically balanced making surgical repair easier but there is propensity for extension through the external anal sphincter and into rectum.

27. **d.** All of the above
    - Muscle cut during episiotomy bulbocavernosus
    - Transverse perineal and puborectalis muscles

28. **a.** 0.5–5%
    The incidence of third- and fourth-degree tears is 0.5–5%.

29. **b.** Endoanal ultrasound (USG)
    Endoanal ultrasound (USG) shows that up to one-third women after first vaginal delivery may develop sphincter injury. Disruption of anal sphincter at delivery may be unrecognized, subsequent endo-anal USG that shows disruption of external anal sphincter and internal anal sphincter.

30. **b.** Elective lower segment cesarean section (LSCS)
    Any vaginal plastic surgery, deep-seated vaginal and rectal tears which are repaired have a tendency of weakening of tear during next delivery if episiotomy is not given. As a safer option elective LSCS is preferred.

REFERENCES

1. Lower genital tract trauma. In: Baskett TF, Calder AA, Arulkumaran S (Eds). Munro Kerr's Operative Obstetrics, 11th edition. Edinburgh: Saunders; 2007. pp. 251-9.
2. Williams JW. Obstetrical Hemorrhage: Injuries to the birth canal. In: Cunningham FG, Leveno KJ, Bloom SL, Dashe JS, Hoffman BL, Casey BM, Spong CY (Eds). Williams Obstetrics, 25th edition. New York: McGraw Hill; 2018. pp. 763-5.

Chapter 51

Term Newborn Infant

Charmila Ayyavoo, S Karthikeyan

QUESTIONS

1. Classic vitamin K deficiency (VKDB) bleeding occurs during:
   a. First week of life
   b. Second week of life
   c. First day of life
   d. First 3 days of life

2. Cesarean section is indicated in diabetic mother if weight of the baby is:
   a. 4 kg
   b. 4.5 kg
   c. 5 kg
   d. 3.5 kg

3. Target preductal oxygen saturation at 5 minutes after birth is:
   a. 60–65%
   b. 65–70%
   c. 80–85%
   d. 85–95%

4. Which one of the following is not a ventilation corrective step in newborn resuscitation?
   a. Mask adjustment
   b. Reposition the head and neck
   c. Suction the mouth and nose
   d. Decrease pressure

5. Which of the following device is not used for delivering positive end-expiratory pressure (PEEP)?
   a. Self-inflating AMBU bag
   b. Flow inflating bag
   c. T-piece resuscitator
   d. None of the above

6. Which one of the following is not a risk factor for hyperbilirubinemia neurotoxicity?
   a. Asphyxia
   b. Albumin <2.5 g/dL
   c. Isoimmune hemolytic disease
   d. Acidosis

7. What is false about caput succedaneum?
   a. Poorly defined margins
   b. Crosses midline and across suture lines
   c. Subperiosteal fluid collection
   d. Resolves spontaneously

8. What is true about Erb's palsy?
   a. Involves nerve roots C6, C7
   b. Diaphragm paralysis does not occur
   c. Grasp reflex is intact
   d. Second most common type of brachial plexus injury

9. What is false about mastitis in mother?
   a. Clinical features include fever, headache, tender, and reddened breast area
   b. Usually affects both breasts
   c. Antibiotics for 10–14 days
   d. Not necessary to discard expressed breastmilk

10. Newborn reaches blood glucose control similar to older children and adults at what age?
    a. 24 hours of life
    b. 1 week of life
    c. 48–72 hours of life
    d. 1 month of life

11. What is the most common cause of nonhereditary sensorineural hearing loss?
    a. Cytomegalovirus (CMV)
    b. Toxoplasmosis
    c. Syphilis
    d. Rubella

12. What is the most frequent surgical cause of polyhydramnios?
    a. Abdominal wall defects
    b. Gastrointestinal obstruction
    c. Diaphragmatic hernia
    d. Anencephaly

13. What is the most common congenital heart disease associated with insulin dependent diabetes?
    a. Tetralogy of Fallot (TOF)
    b. Atrial septal defect (ASD)
    c. Ventricular septal defect (VSD)
    d. Patent ductus arteriosus (PDA)

14. Folic acid should be taken how many months before conception to prevent neural tube defects?
    a. 1 month
    b. 2 months
    c. 3 months
    d. 4 months

15. What is the most frequent cause of mild to moderate early onset thrombocytopenia in well-appearing neonate?
    a. Sepsis
    b. Placental insufficiency
    c. Maternal thrombocytopenia
    d. TORCH infection

16. Which one of the statements is false regarding diabetes in pregnancy?
    a. Most important complication is diabetic embryopathy resulting in congenital anomalies
    b. Folic acid supplementation of 1 mg/day is recommended to reduce the risk of congenital malformation in women with pregestational diabetes
    c. Delivery is planned for 36–37 weeks without any pregnancy complication in gestational diabetes
    d. Route of delivery is determined by USG estimated fetal weight, maternal and fetal conditions, and previous obstetric history

17. A 35-weeks-primi mother diagnosed to have preeclampsia without severe features came to clinic for your opinion. What is your next line of action?
    a. Administer antenatal steroids
    b. Administer intravenous (IV) magnesium sulfate (MgSO$_4$) for neuroprotection
    c. Do elective lower segment cesarean section (LSCS) after evaluating mother and fetus
    d. Evaluate mother and fetus and then decide upon further action

18. Subperiosteal collection of blood resulting from rupture of superficial veins between the skull and periosteum is termed as:
    a. Subgaleal hematoma
    b. Cephalohematoma
    c. Caput succedaneum
    d. Epidural hemorrhage

19. How much percentage difference in birth weight of larger twin weight is defined as fetal growth discordance?
    a. 10%
    b. 20%
    c. 30%
    d. 40%

20. Name of the placenta when splitting of embryo occurs about days 4–7:
    a. Dichorionic diamniotic placenta
    b. Monochorionic diamniotic placenta
    c. Monochorionic monoamniotic placenta
    d. Conjoined twins

21. Premature infants are more prone for hypothermia than term infants because:
    a. Increased subcutaneous fat with less insulative capacity
    b. Increased glycogen stores
    c. Decreased transepidermal water loss
    d. Less developed stores of brown fat

22. What is false about breastfeeding?
    a. Early initiation of breastfeeding within 1 hour of life
    b. Encourage frequent feeding (8–12 feeds per 24 hours) in response to early infant cues
    c. Give formula when direct breastfeeding is not possible
    d. Complementary foods should be introduced around 6 months with continued breastfeeding up to and beyond 2 years

23. During resuscitation of newborn, intubation procedure should be completed within how many seconds?
    a. 20 seconds
    b. 30 seconds
    c. 40 seconds
    d. 60 seconds

24. A term newborn baby is born apneic, you completed initial steps of resuscitation (Flowchart 1). What is the next step?
    a. Start cardiopulmonary resuscitation (CPR)
    b. Start oxygen via prongs
    c. Check heart rate and start positive pressure ventilation (PPV)
    d. Intubate immediately

25. **A term newborn not cried at birth, you completed initial steps of resuscitation and started positive pressure ventilation (PPV) and heartrate was below 60 bpm after five inflations. What is the next step?**
    a. Start cardiopulmonary resuscitation (CPR)
    b. Look for ventilation corrective steps
    c. Give continuous positive airway pressure (CPAP)
    d. Intubate immediately

26. **Factors that do not affect lung maturation are:**
    a. Poorly controlled maternal diabetes
    b. Preterm babies delivered by lower segment cesarean section (LSCS) before onset of labor
    c. Mutation in surfactant protein B
    d. Female sex

27. **Identify the false statement regarding meconium aspiration syndrome (MAS):**
    a. Meconium-stained amniotic fluid (MSAF) occurs more commonly in term or post-term pregnancies
    b. MSAF rarely occurs prior to 34 weeks gestation
    c. Severity of MAS appears to be related to thickness of MSAF
    d. Bag and mask ventilation contraindicated in thick MSAF

28. **What is the most common cause of permanent congenital hypothyroidism (CH)?**
    a. Thyroid dysgenesis
    b. Thyroid dyshormonogenesis
    c. Thyroid-stimulating hormone (TSH) resistance
    d. Central hypothyroidism

29. **What is the most common cause of neonatal seizures?**
    a. Hypoglycemia
    b. Hypocalcemia
    c. Perinatal asphyxia
    d. Intracranial hemorrhage

30. **What is not correct about congenital tuberculosis (TB)?**
    a. Lungs is frequently infected
    b. Hepatic primary complex or a caseating hepatic granuloma is the definitive lesion
    c. Investigation includes examination of placenta or uterine tissue
    d. Initial presentation is similar to that of sepsis

ANSWERS

1. **a.** First week of life
   - Classic" vitamin K deficiency bleeding (VKDB) occurs in newborns during the first week of life. Although the presentation is often mild, blood loss can be significant, and intracranial hemorrhages have been reported.
   - Although estimates differ, the incidence of classic VKDB, in the absence of vitamin K supplementation, is 0.25–1.7%.
   - Early VKDB presents in first 24 hours after birth
   - Late VKDB presents between 2 and 12 weeks after birth

   (Reference: Avery Diseases of Newborn 10th edition, page 317)

2. **b.** 4.5 kg
   The ultrasonography-estimated weight at which an elective cesarean delivery is recommended as a controversial issue, with the American College of Obstetricians and Gynecologists recommending discussion of cesarean delivery at an estimated fetal weight of >4,500 g due to the increased risk of shoulder dystocia.

   (Reference: Cloherty and Stark's Manual of Neonatal Care South Asian edition, page 32)

3. **c.** 80–85%
   Target oxygen saturation:
   - *1 minute:* 60–65%
   - *2 minutes:* 65–70%
   - *3 minutes:* 70–75%
   - *4 minutes:* 75–80%
   - *5 minutes:* 80–85%
   - *10 minutes:* 85–95%

   (Reference: Newborn resuscitation, India 3rd edition, 2019, page 32)

4. **d.** Decrease pressure
   Ventilation corrective steps are (MR SOPA):
   - Mask adjustment
   - Reposition the head and neck
   - Suction the mouth and nose
   - Open the mouth
   - Pressure increase
   - Alternate airway

   (Reference: Textbook of Neonatal Resuscitation, AAP 8th edition, 2020, page 67)

5. **a.** Self-inflating AMBU bag
   Gas does not flow out of the mask unless the bag is being squeezed; a self-inflating bag and mask cannot be used to administer continuous positive airway pressure (CPAP) or free-flow oxygen.
   (Reference: Textbook of Neonatal Resuscitation, AAP 8th edition, 2020, page 49)

6. **b.** Albumin <2.5 g/dL
   Risk factors:
   - Acidosis, albumin level low (<3 g/dL)
   - Blood brain-barrier disruption (example: intracranial hemorrhage, asphyxia, and sepsis)
   - Coombs positive hemolytic anemia
   - Displacers of bilirubin (example: free fatty acid (FFA) from intralipid, ceftriaxone)
   - Encephalopathy (extreme prematurity)

   (Reference: Cloherty and Stark's Manual of Neonatal Care South Asian edition, page 363)

7. **c.** Subperiosteal fluid collection
   Caput succedaneum is a commonly occurring subcutaneous, extraperiosteal fluid collection that is occasionally hemorrhagic. It has poorly defined margins and can extend over the midline and across suture lines. It typically extends over the presenting portion of the scalp and is usually associated with molding. The lesion usually resolves spontaneously without sequelae over the first several days after birth. It rarely causes significant blood loss or jaundice.
   (Reference: Cloherty and Stark's Manual of Neonatal Care South Asian edition, page 79)

8. **c.** Grasp reflex is intact.
   Duchenne-Erb's palsy involves the upper trunks (C5, C6, and occasionally C7) and is the most common type of brachial plexus injury, accounting for approximately 90% of cases. Total brachial plexus palsy occurs in some cases and involves all roots from C5 to T1. Klumpke palsy involves C7/C8-T1 and is the least common.

   Duchenne-Erb's palsy: The arm is typically adducted and internally rotated at the shoulder. There is extension and pronation at the elbow and flexion of the wrist and fingers in the characteristic "Waiter's tip" posture. The deltoid, infraspinatus, biceps, supinator, and brachioradialis muscles and the extensors of the wrist and fingers may be weak or paralyzed. The Moro, biceps, and radial reflexes are absent on the affected side. The grasp reflex is intact. Sensation is variably affected. Diaphragm paralysis occurs in 5% of cases.
   (Reference: Cloherty and Stark's Manual of Neonatal Care South Asian edition, page 86)

9. **b.** Usually affects both breasts
   Inflammatory and/or infectious breast condition—usually affecting only one breast. Signs and symptoms include rapid onset of fatigue, body aches, headache, fever, and tender, reddened breast area. Treatment includes the following: (i) continued breastfeeding on the affected and unaffected breasts; (ii) frequent and efficient milk removal—using an electric breast pump when necessary (it is not necessary to discard expressed breast milk; (iii) appropriate antibiotics for a sufficient period (10-14 days); and (iv) comfort measures to relieve breast discomfort and general malaise (i.e., analgesics, moist heat/massage to the breast).
   (Reference: Cloherty and Stark's Manual of Neonatal Care South Asian edition, page 294)

10. **c.** 48-72 hours of life
    (Reference: Cloherty and Stark's Manual of Neonatal Care South Asian edition, page 323)

11. **a.** Cytomegalovirus (CMV)
    (Reference: Cloherty and Stark's Manual of Neonatal Care South Asian edition, page 1033)

12. **b.** Gastrointestinal obstruction
    (Reference: Cloherty and Stark's Manual of Neonatal Care South Asian edition, page 977)

13. **c.** Ventricular septal defect (VSD)
    (Reference: Cloherty and Stark's Manual of Neonatal Care South Asian edition, page 945)

14. **c.** 3 months
    Folic acid should be taken at least 3 months prior to conception and during first month of pregnancy.
    (Reference: Cloherty and Stark's Manual of Neonatal Care South Asian edition, page 861)

15. **b.** Placental insufficiency
    The most frequent cause of mild-to-moderate, early onset thrombocytopenia in a well-appearing neonate is placental insufficiency, as occurs in infants born to mothers with pregnancy-induced hypertension/preeclampsia or diabetes, or in those with fetal growth restriction (FGR).
    (Reference: Cloherty and Stark's Manual of Neonatal Care South Asian edition, page 653)

16. **c.** Delivery is planned for 36–37 weeks without any pregnancy complication in gestational diabetes.

The most important complication is diabetic embryopathy resulting in congenital anomalies. Congenital anomalies are associated with 50% of perinatal deaths among women with diabetes compared to 25% among women without diabetes. The risk of congenital anomalies is associated with glycemic control at the time of conception. The most common types of anomalies include cardiac malformations and neural tube defects.

Folic acid supplementation of 1 mg/day 3 months prior to conception and continuing to at least 12 weeks into gestation is recommended to reduce the risk of congenital malformations in women with pregestational diabetes.

Delivery is planned for 39–40 weeks, unless other pregnancy complications dictate earlier delivery. Elective delivery after 39 weeks does not require fetal lung maturity (FLM) testing. Indicated delivery before 39 weeks' gestation should be carried out without FLM testing. Route of delivery is determined by ultrasonography-estimated fetal weight, maternal and fetal conditions, and previous obstetric history. The ultrasonography-estimated weight at which an elective cesarean delivery is recommended is a controversial issue, with the American College of Obstetricians and Gynecologists recommending discussion of cesarean delivery at an estimated fetal weight of >4,500 g due to the increased risk of shoulder dystocia.

(Reference: Cloherty and Stark's Manual of Neonatal Care South Asian edition, page 28-32)

17. **d.** Evaluate mother and fetus and then decide upon further action

Fetal indications for delivery include nonreassuring fetal testing. If severe growth restriction and/or oligohydramnios are noted, then further assessment of the fetus is recommended with umbilical artery Doppler studies:

- Maternal indications for delivery include a gestational age ≥37 weeks; thrombocytopenia (<100,000); progressive deterioration in hepatic or renal function; placental abruption; and persistent severe headaches, visual changes, or epigastric pain.
- When early delivery is indicated, it is our practice that vaginal delivery is preferred. Cesarean delivery should be reserved for cases with nonreassuring fetal testing, when further fetal evaluation is not possible, or when a rapidly deteriorating maternal condition mandates expeditious delivery (e.g., HELLP syndrome with decreasing platelet counts, abruption).
- Antenatal steroid (<34 weeks) and intravenous (IV) magnesium sulfate ($MgSO_4$) for neuroprotection (<32 weeks) should be offered, if indicated, in case of preterm delivery to improve the neonatal outcome.

(Reference: Cloherty and Stark's Manual of Neonatal Care South Asian edition, page 39-40)

18. **b.** Cephalohematoma

Caput succedaneum is a commonly occurring subcutaneous, extraperiosteal fluid collection that is occasionally hemorrhagic. It has poorly defined margins and can extend over the midline and across suture lines. It typically extends over the presenting portion of the scalp and is usually associated with molding.

Cephalohematoma is a subperiosteal collection of blood resulting from rupture of the superficial veins between the skull and the periosteum. The lesion is always confined by suture lines and does not cross the midline although can be bilateral over occipital or parietal region.

Subgaleal hematoma is hemorrhage under the aponeurosis of the scalp.

(Reference: Cloherty and Stark's Manual of Neonatal Care South Asian edition, page 79)

19. **b.** 20%

(Reference: Cloherty and Stark's Manual of Neonatal Care South Asian edition, page 148)

20. **b.** Monochorionic diamniotic placenta

Monozygotic pregnancies result from the splitting of a single egg between days 0 and 14 postfertilization. The type of placenta that forms depend on the day of embryo splitting. A dichorionic diamniotic placenta results when early splitting occurs on days 0-3 before chorion formation (which usually occurs about day 3 and before implantation. A monochorionic diamniotic placenta results when splitting occurs about days 4-7 at which time the blastocyst cavity has developed and

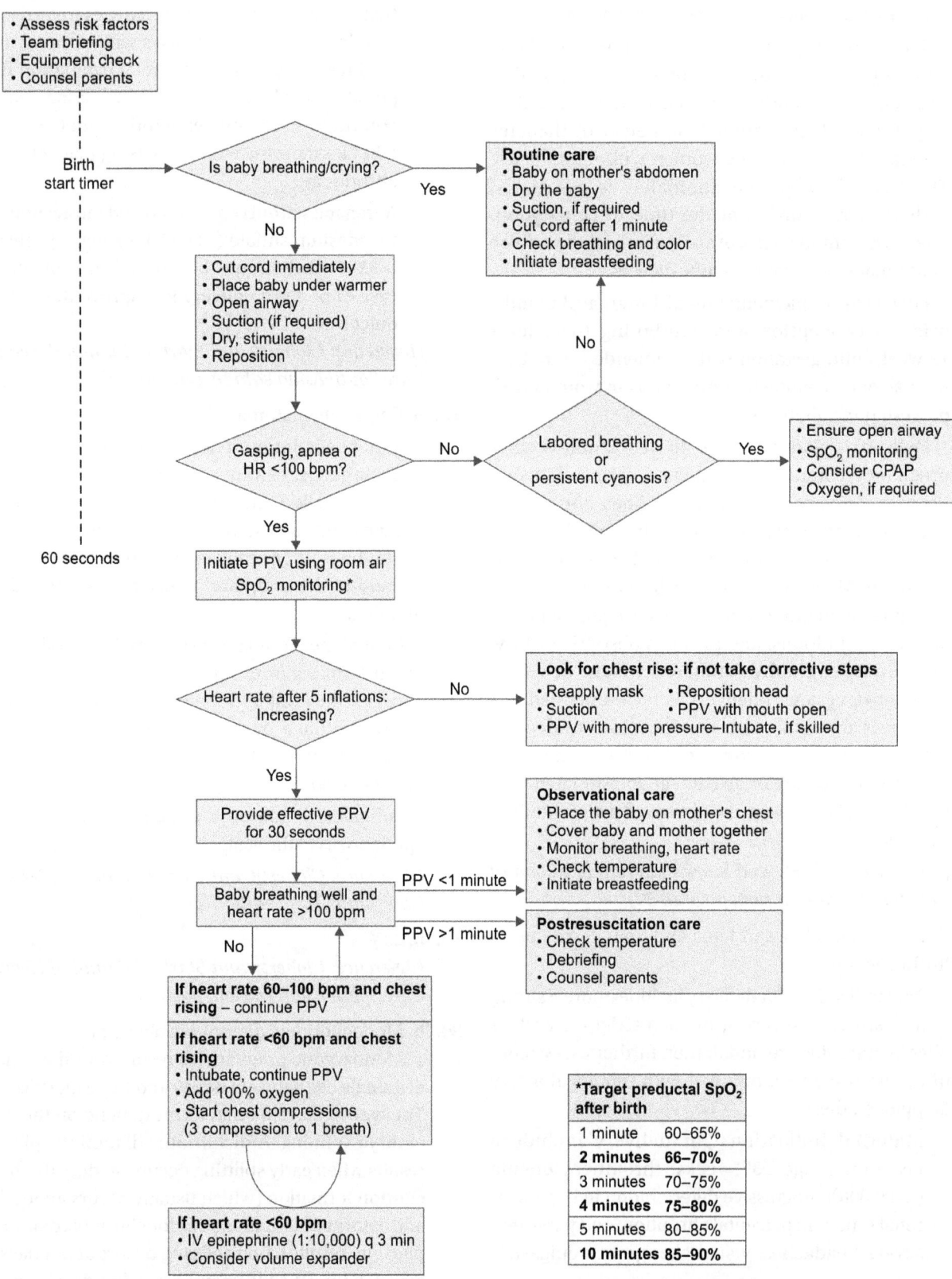

Flowchart 1: Newborn resuscitation: India.

(CPAP: continuous positive airway pressure; HR: heart rate; PPV: positive pressure ventilation)

the chorion has formed. Amnion formation occurs on days 6-8, and splitting of the egg after this time (days 8-13) results in a monochorionic monoamniotic placenta. The frequency of placentation types is 30% dichorionic diamniotic, 70% monochorionic diamniotic, and <1% monochorionic monoamniotic. On day 14 and thereafter, the primitive streak begins to form and late splitting of the embryo at this time results in conjoined twins.
(Reference: Cloherty and Stark's Manual of Neonatal Care South Asian edition, page 145)

21. **d.** Less developed stores of brown fat
    Compared with term infants, premature infants have:
    - A higher ratio of skin surface area to weight
    - Highly permeable skin which leads to increased transepidermal water loss
    - Decreased subcutaneous fat with less insulative capacity
    - Less-developed stores of brown fat and decreased glycogen stores
    - Poor vasomotor control
    - Challenges with adequate caloric intake to provide nutrients for thermogenesis
    - Limited oxygen delivery if pulmonary conditions coexist

    (Reference: Cloherty and Stark's Manual of Neonatal Care South Asian edition, page 203-204)

22. **c.** Give formula when direct breastfeeding is not possible.
    When direct breastfeeding is not possible, instruct the mother to hand express and/or pump to promote milk production.
    Formula should not be given unless medically indicated.
    (Reference: Cloherty and Stark's Manual of Neonatal Care South Asian edition, page 292)

23. **b.** 30 seconds
    (Reference: Newborn Resuscitation, India 3rd edition, 2019, page 75)

24. **c.** Check heart rate and start positive pressure ventilation (PPV)
    (Reference: Newborn Resuscitation, India 3rd edition, 2019, page 11)

25. **b.** Look for ventilation corrective steps
    After five inflations look for chest rise. If there is no chest rise look for ventilation corrective steps (MR SOPA) which are performed after 30 seconds of effective ventilation. If the baby's heart rate is below 60 bpm, start chest compressions coordinated with positive pressure ventilation (PPV).
    (Reference: Newborn Resuscitation, India 3rd edition, 2019, page 11)

26. **d.** Female sex
    - *Maternal diabetes:* Poorly controlled maternal diabetes is associated with respiratory distress syndrome (RDS) due to enhanced production of fetal insulin which inhibits the production of surfactant phospholipids important for surfactant function. Strict glycemic control allows the lungs to mature in a near-normal fashion.
    - Due to the production of endogenous maternal glucocorticoids, it may enhance lung fluid clearance by enhancing sodium reabsorptive properties of epithelial sodium channels (E-NaC). Preterm babies delivered by a cesarean section before the onset of labor have a higher incidence of RDS.
    - Mutations in surfactant-related proteins, specifically surfactant protein B and ABCA3 result in severe RDS typically in term infants from either dysfunctional surfactant or severely limited production, respectively.
    - *Fetal sex:* Male infants are at a higher risk for RDS due to the presence of circulating weak fetal androgens that inhibit the production of surfactant phospholipids.

    (Reference: Cloherty and Stark's Manual of Neonatal Care South Asian edition, page 449)

27. **c.** Severity of meconium aspiration syndrome (MAS) appears to be related to thickness of meconium-stained amniotic fluid (MSAF)
    Severity of MAS appears not to be related to thickness of MSAF. Severe MAS appears to be caused by chronic hypoxia, acidosis, and infection.
    Bag and mask ventilation not contraindicated in MSAF. It is contraindicated only in suspected diaphragmatic hernia and pneumothorax.
    (Reference: Cloherty and Stark's Manual of Neonatal Care South Asian edition, page 476)

28. **a.** Thyroid dysgenesis
    Abnormal thyroid gland development is the cause of permanent congenital hypothyroidism (CH) in about 70% of cases. It includes agenesis, hypoplasia and ectopy.

(Reference: Cloherty and Stark's Manual of Neonatal Care South Asian edition, page 931)

29. **c.** Perinatal asphyxia
    - Perinatal asphyxia accounts for 50–75% of cases.
    - *Intracranial hemorrhage:* 10–15%
    - Acute metabolic disorders, such as hypoglycemia, hypocalcemia, and hypomagnesemia—5%

(Reference: Cloherty and Stark's Manual of Neonatal Care South Asian edition, page 847)

30. **a.** Lungs is frequently infected

    The usual deposits of hematogenous spread follow the path of the umbilical vein. The liver is frequently infected, where a primary focus develops within periportal lymph nodes. The organisms may spread beyond the liver and into the main systemic circulation by the patent foramen ovale or into the pulmonary circulation via the right ventricle. Multiple sites may be seeded initially or seeded secondary to the initial hepatic or pulmonary foci. The definitive lesion of congenital tuberculosis (TB) is the hepatic primary complex with caseating hepatic granulomas:
    - The initial presentation is similar to that of sepsis or a congenital infection and should be suspected if an ill neonate does not respond to empiric antimicrobials and has an otherwise unrevealing evaluation. Hepatosplenomegaly and respiratory distress are the two most common signs and symptoms, followed by fever.
    - Investigation of congenital TB should include examination of placenta or uterine tissue. The placenta should be examined by a pathologist and should be cultured for *Mycobacterium tuberculosis*. If the placenta is not available, the mother should be examined and consider to perform a uterine dilation and curettage because endometrial specimens often yield positive culture results.
    - The infant should be evaluated for microbiologic confirmation of disease by acid-fast bacillus (AFB) smear and culture of body fluids or tissues including gastric aspirates, middle ear fluid, bone marrow, tissue biopsy, and tracheal aspirates. The cerebrospinal fluid (CSF) should also be examined because TB meningitis occurs in one-third of congenital TB cases.

(Reference: Cloherty and Stark's Manual of Neonatal Care South Asian edition, page 770-771)

Chapter 52

Induction of Labor

Rajshree Dayanand Katke, Prachi Yadav

QUESTIONS

1. Which of the following is/are criteria for normal labor?
   a. Spontaneous in onset and at term
   b. Vertex presentation
   c. Natural termination with minimal aids
   d. All of the above

2. Which of the following is/are contraindications for induction of labor?
   a. Abnormally implanted placenta
   b. Cervical cancer
   c. Distorted pelvic anatomy
   d. All of the above

3. What percent of cases of induction of labor in primigravida patients, ultimately cesarean delivery is required?
   a. 10%
   b. 18%
   c. 25%
   d. 30%

4. As per American College of Obstetricians and Gynecologists (ACOG), which of the following is true regarding labor induction in patients with previous lower segment cesarean section (LSCS)?
   a. Misoprostol is used for preinduction cervical ripening or for labor induction in women with a prior uterine incision
   b. Labor induction with oxytocin can be done in previous lower segment cesarean section (LSCS) cases
   c. Amniotomy is contraindicated for augmentation of labor in previous LSCS cases
   d. All of the above

5. Which of the following statement is true regarding Bishop score?
   a. Bishop score >8 conveys a high likelihood for a successful induction
   b. Bishop score ≤6 is considered unfavorable
   c. Bishop score >5 conveys a high likelihood for a successful induction
   d. a + b

6. Which of the following factors are used in modified Bishop scoring system?
   a. Cervical effacement and cervical dilatation
   b. Presenting part station
   c. Cervical length
   d. All of the above

7. Which of the following is a synthetic analog of prostaglandin E2 (PGE2)?
   a. Dinoprostone
   b. Mifepristone
   c. Misoprostol
   d. None of the above

8. Which of the following is contraindication for induction of labor using dinoprostone gel?
   a. Unexplained vaginal bleeding
   b. Six or more prior term pregnancies
   c. Women already receiving oxytocin
   d. All of the above

9. What dose of tablet misoprostol can be used for labor induction recommended?
   a. 25 µg
   b. 50 µg
   c. 100 µg
   d. 200 µg

10. Which of the following statement is or are true regarding labor induction?
    a. Misoprostol used safely at a dose of 200 µg
    b. Intracervical prostaglandin E2 (PGE2) gel in poor Bishop score
    c. 15-methyl-prostaglandin F2α (PGF2α) can be used as a drug of choice
    d. None of the above

11. Which of the following is or are maternal complications associated with labor induction?
    a. Chorioamnionitis
    b. Uterine rupture
    c. Postpartum hemorrhage
    d. All of the above

12. What are the causes of failed induction?
    a. Advanced maternal age and primigravida
    b. Very poor Bishop score
    c. Birth weight >3.5 kg
    d. All of the above

13. What are the indications for induction of labor among following?
    a. Brow presentation
    b. Severe pregnancy induced hypertension at term
    c. Transverse lie
    d. Active genital herpes infection

14. All of the following are used for induction of labor, *except*:
    a. Prostaglandin F2α (PGF2α) tablet
    b. Prostaglandin E1 (PGE1) tablet
    c. Prostaglandin E2 (PGE2) gel
    d. Misoprostol

15. What is the use of partogram in induction of labor?
    a. To see the progress of labor
    b. To see the cervical dilatation
    c. To see the descent of presenting part
    d. All of the above

16. Time interval between alert line and action line is:
    a. 3 hours   b. 4 hours
    c. 1 hour   d. 6 hours

17. What is the mechanism of action of prostaglandin E2 (PGE2) gel?
    a. Stimulates uterine contraction
    b. Acts on collagen present in cervix and softens it
    c. Cervical dilatation
    d. All of the above

18. Which of the following statement is false regarding partograph?
    a. Alert line starts at 4 cm of cervical dilatation as per the World Health Organization (WHO)
    b. Action line is drawn 6 hours to the right and parallel to the alert line
    c. In a normal labor, the partograph (cervical dilatation) should be either on the alert line or to the left of it
    d. When partograph falls in zone 3, case should be reassessed by a senior person

19. Cervical balloon catheter causes cervical ripening by release of which of the following biochemical molecules, *except*?
    a. Interleukin-6 (IL-6)
    b. Interleukin-1 (IL-1)
    c. Matrix metalloproteinase-8 (MMP-8)
    d. Hyaluronic acid synthetase

20. After performing artificial rupture of membranes (ARM), which of the following are to be assessed?
    a. Color of the amniotic fluid
    b. Fetal heart rate (FHR) pattern
    c. Detection of cord prolapse, if any
    d. All of the above

21. Which of the following are potential complications of oxytocin, as a method of induction, *except*?
    a. Water intoxication   b. Uterine tachysystole
    c. Chorioamnionitis   d. Hypotension

22. Which of the following are potential complications of artificial rupture of membrane (ARM), *except*?
    a. Cord prolapse   b. Chorioamnionitis
    c. Vaginal bleeding   d. Hypotension

23. Which of the following is true regarding oxytocin used in induction of labor?
    a. In primigravida five units oxytocin intravenously given [diluted in 1 pint Ringer's lactate (RL) IV fluid solution] for labor augmentation starting with rate of 8 drops/min
    b. Oxytocin is discontinued if the number of contractions persists with a frequency of more than five in a 10-minute period
    c. When oxytocin is stopped, its concentration in plasma rapidly falls because the half-life is approximately 3–5 minutes
    d. All of the above

24. Which of the following is true regarding artificial rupture of the membranes (ARM), *except*?
    a. Umbilical cord prolapse risk is high with engaged head
    b. Artificial rupture of the membranes (ARM) will shorten the induction–delivery interval
    c. Accidental injury to the placenta, cervix can occur during ARM
    d. a + c

25. **Which of the following is a contraindication of induction of labor?**
    a. Heart disease
    b. Chronic renal disease
    c. Intrauterine growth restriction (IUGR)
    d. Rh isoimmunization

26. **Which of the following parameters to be assessed prior to induction of labor?**
    a. *Assess Bishop score:* (Score >6 is favorable)
    b. Perform clinical pelvimetry to assess pelvic adequacy
    c. To ensure fetal gestational age and estimate fetal weight
    d. All of the above

27. **Which of the following is a contraindication of use of prostaglandin in labor?**
    a. Prostaglandin hypersensitivity
    b. Cases with history of previous two lower segment cesarean section (LSCS)
    c. Primigravida
    d. a + b

28. **Which of the following factors are responsible for successful induction of labor?**
    a. Bishop score ≥6 is favorable.
    b. Positive oxytocin sensitivity test
    c. Presence of fetal fibronectin (fFN) in vaginal swab (>50 ng/mL)
    d. All of the above

29. **In low rupture of the membranes (LRM) mechanism of onset of labor are related with:**
    a. Stretching of the cervix
    b. Separation of the membranes leading to liberation of progesterone
    c. Increase of amniotic fluid volume
    d. All of the above

30. **Which of the following is/are indications for induction of labor?**
    a. Rh isoimmunization
    b. Intrauterine death of the fetus
    c. Eclampsia
    d. All of the above

ANSWERS

1. **d.** All of the above
   Labor is called normal if it fulfils the following criteria:
   - Spontaneous in onset and at term
   - Vertex presentation
   - Without undue prolongation
   - Natural termination with minimal aids
   - Without having any complications affecting the health of the mother and/or the baby

2. **d.** All of the above
   Maternal contraindications for induction of labor are:
   - Abnormally implanted placenta
   - Prior uterine incision
   - Active genital herpes infection
   - Contracted or distorted pelvic anatomy
   - Cervical cancer

   Fetal factors as contraindications for induction of labor are:
   - Appreciable macrosomia
   - Severe hydrocephalus
   - Malpresentation
   - Nonreassuring fetal status

3. **b.** 18%
   In 18% of cases of induction of labor in primigravida patients, ultimately cesarean delivery is required.

4. **b.** Labor induction with oxytocin can be done in previous lower segment cesarean section (LSCS) cases.
   The American College of Obstetricians and Gynecologists recommends against the use of prostaglandins for preinduction cervical ripening or for labor induction in women with a prior uterine incision. It recognizes labor induction with oxytocin as an option but it has higher potential rupture rate and lower vaginal birth after cesarean section (VBAC) rate. Amniotomy is often selected to augment labor in previous LSCS cases.

5. **d.** a + b
   Bishop score >8 conveys a high likelihood for a successful induction and a score ≤6 is considered unfavorable.

6. **d.** All of the above
   Factors used in modified Bishop scoring system are as follows:
   - Cervical dilatation
   - Cervical length
   - Station of presenting part
   - Cervical position
   - Cervical consistency

7. **a.** Dinoprostone
   Dinoprostone is a synthetic analog of prostaglandin E2 (PGE2).
   It is available in three forms: (1) A gel, (2) a time-release vaginal insert, and (3) a 20-mg suppository.
   The gel and time-release vaginal insert formulations are indicated only for cervical ripening before labor induction. 20-mg suppository is not indicated for cervical ripening.

8. **d.** All of the above
   Following are contraindication for induction of labor using dinoprostone gel: prior dinoprostone hypersensitivity, suspicion of fetal compromise or cephalopelvic disproportion, unexplained vaginal bleeding, six or more prior term pregnancies, contraindications to vaginal delivery, women already receiving oxytocin, those with a contraindication to oxytocin, or in those who may be endangered by prolonged uterine contractions, for example, those with prior cesarean delivery or uterine surgery.

9. **a.** 25 µg
   Dose of tablet misoprostol can be used for labor induction recommended is 25 µg.

10. **b.** Intracervical prostaglandin E2 (PGE2) gel in poor Bishop score
    In labor induction:
    - Misoprostol used safely at a dose of 25 µg
    - Intracervical prostaglandin E2 (PGE2) gel is used in poor Bishop score.
    - 15-methyl-prostaglandin F2α (PGF2α) is not used for induction of labor.

11. **d.** All of the above
    Maternal complications associated with labor induction are chorioamnionitis, uterine rupture, and postpartum hemorrhage from uterine atony.

12. **a.** Advanced maternal age and primigravida
    Causes of failed induction are as follows:
    - Advanced maternal age
    - Primigravida
    - Very poor Bishop score
    - Birth weight >3.5 kg
    - Body mass index (BMI) >30

13. **b.** Severe pregnancy induced hypertension at term
    The more common indications for induction of labor include membrane rupture without labor, gestational hypertension, oligohydramnios, nonreassuring fetal status, post-term pregnancy, and various maternal medical conditions such as chronic hypertension and diabetes.

14. **a.** Prostaglandin F2α (PGF2α) tablet
    Prostaglandin F2α (PGF2α) tablet is not used for induction of labor.

15. **d.** All of the above
    Uses of partogram in induction of labor are as follows:
    - To see the progress of labor
    - To see the cervical dilatation
    - To see the descent of presenting part

    Assessment of progress of labor and partograph recording:
    - Pulse is recorded every 30 minutes and is marked with a dot (.) in the partograph.
    - Blood pressure is recorded at every 1 hour and is marked with arrows (↕)
    - Temperature is recorded at every 2 hours.
    - Urine output is recorded for volume, protein, or acetone.
    - Any drug (oxytocin or other) when given is recorded in the partograph.

    Abdominal palpation: (a) Uterine contractions as regard the frequency, intensity, and duration are assessed. The number of contractions in 10 minutes and duration of each contraction in seconds are recorded in the partograph.
    Partograph is charted every half an hour as contraction duration <20 seconds (mild); between 20 and 40 seconds (moderate), and >40 seconds (strong).

16. **b.** 4 hours
    Time interval between action line and alert line is 4 hours.

17. **d.** All of the above
    The mechanism of action of prostaglandin E2 (PGE2) gel is as follows:
    - Stimulates uterine contraction.
    - Acts on collagen present in cervix and softens it.
    - Causes cervical dilatation.

18. **b.** Action line is drawn 6 hours to the right and parallel to the alert line.
    In partograph, the alert line starts at 4 cm of cervical dilatation as per World Health Organization (WHO) and ends at 10 cm dilatation (at the rate of 1 cm/hour). The action line is drawn 4 hours to the right

and parallel to the alert line. In a normal labor, the cervicograph (cervical dilatation) should be either on the alert line or to the left of it. When it falls on zone 2, it is abnormal and needs to be critically assessed. When it falls in zone 3, case should be reassessed by a senior person. Decision is to be made either for termination of labor (cesarean section) or for augmentation of labor (amniotomy and/or oxytocin).

19. **b.** Interleukin-1 (IL-1)
Cervical balloon catheter causes cervical ripening with release of the interleukins (IL-6, IL-8), matrix metalloproteinase-8 (MMP-8), and hyaluronic acid synthetase. Balloon volumes used may be low (30 mL) or high (60–80 mL).

20. **d.** All of the above
After the membranes rupture, the following are to be assessed:
- Color of the amniotic fluid
- Status of the cervix
- Station of the head
- Detection of cord prolapse, if any
- Fetal heart rate (FHR) pattern is checked.

21. **c.** Chorioamnionitis
Potential complications of oxytocin as a method of induction are as follows:
- Water intoxication
- Uterine tachysystole
- Hypotension
- Fetal heart rate (FHR) changes

22. **d.** Hypotension
Following are potential complications of artificial rupture of the membranes (ARM):
- Cord prolapse
- Chorioamnionitis
- Infection
- Bleeding

23. **d.** All of the above
Following are contraindications of artificial rupture of the membranes (ARM):
- Woman with human immunodeficiency virus (HIV) infection
- Woman with group B Streptococcus infection
- It is preferably avoided in chronic hydramnios, as there is risk of sudden massive liquor drainage. Sudden uterine decompression may precipitate early placental separation (abruption). In such a case, controlled ARM is to be done.

24. **a.** Umbilical cord prolapse risk is high with engaged head.
In artificial rupture of the membranes (ARM), once the procedure is adopted, there is no scope of retreating from the decision of delivery. Chance of umbilical cord prolapse—the risk is low with engaged head or rupture of membranes with head fixed to the brim. Careful selection of cases with favorable preinduction score will shorten the induction–delivery interval. Meticulous asepsis during the procedure reduces the risk of chorioamnionitis. Care taken during rupture of the membranes minimizes the problem. Liquor amnii embolism can occur during ARM.

25. **a.** Heart disease
Contraindications of induction of labor are as follows: Contracted pelvis, cephalopelvic disproportion, malpresentation (breech, transverse, or oblique lie), previous classical cesarean section or hysterotomy (scarred uterus), uteroplacental factors such as unexplained vaginal bleeding, vasa previa, placenta previa, active genital herpes infection, high-risk pregnancy with fetal compromise, heart disease, pelvic tumor, elderly primigravida with obstetric or medical complications, umbilical cord prolapse, and cervical carcinoma.

26. **d.** All of the above
Parameters to be assessed prior to induction:
- To confirm the indication for induction of labor (IOL)
- Exclude the contraindication of IOL
- *Assess Bishop score:* (Score >6 is favorable)
- Perform clinical pelvimetry to assess pelvic adequacy
- To ensure fetal gestational age
- *To estimate fetal weight:* Clinical and USG
- Ensure fetal lung maturation status
- Ensure fetal presentation and lie confirm fetal well-being

27. **d.** a + b
Contraindications of use of prostaglandin in labor include prior dinoprostone hypersensitivity, previous lower segment cesarean section (LSCS), suspicion of fetal compromise or cephalopelvic disproportion, unexplained vaginal bleeding, six or more prior term pregnancies, and contraindications to vaginal delivery.

28. **d.** All of the above
    - Predictive factors for successful induction of labor are period of gestation, pregnancy nearer the term or post-term—more is the success.
    - Bishop score ≥6 is favorable.
    - Positive oxytocin sensitivity test is favorable for induction of labor (IOL)
    - Cervical ripening is favorable in multiparous and in cases with premature rupture of membranes (PROM). Less responsive in elderly primigravidae or cases with prolonged retention of dead fetus.
    - Presence of fetal fibronectin (fFN) in vaginal swab (>50 ng/mL) favorable for successful IOL
    - Other positive factors: Maternal height >5', normal body mass index (BMI), and estimated fetal weight (EFW) <3 kg

29. **a.** Stretching of the cervix
    In low rupture of the membranes (LRM), mechanism of onset of labor is related with:
    - Stretching of the cervix
    - Separation of the membranes (liberation of prostaglandins)
    - Reduction of amniotic fluid volume

30. **d.** All of the above
    Indications for induction of labor (IOL):
    - Preeclampsia, eclampsia (hypertensive disorders in pregnancy)
    - Maternal medical complications: Diabetes mellitus, chronic renal disease, and cholestasis of pregnancy
    - Postmaturity
    - Abruptio placentae
    - Intrauterine growth restriction (IUGR)
    - Rh isoimmunization
    - Premature rupture of membranes
    - Fetus with a major congenital anomaly
    - Intrauterine death of the fetus
    - Oligohydramnios
    - Polyhydramnios
    - Unstable lie—after correction into longitudinal lie
    - Maternal request

REFERENCES

1. Cunningham FG, Leveno KJ, Dashe JS, Hoffman BL, Spong CY, Casey BM (Eds). Williams Obstetrics, 26th edition. New York: McGraw Hill; 2022.
2. Konar H. DC Dutta's Textbook of Obstetrics, 10th edition. New Delhi: Jaypee Brothers Medical Publishers (P) Ltd.; 2022.

Chapter 53

Operative Obstetrics

Nandita Palshetkar, Rohan Palshetkar

QUESTIONS

1. All of the following are changes that occur to the fetal circulation within minutes of birth, *except* for:
   a. Constriction of the umbilical vessels
   b. Constriction of the ductus venosus
   c. Constriction of the ductus arteriosus
   d. Constriction of the hepatic portal sinus
   e. Closure of the foramen ovale

2. Levels of human chorionic gonadotropin (hCG) in the maternal circulation typically peak at what level and at what gestation age?
   a. 100,000 mIU/mL at 10 weeks
   b. 10,000 mIU/mL at 10 weeks
   c. 10,000 mIU/mL at 20 weeks
   d. 100,000 mIU/mL at 40 weeks

3. Which of the following observations would *not* be expected to be seen on an obstetric ultrasound at 7 weeks gestation?
   a. Chorionic sac
   b. Yolk sac
   c. Embryo with cardiac activity
   d. Physiological bowel herniation

4. Which of the following organisms is the most common cause of early onset neonatal conjunctivitis?
   a. Guillain–Barré syndrome (GBS)
   b. Toxoplasmosis
   c. Chlamydia
   d. Trichomoniasis

5. A 24-year-old G2P1 presents at 36 weeks' gestation in active labor. Her Guillain–Barré syndrome culture is not available. Which of the following represents the most appropriate management in this setting?
   a. Do nothing
   b. Administer Guillain–Barré syndrome chemoprophylaxis empirically
   c. Administer antibiotics only if she develops a fever
   d. Send a GBS perineal culture and wait for the result to decide whether or not to give antibiotics

6. Congenital syndromes related to viral infections are most likely to occur if the mother contracts the illness during which of the following trimesters?
   a. In the first trimester
   b. In the second trimester
   c. In the third trimester
   d. Postpartum

7. A patient presents for her first prenatal visit at 10 weeks' gestation. Her routine prenatal intake laboratory tests reveal that she is not immune to rubella. What should you recommend?
   a. Administer measles-mumps-rubella (MMR) vaccination now
   b. Administer MMR vaccination at 28 weeks
   c. Administer MMR vaccination postpartum
   d. She does not need MMR vaccination

8. Which of the following infections are sexually transmitted?
   a. Human immunodeficiency virus (HIV)
   b. Herpes
   c. Syphilis
   d. Chlamydia infection
   e. All of the above

9. A patient who is a chronic hepatitis B carrier delivers vaginally at 39 weeks' gestation. The baby should receive which of the following therapies on the first day of life?
   a. Hepatitis B immune globulin (HBIG)
   b. Hepatitis B vaccination
   c. Hepatitis B immune globulin and hepatitis B vaccination
   d. None of the above

10. A patient, 12 weeks pregnant, come to the emergency department with abdominal cramping and moderate vaginal bleeding. Speculum examination reveals 2–3 cm cervical dilation. What is the diagnosis?
    a. Threatened abortion
    b. Inevitable abortion
    c. Complete abortion
    d. Missed abortion

11. Which is *not* the predisposing factor for hyperemesis gravidarum (HG)?
    a. Multiple pregnancies
    b. Primi para
    c. First trimester
    d. Malnutrition

12. Which of the following is *correct* about the measurement of uterus fundal height at various stages of gestation in pregnant women?
    a. At 6 weeks, you can feel it in the abdomen
    b. At 12 weeks, it is at the umbilical level
    c. At 20 weeks, it reaches pelvic girdle
    d. At 36 weeks, it felt at lower part of sternum

13. What is the recommended period for taking a postcoital contraceptive pill after unprotected intercourse?
    a. Within a week
    b. Within 4 days
    c. Within 3 days
    d. Within 5 days

14. Reproductive age in women starts when their:
    a. Menstruation starts
    b. Breasts start developing
    c. Body weight increases
    d. Height increases

15. This phase is so named because it is when the follicles in the ovary grow and form a mature egg. Name the phase:
    a. Luteal phase
    b. Follicular phase
    c. Ovulation
    d. Menstruation

16. Which of the following assessment findings of a pregnant lady determine that she is in the second stage of labor?
    a. Artificial rupture of membranes is done
    b. Cervix is dilated completely
    c. Contractions are regular and lasting for 30–45 seconds
    d. Show is noted

17. Which of the following statements about breastfeeding is *correct*?
    a. Breastfed infants have fewer allergies
    b. Women who breastfeed have a lower risk of breast cancer in later life
    c. Breastfed infants gain more weight and gain weight more quickly
    d. Both a and b

18. Which of the following statements about postpartum hemorrhage (PPH) is *true*?
    a. Postpartum hemorrhage should be diagnosed if there is 2,500 mL estimated blood loss after vaginal delivery
    b. Postpartum hemorrhage should be diagnosed if there is a drop in hematocrit of ≥10% after delivery
    c. Postpartum hemorrhage complicates approximately 5% of all deliveries
    d. All of the above

19. Which of the following statements regarding cesarean section delivery is *true*?
    a. Maternal morbidity is significantly increased with cesarean compared with vaginal delivery
    b. Elective cesarean section delivery can be performed before 39 weeks' gestation without documenting fetal lung maturity
    c. Elective surgeries (such as myomectomy) can be performed safely at the time of cesarean section
    d. A desire for permanent sterilization by bilateral tubal ligation is an acceptable indication for cesarean section delivery

20. Nonreassuring elements of intrapartum fetal heart rate monitoring patterns include which of the following?
    a. Minimal or absent variability
    b. Absence of accelerations
    c. Bradycardia or tachycardia
    d. Both a and c

21. A 37-year-old G2P1L1 presents at 40 weeks for elective induction of labor. Her prior delivery was by cesarean section for breech presentation at term. Which of the following methods of inducing labor is absolutely contraindicated in this setting?
    a. Oxytocin
    b. Membrane stripping
    c. Transcervical Foley catheter
    d. Vaginal administration of prostaglandin E2

22. In monozygous twin pregnancy, what type of chorionicity results when the blastocyst divides between days 9 and 12 postconception?
    a. Conjoined twins
    b. Dichorionic/diamniotic placentation
    c. Monochorionic/monoamniotic placentation
    d. Monochorionic/diamniotic placentation

CHAPTER 53: Operative Obstetrics

23. At what gestational age is the amniotic fluid volume at its maximum?
    a. 22 weeks
    b. 26 weeks
    c. 30 weeks
    d. 34 weeks

24. What is the single most useful test in identifying the cause of an as yet unexplained term intrauterine fetal demise?
    a. Serologic testing for antiphospholipid antibody syndrome
    b. Kleihauer-Betke test
    c. Fetal autopsy
    d. Urine toxicology

25. Which of the following medications is *not* associated with central nervous system (CNS) abnormalities?
    a. Valproic acid
    b. Methotrexate
    c. Tegretol
    d. Thalidomide

26. Medications that may be acceptable for use in pregnancy include which of the following FDA categories?
    a. Category A
    b. Category B
    c. Category C
    d. All of the above

27. Which of the following drugs is a known fetal teratogen?
    a. Marijuana
    b. Alcohol
    c. Heroin
    d. Caffeine

28. All of the following pregnancy/neonatal complications are associated with maternal cigarette smoking except one. Which is the exception?
    a. Low birth weight
    b. Sudden infant death syndrome (SIDS)
    c. Preeclampsia
    d. Preterm labor

29. Which of the following agents is a known teratogen in humans?
    a. Vitamin A
    b. Vancomycin
    c. Oral contraceptives
    d. Metronidazole

30. Which of the following medications is recommended most commonly for the treatment of maternal hyperthyroidism in pregnancy?
    a. Carbimazole
    b. Propylthiouracil (PTU)
    c. Levothyroxine
    d. Radioactive iodine

ANSWERS

1. **d.** Constriction of the hepatic portal sinus
   Within minutes of birth, the fetal circulatory system undergoes marked changes, which include constriction of the umbilical vessels, constriction of the ductus arteriosus and ductus venosus, and closure of the foramen ovale. The hepatic portal sinus does not close.

2. **a.** 100,000 mIU/mL at 10 weeks
   Human chorionic gonadotropin is produced by the syncytiotrophoblast and the levels increase in the maternal serum from the moment of implantation. In a singleton pregnancy, levels peak at around 10 weeks of gestation at a concentration of approximately 100,000 mIU/mL.

3. **d.** Physiological bowel herniation
   Sonographic findings of physiologic bowel herniation would be expected to be seen only at 8–12 weeks of gestation. Therefore, on a 7-week ultrasound would not be expected to demonstrate this finding.

4. **c.** Chlamydia
   Several organisms can cause neonatal conjunctivitis, but the most common cause is *Chlamydia trachomatis*. Moreover, many women with chlamydia infection are asymptomatic. For this reason, it is routine practice in the USA to administer erythromycin or silver nitrate prophylaxis to the eyes of all infants within 1 hour of birth.

5. **b.** Administer Guillain-Barré syndrome chemoprophylaxis empirically
   If a patient presents in labor and her GBS perineal carrier status is unknown, she should be treated with intrapartum GBS chemoprophylaxis only if she has one or more of the following risk factors: (1) if she is preterm, (2) if she had a prior infant with GBS sepsis, (3) if she had GBS bacteriuria in the index pregnancy, (4) if she has rupture of membranes >18 hours, or (5) if she has a fever. A GBS culture typically takes 48 hours to perform, so it is too late to send in labor. The rapid GBS test is not reliable; as such, it is not recommended that a rapid GBS test be sent in labor.

6. **a.** In the first trimester
   If a maternal viral illness is contracted in the first trimester, it increases the chance that a congenital syndrome could result from the infection, e.g., if chickenpox is contracted in the first trimester, the chance of the fetus developing congenital varicella syndrome is much higher. If the illness is contracted in the third trimester, it is more likely to result in an infection resembling the childhood infection.

7. **c.** Administer mumps-measles-rubella (MMR) vaccination postpartum

    Mumps-measles-rubella is a live attenuated trivalent vaccine.

    As such, it should not be administered during pregnancy. It should be administered shortly after delivery.

8. **e.** All of the above

    All of the above listed infections (HIV, herpes, syphilis, and chlamydia infection) can be transmitted through sexual intercourse.

9. **c.** Hepatitis B immune globulin and hepatitis B vaccination

    Hepatitis B viral (HBV) infection can be transmitted vertically from mother to infant. To prevent such transmission, infants born to women who have HBV infection should receive HBIG and hepatitis B vaccination on the first day of life. Additional hepatitis B vaccination is required at 6 weeks and 6 months of age. Women with HBV infection can breastfeed.

10. **b.** Inevitable abortion

    Inevitable abortion:
    - In medical terms, it is also known as a spontaneous abortion and pregnancy loss.
    - It is the death of an embryo or fetus before it can survive.
    - The most common symptom of a miscarriage is vaginal bleeding with or without pain.
    - Tissue and clot-like material may leave the uterus and pass through and out of the vagina.
    - About 80% of miscarriages occur in the first 12 weeks of pregnancy.
    - Diagnosis of a miscarriage may involve checking to see if the cervix is open or closed, testing blood levels of human chorionic gonadotropin and an ultrasound.

    Threatened abortion:
    - The term threatened abortion is used when there is vaginal bleeding before 20 weeks gestation.
    - It may be accompanied by abdominal aching or cramping.
    - Incidence is that 25% of pregnant women experience some quantity of vaginal bleeding, of these, 50% ultimately miscarry.

    Complete abortion: It is a completed miscarriage.

    Missed abortion:
    - It is a miscarriage in which the fetus did not form or has died, but the placenta and embryonic tissues are still inside the uterus.
    - It is known more commonly as a missed miscarriage.
    - It is also sometimes called a silent miscarriage.

11. **d.** Malnutrition

    Hyperemesis gravidarum
    - It is a pregnancy complication that is characterized by severe nausea, vomiting, weight loss, and possibly dehydration.
    - Risk factors include the first pregnancy, multiple pregnancies, obesity, prior or family history of HG, trophoblastic disorder, and a history of eating disorders.
    - It tends to occur in the first trimester of pregnancy.

    Malnutrition:
    - It refers to deficiencies, excesses or imbalances ii a person's intake of energy and/or nutrients. It is "a deficiency, excess, or imbalance of energy, protein, and other nutrients" which adversely affects the body's tissues and form.
    - It is estimated that nearly one in three persons globally suffers from at least one form of malnutrition: wasting, stunting, vitamin or mineral deficiency, overweight, obesity, or diet-related noncommunicable diseases
    - *Causes of malnutrition include:*
        - Unsuitable dietary choices
        - Having a low income
        - Difficulty obtaining food
    - *Malnutrition can lead to:*
        - Short- and long-term health problems
        - Slow recovery from wounds and illnesses
        - A higher risk of infection

    Multiple pregnancies:
    - Pregnancy with more than one fetus is called multiple pregnancies.
    - There are two main ways that multiple pregnancies can happen:
        1. One fertilized egg (ovum) splits before it implants in the uterine lining
        2. Two or more separate eggs are fertilized by different sperm at the same time.

    Primi para:
    - A woman who has given birth once is primiparous and is referred to as a primipara.
    - The birth of a child occurs beyond the 20th week of pregnancy or beyond the stage of abortion.

First trimester:
- It is the earliest phase of pregnancy.
- It starts on the first day of the last period and lasts until the end of the 13th week.
- Rapid changes for both mother and baby occur.

12. **d.** At 36 weeks, it felt at lower part of sternum
Fundal height:
- It is the distance between the pubic bone and the top of the uterus during pregnancy.
- It helps healthcare providers to assess whether the baby is growing correctly or not.
- It determines the gestational age and the baby's position in the uterus.

Explanation:
At 36 weeks, it felt in the lower part of the sternum:
- The location of the fundus moves as pregnancy progresses
- At around 36 weeks, fundus reaches the sternum or breastbone
- At 36 weeks, it reaches the highest point
- After 63 weeks, fundal height can decrease because the baby has engaged in the pelvis to prepare for labor or other reasons.

At 6 weeks, you can feel it in the abdomen:
- At 6 weeks pregnant, a baby is the size of a sweet pea.
- The uterus can sometimes be easily flexed at the markedly softened isthmus.
- A cavity that is consistent with pregnancy can be detected within the uterus using ultrasound.
- The feeling of cramping and bloating occurs and the belly feels a little bigger than normal.

At 12 weeks, it is at the umbilical level:
- The uterus is larger than the pelvic area and rises into the abdomen.
- The uterus can be felt above the pubic bone.
- At 12 weeks, babies can open and close their hands and curl their toes.

At 20 weeks, it reaches the pelvic girdle:
- The upper point of the uterus is at the level of the woman's belly button.
- It is the time when fundal height and week of pregnancy begin to match one another.
- At 20 weeks, baby is the size of a banana.
- At 20 weeks pregnant, weight gain is happening slowly.

13. **c.** Within 3 days
Oral contraceptive pills or birth control pills are pills containing a number of hormones that help to prevent unwanted pregnancy.
- Postcoital pills are to be taken within 72 hours of or 3 days of unprotected sex.
- There are mainly three types of oral contraceptive pills:
  1. Combined estrogen-progesterone
  2. Progesterone-only
  3. Continuous or extended use pill

Mechanism of action:
- Progesterone is the hormone that is responsible for pregnancy. Progesterone in the birth control pill mainly inhibits the mechanism of ovulation, which further inhibits follicular development.
- After drug administration, progesterone negative feedback mechanism acts on the hypothalamus and it reduces the action of gonadotropin-releasing hormone and also decreases the level of follicle-stimulating hormone (FSH) and luteinizing hormone.
- These hormonal changes will prevent follicle development.
- Another primary mechanism of action says that progesterone inhibits the ability of sperm to penetrate through the cervix and upper genital tract by changing the normal flora of the cervical mucus.

14. **a.** Menstruation starts
Reproductive age in women:
- In females, the reproductive phase of life begins at puberty (10–12 years of age) and generally lasts till the age of approximately 45–50 years.
- The ova begin to mature with the onset of puberty.
- One ovum matures and is released by one of the ovaries once in about 28–30 days.
- During this period, the wall of the uterus becomes thick so as to receive the egg, in case it is fertilized and begins to develop.
- This results in pregnancy. If fertilization does not occur, the released egg and the thickened lining of the uterus along with its blood vessels are shed off.
- This causes bleeding in women which is called menstruation.
- Menstruation occurs once in about 28–30 days.
- The first menstrual flow begins at puberty and is termed menarche.

- At 45-50 years of age, the menstrual cycle stops.
- The stoppage of menstruation is termed menopause.

15. **b.** Follicular phase

The menstrual period cycle progresses in four main phases:

1. *Menstruation:*
   - In this phase, menstrual fluid consisting of blood, mucus, and the cells of the uterine lining is eliminated through the vaginal opening.
   - It can last anywhere between 2 and 7 days.
2. *Follicular phase:*
   - The follicular phase of the menstrual cycle begins from the first day of the period and lasts up until ovulation
   - In the course of this phase, estrogen levels rise, and the ovaries prepare for the release of an egg for possible fertilization
   - The follicular phase also stimulates the phase where the uterine lining begins to build again
3. *Ovulation:*
   - In this phase, the ovaries release the egg. It travels through the fallopian tubes and implants itself on to the lining along the walls of your uterus.
   - This phase usually occurs around 2 weeks prior to your period.
   - During this process, the estrogen level peaks and drops just shortly after
   - The typical life span of this egg is about 24 hours. Unless it is fertilized by a sperm cell during this window, it dies and is shed along with the uterine lining.
4. *Luteal phase:*
   - The phase that occurs between ovulation and the first day of your period is called the luteal phase.
   - This phase sees a rise in the level of progesterone, required to maintain the thickness of the uterine lining to nurture the fertilized egg.
   - If during that time, pregnancy does not occur, progesterone levels drop.
   - This causes the uterine lining to break down and shed away, along with other menstrual fluid.

16. **b.** Cervix is dilated completely

The second stage of labor refers to the time interval from full cervical dilation (10 cm) to delivery of the fetus, regardless of when the patient started pushing. The normal duration of the second stage of labor for a nulliparous patient is <3 hours with an epidural and <2 hours without an epidural (for a multiparous patient, <2 hours with an epidural and <1 hour without an epidural).

17. **d.** Both a and b

Breastfeeding has many advantages including a decreased risk of allergies in infants who are breastfed for 6 months. It is also known to be protective against the subsequent development of breast cancer.

18. **d.** All of the above

The traditional definition of postpartum hemorrhage is an estimated blood loss after vaginal delivery of 2,500 mL. However, obstetric care providers typically underestimate blood loss by 30-50%. The American Congress of Obstetricians and Gynecologists (ACOG) has therefore recommended that a diagnosis of PPH should be made if: (1) there is a drop in hematocrit of ≥10% after delivery or (2) the patient receives a blood transfusion. PPH complicates approximately 5% of all deliveries.

19. **a.** Maternal morbidity is significantly increased with cesarean compared with vaginal delivery.

Cesarean section delivery is major abdominal surgery and is associated with an increased risk of surgical morbidity compared with vaginal delivery including increased blood loss, infectious morbidity, and venous thromboembolic events.

20. **d.** Both a and c

Decreased variability and an alteration in baseline (bradycardia or tachycardia) are concerning features on intrapartum fetal heart rate monitoring.

21. **d.** Vaginal administration of prostaglandin E2

Prostaglandin medications should be regarded as absolutely contraindicated for cervical ripening at term in the setting of a prior cesarean section delivery.

22. **c.** Monochorionic/monoamniotic placentation

Chorionicity is defined as the arrangement of the placenta/fetal membranes in a multiple pregnancy. In monozygous twins (i.e., identical twins arising from a single embryo), dichorionic/diamniotic placentation results if the embryo divides before day 3 postconception, monochorionic/diamniotic placentation results if the embryo divides between days 4 and 8 postconception, and monochorionic/

monoamniotic placentation if the embryo divides between days 9 and 12 postconception. If division occurs after day 12 postconception, the embryo never completely separates and a conjoined twin pregnancy results.

23. **c.** 30 weeks

    Amniotic fluid volume is maximal at around 30–32 weeks' gestation (800–1,000 mL). Thereafter, amniotic fluid volume decreases slowly to term (400–500 mL) and then more rapidly after 40 weeks.

24. **c.** Fetal autopsy

    Fetal autopsy and pathologic examination of the placenta/fetal membranes are the most valuable tests to identify the cause of a term intrauterine fetal demise. Other tests that may have some value include serologic testing for antiphospholipid antibody syndrome, Kleihauer–Betke test (to identify a large fetal-maternal hemorrhage), and urine toxicology (which may identify maternal drug abuse). Serologic testing for TORCH (toxoplasmosis, rubella, cytomegalovirus, herpes) infections are low yield and not cost-effective.

25. **d.** Thalidomide

    In utero exposure to valproic acid, methotrexate and tegretol have all been associated with central nervous system abnormalities in fetuses, especially neural tube defects.

    Thalidomide has been associated with bilateral limb deficiencies, microtia/anotia (small or absent eyes), cardiac and gastrointestinal anomalies, but *not* CNS abnormalities.

26. **d.** All of the above

    The Food and Drug Administration (FDA) in the USA has defined five risk categories for medication use in pregnancy (A, B, C, D, X). Individual agents are assigned to a risk category according to their risk-benefit ratio. If, in the judgment of the care provider, the benefit to the patient outweighs the risk to the pregnancy, then it is reasonable to prescribe that drug for use in pregnancy. Category X includes drugs that are regarded as absolutely contraindicated in pregnancy, such as radioactive iodine and methotrexate. Interestingly, although oral contraceptives are not teratogenic, they are classified as category X because there is no benefit to being on the combined oral contraceptive pill once you are pregnant; this is a good illustration of the risk–benefit ratio of this classification system.

27. **b.** Alcohol

    Fetal alcohol syndrome (FAS) is the most common preventable cause of congenital learning disability. It is a difficult diagnosis to make antenatally, but is commonly associated with intrauterine growth restriction (IUGR). Marijuana and cigarette smoking are not associated with birth defects.

28. **c.** Preeclampsia

    Maternal cigarette smoking is associated with preterm labor, preterm premature rupture of membranes (PROM), low birth weight, and sudden infant death syndrome. Interestingly, it is protective against the development of preeclampsia (as it is for endometrial cancer and ulcerative colitis flares).

29. **a.** Vitamin A

    Vitamin A is a known human teratogen if taken orally in the first trimester of pregnancy. Topical vitamin A ointments are best avoided in pregnancy, although the risk to the fetus is not well quantified. Oral contraceptives and antibiotics are not generally regarded as being teratogenic (with the exception of tetracyclines, which discolor and weaken developing bones and teeth).

30. **b.** Propylthiouracil

    Both propylthiouracil and methimazole are thioamide medications and are commonly used for the treatment of hyperthyroidism in pregnancy. The former is generally we preferred because it acts both to reduce T4 production and release from the thyroid gland and to prevent conversion of T4 to T3 in peripheral tissues. Methimazole has been associated with aplasia cutis in the offspring, although this association is weak. PTU has been associated with liver disease in the mother.

Chapter 54: Intrauterine Growth Restriction

Priyankur Roy

QUESTIONS

1. **What is one of the solitary parameters for late-onset fetal growth restriction (FGR) (≥32 weeks)?**
   a. Abdominal circumference (AC) or estimated fetal weight (EFW) <5th centile
   b. AC or EFW <3rd centile
   c. AC or EFW <10th centile
   d. AC or EFW <2nd centile

2. **Why is there a call for the inclusion of reduced growth velocity in the definition of fetal growth restriction (FGR) in future guidelines?**
   a. Because fetuses with a >30% reduction in estimated fetal weight (EFW) are likely to have a higher birthweight
   b. Because fetuses with a >30% reduction in estimated fetal weight (EFW) are more likely to be acidotic at birth
   c. Because fetuses with a >30% reduction in EFW have a higher cerebroplacental ratio
   d. Because fetuses with a >30% reduction in EFW are likely to have a higher percentage body fat

3. **What does recent research say about the effectiveness of low-dose aspirin in women identified as high risk during the first trimester?**
   a. Low-dose aspirin has no significant effect on reducing the risk of preeclampsia
   b. Low-dose aspirin leads to a marked reduction in the risk of late-onset preeclampsia
   c. Low-dose aspirin leads to a marked reduction in the risk of early-onset preeclampsia
   d. Low-dose aspirin leads to a marked increase in the risk of early-onset preeclampsia

4. **What does the Canadian guideline suggest regarding the use of heparin to prevent small for gestational age (SGA) fetuses?**
   a. Heparin should be offered in selected women
   b. Heparin is effective in preventing fetal growth restriction (FGR) in all women
   c. Heparin should not be offered to any women
   d. Heparin is particularly effective in women with thrombophilia

5. **What is the role of second trimester uterine artery Doppler velocimetry screening in the general population?**
   a. It has a high predictive value for late-onset fetal growth restriction (FGR) in all women
   b. It has a modest ability to predict late-onset fetal growth restriction (FGR)
   c. It has a significant ability to predict late-onset FGR in high-risk women only
   d. It is not recommended for predicting late-onset FGR

6. **Mrs A, a 28-year-old primi at 30 weeks of gestation, came for her prenatal checkup. She has history of bronchial asthma and is on inhalers and her pregnancy had been smooth until now. However, an ultrasound examination revealed an estimated fetal weight below the 10th percentile for gestational age and there was a reversal of end-diastolic flow in the umbilical artery. She was understandably concerned and asked what the next steps would be.**
   a. Continue the pregnancy to full term without any intervention
   b. Start her on a regimen of dietary supplements and vitamins to improve fetal growth

c. Arrange for immediate delivery of the baby through an emergency cesarean section
d. Admit her for close monitoring and consider early delivery depending on the clinical condition

7. **Which of the following is correct about fundal height measurements?**
   a. Fundal height measurements are not reliable for women with obesity and/or fibroid uterus
   b. Fundal height measurements are always accurate, regardless of maternal weight
   c. Fundal height measurements should always be plotted on a customized chart
   d. Fundal height measurements are an excellent primary screening tool for predicting low birth weight and small for gestational age (SGA)

8. **What does the Growth Assessment Protocol (GAP) aim to achieve?**
   a. It aims to reduce the rate of stillbirth and improve the detection of small for gestational age (SGA) infants before birth
   b. It aims to increase the rate of early delivery for at-risk mothers
   c. It aims to ensure all mothers undergo a third trimester scan
   d. It aims to implement universal use of heparin in pregnancy

9. **What was the conclusion of the Disproportionate Intrauterine Growth Intervention Trial at Term study on the timing of delivery in late-onset fetal growth restriction (FGR)?**
   a. Delivery at 38 weeks may be optimal, unless there are earlier concerns about fetal well-being
   b. Early delivery is always better in cases of suspected FGR
   c. There was no difference between the induction of labor and expectant management groups
   d. Induction at <38 weeks was associated with increased neonatal unit admission

10. **What are the TRUFFLE study findings on the timing of delivery in early-onset fetal growth restriction (FGR)?**
    a. Waiting until late changes occur in the ductus venosus (DV) or abnormal cardiotocography (CTG) is associated with improved outcomes at 2 years of age
    b. Early delivery is always the best option in cases of early-onset FGR
    c. Cardiotocography (CTG) abnormalities have no bearing on the timing of delivery in early-onset FGR
    d. The timing of delivery in early-onset FGR should be determined on a case-by-case basis

11. **What is the controversy regarding defining small for gestational age (SGA) at birth?**
    a. Whether SGA at birth should be defined using customized, population, or ethnic-specific standards
    b. Whether SGA at birth should always be defined using population standards
    c. Whether SGA at birth should be defined using the mother's weight alone
    d. Whether SGA at birth should always be defined using ethnic-specific standards

12. **How does customization of birth weight measurements impact the detection of small for gestational age (SGA) infants?**
    a. It reduces the detection of SGA infants
    b. It does not change the detection rate of SGA infants.
    c. It increases the detection of SGA infants at risk of perinatal death
    d. It has no significant impact on the detection of SGA infants

13. **What does the American College of Obstetricians and Gynecologists (ACOG) guidelines suggest about the use of PAPP-A as a stand-alone screening test for small for gestational age (SGA)?**
    a. It is recommended by all guidelines as a stand-alone screening test for SGA
    b. It is recommended by half of the guidelines as a stand-alone screening test for SGA
    c. No guidelines recommend it as a stand-alone screening test for SGA
    d. It is considered unreliable as a stand-alone screening test for SGA

14. **What is a significant research priority in intrauterine growth restriction (IUGR)?**
    a. The potential benefits and harms of early delivery in late-onset small for gestational age (SGA) pregnancies
    b. The reliability of ultrasound population charts
    c. The necessity of routine late third trimester ultrasound
    d. All of the above

15. Which of the following is true about the use of customized fetal biometry standards?
    a. They may have limited applicability in high-resource settings
    b. They are generated under optimal conditions, excluding pathology
    c. They always account for individual maternal characteristics
    d. They have limited utility in detecting small for gestational age (SGA) infants

16. Why do population ultrasound references have limited generalizability?
    a. They are specific to the population they are generated in
    b. They do not account for maternal ethnicity
    c. They often use routine, hospital-based data
    d. All of the above

17. What is considered a major risk factor for a small for gestational age (SGA) fetus/neonate?
    a. High maternal body mass index (BMI)
    b. Single minor risk factor
    c. A low level (<0.415 MoM) of the first trimester marker PAPP-A
    d. First trimester Down syndrome markers

18. What is the optimal management for a woman with an abnormal uterine artery Doppler at 20–24 weeks of pregnancy?
    a. Immediate delivery
    b. No further monitoring required
    c. Serial ultrasound measurement of fetal size and assessment of well-being with umbilical artery Doppler commencing at 26–28 weeks of pregnancy
    d. Administration of dietary supplements

19. Which intervention has proven to be effective in preventing small for gestational age (SGA) birth in women at high risk of preeclampsia, even though the effect size is small?
    a. Dietary modification   b. Antiplatelet agents
    c. Progesterone   d. Calcium

20. In a severely small for gestational age fetus detected before 23 weeks, especially with normal uterine artery Doppler, which investigation is most appropriate?
    a. Serological screening for cytomegalovirus (CMV) and toxoplasmosis
    b. Testing for syphilis and malaria
    c. Uterine artery Doppler
    d. Karyotyping

21. What is the recommended surveillance tool in the high-risk population for small for gestational age (SGA) fetus?
    a. Cardiotocography (CTG)
    b. Middle cerebral artery (MCA) Doppler
    c. Uterine artery Doppler
    d. Umbilical artery Doppler

22. When should surveillance be repeated in small for gestational age (SGA) fetuses with normal umbilical artery Doppler flow indices?
    a. Daily
    b. Every 14 days
    c. Once a month
    d. Every 7 days

23. Which Doppler should be used for surveillance and timing of delivery in a preterm small for gestational age (SGA) fetus with an abnormal umbilical artery Doppler?
    a. Cardiotocography (CTG)
    b. Middle cerebral artery (MCA) Doppler
    c. Uterine artery Doppler
    d. Ductus venosus Doppler

24. In terms of research priorities related to small for gestational age (SGA) neonates, which area does not need further evaluation according to the text?
    a. The effect of routine third trimester ultrasound assessment of fetal size and umbilical artery Doppler on substantive clinical endpoints
    b. The health economic benefit of investment in maternity services to provide recommendations in this guideline and future health outcomes of the children
    c. Introducing customized symphysis fundal height (SFH) and estimated fetal weight (EFW) charts into clinical practice on substantive clinical endpoints
    d. The effect of antiplatelet agents on women with no risk of delivering a SGA neonate

25. What condition is magnesium sulfate prophylaxis most commonly recommended for in growth-restricted fetuses?
    a. Intrauterine growth restriction (IUGR)
    b. Gestational diabetes
    c. Preterm labor
    d. Hypertensive disorders in pregnancy

CHAPTER 54: Intrauterine Growth Restriction

26. According to the provided information, what is the recommended gestational age threshold for initiating magnesium sulfate prophylaxis?
    a. <32–33 weeks
    b. <32 weeks
    c. <30 weeks
    d. <29 weeks

27. Why is the identification of fetal growth restriction (FGR) not always straightforward?
    a. Because a single biometric measurement of fetal size is usually sufficient for evaluation
    b. Because additional biophysical tools and evaluations are not necessary
    c. Because a single biometric measurement of fetal size is often not sufficient for evaluation
    d. Because there is a single phenotype of FGR that can easily be diagnosed

28. Once the diagnosis of fetal growth restriction (FGR) has been made, what is the recommended course of action?
    a. Multimodality assessment including Doppler velocimetry, computerized cardiotocography (cCTG), and biophysical profile (BPP)
    b. Immediate delivery of the fetus
    c. Immediate surgical intervention
    d. No specific action is needed

29. What is the major difference between early-onset and late-onset fetal growth restriction (FGR)?
    a. Early-onset FGR is associated more strongly with abnormal trophoblastic invasion and placental insufficiency
    b. Late-onset FGR is associated more strongly with abnormal trophoblastic invasion and placental insufficiency
    c. Both early-onset and late-onset FGR present severe prematurity
    d. There is no significant difference between early-onset and late-onset FGR

30. What is the current challenge in the management of fetal growth restriction (FGR) pregnancies?
    a. Lack of technologies and tools for differentiating between SGA and FGR
    b. Uncertainty about the feasibility of therapeutic intervention in FGR
    c. Doppler evaluation of cerebral blood-flow redistribution is not beneficial
    d. There is clear evidence on all aspects of management of FGR

ANSWERS

1. **b.** AC or EFW <3rd centile
   Either an abdominal circumference (AC) or an estimated fetal weight (EFW) falling below the 3rd centile are solitary parameters for late-onset FGR.

2. **b.** Because fetuses with a >30% reduction in estimated fetal weight (EFW) are more likely to be acidotic at birth.
   The fetuses with a >30% reduction in EFW are more likely to be acidotic at birth, have an abnormal cerebroplacental ratio, and lower body fat percentage. This information supports the inclusion of reduced growth velocity in FGR definitions.

3. **c.** Low-dose aspirin leads to a marked reduction in the risk of early-onset preeclampsia
   Recent studies have demonstrated a significant reduction in the risk of early-onset preeclampsia in women identified as high risk during the first trimester and treated with low-dose aspirin in the evening.

4. **a.** Heparin should be offered in selected women.
   The Canadian guideline, according to the chapter, recommends offering heparin to selected women. However, it's important to note that it is not effective in preventing FGR in women with severe or early-onset FGR or thrombophilia.

5. **b.** It has a modest ability to predict late-onset fetal growth restriction (FGR).
   The second trimester uterine artery Doppler velocimetry screening has a modest ability to predict late-onset FGR in the general population, but its predictive value is limited, and a normal test may rule out FGR in women with a baseline increase in risk.

6. **d.** Admit her for close monitoring and consider early delivery depending on the clinical condition
   The finding of reversal of end-diastolic flow in the umbilical artery in a fetus with intrauterine growth restriction (IUGR) is concerning. It is associated with significant risks including stillbirth, neonatal death, and long-term neurodevelopmental complications. Management usually involves close fetal surveillance, ideally in a hospital setting. Depending on the gestational age, the severity of the Doppler abnormalities, and the presence of any additional signs of fetal compromise, early delivery might be necessary, balancing the risks of prematurity with

the risks of a hostile in utero environment. The other options are not optimal: (a) Risks severe fetal complications or stillbirth, (b) would not reverse severe placental insufficiency that led to reversed end-diastolic flow, (c) immediate delivery may not be necessary and could lead to complications associated with prematurity if the baby's condition remains stable under close monitoring.

7. **a.** Fundal height measurements are not reliable for women with obesity and/or fibroid uterus.

    Guidelines recommend considering ultrasound scans in women with obesity, multiple gestations, and/or a fibroid uterus, as fundal height measurements are not reliable in these cases.

8. **a.** It aims to reduce the rate of stillbirth and improve the detection of small for gestational age (SGA) infants before birth

    The Growth Assessment Protocol (GAP), a UK initiative, is designed to standardize the measurement of fundal height and plotting on customized growth charts, aiming to improve detection of SGA infants before birth and optimize management. This program has been associated with an increased detection of SGA babies and a reduction in stillbirth.

9. **a.** Delivery at 38 weeks may be optimal, unless there are earlier concerns about fetal well-being.

    The Disproportionate Intrauterine Growth Intervention Trial at Term study suggests that delivery at 38 weeks may be optimal for babies with suspected fetal growth restriction (FGR), unless there are earlier concerns about fetal well-being.

10. **a.** Waiting until late changes occur in the ductus venosus (DV) or abnormal cardiotocography (CTG) is associated with improved outcomes at 2 years of age.

    The TRUFFLE study on management of preterm FGR suggested that waiting until late changes occur in the DV or abnormal CTG is associated with improved outcomes at 2 years of age.

11. **a.** Whether SGA at birth should be defined using customized, population, or ethnic-specific standards.

    There is a significant controversy over whether small for gestational age (SGA) at birth should be defined using customized, population, or ethnic-specific standards, and which population standard is best suited for international comparisons.

12. **c.** It increases the detection of SGA infants at risk of perinatal death

    The customization of birth weight measurements, which adjusts for maternal height, weight, parity, and ethnicity increases the detection of small for gestational age (SGA) infants at risk of perinatal death.

13. **c.** No guidelines recommend it as a stand-alone screening test for SGA

    According to the text, no guidelines recommend PAPP-A as a stand-alone screening test for small for gestational age (SGA), although some consider low PAPP-A in the first trimester a major risk factor for SGA.

14. **d.** All of the above

    All of these are key areas of research priority including the potential benefits and harms of early delivery in late-onset small for gestational age (SGA) pregnancies, the reliability of ultrasound population charts, and the necessity of routine late third-trimester ultrasound.

15. **b.** They are generated under optimal conditions, excluding pathology.

    Customized fetal biometry standards are developed under optimal conditions, excluding pathological influences. They are intended for general use, but as the text notes, may have limited applicability in low-resource settings.

16. **d.** All of the above

    The text notes that population ultrasound references are specific to the population they are generated in and often do not account for factors like maternal ethnicity. They also often use routine, hospital-based data, which adds to their limitations.

17. **c.** A low level (<0.415 MoM) of the first trimester marker PAPP-A

    According to the text, a low level of the first trimester marker PAPP-A should be considered a major risk factor for the delivery of a small for gestational age (SGA) neonate. This marker can assist in early identification of pregnancies that may be at risk of adverse outcomes related to fetal growth restriction.

18. **c.** Serial ultrasound measurement of fetal size and assessment of well-being with umbilical artery Doppler commencing at 26–28 weeks of pregnancy

The text recommends that women with an abnormal uterine artery Doppler at 20–24 weeks should be referred for serial ultrasound measurements of fetal size and umbilical artery Doppler studies starting from 26–28 weeks of gestation. This is important for close monitoring of fetal growth and well-being.

19. **b.** Antiplatelet agents
    That antiplatelet agents may be effective in preventing small for gestational age (SGA) birth in women at high risk of preeclampsia. While the effect size may be small, it is still beneficial and recommended in the prevention of SGA births in high-risk pregnancies.

20. **d.** Karyotyping
    In the case of a severely small for gestational age (SGA) fetus with structural anomalies or those detected before 23 weeks, especially if the uterine artery Doppler is normal, karyotyping should be offered. This can provide important information about genetic conditions that may be contributing to the SGA status.

21. **d.** Umbilical artery Doppler
    In a high-risk population, umbilical artery Doppler has been shown to reduce perinatal morbidity and mortality. Hence, it should be the primary surveillance tool in the small for gestational age (SGA) fetus.

22. **b.** Every 14 days
    When umbilical artery Doppler flow indices are normal, it is reasonable to repeat surveillance every 14 days. This allows for close monitoring of fetal growth and well-being.

23. **d.** Ductus venosus Doppler
    In a preterm small for gestational age (SGA) fetus with abnormal umbilical artery Doppler, ductus venosus Doppler should be used for surveillance and used to time delivery. This is due to its moderate predictive value for acidemia and adverse outcome.

24. **d.** The effect of antiplatelet agents on women with no risk of delivering a SGA neonate
    The text does not mention the need for research on the effect of antiplatelet agents on women with no risk of delivering a small for gestational age (SGA) neonate. The focus of the research priorities is on those with a high risk of delivering a SGA neonate.

25. **a.** Intrauterine growth restriction (IUGR)
    Magnesium sulfate prophylaxis is often recommended for growth-restricted fetuses to provide neuroprotection and reduce the risk of neurological complications associated with preterm birth.

26. **d.** It is recommended in the gestational age of 24 to 32 weeks for initiating the magnesium sulfate prophylaxis.
    The exact gestational age threshold for initiating magnesium sulfate prophylaxis is not mentioned in the given text. The information only mentions that the suggested time of commencement varies among different guidelines and studies, but the specific gestational age thresholds are not provided. Therefore, further information would be needed to answer this question accurately.

27. **c.** Because a single biometric measurement of fetal size is often not sufficient for evaluation
    The diagnosis of fetal growth restriction (FGR) is not straightforward as it requires not just a single biometric measurement of fetal size, but also additional biophysical tools and evaluations. The complexity increases due to the existence of two significantly different FGR phenotypes—early-onset and late-onset FGR.

28. **a.** Multimodality assessment including Doppler velocimetry, computerized cardiotocography (cCTG), and biophysical profile (BPP)
    Upon diagnosis of fetal growth restriction (FGR), multimodality assessment is recommended. This can include Doppler velocimetry, cCTG, and BPP. These assessments are necessary to closely monitor the condition of the fetus.

29. **a.** Early-onset FGR is associated more strongly with abnormal trophoblastic invasion and placental insufficiency.
    Early-onset fetal growth restriction (FGR) is more strongly associated with abnormal trophoblastic invasion and placental insufficiency. It poses a high risk of perinatal mortality, morbidity, and long-term adverse outcomes. On the other hand, late FGR usually presents a milder clinical picture and is not associated with severe prematurity, but it can still lead to significant morbidity.

30. **b.** Uncertainty about the feasibility of therapeutic intervention in FGR
    The passage mentions that a significant challenge in the management of fetal growth restriction (FGR) pregnancies is determining whether therapeutic

intervention in FGR will ever be feasible. Moreover, current tools and technologies might not be adequate in differentiating between small for gestational age (SGA) and FGR.

REFERENCES

1. Royal College of Obstetricians and Gynaecologists. Small-for-Gestational-Age Fetus, Investigation and Management (Green-top Guideline No. 31). London: RCOG; 2014.
2. Spencer K, Cowans NJ, Avgidou K, Molina F, Nicolaides KH. First-trimester biochemical markers of aneuploidy and the prediction of small-for-gestational age fetuses. Ultrasound Obstet Gynecol. 2008;31(1):15-9.
3. Chien PF, Owen P, Khan KS. Validity of ultrasound estimation of fetal weight. Obstet Gynecol. 2000;95:856-60.
4. Robson SC, Gallivan S, Walkinshaw SA, Vaughan J, Rodeck CH. Ultrasonic estimation of fetal weight; use of targeted formulas in small for gestational age fetuses. Obstet Gynecol. 1993;82:359-64.
5. Hadlock FP, Harrist RB, Sharman RS, Deter RL, Park SK. Estimation of fetal weight with the use of head, body and femur measurements–a prospective study. Am J Obstet Gynecol. 1985;151(3):333-7.
6. Royal College of Obstetricians and Gynaecologists. Antenatal corticosteroids to reduce neonatal morbidity and mortality (Greentop Guideline no. 7). London: RCOG; 2010.

Chapter 55: Imaging in Obstetrics

Vandana Bansal, Meera Jayaprakash

QUESTIONS

1. **Ultrasound machine was invented by:**
   a. John Logie Baird
   b. Wilhelm Röntgen
   c. Christian Doppler
   d. Ian Donald

2. **Ultrasound waves are:**
   a. Light waves
   b. Sound waves
   c. Piezoelectric crystals
   d. Radiofrequency waves

3. **ALARA is short for:**
   a. As less as routinely assessed
   b. As low as reasonably achievable
   c. As less as reasonable assessment
   d. As low as randomly assigned

4. **With respect to a high frequency transducer, true statement is:**
   a. Penetration is more
   b. Resolution is better
   c. Can be used easily in obese patients
   d. Curvilinear probe usually has higher frequency than transvaginal probe

5. **Most preferred Doppler indices in the present day is/are:**
   a. Systolic/diastolic (S/D) ratio
   b. Resistive index (RI)
   c. Pulsatility index (PI)
   d. All the above

6. **B-mode stands for:**
   a. Basic mode
   b. Black-and-white mode
   c. Brauckmann mode
   d. Brightness mode

7. **Ultrasound transducers use:**
   a. Piezoelectric crystal
   b. Silicon chip
   c. Semiconductors
   d. Sound-emitting diodes

8. **Fourth dimension in 4D scan is:**
   a. X-axis
   b. Z-axis
   c. Space
   d. Time

9. **In Natal Diagnostic Technique PCPNDT (Pre-Conception and Pre-Natal Diagnostic Techniques) act, all are true, *except*:**
   a. Offence under the act is noncompoundable and noncognizable
   b. Wearing of apron and ID card is mandatory for all staff
   c. All F-forms should be duly signed by the registered owner of the ultrasound machine
   d. If a registered center acquires a new machine, the new machine is also required to be registered with the district/appropriate authority

10. **First trimester nuchal translucency scan is done between:**
    a. 6 and 9.6 weeks of gestation
    b. 7 and 10.6 weeks of gestation
    c. 11 and 13.6 weeks of gestation
    d. None of the above

11. **Increased nuchal translucency (NT) refers to all, *except*:**
    a. Nuchal translucency (NT) >2 mm
    b. NT >3.5 mm
    c. NT >95th centile for gestational age
    d. NT >4 mm

12. **At nuchal translucency (NT) scan, we can screen for all the following, *except*:**
    a. Congenital anomalies
    b. Preeclampsia
    c. Fetal anemia
    d. Patau syndrome

13. **Open neural tube defect in fetus can be suspected by all, *except*:**
    a. Polyhydramnios
    b. Tachycardia
    c. Lemon sign
    d. Banana sign

14. Fetal hydrops can be due to all, *except*:
    a. Chromosomal anomaly
    b. Rh isoimmunization
    c. Tracheoesophageal fistula
    d. Single-gene disorders

15. Double-bubble sign is seen in:
    a. Congenital hypertrophic pyloric stenosis
    b. Holoprosencephaly
    c. Fetal akinesia deformation sequence (FADS)
    d. Duodenal atresia

16. Cardiac rhabdomyoma is a feature of:
    a. Congenital adrenal hyperplasia
    b. Neurofibromatosis 1 and 2
    c. Mucopolysaccharidosis type 7
    d. Tuberous sclerosis

17. A patient G2P1L1 is pregnant at 12 weeks. The first child is having sickle cell disease. The wrong statement in the following is:
    a. It follows the rules of Mendelian genetics
    b. The present pregnancy and the subsequent two pregnancies are unlikely to be affected as only one in four children are affected and next three will be carriers or normal
    c. It is an autosomal recessive single gene causing a point missense mutation
    d. It can affect boys and girls equally and hence sex determination is not indicated

18. A patient has been dated 19 weeks by the first trimester scan. When she comes for anomaly scan, we find that the fetal biometry corresponds to 16 weeks. What is the most appropriate line of management?
    a. Continue the anomaly scan and assess for fetal growth restriction
    b. Call her back after 3–4 weeks for anomaly scan as it is too early
    c. Redo the dating scan as the first scan may be wrong
    d. Do an interval scan now followed by an anomaly scan after 3–4 weeks

19. A patient is diagnosed with exencephaly at 13 weeks of gestation. What is the best line of management?
    a. Counseling the patient and letting then take an informed decision to continue the pregnancy
    b. Termination of pregnancy as it is a lethal anomaly.
    c. Continue the pregnancy till term as it is a correctable anomaly
    d. Follow-up scan to determine if the fetus develops anencephaly or not, and then decide

20. Fetal anemia can be determined by all, *except*:
    a. Liley's curve
    b. Queenan chart
    c. Mari chart
    d. Kleihauer-Betke test

21. A 38-year-old patient conceived with in vitro fertilization (IVF) (self-oocytes) has done her first trimester scan at 12 weeks and a dual marker test at 13 weeks of gestation. The combined risk of trisomy 21 has come 1:6. At present, she is 13.5 weeks of gestation. What is the next line of management?
    a. Repeat the nuchal translucency (NT) scan and dual marker immediately
    b. Offer chorionic villus sampling for karyotype
    c. Noninvasive prenatal screening as maternal age is >35 years
    d. Quadruple marker for sequential screening with genetic sonogram at 16 weeks

22. Common vessels insonated for fetal color Doppler include the following, *except*:
    a. Umbilical artery
    b. Ductus arteriosus
    c. Ductus venosus
    d. Middle cerebral artery

23. The angle of insonation of middle cerebral artery for fetal anemia should be close to:
    a. 0 degrees
    b. 30 degrees
    c. 60 degrees
    d. 90 degrees

24. Classification for twin-to-twin transfusion is:
    a. Doppler classification
    b. Quintero classification
    c. Liley's classification
    d. De Niro classification

25. Second trimester soft markers for aneuploidy include all, *except*:
    a. Increased nuchal translucency (NT)
    b. Ventriculomegaly
    c. Renal pyelectasis >4 mm
    d. Aberrant right subclavian artery

26. Ductus venosus A wave reversal may be seen in all, *except*:
    a. Aneuploidy
    b. Cardiac anomaly
    c. Fetal acidosis
    d. Fetal brain sparing effect

27. Hydrocephalus may be seen in all, *except*:
    a. Open neural tube defect
    b. Holoprosencephaly
    c. Aqueductal stenosis
    d. Intraventricular hemorrhage

28. **EXIT procedure may be done in all, *except*:**
    a. Large fetal goiter
    b. Removal of fetal endotracheal occlusion (FETO) plug
    c. Chorioangioma with polyhydramnios
    d. Congenital high airway obstruction syndrome (CHAOS)

29. **Causes of anhydramnios include:**
    a. Open neural tube defect
    b. Bilateral renal agenesis
    c. Fetal anal atresia
    d. Ciliary dyskinesia and Kartagener syndrome

30. **In twin gestation, liquor assessment is done by:**
    a. Four-quadrant amniotic fluid index (AFI)
    b. Deepest vertical pocket
    c. Infolding of intertwin membrane
    d. None of the above

31. **In twin gestation with last menstrual period (LMP) unknown, dating is done using:**
    a. Crown–rump length (CRL) of the larger twin
    b. Crown–rump length of the smaller twin
    c. Average crown–rump length of both twins
    d. Two-thirds of CRL of smaller twin + one-third of CRL of larger twin

32. **Twin reversed arterial perfusion is seen in:**
    a. Stage IV fetal growth restriction in twins
    b. Severe twin-to-twin transfusion syndrome
    c. Some monochorionic twins
    d. Twin anemia-polycythemia sequence

ANSWERS

1. **d.** Ian Donald
   The ultrasound machine was invented by Ian Donald and Tom Brown based on a machine used to detect defects in industrial ships.
   [Reference: Donald I, Macvicar J, Brown TG. Investigation of abdominal masses by pulsed ultrasound. Lancet. 1958;1(7032):1188-95]

2. **b.** Sound waves
   As the name suggests, ultrasound waves are sound waves. Ultrasound and Doppler are based on the scattering of sound energy by interfaces of materials with different properties as per the laws of acoustic physics.
   [Reference: Merritt CRB. Physics of ultrasound. In: Rumack CM, Wilson SR, Charboneau JW, Levine D (Eds). Diagnostic Ultrasound, 4th edition. Philadelphia, PA: Elsevier Mosby; 2011]

3. **b.** As low as reasonably achievable
   Even though ultrasound is reasonably safe and does not produce dramatic adverse effects in human embryos and fetuses, we have to reduce the mechanical effects of ultrasound scanning and Doppler by restricting ourselves to the lowest possible intensities and the lowest possible acoustic exposures. The full form of ALARA is "as low as reasonably achievable".
   [Reference: Merritt CRB. Physics of ultrasound. In: Rumack CM, Wilson SR, Charboneau JW, Levine D (Eds). Diagnostic Ultrasound, 4th edition. Philadelphia, PA: Elsevier Mosby; 2011]

4. **b.** Resolution is better
   Higher frequencies give better resolution. Lower frequencies can be used to image deeper structures.
   [Reference: Merritt CRB. Physics of ultrasound. In: Rumack CM, Wilson SR, Charboneau JW, Levine D (Eds). Diagnostic Ultrasound, 4th edition. Philadelphia, PA: Elsevier Mosby; 2011]

5. **c.** Pulsatility index (PI)
   S/D or systolic/diastolic ratio is the ratio of peak systolic velocity (PSV) to end diastolic velocity (EDV). Resistive index (RI) = (PSV − EDV)/PSV. Pulsatility index (PI) = (PSV − EDV)/Mean. In situations where end diastolic velocity is zero or negative, the S/D ratios or RI cannot be a good marker, especially in cases of fetal growth restriction where the umbilical arteries can have absent or reversed end-diastolic flow. Hence, nowadays, PI is considered as the denominator is the mean velocity that can be calculated in real-time on the ultrasound machines.
   [Reference: Rivaz M, Meyer NL, Uhlmann RA, Mari G. Fetal surveillance: Doppler assessment of pregnancy and biophysical profile. In: Rumack CM, Wilson SR, Charboneau JW, Levine D (Eds). Diagnostic Ultrasound, 4th edition. Philadelphia, PA: Elsevier Mosby; 2011]

6. **d.** Brightness mode
   The mainstay of imaging with ultrasound is provided by real-time, gray scale, B-mode display, in which variations in display intensity or brightness are used to indicate reflected signals of differing amplitude.
   [Reference: Merritt CRB. Physics of ultrasound. In: Rumack CM, Wilson SR, Charboneau JW, Levine

D (Eds). *Diagnostic Ultrasound, 4th edition.* Philadelphia, PA: Elsevier Mosby; 2011]

7. **a.** Piezoelectric crystal
   Ultrasound transducers use piezoelectricity, a principle discovered by Pierre and Jacques Curie in 1880. Piezoelectric materials can respond to an electric field by changing shape.
   [Reference: Merritt CRB. Physics of ultrasound. In: Rumack CM, Wilson SR, Charboneau JW, Levine D (Eds). *Diagnostic Ultrasound, 4th edition.* Philadelphia, PA: Elsevier Mosby; 2011]

8. **d.** Time
   With four-dimensional (4D) ultrasound, the user can see a 3D view in real-time.
   [Reference: Kurjak A, Miskovic B, Andonotopo W, Stanojevic M, Azumendi G, Vrcic H. How useful is 3D and 4D ultrasound in perinatal medicine? *J Perinat Med.* 2007;35(1):10-27]

9. **c.** All F-forms should be duly signed by the registered owner of the ultrasound machine.
   All F-forms should be signed by the person conducting ultrasonography on the pregnant woman.
   [Reference: The Act No. 57 of 1994 Pre-Conception and Pre-Natal Diagnostic Techniques, (Prohibition of Sex Selection) and rules 1996 (Regulation and Prevention) as amended vide Act No. 14 of 2003 enacted by the Parliament of Republic of India]

10. **c.** 11 to 13.6 weeks is the gestational age for performing Nuchal Translucency scan in pregnancy
    [Reference: Nicolaides KH. Screening for fetal aneuploidies at 11 to 13 weeks. *Prenat Diagn.* 2011;31(1):7-15]

11. **a.** Nuchal translucency (NT) >2 mm
    A cut-off of 3 mm or an NT >95th centile for gestational age is usually used as the definition of an increased NT.
    [Reference: Nicolaides KH, Azar G, Byrne D, Mansur C, Marks K. Fetal nuchal translucency: ultrasound screening for chromosomal defects in first trimester of pregnancy. *BMJ.* 1992;304(6831):867-9]

12. **c.** Fetal anemia
    Screening for fetal anemia in Rh isoimmunized pregnancies using middle cerebral artery peak systolic velocity (MCA PSV) begins at 18 weeks of gestation.
    [Reference: Mari G, Deter RL, Carpenter RL, Rahman F, Zimmerman R, Moise KJ Jr, et al. Noninvasive diagnosis by Doppler ultrasonography of fetal anemia due to maternal red-cell alloimmunization. Collaborative Group for Doppler Assessment of the Blood Velocity in Anemic Fetuses. *N Engl J Med.* 2000;342(1):9-14]

13. **b.** Tachycardia
    Polyhydramnios and the lemon sign and banana signs are associated with open neural tube defects.
    [Reference: Barnewolt CE, Rumack CM. The pediatric spinal canal. In: Rumack CM, Wilson SR, Charboneau JW, Levine D (Eds). *Diagnostic Ultrasound, 4th edition.* Philadelphia, PA: Elsevier Mosby; 2011]

14. **c.** Tracheoesophageal fistula
    Immune fetal hydrops is seen in Rh isoimmunization. Nonimmune hydrops can be seen in chromosomal anomalies, cardiac anomalies, single-gene defects, and many other abnormalities. Hydrops is not seen in fetuses with tracheoesophageal fistulas.
    [Reference: Levine D. Fetal hydrops. In: Rumack CM, Wilson SR, Charboneau JW, Levine D (Eds). *Diagnostic Ultrasound, 4th edition.* Philadelphia, PA: Elsevier Mosby; 2011]

15. **d.** Duodenal atresia
    Double-bubble sign is seen in duodenal atresia. The two bubbles should be seen across the midline.
    [Reference: Abbott JF. The fetal abdominal wall and gastrointestinal tract. In: Rumack CM, Wilson SR, Charboneau JW, Levine D (Eds). *Diagnostic Ultrasound, 4th edition.* Philadelphia, PA: Elsevier Mosby; 2011]

16. **d.** Tuberous sclerosis
    Fetal rhabdomyomas are associated with tuberous sclerosis.
    [Reference: Bader RS, Chitayat D, Kelly E, Ryan G, Smallhorn JF, Toi A, et al. Fetal rhabdomyoma: prenatal diagnosis, clinical outcome, and incidence of associated tuberous sclerosis complex. *J Pediatr.* 2003;143(5):620-4]

17. **b.** The present pregnancy and the subsequent two pregnancies are unlikely to be affected as only one in four children are affected and next three will be carriers or normal.
    Sickle cell disease follows the rules of Mendelian genetics. It is an autosomal recessive disease. If the first child has sickle cell disease, it is likely that the parents are carriers of the sickle cell trait. In each pregnancy, the risk of having a child affected by sickle cell disease is 25%.

[Reference: Bapa PDI, Lewis LH, Neeraj K, et al. Sickle Cell Disease-Genetics, Pathophysiology, Clinical Presentation and Treatment: Int J Neonatal Screen. 2019;5(2):20]

18. **a.** Continue the anomaly scan and assess for fetal growth restriction

   Ultrasound dating of pregnancy is most accurate in the first trimester using the crown–rump length. The pregnancy should not be redated after an accurate scan has been performed earlier and is available for comparison.
   [Reference: Callen PW, Norton ME. Obstetric ultrasound examination. In: Norton ME, Scoutt LM, Feldstein VA, Callen PW (Eds). Callen's Ultrasonography in Obstetrics and Gynecology, 6th edition. Philadelphia: Elsevier; 2017]

19. **b.** Termination of pregnancy as it is a lethal anomaly. Exencephaly is part of the acrania-exencephaly-anencephaly sequence. This is a uniformly fatal abnormality and termination of pregnancy should be offered as such fetuses invariably develop anencephaly. The cranial vault is not visualized in exencephaly and the intracranial contents appear freely floating in the amniotic fluid.
   [Reference: Trudell AS, Odibo AO. Evaluation of fetal anatomy in the first trimester. In: Norton ME, Scoutt LM, Feldstein VA, Callen PW (Eds). Callen's Ultrasonography in Obstetrics and Gynecology, 6th edition. Philadelphia: Elsevier; 2017]

20. **d.** Kleihauer-Betke test
   Kleihauer-Betke test is a test for fetomaternal hemorrhage. All the other charts are used to determine the degree of fetal anemia, whereas Kleihauer-Betke test quantifies the amount of fetomaternal hemorrhage.
   [Reference: Levine D. Fetal hydrops. In: Rumack CM, Wilson SR, Charboneau JW, Levine D (Eds). Diagnostic Ultrasound, 4th edition. Philadelphia, PA: Elsevier Mosby; 2011]

21. **b.** Offer chorionic villus sampling for karyotype
   1:6 is high risk for Down syndrome and requires diagnostic testing.
   [Reference: American College of Obstetricians and Gynecologists' Committee on Practice Bulletins—Obstetrics; Committee on Genetics; Society for Maternal-Fetal Medicine. Screening for Fetal Chromosomal Abnormalities: ACOG Practice Bulletin, Number 226. Obstet Gynecol. 2020;136(4):e48-e69]

22. **b.** Ductus arteriosus
   Fetal umbilical artery and middle cerebral artery are commonly evaluated in the management of fetal growth restriction. Ductus venosus is commonly evaluated in the first trimester scan. Ductus arteriosus is not a part of fetal color Doppler evaluation.
   [Reference: Lees CC, Romero R, Stampalija T, Dall'Asta A, DeVore GA, Prefumo F, et al. Clinical Opinion: The diagnosis and management of suspected fetal growth restriction: an evidence-based approach. Am J Obstet Gynecol. 2022;226(3):366-78]

23. **a.** 0 degrees
   While evaluating the middle cerebral artery for fetal anemia, the insonating beam must be parallel to the vessel to accurately reflect the true velocity of blood flow. Thus the angle of insonation should be zero.
   [Reference: Mlynarczyk M, Romary L, Abuhamad AZ. Role of Doppler sonography in obstetrics. In: Norton ME, Scoutt LM, Feldstein VA, Callen PW (Eds). Callen's Ultrasonography in Obstetrics and Gynecology, 6th edition. Philadelphia: Elsevier; 2017]

24. **b.** Quintero classification
   Quintero classification has established the diagnostic criteria and classification of twin-to-twin transfusion syndrome.
   [Reference: Quintero RA, Morales WJ, Allen MH, Bornick PW, Johnson PK, Kruger M. Staging of twin-twin transfusion syndrome. J Perinatol. 1999;19(8 Pt 1):550-5]

25. **a.** Increased nuchal translucency (NT)
   Soft markers are evaluated in the second trimester. NT is a parameter measured in the first trimester.
   [Reference: Agathokleous M, Chaveeva P, Poon LC, Kosinski P, Nicolaides KH. Meta-analysis of second-trimester markers for trisomy 21. Ultrasound Obstet Gynecol. 2013;41(3):247-61]

26. **d.** Fetal brain sparing effect
   Ductus venosus A wave reversal may be a feature in aneuploidy and certain cardiac abnormalities. It is also seen in fetuses at high risk of fetal acidosis. Fetal brain sparing effect is a feature of late-onset fetal growth restriction and depends upon the pulsatility index of the fetal middle cerebral artery and the cerebroplacental ratio.
   [Reference: Lees CC, Romero R, Stampalija T, Dall'Asta A, DeVore GA, Prefumo F, et al. Clinical Opinion: The

diagnosis and management of suspected fetal growth restriction: an evidence-based approach. Am J Obstet Gynecol. 2022;226(3):366-78]

27. **b.** Holoprosencephaly
Hydrocephalus or severe ventriculomegaly is a feature of fetal open neural tube defects and aqueductal stenosis, and may be seen in fetal intraventricular hemorrhage. In holoprosencephaly, there are varying degrees of noncleavage of the fetal brain. Hydrocephalus is not a feature of holoprosencephaly.
[Reference: Toi A, Levine D. The fetal brain. In: Rumack CM, Wilson SR, Charboneau JW, Levine D (Eds). Diagnostic Ultrasound, 4th edition. Philadelphia, PA: Elsevier Mosby; 2011]

28. **c.** Chorioangioma with polyhydramnios
The EXIT procedure is used to secure the airway of the fetus at the time of delivery when the uteroplacental circulation is still active. Chorangioma does not interfere with the fetal airway.
[Reference: Marwan A, Crombleholme TM. The EXIT procedure: principles, pitfalls, and progress. Semin Pediatr Surg. 2006;15(2):107-15]

29. **b.** Bilateral renal agenesis
Fetal bilateral renal agenesis causes anhydramnios from the second trimester as the fetal kidneys produce amniotic fluid from the 16th week onward.
[Reference: Fong KW, Robertson JE, Maxwell CV. The fetal urogenital tract. In: Rumack CM, Wilson SR, Charboneau JW, Levine D (Eds). Diagnostic Ultrasound, 4th edition. Philadelphia, PA: Elsevier Mosby; 2011]

30. **b.** Deepest vertical pocket
The deepest vertical pocket (DVP) of fluid in centimeters in each amniotic sac is used to estimate amniotic fluid volume in twins. DVP of 2 cm or less is defined as oligohydramnios and >8 cm is defined as polyhydramnios.
[Reference: Magann EF, Sandlin AT. Amniotic fluid volume in fetal health and disease. In: Norton ME, Scoutt LM, Feldstein VA, Callen PW (Eds). Callen's Ultrasonography in Obstetrics and Gynecology, 6th edition. Philadelphia: Elsevier; 2017]

31. **a.** Crown–rump length (CRL) of the larger twin
Although the CRL of the smaller twin is more accurate in gestational age estimation, using the CRL of the larger twin reduces the risk of underestimating early-onset fetal growth restriction (FGR).
[Reference: Chaudhuri K, Su LL, Wong PC, Chan YH, Choolani MA, Chia D, et al. Determination of gestational age in twin pregnancy: Which fetal crown-rump length should be used? J Obstet Gynaecol Res. 2013;39(4):761-5]

32. **c.** Some monochorionic twins
TRAP syndrome is a complication of monochorionic twin gestations whereby one of the twins perfuses the other acardiac fetus. The arterial flow in the acardiac fetus is reversed.
[Reference: Chalouhi GE, Stirnemann JJ, Salomon LJ, Essaoui M, Quibel T, Ville Y. Specific complications of monochorionic twin pregnancies: twin-twin transfusion syndrome and twin reversed arterial perfusion sequence. Semin Fetal Neonatal Med. 2010;15(6):349-56]

Chapter 56: Anesthesia and Analgesia in Obstetrics

Sukriti Atram, Ruchika Garg

QUESTIONS

1. Amino-amide local anesthetics include all, *except:*
   a. Lidocaine
   b. Bupivacaine
   c. Ropivacaine
   d. Procaine

2. First drug of choice for spinal-induced hypotension for cesareans section:
   a. Mephentermine
   b. Ephedrine
   c. Phenylephrine
   d. Dopamine

3. Mrs Rita posted for emergency cesarean section for transvers lie presentation. Which of the most appropriate blood tests before initiating neuraxial analgesia in patient taking subcutaneous heparin for deep venous thrombosis (DVT)?
   a. Hemoglobin/hematocrit
   b. Activated partial thromboplastin time (aPTT)
   c. Antibody screen (type and screen)
   d. Platelet count

4. After administration of 20 mL of lidocaine 2% + 1:400,000 epinephrine + bicarbonate via epidural catheter in the operating room, the patient suddenly becomes unresponsive. First line of important tasks which is the most appropriate next step?
   a. Deliver the infant
   b. Ventilate the patient
   c. Administer lipid emulsion
   d. Check the blood glucose

5. Needle causes less chances of postdural puncture headache (PDPH):
   a. 25 G needle
   b. 24 G needle
   c. 26 G needle
   d. 23 G needle

6. Labor analgesia is recommended in which stage of labor?
   a. First stage of labor
   b. Second stage of labor
   c. Third stage of labor
   d. Maternal request

7. All are the symptoms of postdural puncture headache (PDPH), *except:*
   a. Neck stiffness
   b. Nausea
   c. Photophobia
   d. Hypertension

8. Nonpharmacological labor analgesia techniques are, *except:*
   a. Hypnosis
   b. Breathing exercise
   c. Massage
   d. Bupivacaine

9. An obese 102 kg parturient is more likely to have complication than a normal obstetric patient to be taken for general anesthesia.
   a. Difficulty of tracheal intubation
   b. Hypoxemia during induction of general anesthesia
   c. Hypertension
   d. Increased incidence of venous thromboembolism

10. The conditions which significantly increase maternal mortality rates:
    a. Asthma
    b. Pulmonary hypertension
    c. Mitral valve prolapse
    d. Sickle cell disease

11. Epidural analgesia during labor is contraindicated in women with:
    a. Cardiac conditions that lead to a fixed cardiac output
    b. Untreated streptococcal pneumonia
    c. Coagulopathy
    d. Multiple sclerosis

12. Which of the following is/are true regarding Entonox?
    a. It is the most popular analgesic for labor in the UK
    b. Nitrous oxide passes readily across the placenta
    c. It is rapidly excreted by the newborn lungs
    d. It has been shown to have little apparent effect on Apgar scores

13. **The neonatal effects of meperidine given for labor analgesia:**
    a. Are most severe if it is given 3 hours or more before delivery
    b. Are slight if it is given only during the last hour of labor
    c. Include respiratory depression
    d. Include a reduction in umbilical artery pH and base excess

14. **Which of the following describes the proper intubation technique for a pregnant female undergoing general anesthesia?**
    a. Rapid sequence induction
    b. Awake fiber-optic intubation
    c. Regular induction, but have GlideScope ready is needed
    d. Perform all cases with Laryngeal mask airways (LMAs) due to airway difficulty

15. **Which nonparticulate antacid is commonly given to pregnant patients undergoing general anesthesia?**
    a. Metoclopramide
    b. Bicitra
    c. Calcium carbonate
    d. Pepcid

16. **For cesarean section with epidural in place, you want to achieve a sensory blockade at what level?**
    a. T6
    b. T2
    c. T4
    d. T8

17. **The application of backward pressure on the cricoid cartilage to occlude the esophagus. This maneuver prevents aspiration of gastric contents during induction of anesthesia and in resuscitation of emergency victims when intubation is delayed or not possible.**
    a. Salinger's maneuver
    b. Sellar's maneuver
    c. Sellick's maneuver
    d. Seligman's maneuver

18. **All obstetric patients going for a C-section are considered to have full stomach regardless of how long they have been NPO.**
    a. True
    b. False

19. **Mrs Maya posted for elective lower segment cesarean section (LSCS) posted at 8 AM. She was asked to be nil by mouth (NBM) overnight. She had one glass of water at 4 AM in the morning.**
    a. Defer surgery by 2 hours
    b. Defer surgery by 4 hours
    c. Give all available aspiration prophylaxis medication and taken as aspiration consent
    d. Can do surgery at scheduled time without high risk of aspiration

20. **Which of the following does contribute to increases risk of aspiration during anesthesia for pregnant patients?**
    a. Increased intragastric pressure
    b. Decrease esophageal sphincter tone
    c. Delayed gastric emptying
    d. All the above contribute

21. **What are the most common precipitating events leading to adverse outcome in obstetric anesthesia under general anesthesia?**
    a. Respiratory events
    b. Neurological events
    c. Abnormal fetal presentation
    d. Cardiac events

22. **Why one must avoid nitrous oxide during pregnancy?**
    a. N_2O diffuses into and expands uterus, increasing risk for uterine rupture
    b. Nitrous oxide causes fetal bradycardia and increasing risk of spontaneous abortion
    c. N_2O interferes with folic acid metabolism, thus impairing DNA synthesis
    d. All of the above

23. **What is MAC in anesthesia?**
    a. Minimum alveolar concentration
    b. Maximum alveolar concentration
    c. Maximum airway complication
    d. Minimum airway complication

24. **The concentration of epinephrine that is optimal for hemostasis is:**
    a. 1:50,000
    b. 1:150,000
    c. 1:100,000
    d. 1:200,000

25. A 40-week-pregnant patient with no relevant prior history was admitted in the labor ward during first stage labor and requested epidural analgesia at 3 cm of dilation. An epidural catheter was sited and started a patient-controlled epidural analgesia (PCEA) with bupivacaine 0.1% and fentanyl 2 μg/mL, with a 6-6-8 regimen (6 mL/hour infusion plus 6 mL boluses at request with 8 minutes lockout). The patient requested three extra boluses during the course of labor. At 7 cm of dilation, the obstetrician reported that due to a persistent type II fetal record (nonreassuring fetal heart rate), the

patient needs a cesarean section. Regarding the anesthetic plan, it is correct that:
a. It constitutes a grade 1 cesarean section, so the most advisable plan is to administer general anesthesia
b. The requirement for extra manual boluses of epidural analgesia by the patient is a predictor of failure to convert to surgical epidural anesthesia
c. If the patient shows effective epidural analgesia during labor, the success rate when using the catheter for surgical anesthesia is almost 100%
d. Performing a spinal technique after a failed epidural analgesia is always the safest and most reliable option for a cesarean section

26. Succinylcholine will normally last longer during pregnancy.
a. True   b. False

27. Which of the following patient is contraindicated for spinal anesthesia?
a. Patient who is terrified of general anesthesia
b. Patient with a known difficult airway
c. Patient with aortic stenosis
d. Patient with history of asthma and bronchitis

28. Which of the following is not an appropriate treatment for postdural puncture headache?
a. Blood patch, at same interspace prior epidural was performed
b. Intravenous (IV) caffeine
c. Oral/IV hydration
d. Maintaining patient in upright position on bed rest

29. Which of the following is not true of respiratory changes during pregnancy?
a. Larger endotracheal tube
b. Decrease functional residual capacity (FRC)
c. O_2 dissociation curve shifts to right
d. Respiratory alkalosis may be normal

30. Spinal and epidural anesthesia are known to decrease uterine blood flow.
a. True   b. False

31. What is the leading cause of maternal death under general anesthesia?
a. Aspiration
b. Uterine rupture and hemorrhage
c. Amniotic fluid embolism
d. Myocardial infarction

32. What is the optimal surgical position for a patient undergoing C-section to prevent hypotension?
a. Reverse Trendelenburg
b. Supine and slightly lateral
c. Trendelenburg
d. Lithotomy

33. You are now going in for an emergent C-section for Mrs Rita, no time to an epidural you must do general anesthesia (GA). Mrs Rita had premature rupture of membrane at 28 weeks and has been on a magnesium drip to stop contractions. How will this affect your anesthetic technique?
a. Patient is prone to electrolyte imbalances and cardiac arrhythmias
b. Must keep FiO_2 low to prevent pulmonary alveolitis
c. Patient is at increased risk of bleeding since magnesium will cause a low plate count
d. Duration of action of muscle relaxant will be prolonged

34. The fetus is most sensitive to anesthesia drugs during which trimester?
a. Equally sensitive during all trimesters
b. Second trimester
c. Third trimester
d. First trimester

35. Postoperative analgesia after a cesarean section under spinal anesthesia, choose the correct alternative:
a. Analgesic management is similar to cesarean sections under general anesthesia
b. Hourly respiratory rate monitoring is recommended for the first 12 hours after cesarean section in all patients receiving intrathecal morphine, regardless of the dose administered
c. The transverse abdominis plane block (TAP block) is an effective alternative to intrathecal morphine and avoids its potential adverse effects
d. The dose of intrathecal morphine is associated with the duration of the effect and not with the analgesic quality

36. Which of the following drugs cross the placenta, *except*:
a. Metoclopramide   b. Ephedrine
c. Glycopyrrolate   d. Fentanyl

37. All can be seen in ketamine anesthesia, *except*:
a. Hypertension   b. Hallucinations
c. Bronchospasm   d. Analgesia

38. **Best uterine relaxation is seen with:**
    a. Chloroform
    b. Nitrous oxide
    c. Ether
    d. Halothane

39. **Magnesium sulfate for the treatment of eclampsia/preeclampsia may cause all of the following, *except*:**
    a. Cardiac arrest
    b. Renal failure
    c. Respiratory depression
    d. Hyperreflexia

ANSWERS

1. **d.** Procaine
   Amino-ester local anesthetics contain an amide bond between the aromatic ring and the hydrocarbon chain. Commonly used amino-ester anesthetics include procaine, chloroprocaine, tetracaine, and cocaine (cocaine is not commonly administered to parturients due to teratogenicity). Amino-amide local anesthetics have an amide group linking the aromatic ring and the hydrocarbon chain. Lidocaine, bupivacaine, levobupivacaine, ropivacaine, and mepivacaine are examples of amino-amides.
   [References: Suresh MS, Segal BS, Preston RL, Fernando R, Mason CL (Eds). Shnider and Levinson's Anesthesia for Obstetrics, 5th edition. Philadelphia, PA: Lippincott Williams & Wilkins; 2013; Santos AC, Epstein JN, Chaudhuri K (Eds). Obstetric Anesthesia. New York: McGraw-Hill Education; 2015]

2. **c.** Phenylephrine
   For decades, ephedrine was considered to be the best vasopressor for the management of maternal hypotension. However, its use has been reported to be associated with a fivefold increased risk of fetal acidosis than phenylephrine. At present, phenylephrine is the vasopressor of choice for preventing and treating spinal-induced hypotension (SIH) at cesarean section.
   Author: Ebru Biricik, Hakkı Ünlügenç
   Ephedrine was considered the vasopressor of choice to manage hypotension caused by neuraxial anesthesia in pregnancy; however, prophylactic or therapeutic phenylephrine in boluses or as an infusion is not only effective in reducing hypotension but also has less transfer to the fetus and results in less fetal acidosis than ephedrine.
   [Reference Obstetric care consensus no. 1: safe prevention of the primary cesarean delivery. Obstet Gynecol. 2014;123(3):693-711]

3. **d.** Platelet count
   Heparin has been studied extensively and is considered very safe during pregnancy. Heparin is usually administered during the first and third trimesters of pregnancy. Heparin 5,000–7,500 units subcutaneously every 12 hours during the first trimester, 7,500–10,000 units subcutaneously every 12 hours during the second trimester, and 10,000 units subcutaneously every 12 hours during the third trimester may be given for thromboprophylaxis during pregnancy. An initial loading dose of 5,000–10,000 units of intravenous unfractionated heparin should be started immediately following the diagnosis of acute pulmonary embolism. Following the initial loading, an infusion of 18 U/kg should be started for maintenance. The activated partial thromboplastin time (aPTT) should be monitored 6 hours after injection and maintained in the therapeutic range of 1.5–2.5 times baseline. For maintenance, subcutaneous injections of 10,000 IU may be given two times daily throughout pregnancy until just prior to delivery. Following delivery, warfarin can be started to achieve an international normalized ratio (INR) of 2–3 for at least 6–8 weeks postpartum. Heparin-induced thrombocytopenia is seen in approximately 3% of patients receiving unfractionated heparin.
   (Reference: Beaulieu MD, Fabia J, Leduc B, Brisson J, Bastide A, Blouin D, et al. The reproducibility of intrapartum cardiotocogram assessments. Can Med Assoc J. 1982;127:214-6)

   Type I thrombocytopenia, believed to be caused by platelet aggregation, occurs quickly usually within 3–4 days of starting treatment, and is usually reversible. Heparin treatment may be continued and the thrombocytopenia is usually self-limiting. Type II thrombocytopenia usually occurs within 5–14 days after starting treatment and is immunoglobulin mediated and occurs in 1–3% of nonpregnant patients. Significant morbidity from arterial thrombosis and venous thrombosis may occur in untreated heparin-induced thrombocytopenia. Therefore, platelet count should be monitored closely during the first 2 weeks of treatment.
   [Reference: Beaulieu MD, Fabia J, Leduc B, Brisson J, Bastide A, Blouin D, et al. The reproducibility of intrapartum cardiotocogram assessments. Can Med Assoc J 1982;127:214-6; Blix E, Sviggum O, Koss KS, et al. Inter-observer variation in assessment of 845 labour

admission tests: comparison between midwives and obstetricians in the clinical setting and two experts. BJOG. 2003;10(1):1-5]

4. **b.** Ventilate the patient
Systemic toxicity often occurs after inadvertent intravascular injection or by absorption of local anesthetic from a regional or local injection site. The signs and symptoms of toxicity progress in a typical manner starting with drowsiness, perioral numbness, and tinnitus. These central nervous system (CNS) symptoms progress to muscle twitching and generalized convulsions, coma, respiratory arrest, and cardiovascular collapse. Cardiovascular effects arise both from the CNS and the direct dose-dependent inhibition of cardiac sodium-gated ion channels. The cardiac disturbances include QRS prolongation, PR prolongation, and dysrhythmias including ventricular fibrillation. Local anesthetics differ in their cardiotoxic profiles. Lidocaine rarely causes ventricular dysrhythmias, whereas bupivacaine accumulates in cardiac tissues and has the most severe cardiac effects. The use of incremental injection, frequent aspiration, test doses, and reduced local anesthetic concentration may account for the decreased incidence of local anesthetic toxicity in pregnancy. However, local anesthetic systemic toxicity has been recognized for decades as an important potential cause of maternal mortality.

Treatment of systemic toxicity rapid treatment of convulsions and cardiotoxicity is needed to improve patient outcomes and survival. Hypoxemia and acidosis exacerbate CNS and cardiac toxicity, so, aggressive airway and respiratory management are necessary. Seizures should be treated with benzodiazepines with or without muscle relaxants to reduce acidosis due to convulsions and allow easier control of the airway. In addition to advanced cardiac life support, intralipid 20% is the treatment of choice for cardiotoxicity related to bupivacaine or ropivacaine intoxication. See checklist for treatment of local anesthetic systemic toxicity.

[Reference: Santos AC, Epstein JN, Chaudhuri K (Eds). Obstetric Anesthesia. New York: McGraw-Hill Education; 2015]

Weinberg emphasizes the "primacy of airway management" in the treatment of local anesthetic toxicity. In vitro data indicate that hypoxemia and acidosis enhance bupivacaine associated myocardial depression and bradyarrythmogenic effects. Likewise, in animals, severe hypoxia augments both CNS and cardiovascular toxicity from bupivacaine; it also increases the likelihood that bupivacaine will induce arrhythmias before seizures (it is noted that severe hypocapnia may prolong the arrhythmogenic period and so maintaining normocapnia is recommended). Therefore, it is of paramount importance to control seizure activity, so as to gain airway control and ensure oxygenation and ventilation, as well as ameliorate the metabolic acidosis that may accompany generalized tonic-clonic seizures.

[References: Suresh MS, Segal BS, Preston RL, Fernando R, Mason CL (Eds). Shnider and Levinson's Anesthesia for Obstetrics, 5th edition. Philadelphia, PA: Lippincott Williams & Wilkins; 2013; Santos AC, Epstein JN, Chaudhuri K (Eds). Obstetric Anesthesia. New York: McGraw-Hill Education; 2015]

5. **c.** 26 G needle
The needle gauge is the other major determinant for developing a headache. As one might expect, the larger bore the needle, the more cerebrospinal fluid (CSF) leakage, which, in turn, leads to a more significant headache **(Table 1)**.

TABLE 1: Effect of gauge and type of needle on incidence of PDPH.

Gauge/type of spinal	Incidence of postdural
18-gauge Tuohy	70–80
22-gauge Quincke	20–40
25-gauge Quincke	10–15
22-gauge pencil point	1–2
25-gauge pencil point	<1

(PDPH: postdural puncture headache)
Source: Data from Cesarini M, Torrielli R, Lahaye F, Mene JM, Cabiro C. Sprotte needle for intrathecal anaesthesia for caesarean section: incidence of postdural puncture headache. Anaesthesia. 1990;45(8):656-8.

Smaller needle size: A smaller needle size is associated with reduced frequency of PDPH. However, if there is unrecognized dural puncture due to a slower flow from very small gauge needles, there could be multiple dural punctures, a greater failure rate, and this could increase the incidence of PDPH.

[References: Suresh MS, Segal BS, Preston RL, Fernando R, Mason CL (Eds). Shnider and Levinson's Anesthesia for Obstetrics, 5th edition. Philadelphia, PA: Lippincott Williams & Wilkins; 2013; Santos AC, Epstein JN, Chaudhuri K (Eds). Obstetric Anesthesia. New York: McGraw-Hill Education; 2015]

6. **d.** Maternal request

American Society of Anesthesiologists (ASA) guidelines note that maternal request for labor pain relief is sufficient justification for epidural initiation and the timing should not depend on an arbitrary cervical dilation.

[Reference: Practice Guidelines for Obstetric Anesthesia: An Updated Report by the American Society of Anesthesiologists Task Force on Obstetric Anesthesia and the Society for Obstetric Anesthesia and Perinatology. Anesthesiology. 2016;124(2):270-300]

7. **d.** Hypertension

The headache is classically located over the occipital or frontal regions. It is frequently accompanied by neck tension, tinnitus, diplopia, photophobia, nausea, and vomiting. The most diagnostic feature of PDPH is that it changes with position. The symptoms improve in the supine position and are exacerbated in the erect position (sitting or standing).

[Reference: Reed AP, Yudkowitz FS. Clinical Cases in Anesthesia. Philadelphia: Elsevier; 2014]

8. **d.** Bupivacaine

Hypnosis has been used both as a relaxation technique and for management of pain during labor. When hypnosis was compared with standard care, no evidence was found that pain was less with the use of hypnosis, nor was evidence found for a difference in satisfaction with pain relief.

[Reference: Smith CA, Levett KM, Collins CT, Dahlen HG, Ee CC, Suganuma M. Massage, reflexology and other manual methods for pain management in labour. Cochrane Database Syst Rev. 2018;3(3):CD009290]

Other nonpharmacologic techniques include the breathing techniques described by Lamaze, the Leboyer technique, the Bradley method, transcutaneous nerve stimulation, hydrotherapy, presence of a support person, intradermal water injections, and biofeedback.

[References: Declercq ER, Sakala C, Corry MP, Applebaum S. Listening to Mothers II: Report of the Second National U.S. Survey of Women's Childbearing Experiences: Conducted January-February 2006 for Childbirth Connection by Harris Interactive® in partnership with Lamaze International. J Perinat Educ. 2007;16(4):9-14]

9. **a.** Difficulty of tracheal intubation

When general anesthesia is required, a thorough airway assessment is of utmost importance, as the incidence of difficult laryngoscopy in the obstetric population has been reported to be >8%, with a reported incidence of 1 in 390 for failed intubations. Multiple aspects of obesity and pregnancy including airway edema, enlarged breasts, greater anteroposterior chest diameter, and larger neck circumference, make difficult airway more likely, and difficult intubation is significantly associated with greater body mass index (BMI).

[References: Honarmand A, Safavi MR. Prediction of difficult laryngoscopy in obstetric patients scheduled for caesarean delivery. Eur J Anaesthesiol. 2008;25(9):714-20; Kinsella SM, Winton AL, Mushambi MC, Ramaswamy K, Swales H, Quinn AC, et al. Failed tracheal intubation during obstetric general anaesthesia: a literature review. Int J Obstet Anesth. 2015;24(4):356-74; Hirmanpour A, Safavi M, Honarmand A, Jabalameli M, Banisadr G. The predictive value of the ratio of neck circumference to thyromental distance in comparison with four predictive tests for difficult laryngoscopy in obstetric patients scheduled for caesarean delivery. Adv Biomed Res. 2014;3:200]

10. **b.** Pulmonary hypertension

Pulmonary hypertension (PH) among pregnant women carries a high mortality risk for both the mother and fetus, with some data suggesting that the maternal mortality rate is as high as 30-56%.

[Reference: Weiss BM, Zemp L, Seifert B, Hess OM. Outcome of pulmonary vascular disease in pregnancy: a systematic overview from 1978 through 1996. J Am Coll Cardiol. 1998;31(7):1650-7]

11. **c.** Coagulopathy

Epidural analgesia is a commonly employed technique of providing pain relief during labor. The number of parturients given intrapartum epidural analgesia is reported to be over 50% at many institutions in the United States. The procedure has few contraindications, the primary ones being patient refusal, maternal hemorrhage, and coagulopathy.

[Reference: Vincent RD Jr, Chestnut DH. Epidural analgesia during labor. Am Fam Physician. 1998;58(8):1785-92]

12. **d.** It has been shown to have little apparent effect on Apgar scores

In the United Kingdom and Europe, a mixture of 50% nitrous oxide and 50% oxygen (Entonox) is used extensively. Nitrous oxide has a low blood-gas partition coefficient and accordingly, a rapid-onset and offset of action. It is self-administered through a mouthpiece incorporating a two-stage reducing and on-demand valve. Should the mother become drowsy, the delivery system will be released before unconsciousness occurs. Entonox needs to be inhaled for at least 45 seconds to achieve maximum analgesic effect, so deep inhalation must start as soon as the contraction is first felt. It may cause disorientation, drowsiness, and nausea in some mothers. However, it does relieve labor pain to some degree, and it is easy to use, inexpensive, has minimal accumulation with intermittent use, and is safe for mother and fetus.
[Reference: Santos AC, Epstein JN, Chaudhuri K (Eds). Obstetric Anesthesia. New York: McGraw-Hill Education; 2015]

13. **c.** Include respiratory depression

Meperidine, a commonly used opioid, can be given in doses of 10-25 mg intravenously or 25-50 mg intramuscularly, usually up to a total of 100 mg. Maximal maternal and fetal respiratory depression is seen in 10-20 minutes following intravenous administration and in 1-3 hours following intramuscular administration. Consequently, meperidine is usually administered early in labor when delivery is not expected for at least 4 hours.
[Reference: Butterworth JF IV, Mackey DC, Wasnick JD. Morgan and Mikhail's Clinical Anesthesiology, 7th edition. New York: McGraw Hill; 2022]

14. **a.** Rapid sequence induction

General indications—rapid sequence induction and intubation (RSII) should be considered for the patient who is at increased risk of aspiration with induction of anesthesia. This includes the patient with a full stomach, gastrointestinal pathology, increased abdominal pressure, or pregnancy after 20 weeks gestation RSII for anesthesia:
[Reference: Berkow LC, Hagberg CA, Crowley M. (2023). Rapid sequence induction and intubation (RSII) for anesthesia. [online] Available from: https://medilib.ir/uptodate/show/94214 (Last accessed December, 2023)]

After careful preoxygenation, a rapid sequence induction of anesthesia with cricoid pressure should be employed. The aim of cricoid pressure is to compress the esophagus, or perhaps more accurately the cricopharyngeal muscle against the body of C6 and thereby prevents gastric contents from passing into the oropharynx.
[References: Suresh MS, Segal BS, Preston RL, Fernando R, Mason CL (Eds). Shnider and Levinson's Anesthesia for Obstetrics, 5th edition. Philadelphia, PA: Lippincott Williams & Wilkins; 2013; Santos AC, Epstein JN, Chaudhuri K (Eds). Obstetric Anesthesia. New York: McGraw-Hill Education; 2015]

15. **b.** Bicitra

Oral antacids should be mandatory before the induction of anesthesia for all parturients. Thirty milliliters of 0.3 mol/L sodium citrate, administered 1 hour before induction of anesthesia for cesarean delivery, maintained gastric pH at >2.5 until the end of surgery. Metoclopramide, a dopamine antagonist, increases lower esophageal sphincter (LES) tone, is a prokinetic, sensitizes gastric muscle to the effects of acetylcholine and has central antiemetic effects. It can have significant effects on gastric volume as early as 15 minutes after administration. Histamine (H) receptor antagonists, such as cimetidine and ranitidine, decrease basal gastric acid secretion and volume within 60-90 minutes, but have no effect on acid already secreted into the stomach. Oral cimetidine, 400 mg given 3-4 hours preoperatively, followed by oral antacid 1-2 hours before induction, has been shown to be more efficacious than either agent alone.
[Reference: Healy TEJ, Knight PR. Wylie and Churchill-Davidson's A Practice of Anesthesia, 7th edition. New York, NY: CRC Press; 2003]

16. **c.** T4

Epidural drugs for surgical anesthesia: An upper sensory block at the level of T10 is often desired for epidural labor analgesia using a combination of low-concentration local anesthetics (Las) (bupivacaine 0.0625-0.1% or ropivacaine 0.08-0.1%) and lipid-soluble opioids such as fentanyl or sufentanil. Conversion to surgical anesthesia requires a dense

sensory and motor blockade. A sensory block extending from sacral segments to the T4 level is desirable for cesarean delivery (CD). The absence of touch sensation at the T6 level indicates an adequate block to proceed without pain or discomfort in most cases. Motor block in the lumbosacral segments is commonly assessed by the Bromage scale. For epidural conversion to CD anesthesia, 15–20 mL of high-concentration LAs combined with 1 or more adjuvants is usually required to achieve an adequate block.
[Reference: Mogal SS, Madapu M. (2022). Conversion of Labour Epidural Analgesia to Anaesthesia for Caesarean Delivery. (online) Available from: https://resources.wfsahq.org/atotw/conversion-of-labour-epidural-analgesia-to-anaesthesia-for-caesarean-delivery/ (Last accessed December, 2023)]

17. **c.** Sellick's maneuver
To avoid aspiration of gastric contents in preparation for intubation, Sellick proposed a method of esophageal compression. The eponymously named "Sellick maneuver" is now commonly referred to as cricoid pressure. This method has been widely adopted and thoroughly investigated following its introduction in 1961. Arguably one of its most distinctive features is that it has become an integral part of rapid sequence intubation along with preoxygenation and short induction to intubation interval.

Cricoid pressure has been shown to attenuate the incidence of aspiration mostly through compression of the cricoid cartilage posteriorly. The cricoid cartilage is a hard, ring-like structure inferior to the cricothyroid cartilage at level C6. Sellick documented that this compression occludes the esophagus at C5, whereas other studies, aided by advanced imaging technologies, have specified the postcricoid hypopharynx as the likely target. The postcricoid hypopharynx includes the cricopharyngeus as a component of the upper esophageal sphincter.
[Reference: Chaney B, Brady MF. Sellick Maneuver. In: StatPearls [Internet]. Treasure Island (FL): StatPearls Publishing; 2023]

18. **a.** True
The changing position of the stomach during pregnancy shifts the intra-abdominal segment of the esophagus toward the thorax in many pregnant women. This leads to a decrease in the tone of the lower esophageal high pressure area, which normally prevents reflux of stomach contents. Hence, pulmonary aspiration risk occurs. The risk is higher during anesthesia induction and tracheal intubation. Therefore, rapid sequence induction is recommended.
[Reference: Saracoglu KG, Cakmak G, Saracoglu A. (2020). Airway Management During Pregnancy and Labor. (online) Available from: https://www.intechopen.com/chapters/75356 (Last accessed December, 2023)]

19. **d.** Can do surgery at scheduled time without high risk of aspiration
Clear liquids may be ingested for up to 2 hours before procedures requiring general anesthesia, regional anesthesia, or procedural sedation and analgesia. These liquids should not include alcohol.

A light meal or nonhuman milk may be ingested for up to 6 hours before elective procedures requiring general anesthesia, regional anesthesia, or procedural sedation and analgesia. Additional fasting time (e.g., 8 or more hours) may be needed in cases of patient intake of fried foods, fatty foods, or meat. Consider both the amount and type of foods ingested when determining an appropriate fasting period. Since nonhuman milk is similar to solids in gastric emptying time, consider the amount ingested when determining an appropriate fasting period.
[References: American Society of Anesthesiologists Committee. Practice guidelines for preoperative fasting and the use of pharmacologic agents to reduce the risk of pulmonary aspiration: application to healthy patients undergoing elective procedures: an updated report by the American Society of Anesthesiologists Committee on Standards and Practice Parameters. Anesthesiology. 2011;114(3):495-511; Practice Guidelines for Preoperative Fasting and the Use of Pharmacologic Agents to Reduce the Risk of Pulmonary Aspiration: Application to Healthy Patients Undergoing Elective Procedures: An Updated Report by the American Society of Anesthesiologists Task Force on Preoperative Fasting and the Use of Pharmacologic Agents to Reduce the Risk of Pulmonary Aspiration. Anesthesiology. 2017;126(3):376-93]

20. **d.** All the above contribute
As pregnancy progresses, the stomach is increasingly displaced upward by the gravid uterus leading to

altered axis and increased intragastric pressure. This combined with decreased esophageal sphincter tone leads to the symptoms of heartburn in pregnancy, essentially the cephalad passage of acidic gastric content. In the nonlaboring term parturient, gastric emptying itself is not delayed. In the laboring patient in whom there may be the additive effects from anxiety and pain of labor, gastric emptying is delayed. Gastric emptying is also delayed in women who have received opiates by any route including the epidural or subarachnoid route. This results in an increased risk of aspiration. The incidence of aspiration, leading to Mendelson's syndrome (acid aspiration leading to an inflammatory response of the lung parenchyma causing a chemical pneumonia), is declining. Oral intake is normal.
[Reference: Bedson R, Riccoboni A. Physiology of pregnancy: clinical anaesthetic implications. Contin Educ Anaesth Crit Care Pain. 2014;14(2):69-72]

21. a. Respiratory events
Deaths associated with general anesthesia are generally related to airway problems, such as inability to intubate, inability to ventilate, or aspiration pneumonitis.
[Reference: Butterworth JF IV, Mackey DC, Wasnick JD. Morgan and Mikhail's Clinical Anesthesiology, 7th edition. New York: McGraw Hill; 2022]

22. c. N_2O interferes with folic acid metabolism, thus impairing DNA synthesis
By irreversibly oxidizing the cobalt atom in vitamin B_{12}, nitrous oxide inhibits enzymes that are vitamin B_{12} dependent. These enzymes include methionine synthase, which is necessary for myelin formation, and thymidylate synthase, which is necessary for DNA synthesis. Prolonged exposure to anesthetic concentrations of nitrous oxide can result in bone marrow depression (megaloblastic anemia) and even neurologic deficiencies (peripheral neuropathies). Because of possible teratogenic effects, nitrous oxide is often avoided in pregnant patients who are not yet in the third trimester. Nitrous oxide may also alter the immunologic response to infection by affecting chemotaxis and motility of polymorphonuclear leukocytes.
[Reference: Butterworth JF IV, Mackey DC, Wasnick JD. Morgan and Mikhail's Clinical Anesthesiology, 7th edition. New York: McGraw Hill; 2022]

Mechanism of nitrous oxide teratogenicity is not fully understood, it has been shown to inactivate methionine synthase via oxidation of vitamin B_{12}, which could lead to decreased DNA synthesis in the developing embryo.
[Reference: Healy TEJ, Knight PR. Wylie and Churchill-Davidson's A Practice of Anesthesia, 7th edition. New York, NY: CRC Press; 2003]

23. a. Minimum alveolar concentration
In 1963, the term minimum alveolar concentration (MAC) was introduced as an index of comparison in order to allow the potency of the different inhalational anesthetics to be compared. The MAC was further defined in 1964 as the MAC of inhaled anesthetic, at steady state, required to prevent movement in 50% of patients exposed to a painful stimulus. The MAC is useful both as a guide for the administration of inhalational anesthetics and as an index for comparing the potency of different inhalational anesthetic agents. Alveolar concentration is used as an approximation of brain anesthetic tension. Various factors have been found to affect the MAC. Anesthetic requirements are reduced by hypothermia, and it has been observed that humans enter into a "narcotic state" at temperatures below 30°C. The administration of narcotics, sedatives, or tranquilizers also reduces the MAC.
[Reference: Healy TEJ, Knight PR. Wylie and Churchill-Davidson's A Practice of Anesthesia, 7th edition. New York, NY: CRC Press; 2003]

24. d. 1:200,000
Recommend using an epinephrine concentration of 1:200,000 or 1:400,000 to provide optimal initial hemostasis while minimizing potential side effects.
[Reference: Dunlevy TM, O'Malley TP, Postma GN. Optimal concentration of epinephrine for vasoconstriction in neck surgery. Laryngoscope. 1996;106(11):1412-4]

25. b. The requirement for extra manual boluses of epidural analgesia by the patient is a predictor of failure to convert to surgical epidural anesthesia.

Additional unscheduled boluses of epidural analgesia to treat pain during labor have been found to be one of the most important risk factors for catheter failure. Indeed, a meta-analysis showed a threefold greater probability of catheter failure in patients who required additional boluses compared to those who did not [conversion failure of 16.4% vs. 4.6%, respectively; odds ratio (OR): 3, 2; 95% confidence interval (CI): 1.8–5.5].[1] Two other risk factors associated with epidural catheter failure are the insertion of an epidural catheter by nonobstetric anesthesiologists and the urgency of cesarean section.[2] Other factors studied such as the use of combined spinal-epidural (CSE) versus traditional epidural, duration of labor, cervical dilation, and patient weight, do not appear to be relevant risk factors according to the current evidence.[1]

[References: 1. Bauer ME, Kountanis JA, Tsen LC, Greenfield ML, Mhyre JM. Risk factors for failed conversion of labor epidural analgesia to cesarean delivery anesthesia: a systematic review and meta-analysis of observational trials. Int J Obstet Anesth. 2012;21(4):294-309.
2. Mankowitz SK, Gonzalez Fiol A, Smiley R. Failure to Extend Epidural Labor Analgesia for Cesarean Delivery Anesthesia: A Focused Review. Anesth Analg. 2016;123(5):1174-80]

26. **a.** True

Plasma cholinesterase activity reduces from the 10th week of pregnancy to a maximal reduction on the third postpartum day where levels may be 33% less than the nonpregnant state. This is partly due to the hemodilution effect and partly due to reduced synthesis by the liver. This is usually insignificant in the fit parturient, so drug doses do not need to be adjusted. Activity has to be reduced by 50% for there to be increased sensitivity to succinylcholine.

[Reference: Bedson R, Riccoboni A. Physiology of pregnancy: clinical anaesthetic implications. Contin Educ Anaesth Crit Care Pain. 2014;14(2):69-72]

27. **c.** Patient with aortic stenosis

There are major known contraindications to neuraxial anesthesia (spinal and epidural). The absolute contraindications are lack of consent from the patient, elevated intracranial pressure (ICP), primarily due to intracranial mass and infection at the site of the procedure (risk of meningitis).

Relative contraindications are:
- Preexisting neurological diseases (particularly those that wax and wane, e.g., multiple sclerosis)
- Severe dehydration (hypovolemia) due to the risk of hypotension—risk factors for hypotension include hypovolemia, age >40–50 years, emergency surgery, obesity, chronic alcohol consumption, and chronic hypertension.
- Thrombocytopenia or coagulopathy (especially with epidural anesthesia due to the risk of epidural hematoma)
- Other relative contraindications are severe mitral and aortic stenosis and left ventricular outflow obstruction as seen with hypertrophic obstructive cardiomyopathy.

[References: 1. Hartmann B, Junger A, Klasen J, Benson M, Jost A, Banzhaf A, Hempelmann G. The incidence and risk factors for hypotension after spinal anesthesia induction: an analysis with automated data collection. Anesth Analg. 2002;94(6):1521-9, table of contents.
2. Carpenter RL, Caplan RA, Brown DL, Stephenson C, Wu R. Incidence and risk factors for side effects of spinal anesthesia. Anesthesiology. 1992;76(6):906-16]

28. **d.** Maintaining patient in upright position on bed rest

Treatment/management: Initial symptom management with simple analgesics, oral or intravenous hydration, and avoidance of the upright position may often be effective. PDPH symptoms can resolve spontaneously within 1–2 weeks in over two-thirds of patients. In many cases, symptoms are severe and persistent and require intervention.

There is some evidence to support the use of oral or intravenous caffeine (300–500 mg in 1 L of intravenous fluid over 1 hour) for PDPH, although effects may be transient with high failure and recurrence rates.

Specific treatment of the dura leak may not be required in all cases since spontaneous resolution typically occurs within days to weeks. However, prolonged symptoms and complications have been reported when treatment is not pursued.

The idea of using blood to patch a hole in the dura was described in 1960 by Dr James Gorley, a surgeon from Pennsylvania. He described placing small volumes of blood outside the dura to treat PDPH, with very good results. This later became the concept for the epidural blood patch.

[Reference: Plewa MC, McAllister RK. Postdural Puncture Headache. In: StatPearls (Internet). Treasure Island (FL): StatPearls Publishing; 2023]

29. **a.** Larger endotracheal tube

Engorgement of the respiratory mucosa during pregnancy predisposes the upper airways to trauma, bleeding, and obstruction. Gentle laryngoscopy and

smaller endotracheal tubes (6–6.5 mm) should be employed during general anesthesia.
[Reference: Butterworth JF IV, Mackey DC, Wasnick JD. Morgan and Mikhail's Clinical Anesthesiology, 7th edition. New York: McGraw Hill; 2022]

30. **b.** False
Spinal and epidural anesthesia typically do not decrease uterine blood flow except when arterial hypotension occurs. Moreover, uterine blood flow during labor may actually improve in preeclamptic patients following epidural anesthesia; a reduction in circulating endogenous catecholamines likely decreases uterine vasoconstriction. The addition of dilute concentrations of epinephrine to local anesthetic solutions does not appreciably alter uterine blood flow. Intravascular uptake of the epinephrine from the epidural space may result in only minor systemic β-adrenergic effect.
[Reference: Butterworth JF IV, Mackey DC, Wasnick JD. Morgan and Mikhail's Clinical Anesthesiology, 7th edition. New York: McGraw Hill; 2022]

31. **a.** Aspiration
Pulmonary aspiration of gastric contents and failed endotracheal intubation are the major causes of maternal morbidity and mortality associated with general anesthesia.
[Reference: Butterworth JF IV, Mackey DC, Wasnick JD. Morgan and Mikhail's Clinical Anesthesiology, 7th edition. New York: McGraw Hill; 2022]

32. **a.** Supine and slightly left tilt
A number of measures for the prevention and treatment of spinal block-induced hypotension are used in clinical practice, such as preloading and coloading with crystalloid and/or colloid infusion, wrapping of lower limbs with compression stockings or bandages, administering an optimal dose of local anesthetic and achieving an optimal spinal block level, left tilt positioning, and administering inotropes and vasopressors.
[Reference: Šklebar I, Bujas T, Habek D. Spinal anaesthesia-induced hypotension in obstetrics: prevention and therapy. Acta Clin Croat. 2019;58(Suppl 1):90-5]

33. **d.** Duration of action of Muscle relaxant will be prolong
Enhancement of vecuronium-induced muscle relaxation by magnesium sulfate can be attributed partly to synergism between magnesium sulfate and nondepolarizing muscle relaxants at adult muscle-type acetylcholine receptors.
[Reference: Wang H, Liang QS, Cheng LR, Li XH, Fu W, Dai WT, et al. Magnesium sulfate enhances nondepolarizing muscle relaxant vecuronium action at adult muscle-type nicotinic acetylcholine receptor in vitro. Acta Pharmacol Sin. 2011;32(12):1454-9]

34. **d.** First trimester
The first trimester (up to week 12 of gestation) is a highly sensitive period for embryonic or fetal development, with increased susceptibility to toxicity from xenobiotics. This increased risk of fetotoxicity is largely attributed to the immaturity of the mechanisms and structure of the maternal-fetal circulatory exchange. The barrier function provided by the placenta forms the core of the regulatory and filtration capabilities, affecting medications administered to or consumed by the parturient.
[Reference: Shin J. Anesthetic Management of the Pregnant Patient: Part 2. Anesth Prog. 2021;68(2): 119-127]

35. **d.** The dose of intrathecal morphine is associated with the duration of the effect and not with the analgesic quality.
Although there is a variety of reported intrathecal morphine doses (spinal morphine 50–250 μg) and adverse effects will depend on it, analgesia quality will be similar except for analgesia duration, which will range from approximately 14–36 hours.[1,2]

Doses over 100 μg (up to 250 μg) will extend the time to the first analgesic requirement by 4.5 hours compared to doses between 50 and 100 μg.[3] It is also important to consider other common adverse effects of opioids. After intrathecal morphine 100 μg, 43% will experience pruritus, 12% will have vomiting, and 10% will have postoperative nausea.[2]
[References: 1. Carvalho B, Butwick AJ. Postcesarean delivery analgesia. Best Pract Res Clin Anaesthesiol. 2017 Mar;31(1):69-79. (Crossref) 44. Sumikura H, Niwa H, Sato M, Nakamoto T, Asai T, Hagihira S. Rethinking general anesthesia for cesarean section. J Anesth. 2016;30(2):268-73.
2. Dahl JB, Jeppesen IS, Jørgensen H, Wetterslev J, Møiniche S. Intraoperative and postoperative analgesic efficacy and adverse effects of intrathecal opioids in patients undergoing cesarean section with spinal

anesthesia: a qualitative and quantitative systematic review of randomized controlled trials. Anesthesiology. 1999;91(6):1919-27.
3. Sultan P, Halpern SH, Pushpanathan E, Patel S, Carvalho B. The Effect of Intrathecal Morphine Dose on Outcomes After Elective Cesarean Delivery: A Meta-Analysis. Anesth Analg. 2016;123(1):154-64]

36. **c.** Glycopyrrolate
Most commonly used anesthetic adjuncts also readily cross the placenta. Thus, maternally administered ephedrine, β-adrenergic blockers (such as labetalol and esmolol), vasodilators, phenothiazines, antihistamines (H1 and H2), and metoclopramide are transferred to the fetus. Atropine and scopolamine, but not glycopyrrolate, cross the placenta; the latter's quaternary ammonium (ionized) structure results in only limited transfer.
(Reference: Butterworth JF IV, Mackey DC, Wasnick JD. Morgan and Mikhail's Clinical Anesthesiology, 7th edition. New York: McGraw Hill; 2022)

Glycopyrrolate—following administration of intravenous glycopyrrolate (0.025 mg/kg) to a pregnant ewe, an F/M ratio of 0.13 was reported, indicating that glycopyrrolate does not cross the placenta to any significant degree
[Reference: Suresh MS, Segal BS, Preston RL, Fernando R, Mason CL (Eds). Shnider and Levinson's Anesthesia for Obstetrics, 5th edition. Philadelphia, PA: Lippincott Williams & Wilkins; 2013; Santos AC, Epstein JN, Chaudhuri K (Eds). Obstetric Anesthesia. New York: McGraw-Hill Education; 2015]

37. **c.** Bronchospasm
Ketamine is as effective as halothane or enflurane in preventing experimentally induced bronchospasm. The mechanism for this effect is probably a result of the sympathomimetic response to ketamine.

Ketamine is a bronchial smooth muscle relaxant. When it is given to patients with reactive airway disease and bronchospasm, pulmonary compliance is improved. Ketamine is as effective as halothane or enflurane in preventing experimentally induced bronchospasm. The mechanism for this effect is probably a result of the sympathomimetic response to ketamine, but there are isolated bronchial smooth muscle studies showing that ketamine can directly antagonize the spasmogenic effects of carbachol and histamine. Owing to its bronchodilating effect, administration of ketamine can treat status asthmaticus unresponsive to conventional therapy.
[Reference: Gropper MA, Eriksson LI, Fleisher LA, Wiener-Kronish JP, Cohen NH, Leslie K. Miller's Anesthesia, 9th edition. Philadelphia: Elsevier Health Sciences; 2019]

38. **d.** Halothane
Its specific action in relaxing uterine muscle is sometimes of value, as in external cephalic version, in operative delivery when manipulations are hindered by uterine hypertonicity, occasionally in manual removal of the placenta and in acute inversion of the uterus.

Halothane is rarely indicated in operations for the removal of retained products of conception. It is emphasized that the relaxation obtained, unless carefully controlled, may fail to respond to ergometrine and oxytocic posterior pituitary extract. Halothane is not recommended for obstetrical anesthesia except when uterine relaxation is needed.
[Reference: Crawford JS. The place of halothane in obstetrics. Br J Anaesth. 1962;34:386-90]

39. **d.** Hyperreflexia
Symptoms and signs of hypermagnesemia:
- Nausea and flushing
- Somnolence
- Double vision
- Slurred speech
- ↓ Patellar reflexes – first sign >5 mmol/L
- Respiratory depression >6 mmol/L
- Respiratory arrest 6.3–7.1 mmol/L
- Cardiac arrest at 12.5–14.6 mmol/L

Magnesium may work by prevention of cerebral vasospasm through the block of Ca^{2+} influx via N-methyl-D-aspartate (NMDA) glutamate channels.
(Reference: Barker JM, Mills SJ, Maguire SL, Lalkhen AG, McGrath BA, Thomson H. The Clinical Anaesthesia Viva Book, 2nd edition. UK: Cambridge University Press; 2009)

Chapter 57

HIV in Pregnancy

Arun Kumar Dora, Prabhat Agrawal

QUESTIONS

1. A pregnant women at first trimester attended a secondary-level healthcare center. Her standard antibody–antigen combined test for human immunodeficiency virus (HIV) was negative. After 6 months at third trimester, she started her consultation at a tertiary-level hospital. Which one of the following is false?
   a. Repeat HIV testing in the third trimester is recommended in those receiving care in facilities that have an HIV incidence of ≥1 case per 1,000 pregnant women per year
   b. Repeat HIV testing is recommended for pregnant people with a sexually transmitted infection
   c. Partners of all pregnant people need not be referred for HIV testing when their status is unknown
   d. Expedited HIV testing should be performed during labor or delivery for those who tested negative early in pregnancy but are at increased risk of HIV infection and were not retested in the third trimester

2. Partner of a pregnant women is HIV-positive. His HIV RNA level is 2,000 copies/mL. Which statement about the pre-exposure prophylaxis (PrEP) for the pregnant women is not correct?
   a. PrEP is recommended
   b. Tenofovir disoproxil fumarate/emtricitabine (TDF/FTC) is Food and Drug Administration (FDA)-approved for PrEP of pregnant women
   c. Long-acting injectable cabotegravir (CAB-LA) is the preferred drug
   d. Patients should be counseled to use additional HIV prevention strategies (e.g., condoms) for the first 20 days after initiating FDA-approved pre-exposure prophylaxis

3. A newlywed couple, of which the husband is HIV-positive, came for preconceptional counseling. Which of the following statements is not correct?
   a. They should try for conception if two recorded measurements of plasma viral loads of the husband are below the limits of detection at least 3 months apart
   b. Both persons should be screened and treated for genital tract infections before attempting to conceive
   c. Partner without HIV should not take pre-exposure prophylaxis (PrEP) if the partner with HIV has achieved viral suppression
   d. Administration of antiretroviral PrEP to the partner without HIV reduces the risk of sexual acquisition of HIV

4. Human immunodeficiency virus drug resistance testing should be conducted in all, *except:*
   a. Before initiating antiretroviral therapy (ART) in antiretroviral (ARV)-naive pregnant people who have not been previously tested for ARV drug resistance
   b. Before initiating ART in ARV-experienced pregnant people
   c. Before modifying ARV regimens for people with HIV who become pregnant while receiving ARV drugs
   d. When the HIV RNA level is 40 copies/mL

5. If zidovudine resistance is found in a pregnant woman with HIV then which of the following is correct regarding intrapartum therapy?
   a. Zidovudine can be given to prevent vertical transmission
   b. Zidovudine need not be given if she is taking antiretroviral treatment
   c. Zidovudine need not be given if CD4 count is >200 cells/cm^3

d. Injectable long-acting cabotegravir (CAB-LA) should be given

6. **Pregnant women with HIV should initiate antiretroviral treatment if:**
   a. HIV RNA level is >1,000 copies/mL
   b. CD4 count is <200 cells/mm^3
   c. Both (a) and (b) present
   d. Initiate antiretroviral treatment irrespective of HIV RNA and CD4 count

7. **Human immunodeficiency virus viral suppression is called undetectable levels when:**
   a. HIV RNA level is <1,000 copies/mL
   b. HIV RNA level is <400 copies/mL
   c. HIV RNA level is <50 copies/mL
   d. CD4 count is >200 cells/cm^3

8. **Preferred drugs or combinations in antiretroviral for a pregnant women are all, *except*:**
   a. Dual-nucleoside reverse transcriptase inhibitor combination
   b. Darunavir/cobicistat
   c. Ritonavir-boosted protease inhibitor
   d. Integrase strand transfer inhibitor

9. **For HIV/hepatitis B virus (HBV) coinfection in pregnancy which of the following is not correct?**
   a. Pregnant people with HBV/HIV coinfection who are receiving antiretroviral therapy (ART) should be counselled about signs and symptoms of liver toxicity
   b. Liver transaminases should be assessed 1 month after initiating ART and at least every 3 months thereafter during pregnancy
   c. Within 12 hours of birth, infants born to people with HBV should receive hepatitis B immune globulin and the first dose of the HBV vaccine series
   d. HBV/HIV coinfection is an independent indication for cesarean delivery

10. **In an 8 weeks' pregnant woman with HIV and hepatitis C virus (HCV) coinfection which one of the following is not correct?**
    a. In all patients of HCV during pregnancy treatment for HCV should be started as soon as possible
    b. HCV RNA and liver function tests should be checked at initiation of prenatal care to assess risk of HCV perinatal transmission and severity of liver disease
    c. Should be tested for hepatitis B surface antigen during each pregnancy, preferably in the first trimester, even if vaccinated or tested previously
    d. Who have not already received the hepatitis A virus (HAV) vaccine series should be screened for immunity to HAV

11. **Regarding HIV-2 infection in pregnancy, which one of the following is correct?**
    a. All infants born to people with HIV-2 infection (without HIV-1 infection) should receive a 4-week zidovudine (ZDV) prophylactic regimen
    b. Raltegravir is not recommended
    c. Non-nucleoside reverse transcriptase inhibitors and enfuvirtide should be used
    d. Dolutegravir is not recommended

12. **A woman with 6 weeks' pregnancy tested positive for antigen–antibody combination HIV test. Her HIV RNA level is 5,000 copies/mL. Differentiation test revealed HIV-1 infection. Which of the following statements is not correct?**
    a. In people with early HIV infection, baseline genotypic resistance testing is not necessary
    b. No further confirmatory test for HIV infection is needed
    c. Antiretroviral can be started pending the drug resistance testing report
    d. When early (acute and recent) HIV infection is suspected during pregnancy, the postpartum period, or breastfeeding, a plasma HIV RNA test should be obtained in conjunction with an antigen/antibody immunoassay test

13. **In a woman with term pregnancy in second stage labor, antigen–antibody combination test was positive. The HIV RNA level was tested and found to be 1,500 copies/mL. Which of the following statement is not correct?**
    a. HIV-1/HIV-2 antibody differentiation test not necessary
    b. Intrapartum intravenous zidovudine should be administered
    c. Cesarean section is preferred
    d. Antiretroviral treatment is necessary

14. **Intravenous intrapartum zidovudine is not required for people who meet the following criteria(s):**
    a. Are receiving antiretroviral therapy
    b. Have HIV RNA <50 copies/mL within 4 weeks of delivery
    c. Adherent to their antiretroviral regimen
    d. All the above three must be fulfilled

15. In 38 weeks and 1 day pregnancy with HIV 1 infection, not in labor, the HIV RNA level is 800 copies/mL; which of the following is not correct?
    a. Induction of labor can be done for HIV infection as an indication
    b. Planned cesarean section is not necessary without any other indication
    c. Intrapartum zidovudine is indicated
    d. Duration of ruptured membranes is not associated with an increased risk of perinatal transmission

16. In an HIV-positive woman, the following is/are intrapartum considerations.
    a. Fetal scalp electrodes for fetal monitoring should be avoided, particularly when maternal HIV RNA is not suppressed
    b. Artificial rupture of membranes and operative vaginal delivery should be avoided, if possible, in those with HIV RNA ≥50 copies/mL
    c. Methyl ergometrine should be avoided if the patient is taking a protease inhibitor
    d. All of the above

17. Achieving and maintaining viral suppression through antiretroviral therapy (ART) during pregnancy and postpartum decreases breastfeeding transmission risk to less than:
    a. 1%
    b. 5%
    c. 7%
    d. 10%

18. Regarding breastfeeding in HIV-positive woman, which of the following is not correct?
    a. People with HIV should receive evidence-based, patient-centered counseling to support shared decision-making about infant feeding
    b. Individuals with HIV who are on antiretroviral therapy with a sustained undetectable viral load and who choose to breastfeed should be counseled for formula feed
    c. Replacement feeding with properly prepared formula or pasteurized donor human milk from a milk bank eliminates the risk of postnatal HIV transmission to the infant
    d. In nutritionally deprived countries, exclusive breastfeeding is recommended

19. Regarding vertical transmission to the fetus, which is the primary determinant of transmission?
    a. Maternal plasma viral load
    b. Maternal CD4 count
    c. Proper antenatal management
    d. Mode of delivery

20. For sexual transmission, the viral HIV envelope binds to mucosal dendritic cells. These cells then present the viral particle to:
    a. Macrophages
    b. Plasma cells
    c. CD8 T cells
    d. CD4 T cells

21. The incubation period for HIV from exposure to clinical disease averages:
    a. 3–6 months
    b. 6–12 months
    c. 1–5 days
    d. 3–6 weeks

22. Antiretroviral resistance testing is done if the viral load is at least:
    a. Less than 50 copies/mL
    b. 50–100 copies/mL
    c. 100–200 copies/mL
    d. 500–1,000 copies/mL

23. Which of the following statement is wrong?
    a. Antiretroviral therapy (ART) is recommended for all pregnant women with HIV infection
    b. ART should be initiated as early in pregnancy as possible
    c. Treatment reduces the risk of perinatal transmission regardless of CD4 T-cell count or HIV RNA level
    d. At least two antiretroviral agents are used in pregnancy

24. A second gravida at 38 weeks of pregnancy with HIV RNA level of 1,700 copies/mL attended the antenatal outpatient department (OPD). What is the recommended action plan?
    a. Induction of labor on the same day
    b. Induction of labor at 40 weeks of pregnancy
    c. Wait for spontaneous onset of labor till 42 weeks
    d. Cesarean section on the same day

25. A 38-week HIV-positive pregnant women with HIV RNA load of 750 copies/mL came in early labor. The consultant checked the antiretroviral drugs, the women is taking. It was found that she is taking the drugs regularly. Injection zidovudine was started for the patient. She undergone cesarean section with HIV positivity being the indication. Which management is wrong here?
    a. Starting of injection zidovudine
    b. Cesarean section with HIV infection being the indication
    c. Both (a) and (b)
    d. None of (a) and (b)

26. **Which statement regarding intrapartum management in a HIV-positive women is wrong?**
    a. Zidovudine is used
    b. Infusion should be started at least 12 hours before scheduled caesarean section
    c. Zidovudine dosing is 2 mg/kg intravenous (IV) load over 1 hour, then 1 mg/kg/h until delivery
    d. Zidovudine should be given if HIV RNA load is >50 copies/mL

27. **Which antiretroviral drug is recommended in pregnancy?**
    a. Didanosine
    b. Stavudine
    c. Lamivudine
    d. Full-dose ritonavir

28. **Adequate viral response is?**
    a. At least a 1-log viral load decline within 1–4 weeks after starting therapy
    b. At least a 1-log viral load decline within 2 months after starting therapy
    c. At least a 2-log viral load decline within 1–4 weeks after starting therapy
    d. None of the above

29. **Regarding a HIV-positive woman delivered by cesarean section, which of the following statement is wrong.**
    a. In nutritionally deprived countries breastfeeding is recommended
    b. Antiretroviral therapy (ART) treatment is continued lifelong
    c. For the planning of next pregnancy, she should be receiving ART and have a viral load below 1,200 copies/mL before conception
    d. When ART is available, repeated pregnancy in a healthy woman with HIV has no significant effect on disease progression

30. **If the husband is HIV-positive and the wife is HIV-negative, which of the following is not a method to prevent horizontal transmission?**
    a. Artificial reproductive technologies should be avoided
    b. Use of antiretroviral therapy to achieve viral suppression in the infected partner
    c. Use of pre-exposure prophylaxis in seronegative partner
    d. Use of barrier contraceptive

ANSWERS

1. **c.** Partners of all pregnant people need not be referred for HIV testing when their status is unknown.
   [Reference: U.S. Department of Health and Human Services, Panel on Treatment of Pregnant Women with HIV Infection and Prevention of Perinatal Transmission. (2023). Recommendations for the Use of Antiretroviral Drugs During Pregnancy and Interventions to Reduce Perinatal HIV Transmission in the United States. (online) Available from: https://clinicalinfo.hiv.gov/en/guidelines/perinatal/whats-new (Last accessed December, 2023)]

2. **c.** Tenofovir disoproxil fumarate/emtricitabine (TDF/FTC) is currently the US Food and Drug Administration (FDA)-approved pre-exposure prophylaxis (PrEP) option for HIV prevention with known safety and efficacy data in people with receptive vaginal exposure and with demonstrated safety in pregnancy. People who become pregnant while using TDF/FTC as PrEP can continue PrEP throughout their pregnancy. Risk for HIV acquisition should be reassessed, and people should be counseled regarding benefits and risks of PrEP use in pregnancy.

   Long-acting injectable cabotegravir (CAB-LA) is FDA-approved for people with vaginal exposure to HIV. For people with PrEP indications in pregnancy, CAB-LA dosing, efficacy, and safety remain unknown. If a person receiving cabotegravir PrEP becomes pregnant, the limited available safety data and long half-life of CAB should be discussed with the patient with shared decision-making, and the patient may benefit from expert consultation.

   Patients should be counseled to use additional HIV prevention strategies (e.g., condoms) for the first 20 days after initiating TDF/FTC PrEP and for 28 days after last potential vaginal exposure.
   [Reference: U.S. Department of Health and Human Services, Panel on Treatment of Pregnant Women with HIV Infection and Prevention of Perinatal Transmission. (2023). Recommendations for the Use of Antiretroviral Drugs During Pregnancy and Interventions to Reduce Perinatal HIV Transmission in the United States. (online) Available from: https://clinicalinfo.hiv.gov/en/guidelines/perinatal/whats-new (Last accessed December, 2023)]

3. **c.** When partners with different HIV statuses attempt conception, the partner without HIV can choose to

take PrEP even if the partner with HIV has achieved viral suppression.
[Reference: U.S. Department of Health and Human Services, Panel on Treatment of Pregnant Women with HIV Infection and Prevention of Perinatal Transmission. (2023). Recommendations for the Use of Antiretroviral Drugs During Pregnancy and Interventions to Reduce Perinatal HIV Transmission in the United States. (online) Available from: https:// clinicalinfo.hiv.gov/en/guidelines/perinatal/whats-new (Last accessed December, 2023)]

4. **d.** Human immunodeficiency virus drug resistance testing (genotypic testing and, if indicated, phenotypic testing) should be reviewed in conjunction with antiretroviral (ARV) history (if prior results are available) and performed during pregnancy in those whose HIV RNA levels are above the threshold for resistance testing (usually >500 copies/mL to 1,000 copies/mL but may be possible for HIV RNA >200 to ≤500 copies in some laboratories).

   Human immunodeficiency virus drug resistance testing (genotypic and, if indicated, phenotypic) should be performed in persons with HIV whose HIV RNA levels are above the threshold for resistance testing (i.e., >200 to 1,000 copies/mL). For people with confirmed HIV RNA levels >200 but <1,000 copies/mL, drug resistance testing may be unsuccessful but should still be considered.
   [Reference: U.S. Department of Health and Human Services, Panel on Treatment of Pregnant Women with HIV Infection and Prevention of Perinatal Transmission. (2023). Recommendations for the Use of Antiretroviral Drugs During Pregnancy and Interventions to Reduce Perinatal HIV Transmission in the United States. (online) Available from: https:// clinicalinfo.hiv.gov/en/guidelines/perinatal/whats-new (Last accessed December, 2023)]

5. **a.** Documented zidovudine (ZDV) resistance does not affect the indications for use of intrapartum intravenous ZDV.

   Intravenous ZDV is not required for people who meet all of the following three criteria: (1) Are receiving antiretroviral therapy (ART), (2) have human immunodeficiency virus RNA <50 copies/mL within 4 weeks of delivery, and (3) are adherent to their antiretroviral (ARV) regimen.
   [Reference: U.S. Department of Health and Human Services, Panel on Treatment of Pregnant Women with HIV Infection and Prevention of Perinatal Transmission. (2023). Recommendations for the Use of Antiretroviral Drugs During Pregnancy and Interventions to Reduce Perinatal HIV Transmission in the United States. (online) Available from: https:// clinicalinfo.hiv.gov/en/guidelines/perinatal/whats-new (Last accessed December, 2023)]

6. **d.** All pregnant people with HIV should initiate antiretroviral therapy (ART) as early in pregnancy as possible, regardless of their HIV RNA level or CD4 T lymphocyte count, to maximize their health and prevent perinatal HIV transmission and secondary sexual transmission.
   [Reference: U.S. Department of Health and Human Services, Panel on Treatment of Pregnant Women with HIV Infection and Prevention of Perinatal Transmission. (2023). Recommendations for the Use of Antiretroviral Drugs During Pregnancy and Interventions to Reduce Perinatal HIV Transmission in the United States. (online) Available from: https:// clinicalinfo.hiv.gov/en/guidelines/perinatal/whats-new (Last accessed December, 2023)]

7. **c.** In addition to benefiting an individual's health and preventing HIV transmission to sexual partners, the goal of antiretroviral therapy during pregnancy is to achieve and maintain HIV viral suppression to undetectable levels (HIV RNA <50 copies/mL) to reduce the risk of perinatal transmission.
   [Reference: U.S. Department of Health and Human Services, Panel on Treatment of Pregnant Women with HIV Infection and Prevention of Perinatal Transmission. (2023). Recommendations for the Use of Antiretroviral Drugs During Pregnancy and Interventions to Reduce Perinatal HIV Transmission in the United States. (online) Available from: https:// clinicalinfo.hiv.gov/en/guidelines/perinatal/whats-new (Last accessed December, 2023)]

8. **b.** Antiretroviral (ARV) regimens that are preferred for the treatment of pregnant people with HIV who are ARV-naive include a dual-nucleoside reverse transcriptase inhibitor combination [abacavir plus lamivudine (3TC), tenofovir disoproxil fumarate plus either emtricitabine (FTC) or 3TC, or tenofovir alafenamide plus either FTC or 3TC] and either a ritonavir-boosted protease inhibitor (darunavir/

ritonavir) or an integrase strand transfer inhibitor (dolutegravir).

DRV/c (darunavir/cobicistat), EVG/c (elvitegravir/cobicistat), and ATV/c (atazanavir/cobicistat) [DRV/c, DRV/r (ritonavir), ATV/c] *are not recommended* for use in pregnancy because of pharmacokinetic (PK) changes that pose a risk for low drug levels and viral rebound in the second and third trimesters. However, in cases where virologically suppressed pregnant people present to care on regimens that include these drugs, these drug combinations can be continued with frequent viral load monitoring or can be switched to a recommended or alternative agent.

[Reference: Table 7. Situation-Specific Recommendations for Use of Antiretroviral Drugs in Pregnant People and Nonpregnant People Who Are Trying to Conceive. (online) Available from: https://clinicalinfo.hiv.gov/en/guidelines/perinatal/recommendations-arv-drugs-pregnancy-situation-specific-conceive-full (Last accessed December, 2023)].
[U.S. Department of Health and Human Services, Panel on Treatment of Pregnant Women with HIV Infection and Prevention of Perinatal Transmission. (2023). Recommendations for the Use of Antiretroviral Drugs During Pregnancy and Interventions to Reduce Perinatal HIV Transmission in the United States. (online) Available from: https://clinicalinfo.hiv.gov/en/guidelines/perinatal/whats-new (Last accessed December, 2023)]

9. **d.** Pregnant people with hepatitis B virus (HBV)/HIV coinfection who are receiving antiretroviral therapy (ART) should be counseled about signs and symptoms of liver toxicity, and liver transaminases should be assessed 1 month after initiating ART and at least every 3 months thereafter during pregnancy.

HBV/HIV coinfection is not an independent indication for cesarean delivery.

Within 12 hours of birth, infants born to people with HBV should receive hepatitis B immune globulin and the first dose of the HBV vaccine series.
[Reference: U.S. Department of Health and Human Services, Panel on Treatment of Pregnant Women with HIV Infection and Prevention of Perinatal Transmission. (2023). Recommendations for the Use of Antiretroviral Drugs During Pregnancy and Interventions to Reduce Perinatal HIV Transmission in the United States. (online) Available from: https://clinicalinfo.hiv.gov/en/guidelines/perinatal/whats-new (Last accessed December, 2023)]

10. **a.** For people who are known to be hepatitis C virus (HCV) antibody-positive, HCV RNA and liver function tests should be checked at initiation of prenatal care to assess risk of HCV perinatal transmission and severity of liver disease.

Pregnant people, including those with HIV/HCV coinfection, should be tested for hepatitis B surface antigen during each pregnancy, preferably in the first trimester, even if vaccinated or tested previously. If they are negative and lack evidence of immunity, they should receive the hepatitis B virus vaccine series.

Currently, treatment of HCV during pregnancy is not recommended (unless part of an approved experimental protocol) because of the lack of safety data on the use of HCV direct-acting antiviral agents in persons who are pregnant. If considering initiating HCV treatment in a pregnant person with HCV/HIV coinfection, consultation with an expert in HIV and HCV is strongly recommended.

Hepatitis C virus treatment with direct-acting antiviral agents should be recommended and offered for people with HCV postpartum.
[Reference: U.S. Department of Health and Human Services, Panel on Treatment of Pregnant Women with HIV Infection and Prevention of Perinatal Transmission. (2023). Recommendations for the Use of Antiretroviral Drugs During Pregnancy and Interventions to Reduce Perinatal HIV Transmission in the United States. (online) Available from: https://clinicalinfo.hiv.gov/en/guidelines/perinatal/whats-new (Last accessed December, 2023)]

11. **a.** Pregnant people with HIV-2 infection should be treated based on the guidelines for HIV-1 mono-infection but using antiretroviral (ARV) drugs that are active against HIV-2. Non-nucleoside reverse transcriptase inhibitors (NRTIs) and enfuvirtide are not active against HIV-2 and should not be used.

Dolutegravir, raltegravir, or darunavir/ritonavir plus a dual-NRTI backbone of abacavir plus lamivudine (3TC), or tenofovir disoproxil fumarate or tenofovir alafenamide plus emtricitabine or 3TC are recommended for treating HIV2 mono-infection in pregnant people and in people who are trying to conceive (AIII). Zidovudine (ZDV) plus 3TC can be used as an alternative dual-NRTI backbone.

All infants born to people with HIV-2 infection (without HIV-1 infection) should receive a 4-week ZDV prophylactic regimen.

[Reference: U.S. Department of Health and Human Services, Panel on Treatment of Pregnant Women with HIV Infection and Prevention of Perinatal Transmission. (2023). Recommendations for the Use of Antiretroviral Drugs During Pregnancy and Interventions to Reduce Perinatal HIV Transmission in the United States. (online) Available from: https://clinicalinfo.hiv.gov/en/guidelines/perinatal/whats-new (Last accessed December, 2023)]

12. **a.** All pregnant and breastfeeding people with early HIV infection should start antiretroviral therapy (ART) as soon as possible for their own health and to reduce the risk of perinatal or horizontal HIV transmission, with the goal of rapidly suppressing plasma HIV RNA below detectable levels.

In people with early HIV infection, baseline genotypic resistance testing should be performed simultaneously with initiation of ART and the regimen should be adjusted, if necessary, to optimize virologic response.

[Reference: U.S. Department of Health and Human Services, Panel on Treatment of Pregnant Women with HIV Infection and Prevention of Perinatal Transmission. (2023). Recommendations for the Use of Antiretroviral Drugs During Pregnancy and Interventions to Reduce Perinatal HIV Transmission in the United States. (online) Available from: https://clinicalinfo.hiv.gov/en/guidelines/perinatal/whats-new (Last accessed December, 2023)]

13. **a.** Pregnant people who present in labor with unknown HIV status and people with increased risk of HIV infection who were not retested in the third trimester should undergo expedited antigen/antibody HIV testing.

If results are positive, an HIV-1/HIV-2 antibody differentiation test and an HIV-1 RNA assay should be done as soon as possible, and intravenous (IV) zidovudine (ZDV) should be initiated pending the result of the differentiation test.

For individuals with HIV RNA >1,000 copies/mL or unknown HIV RNA near the time of delivery (within 4 weeks of delivery), intrapartum IV ZDV should be administered.

[Reference: U.S. Department of Health and Human Services, Panel on Treatment of Pregnant Women with HIV Infection and Prevention of Perinatal Transmission. (2023). Recommendations for the Use of Antiretroviral Drugs During Pregnancy and Interventions to Reduce Perinatal HIV Transmission in the United States. (online) Available from: https://clinicalinfo.hiv.gov/en/guidelines/perinatal/whats-new (Last accessed December, 2023)]

14. **d.** Intravenous (IV) zidovudine (ZDV) may be considered for people with HIV RNA ≥50 copies/mL and ≤1,000 copies/mL within 4 weeks of delivery (BII). Data are insufficient to determine whether the administration of IV ZDV to people with HIV RNA levels between 50 copies/mL and 1,000 copies/mL provides any additional protection against perinatal HIV transmission. This decision can be made on a case-by-case basis, taking into consideration their recent antiretroviral.

[Reference: U.S. Department of Health and Human Services, Panel on Treatment of Pregnant Women with HIV Infection and Prevention of Perinatal Transmission. (2023). Recommendations for the Use of Antiretroviral Drugs During Pregnancy and Interventions to Reduce Perinatal HIV Transmission in the United States. (online) Available from: https://clinicalinfo.hiv.gov/en/guidelines/perinatal/whats-new (Last accessed December, 2023)]

15. **a.** In pregnant people with HIV RNA levels ≤1,000 copies/mL, if scheduled cesarean delivery or induction of labor is indicated for non-HIV-related reasons, it should be performed at the standard time for obstetric indications. Labor should not be induced to prevent perinatal HIV transmission.

In pregnant people on ART with HIV RNA ≤1,000 copies/mL, the duration of ruptured membranes is not associated with an increased risk of perinatal transmission and is not an indication for cesarean delivery to prevent HIV transmission.

Scheduled cesarean delivery performed solely for the prevention of perinatal HIV transmission in those receiving ART with HIV RNA ≤1,000 copies/mL near the time of delivery is not recommended given the low rate of perinatal transmission in this group.

[Reference: U.S. Department of Health and Human Services, Panel on Treatment of Pregnant Women with HIV Infection and Prevention of Perinatal Transmission. (2023). Recommendations for the Use of Antiretroviral Drugs During Pregnancy and Interventions to Reduce Perinatal HIV Transmission *in the United States. (online) Available from: https:// clinicalinfo.hiv.gov/en/guidelines/perinatal/whats-new (Last accessed December, 2023)]*

16. **d.** Fetal scalp electrodes for fetal monitoring should be avoided, particularly when maternal HIV RNA is not suppressed (≥50 copies/mL) or is unknown because of the potential risk of HIV transmission.

    Artificial rupture of membranes and operative vaginal delivery with forceps or a vacuum extractor should follow standard obstetric indications but should be avoided, if possible, in those with HIV RNA ≥50 copies/mL.

    In patients who are receiving a cytochrome P450 (CYP) 3A4 enzyme inhibitor (e.g., a protease inhibitor or cobicistat), methergine should be used only if no alternative treatments for postpartum hemorrhage are available and the need for pharmacologic treatment outweighs the risks. If methergine is used, it should be administered at the lowest effective dose for the shortest possible duration.
    [Reference: U.S. Department of Health and Human Services, Panel on Treatment of Pregnant Women with HIV Infection and Prevention of Perinatal Transmission. (2023). Recommendations for the Use of Antiretroviral Drugs During Pregnancy and Interventions to Reduce Perinatal HIV Transmission in the United States. (online) Available from: https:// clinicalinfo.hiv.gov/en/guidelines/perinatal/whats-new (Last accessed December, 2023)]

17. **a.** Achieving and maintaining viral suppression through antiretroviral therapy (ART) during pregnancy and postpartum decreases breastfeeding transmission risk to <1%, but not zero.
    [Reference: U.S. Department of Health and Human Services, Panel on Treatment of Pregnant Women with HIV Infection and Prevention of Perinatal Transmission. (2023). Recommendations for the Use of Antiretroviral Drugs During Pregnancy and Interventions to Reduce Perinatal HIV Transmission in the United States. (online) Available from: https:// clinicalinfo.hiv.gov/en/guidelines/perinatal/whats-new (Last accessed December, 2023)]

18. **b.** Replacement feeding with properly prepared formula or pasteurized donor human milk from a milk bank eliminates the risk of postnatal HIV transmission to the infant.

    Replacement feeding with formula or banked pasteurized donor human milk is recommended to eliminate the risk of HIV transmission through breastfeeding when people with HIV are not on antiretroviral therapy (ART) and/or do not have a suppressed viral load during pregnancy (at a minimum throughout the third trimester) as well as at delivery.

    Individuals with HIV who are on ART with a sustained undetectable viral load and who choose to breastfeed should be supported in this decision

    In nutritionally deprived countries, where infectious disease and malnutrition are primary causes of infant death, the World Health Organization (2016) recommends exclusive breastfeeding during the first 6–12 months.
    [Reference: U.S. Department of Health and Human Services, Panel on Treatment of Pregnant Women with HIV Infection and Prevention of Perinatal Transmission. (2023). Recommendations for the Use of Antiretroviral Drugs During Pregnancy and Interventions to Reduce Perinatal HIV Transmission in the United States. (online) Available from: https:// clinicalinfo.hiv.gov/en/guidelines/perinatal/whats-new (Last accessed December, 2023)]
    [Sexually transmitted infections. In: Cunningham F, Leveno KJ, Dashe JS, Hoffman BL, Spong CY, Casey BM (Eds). Williams Obstetrics, 26th edition. New York: McGraw Hill; 2022]

19. **a.** For human immunodeficiency viruses, which are HIV-1 and HIV-2, sexual intercourse is the main mode of transmission. The virus can be passed by blood, and infected mothers may infect their fetuses during labor and delivery or by breast milk. The primary determinant of transmission is the maternal plasma viral load.
    [Reference: Sexually transmitted infections. In: Cunningham F, Leveno KJ, Dashe JS, Hoffman BL, Spong CY, Casey BM (Eds). Williams Obstetrics, 26th edition. New York: McGraw Hill; 2022]

20. **d.** For sexual transmission, the viral HIV envelope binds to mucosal dendritic cells. These cells then present the viral particle to specific T lymphocytes. These lymphocytes are defined phenotypically by their cluster of differentiation 4 (CD4) glycoprotein surface antigens. The CD4 site serves as a receptor for the virus. Once infected, CD4 T lymphocytes are gradually

depleted, which creates an immunodeficiency that is characterized by low serum CD4 counts.
[Reference: Sexually transmitted infections. In: Cunningham F, Leveno KJ, Dashe JS, Hoffman BL, Spong CY, Casey BM (Eds). Williams Obstetrics, 26th edition. New York: McGraw Hill; 2022]

21. **d.** The incubation period from exposure to clinical disease averages 3-6 weeks. Acute HIV infection is similar to many other viral syndromes and usually lasts <10 days.
[Reference: Sexually transmitted infections. In: Cunningham F, Leveno KJ, Dashe JS, Hoffman BL, Spong CY, Casey BM (Eds). Williams Obstetrics, 26th edition. New York: McGraw Hill; 2022]

22. **d.** Plasma HIV RNA quantification, which establishes the "viral load" value, and antiretroviral resistance testing are to be done if the viral load is at least 500-1000 copies/mL.
[Reference: Sexually transmitted infections. In: Cunningham F, Leveno KJ, Dashe JS, Hoffman BL, Spong CY, Casey BM (Eds). Williams Obstetrics, 26th edition. New York: McGraw Hill; 2022]

23. **d.** Antiretroviral therapy is recommended for all pregnant women with HIV infection, and it should be initiated as early in pregnancy as possible. Treatment reduces the risk of perinatal transmission regardless of CD4 T-cell count or HIV RNA level. Regimen adherence is emphasized to help prevent viral drug resistance. Gravidas are treated with at least three antiretroviral agents.
[Reference: Sexually transmitted infections. In: Cunningham F, Leveno KJ, Dashe JS, Hoffman BL, Spong CY, Casey BM (Eds). Williams Obstetrics, 26th edition. New York: McGraw Hill; 2022]

24. **d.** If HIV RNA level >1,000 copies/mL or is unknown but labor or rupture of membranes (ROM) has ensued, benefits of cesarean delivery are unclear and labor plans are individualized.
  If HIV RNA level <1,000 copies/mL, vaginal delivery is permitted.
  If HIV RNA level >1,000 copies/mL or unknown, plan caesarean delivery at 38 weeks of gestation
[Reference: Sexually transmitted infections. In: Cunningham F, Leveno KJ, Dashe JS, Hoffman BL, Spong CY, Casey BM (Eds). Williams Obstetrics, 26th edition. New York: McGraw Hill; 2022]

25. **b.** If HIV RNA level >1,000 copies/mL or is unknown but labor or rupture of membranes (ROM) has ensued, benefits of cesarean delivery are unclear and labor plans are individualized.
  If HIV RNA level <1000 copies/mL, vaginal delivery is permitted.
  If HIV RNA level >1000 copies/mL or unknown plan caesarean delivery at 38 weeks of gestation
  Start intravenous zidovudine unless the following criteria are met: Taking a prescribed oral antiretroviral therapy regimen, HIV RNA level <50 copies/mL at 34-36 weeks of gestation, or 3-4 weeks before delivery.
[Reference: Sexually transmitted infections. In: Cunningham F, Leveno KJ, Dashe JS, Hoffman BL, Spong CY, Casey BM (Eds). Williams Obstetrics, 26th edition. New York: McGraw Hill; 2022]

26. **b.** Infusion should be started at least 3 hours before the scheduled cesarean section.
  Dosing is 2 mg/kg intravenous load over 1 hour, then 1 mg/kg/h until delivery.
  Intrapartum zidovudine is indicated if HIV RNA level is >50 copies/mL.
[Reference: Sexually transmitted infections. In: Cunningham F, Leveno KJ, Dashe JS, Hoffman BL, Spong CY, Casey BM (Eds). Williams Obstetrics, 26th edition. New York: McGraw Hill; 2022]

27. **c.** Didanosine, stavudine, and full-dose ritonavir, which differs from ritonavir-boosted agents, are exceptions due to pregnancy toxicity but not teratogenicity. The lopinavir/ritonavir combination is no longer recommended based on risks for preterm and small-for-gestational-age neonates.
[Reference: Sexually transmitted infections. In: Cunningham F, Leveno KJ, Dashe JS, Hoffman BL, Spong CY, Casey BM (Eds). Williams Obstetrics, 26th edition. New York: McGraw Hill; 2022]

28. **a.** Most patients with adequate viral response have at least a 1-log viral load decline within 1-4 weeks after starting therapy. Newer integrase inhibitors rapidly decrease viral loads and are useful for women presenting late to prenatal care.
[Reference: Sexually transmitted infections. In: Cunningham F, Leveno KJ, Dashe JS, Hoffman BL, Spong CY, Casey BM (Eds). Williams Obstetrics, 26th edition. New York: McGraw Hill; 2022]

29. **c.** Vertical transmission rates rise with breastfeeding, and it generally is not recommended for women with

HIV infection in the United States, where formula is readily available (Committee on Pediatric AIDS, 2013). In nutritionally deprived countries, where infectious disease and malnutrition are primary causes of infant death, the World Health Organization (2016) recommends exclusive breastfeeding during the first 6-12 months. The Panel on Treatment of Pregnant Women with HIV Infection and Prevention of Perinatal Transmission (2021) strongly recommends that antiretroviral therapy (ART) regimens not be discontinued postpartum but continued lifelong for the advantages of viral suppression. Ideally, all those planning pregnancy should be receiving ART and have a viral load below detectable levels before conception. As one benefits, interpregnancy viral load suppression is associated with less vertical transmission in a subsequent pregnancy (French, 2014; Stewart, 2014). Reassuringly, for those seeking subsequent pregnancy, when ART is available, repeated pregnancy in a healthy woman with HIV has no significant effect on disease progression (Calvert, 2015).

[Reference: Sexually transmitted infections. In: Cunningham F, Leveno KJ, Dashe JS, Hoffman BL, Spong CY, Casey BM (Eds). Williams Obstetrics, 26th edition. New York: McGraw Hill; 2022]

30. **a.** For adults without HIV infection but with risks for HIV acquisition, the USPSTF (United States Preventive Services Task Force) (2019b) recommends offering pre-exposure prophylaxis (PrEP) to decrease the risk of acquiring HIV.

    Current guidance from the Centers for Disease Control and Prevention (CDC) (2018b) emphasizes the use of antiretroviral therapy to achieve viral suppression in the infected partner and barrier used as primary methods of preventing horizontal transmission. However, PrEP for the HIV-negative partner is considered, including during pregnancy to reduce the risk of HIV acquisition and also vertical transmission.

    [Reference: Sexually transmitted infections. In: Cunningham F, Leveno KJ, Dashe JS, Hoffman BL, Spong CY, Casey BM (Eds). Williams Obstetrics, 26th edition. New York: McGraw Hill; 2022]

Chapter 58: Principles of Drugs in Pregnancy and Categories of Drugs (Category B)

Jayashree V Kanavi

QUESTIONS

1. **Food and Drug Organization (FDA) pregnancy risk category B for drugs means:**
   a. No risk in human studies
   b. No risk in animal studies
   c. Risk cannot be ruled out.
   d. Evidence of risk, potential benefits of the drug may outweigh the risks

2. **Which of the statements is true?**
   a. FDA pregnancy risk category replaced the PLLR (Pregnancy and Lactation Labeling Final Rule)
   b. PLLR uses A, B, C, D, and X letter categories
   c. The PLLR officially took effect in 2015
   d. Females and males of reproductive potential are part of FDA pregnancy risk category

3. **Which of the antibiotic is FDA pregnancy category B?**
   a. Amoxicillin
   b. Ciprofloxacin
   c. Doxycycline
   d. Gentamycin

4. **Famotidine belongs to FDA pregnancy category:**
   a. A
   b. B
   c. C
   d. D

5. **A women with 16 weeks' pregnancy visits a dental clinic for toothache where she got a prescription of nonsteroidal anti-inflammatory drug (NSAID) for the management of pain. But she is worried about the fetal risk. How will you counsel her?**
   a. NSAIDs carry no risk for the fetus throughout pregnancy
   b. NSAIDs belong to A category and are very safe during all trimesters
   c. First and second trimester NSAIDs belong to B category but should be restricted in third trimester
   d. NSAIDs should not be used during pregnancy

6. **A young women with polycystic ovarian disease (PCOD) conceives when she was on treatment with metformin. She is concerned about the effect of drug on the fetus. How will you counsel her?**
   a. Metformin is safe drug in pregnancy and belongs to the category B drugs
   b. Metformin should not be taken if a woman is planning for pregnancy
   c. American College of Obstetricians and Gynecologists (ACOG) recommends metformin as first line of drug to manage gestational diabetes mellitus (GDM)
   d. Termination of pregnancy is advised as metformin may cause skeletal malformations

7. **Lispro insulin which is a rapid-acting insulin belongs to FDA category _____ drug.**
   a. A
   b. B
   c. C
   d. D

8. **Low-molecular-weight heparin belongs to FDA category _____ drug.**
   a. A
   b. B
   c. C
   d. D

9. **Choice of anticoagulants during first trimester of pregnancy are all, *except*:**
   a. Unfractionated heparin (UFH)
   b. Low-molecular-weight heparin (LMWH)
   c. Warfarin
   d. Fondaparinux

10. A women is on tablet sulfasalazine for her rheumatoid arthritis. She visits prenatal clinic for prenatal counseling. The counseling to be given is ____
    a. She can continue the drug as it is safe during pregnancy and belongs to FDA category B drug
    b. The drug should be discontinued as it poses potential risk for the fetus
    c. Change to other immunosuppressants
    d. Pregnancy should be avoided

11. A 12-week pregnant lady comes with varicella and gets a prescription of acyclovir with the explanation of ____
    a. Acyclovir carries more maternal benefit compared to fetal risk
    b. Acyclovir is quite safe in pregnancy and belongs to FDA category B
    c. Acyclovir is contraindicated in pregnancy
    d. She cannot continue the pregnancy

12. Acetaminophen belongs to FDA category ____ drug.
    a. A   b. B
    c. C   d. D

13. Which of the following drug belongs to FDA category B?
    a. Clindamycin   b. Amikacin
    c. Doxycycline   d. Streptomycin

14. Cephalosporins belong to FDA category ____ drug.
    a. A   b. B
    c. C   d. D

15. A pregnant women who is suffering with severe gastritis has got a prescription for pantoprazole. She is worried whether she can take the tablet. What is the effect of the drug on the fetus. How will you counsel her?
    a. There is no need to take tablet as gastritis is due to the pregnancy
    b. She should not take the tablet as it is harmful for the fetus
    c. She can try with dietary modifications
    d. She can take the tablet as it is safe during pregnancy and belongs to FDA category B

16. Which of the following statements is true?
    i. Enoxaparin is quite safe in pregnancy and belongs to FDA category B.
    ii. Phenytoin is the drug of choice for an epileptic woman during pregnancy
    iii. Metformin can be used to control the sugars in the case of gestational diabetes mellitus.
    iv. Warfarin is category D drug but still can be used during pregnancy in a lower dose.
    a. i, ii   b. ii, iii
    c. iii, iv   d. i, iii, iv

17. Antiphospholipid syndrome (APS) during pregnancy leads to adverse outcomes, mainly preeclampsia, intrauterine growth restriction (IUGR), abruption, and there is increased risk of fetal demise. Which of the following therapies is recommended for APS during pregnancy?
    a. Immunosuppressants
    b. Corticosteroids
    c. Anticoagulants
    d. Antimalarial drugs

18. Influenza vaccine is recommended for all pregnant women in the second and third trimesters during influenza season.
    a. True   b. False

19. Food and Drug Administration has decided to replace the A, B, C, D, and X risk categories with narrative sections, as a part of Pregnancy and Lactation Labeling Final Rule.
    a. True   b. False

20. A women, who is having mitral stenosis and is on penicillin prophylaxis, has come for prenatal counseling and is worried whether she can continue the prophylaxis before and during pregnancy.
    a. She should stop penicillin prophylaxis 3 months before the conception
    b. She should change the drug used for prophylaxis
    c. Penicillin can be taken during pregnancy
    d. Penicillin is a known teratogenic drug

21. A 10-week pregnant woman with upper respiratory tract infection (URTI) has got prescription of tablet cephalexin from a general practitioner. She is worried about the effects of the drug on the growing fetus. Which of the following statements is correct?
    a. She should not take the drug as it is a teratogenic drug during first trimester
    b. She should outweigh the maternal benefit to fetal risk and take the drug
    c. She can take the drug as it is quite safe during pregnancy
    d. The drug increases the chance of abortion

22. **First- and second-generation antihistamines do not appear to increase fetal risk in any trimester.**
    a. True
    b. False

23. **Acetaminophen should not be used in pregnancy as it increases fetal risk in first trimester.**
    a. True
    b. False

24. **A pregnant women requires a procedure under local anesthesia using lignocaine.**
    a. She can undergo the procedure as lignocaine is safe during pregnancy
    b. She should postpone the procedure until she delivers the baby
    c. Procedure can be done without using local anesthesia
    d. Lignocaine acts as teratogenic drug and belongs to category D, according to FDA classification

25. **The vaccine considered safe during pregnancy are all, *except*:**
    a. Tdap vaccine
    b. Influenza vaccine
    c. COVID vaccine
    d. Rubella vaccine

26. **Which of the following vaccine is routinely not administered during pregnancy, but reserved for the situations in which the woman or fetus are at the significant risk of exposure?**
    a. Tetanus toxoid vaccine
    b. Influenza vaccine
    c. Typhoid vaccine
    d. Rubella vaccine

27. **Clotrimazole belongs to FDA drug category:**
    a. A
    b. B
    c. C
    d. D

28. **Cetrizine, a second-generation antihistamine, belongs to FDA drug category:**
    a. A
    b. B
    c. C
    d. D
    e. X

29. **Which of the antihypertensives belong to FDA category B drug?**
    a. Labetalol
    b. Nifedipine
    c. Hydralazine
    d. Methyldopa

30. **During pregnancy cardiac output and glomerular filtration rate all go up by 20–50% peak during the third trimester around 32–34 weeks, hence for the drugs which are excreted through renal system, doses recommended should be one and half times more than the nonpregnant status.**
    a. True
    b. False

ANSWERS

1. **b.** No risk in animal studies
2. **c.** The PLLR (Pregnancy and Lactation Labeling Final Rule) officially took effect in 2015.
3. **a.** Amoxicillin
4. **b.** B category
5. **c.** Nonsteroidal anti-inflammatory drugs (NSAIDs) in the first and second trimesters is considered to be category B but become category D in the third trimester. Hence, should be avoided in the third trimester.
6. **a.** Metformin is safe drug in pregnancy and belongs to Food and Drug Organization (FDA) category B drugs.
7. **b.** B category
8. **b.** B category
9. **c.** Warfarin
10. **a.** Sulfasalazine is an immunologic agent for which human data suggest low risk. It belongs to category B drug.
11. **b.** Acyclovir is quite safe in pregnancy and belongs to FDA category B.
12. **b.** B category
13. **a.** Clindamycin
14. **b.** B category
15. **d.** She can take the tablet as it is safe during pregnancy and belongs to FDA category B.
16. **d.** Enoxaparin belongs to category B and can be used in all trimesters. Use of metformin is debatable, but it is approved as FDA category B drug. Warfarin even though belongs to FDA category D, and outweighing maternal benefits it can be used in pregnancy in doses <5 mg.
17. **c.** Anticoagulants
18. **a.** True
19. **a.** True; in 2015 the FDA replaced the former pregnancy risk letter categories on prescription and biological drug labeling with new information to make meaningful to both patients and healthcare providers
20. **c.** Penicillin belongs to category B drug and is safe during pregnancy.

21. **c.** She can take the drug as it belongs to cephalosporin group of antibiotics which belongs to FDA category B and does not have any adverse outcome over the fetus or pregnancy.
22. **a.** True
23. **b.** False
24. **a.** It belongs to FDA category B.
25. **d.** Rubella vaccine is an attenuated live-virus vaccine and may cause subclinical placental and fetal infection.
26. **c.** Tetanus and influenza vaccines are recommended during pregnancy routinely. Typhoid vaccine can be administered only if pregnant woman and fetus are at significant risk of exposure to typhoid. Rubella vaccine is a live attenuated vaccine, and is contraindicated during pregnancy.
27. **b.** (B)
28. **b.** (B)
29. **d.** Labetalol, Nifedipine and hydralazine belong to category C.
30. **b.** False

REFERENCES

1. Brigg GG, Freeman RK, Tower CV, Forinash AB. Brigg's Drugs in Pregnancy and Lactation: A Reference Guide to Fetal and Neonatal Risk, 12th edition. United States: Wolters Kluwer Health; 2021; Publisher: Lippincott Williams & Wilkins (LWW) ISBN: 978-1-97-516237-5
2. United States Food and Drug Administration. (2021). Pregnancy and Lactation Labeling (Drugs) Final Rule. [online] Available from: http://www.fda.gov/Drugs/DevelopmentApprovalProcess/DevelopmentResources/Labeling/ucm093307.htm [Last accessed December, 2023].
3. ACOG Practice Bulletin No. 190: Gestational Diabetes Mellitus. Obstet Gynecol. 2018;131(2):e49-e64.
4. Royal College of Obstetricians & Gynaecologists. (2015). Reducing the Risk of Thrombosis and Embolism during Pregnancy and the Puerperium (Green-top Guideline No. 37a). [online] Available from: https://www.rcog.org.uk/media/m4mbpjwi/gtg-no37a-2015_amended-2023.pdf [Last accessed December, 2023].
5. Cunningham FG, Leveno KJ, Dashe JS, Hoffman BL, Spong CY, Casey BM. Williams Obstetrics, 26th edition. United States: McGraw Hill; 2022.
6. Leek JC, Arif H. Pregnancy Medications. 2023 Jul 24. In: StatPearls [Internet]. Treasure Island (FL): StatPearls Publishing; 2023 Jan–. PMID: 29939635.

Chapter 59: Neurological Disorders in Pregnancy

Aruna M Biradar, Sangamesh S Mathapati

QUESTIONS

1. **Multiple sclerosis relapse occurs in:**
   a. First trimester
   b. Second trimester
   c. Third trimester
   d. 6 months postpartum

2. **Topiramate is associated with following teratogenicity when mother receives during in first trimester:**
   a. Oral clefts
   b. Club foot
   c. Congenital cataract
   d. Congenital heart defects

3. **Pregnant women with history of migraine are at increased risk of all, *except*:**
   a. Preeclampsia
   b. Gestational hypertension
   c. Ischemic stroke
   d. Gestational diabetic mellitus

4. **Drug of choice for generalized tonic-clonic seizure (GTCS) in pregnancy is:**
   a. Lamotrigine
   b. Sodium valproate
   c. Levetiracetam
   d. Carbamazepine

5. **Regarding prepregnancy counseling of the patients with epilepsy all are false, *except*:**
   a. Stop medication according to seizures frequency
   b. Increase to polytherapy where ever possible
   c. Medication can be stopped if patient has no seizures for last 2 years
   d. Preconceptional folic acid with 1 mg

6. **Postpartum management of patients with epilepsy includes:**
   a. Postpartum drug doses should be increased
   b. Breastfeeding is contraindicated
   c. Contraception pill better used with antiepileptic medication
   d. Intrauterine contraceptive device (IUCD) can be used

7. **In a women with a space-occupying lesions:**
   a. Regional anesthesia is useful during labor
   b. Labor may lead to dangerous increase in intracranial pressure
   c. Spinal anesthesia may be used for lower-segment cesarean section (LSCS)
   d. Combined neurosurgical and obstetric interventions have been reported

8. **Concerning the anesthetic management of a parturient with raised intracranial pressure:**
   a. A rise in intracranial pressure will compromise cerebral perfusion pressure
   b. Esmolol is the preferred drug to prevent a hypertensive response to laryngoscopy
   c. Mean arterial pressure should be maintained below 80 mm Hg
   d. Nitrous oxide can increase intracranial pressure
   e. Treatment with mannitol does not compromise uterine perfusion

9. **Regarding specific neurological conditions:**
   a. A temperature rise can cause exacerbation of MS
   b. The pregnancy in multiple sclerosis (MS) [(PRIMS) pregnancy in multiple sclerosis] study showed no difference in relapse rate in MS parturient receiving epidural analgesia
   c. Epilepsy is the most common coexisting neurological disorder in pregnancy
   d. Major obstetric hemorrhage is a risk factor for cerebral venous thrombosis (CVT)
   e. Spinal anesthesia is contraindicated in parturients with benign intracranial hypertension

10. **Which neurological disorder in pregnancy is characterized by high blood pressure, swelling, and proteinuria potentially leading to seizures?**
    a. Multiple sclerosis
    b. Guillain-Barré syndrome
    c. Preeclampsia
    d. Migraine

11. Which of the following neurological conditions is considered an autoimmune disorder and can have relapses during pregnancy?
    a. Epilepsy
    b. Parkinson's disease
    c. Myasthenia gravis
    d. Alzheimer's disease

12. During pregnancy, women with epilepsy may be at risk of certain complications due to antiepileptic medications. Which of the following is a potential risk associated with these medications?
    a. Decreased risk of preterm labor
    b. Increased risk of congenital malformations
    c. Lower risk of gestational diabetes
    d. Reduced risk of preeclampsia

13. A pregnant woman presents with sudden onset of facial drop, arm weakness, and slurred speech. What neurological disorder should be suspected in this case?
    a. Bell's palsy
    b. Transient ischemic attack (TIA)
    c. Migraine with aura
    d. Cluster headache

14. Which neurological disorder in pregnancy is characterized by numbness, tingling, and weakness that typically starts in the legs and can ascend to involve the arms and respiratory muscles?
    a. Guillain-Barré syndrome
    b. Multiple sclerosis
    c. Myasthenia gravis
    d. Parkinson's disease

15. A pregnant woman complains of severe, recurrent headaches accompanied by nausea, vomiting, and sensitivity to light and sound. What is the likely diagnosis?
    a. Cluster headache
    b. Tension headache
    c. Migraine
    d. Sinusitis

16. A pregnant woman experiences sudden loss of consciousness and convulsions. What is the most likely cause of these symptoms during pregnancy?
    a. Migraine
    b. Syncope
    c. Epileptic seizure
    d. Myasthenia crisis

17. Which neurological disorder in pregnancy is characterized by involuntary movements, psychiatric symptoms, and cognitive impairment?
    a. Parkinson's disease
    b. Huntington's disease
    c. Essential tremor
    d. Amyotrophic lateral sclerosis (ALS)

18. A pregnant woman develops vision problems, including blurred or double vision. Which neurological disorder is associated with these visual disturbances?
    a. Multiple sclerosis
    b. Myasthenia gravis
    c. Guillain-Barré syndrome
    d. Alzheimer's disease

19. What is the favored treatment by obstetricians for the prevention of eclamptic seizures among pregnant women with epilepsy during their last trimester of pregnancy or soon after delivery?
    a. Magnesium sulfate
    b. Phenytoin
    c. (a) or (b)
    d. None of the above

20. A 28-year-old woman attends the mental health antenatal clinic at 12 weeks for the booking assessment. This is her first pregnancy. Which condition gives her the highest risk of puerperal psychosis?
    a. Anorexia nervosa
    b. Bipolar affective disorder
    c. Moderate depression
    d. Obsessive compulsive disorder
    e. Recurrent anxiety

21. The serum levels of magnesium sulfate at which respiratory depression is seen in?
    a. 4–7 mEq/L
    b. 7–9 mEq/L
    c. 9–11 mEq/L
    d. 12–15 mEq/L

22. The mechanism of action of magnesium sulfate is:
    a. Ability to block neuromuscular transmission by decreasing acetylcholine (Ach) release
    b. Opposing calcium-dependent arterial constriction thereby relieving spasm
    c. Both (a) and (b)
    d. None

23. Posterior reversible encephalopathy syndrome (PRES) predominantly affects which regions of the brain?
    a. Anterior region of the brain
    b. Left hemisphere
    c. Posterior brain regions
    d. Right hemisphere

24. **Which imaging modality is typically used to diagnose PRES?**
    a. Electroencephalogram
    b. Magnetic resonance imaging
    c. Computed tomography scan
    d. X-ray

25. **Postpartum psychosis is a severe mental health condition that occurs after childbirth. At what approximate time frame does it typically develop?**
    a. During the first trimester of pregnancy
    b. Immediately after childbirth (within the first 48 hours)
    c. Within the first week after childbirth
    d. Around 6 months after childbirth

26. **Which of the following factors is NOT considered a risk factor for developing postpartum psychosis?**
    a. Previous history of postpartum depression
    b. Multigravida
    c. Family history of bipolar disorder
    d. A personal history of bipolar disorder or schizophrenia

27. **Which of the following best describes the primary characteristics of multiple sclerosis?**
    a. Impaired vision
    b. Progressive muscle weakness
    c. Elevated blood pressure
    d. Recurrent episodes of neurological dysfunction

28. **Which is the most common maternal peripheral nerve to be injured during labor?**
    a. Common peroneal nerve
    b. Median nerve
    c. Femoral nerve
    d. Anterior tibial nerve

29. **Which of the following regimens can be used for epidural based-labor analgesia?**
    a. Intermittent bolus techniques
    b. Patient-controlled epidural analgesia
    c. Both of the above
    d. None of the above

ANSWERS

1. **d.** Multiple sclerosis is the demyelinating disease that affects the central nervous system at different levels at varying times. It is a relatively common neurological disorder peaking at the age of 30 years. The exacerbation is reported to increase by 20%–40% during the first 6 months after delivery.
   (Reference: James D, Steer PJ, Weiner CP, Gonik B, Robson SC. High Risk Pregnancy Management Options, 5th edition. Cambridge: Cambridge University Press; 2018. p. 1305)

2. **a.** Topiramate is a medication used to manage and treat epilepsy and migraine. It is the second-generation antiepileptic drug. Also comes in the brand name Topamax. It is and Food and Drug Administration (FDA)-approved to treat epilepsy as monotherapy or adjunctive therapy. About 2-3% (15-20 fold higher than expected) of the pregnant women taking this medication will have teratogenic effect, i.e., oral cleft.
   Topiramate: Abnormalities described- Clefts. Affected 2-3% (15-20 fold higher than expected).
   (Table 60-2 Teratogenicity effects of common anticonvulsant medications)
   (Reference: Cunningham FG, Leveno KJ, Bloom SL, Dashe JS, Hoffman BL, Casey BM, et al. Williams Obstetrics, 25th edition. United States: McGraw Hill; 2018)

3. **d.** Migraine describes a periodic incapacitating neurological disorder with episodic attacks of severe headache and autonomic nervous system dysfunction. The prevalence of migraine in the first trimester of pregnancy is 2%. Pregnant women with migraine are at increased risk of preeclampsia, gestational hypertension, preterm birth and cardiovascular morbidities, and ischemic stroke.
   (Reference: Cunningham FG, Leveno KJ, Bloom SL, Dashe JS, Hoffman BL, Casey BM, et al. Williams Obstetrics, 25th edition. United States: McGraw Hill; 2018)

4. **c.** Carbamazepine (CBZ) blood levels remain steady during pregnancy making unnecessary to monitor them.
   On the contrary, both levetiracetam (LEV) and lamotrigine (LTG) were subject to metabolism changes during pregnancy, and therefore, EURAP recommends their monthly monitoring in order to adjust drug dosages and to ensure efficacy on seizures control. Estrogens are known to increase up to 200% the renal clearance of LTG, especially in the third trimester thus causing the drug to be less effective

during pregnancy. An increase of drug dosage was carried out due to poor seizure control in 36.6% of women on LTG, in 13.79% of women on CBZ, and in no patient on LEV monotherapy. Thus making LEV a drug of choice in pregnancy.
[Reference: Mari L, Placidi F, Romigi A, Tombini M, Del Bianco C, Ulivi M, et al. Levetiracetam, lamotrigine and carbamazepine: which monotherapy during pregnancy? Neurol Sci. 2022;43(3):1993-2001]

5. **b.** In women with epilepsy oral folic acid supplementation with 0.4 mg/day is begun at least 1 month before conception. For women with personal history or first- or second-degree relative with neural tube defects the appropriate dose is 5 mg/day.

   Ideally lowest level of free, unbound drug will maintain optimal seizure control. Individuals who have been seizure-free for >2 years are potential candidates to discontinue the antiepileptic drugs.
   (Reference: James D, Steer PJ, Weiner CP, Gonik B, Robson SC. High Risk Pregnancy Management Options, 5th edition. Cambridge: Cambridge University Press; 2018. p. 1278)

6. **d.** Many forms of contraception are available to women with epilepsy. The most common reversible contraceptive methods include oral contraceptives, the dermal patch, depot medroxyprogesterone acetate injection, vaginal rings that contain hormonal steroids with combined progesterone and estrogen or progesterone alone, copper T intrauterine device (IUD) or levonorgestrel IUD, spermicides, and mechanical barriers such as condoms or a diaphragm.

   Long-acting reversible contraceptives such as contraceptive implants and IUDs have the lowest contraceptive failure rates of around 1%. Oral hormonal contraceptives are almost exclusively absorbed through the intestines, and many of them are metabolized to an inactive compound by the cytochrome P450 P3A4 (CYP3A4) enzyme. Antiseizure medications that are CYP3A4 enzyme inducers accelerate hepatic metabolism of both the estrogenic and progestogenic components of systemic hormonal contraceptives. They decrease the duration and intensity of contraceptive's efficacy by reducing their circulating levels and cause potential contraceptive failure. Women with epilepsy should be encouraged to breastfeed their children irrespective of antiseizure medication treatment.

[Reference: Li Y, Meador KJ. Epilepsy and Pregnancy. Continuum (Minneap Minn). 2022;28(1):34-54]

7. **b.** Intracranial space-occupying lesions rarely present during pregnancy. The physiological changes of pregnancy may increase the rate of tumor growth, while labor alters intracranial pressure (ICP). During pregnancy the increase in cardiac output, blood volume, and salt and water retention may exacerbate cerebral edema or increase the size of a vascular tumor. In labor cardiac output increases further and systolic blood pressure peaks with each contraction resulting in fluctuations in cerebral blood flow that can precipitate bleeding into a tumor in the presence of impaired cerebral autoregulation. Intracranial pressure normally increases during contractions and may reach over 70 cmH$_2$O whilst pushing in the second stage.

   These changes may be significant if cerebral compliance is already reduced.
[Reference: Smith IF, Skelton V. An unusual intracranial tumour presenting in pregnancy. Int J Obstet Anesth. 2007;16(1):82-5]

8. **b.** Esmolol (esmolol hydrochloride) is an intravenous cardioselective beta-1 adrenergic antagonist. It is used in various settings, including urgent care, perioperatively, and postoperatively. It is indicated in sinus tachycardia, where a rapid rate requires intervention secondary to other comorbidities. Esmolol is FDA-approved for tachycardia and hypertension induced by intubation. Esmolol is rapidly absorbed, the onset of action is within 60 seconds, and it maintains a steady state within 5 minutes of initiation of infusion. A steady state is achieved at the 2-minute if a loading dose is administered. The drug has a 9-minute half-life and rapid renal clearance.
[Reference: Pevtsov A, Kerndt CC, Ahmed I, Fredlund KL. Esmolol. In: StatPearls (Internet). Treasure Island (FL): StatPearls Publishing; 2023].

9. **c.** Neurological disorders in pregnancy can be pregnancy-related or can be caused by exacerbation of a preexisting neurological condition or sometimes may even be detected for the first time during pregnancy in which it might be an incidental finding. They present with excruciating headache, recurrent seizures, altered sensorium, fever, coma,

visual disturbances, paresthesias, ataxia, and speech disturbances. The most common neurological disorder seen during pregnancy is epilepsy with the incidence being 3-5 per 1,000 births.
[Reference: Renukesh S, Rai L. Neurological Disorders Complicating Pregnancy—Focus on Obstetric Outcome. J Clin Diagn Res. 2016;10(12):QC06-QC09]

10. **c.** Preeclampsia and related hypertensive disorders of pregnancy affect up to 10% of pregnancies. Neurological complications are common and neurologists often become involved in the care of obstetric patients with preeclampsia. Neurological symptoms are early and include disease-defining features of preeclampsia. Neurological complications of preeclampsia may include headaches, visual symptoms, cerebral edema, seizures, or acute cerebrovascular disorders such as intracerebral hemorrhage or reversible cerebral vasoconstriction syndrome.
[Reference: Miller EC, Vollbracht S. Neurology of Preeclampsia and Related Disorders: an Update in Neuro-obstetrics. Curr Pain Headache Rep. 2021;25(6):40]

11. **c.** It is an autoimmune-mediated neuromuscular disorder, which is more common in women. Incidence peaks in their 20s and 30s. The greatest period of risk is within the first year following diagnosis. Thus postponing pregnancy until improvement is reasonable. Acute onset or exacerbation of myasthenia gravis demands hospitalization and supportive care. Fatigue, most common with pregnancies, is exacerbated and the expanding uterus may compromise respiration.
[References: Bansal R, Goyal MK, Modi M. Management of myasthenia gravis during pregnancy. Indian J Pharmacol. 2018;50(6):302-8.
Cunningham FG, Leveno KJ, Dashe JS, Hoffman BL, Spong CY, Casey BM. Williams Obstetrics, 26th edition. United States: McGraw Hill; 2022]

12. **b.** All women with epilepsy of childbearing age should receive preconception counseling and should be encouraged to start planning for a pregnancy at least 1-2 years in advance. First, women should be aware that all antiseizure drugs increase the risk of birth defects, and that valproate (valproic acid, divalproex acid) has the highest risk and should be avoided in pregnancy.
[References: Cunningham FG, Leveno KJ, Bloom SL, Dashe JS, Hoffman BL, Casey BM, et al. Williams Obstetrics, 25th edition. United States: McGraw Hill; 2018.
Patel T, Grindrod K. Antiseizure drugs for women with epilepsy: Before, during, and after pregnancy. Can Fam Physician. 2020;66(4):266-9]

13. **b.** [Reference: Grear KE, Bushnell CD. Stroke and pregnancy: clinical presentation, evaluation, treatment, and epidemiology. Clin Obstet Gynecol. 2013;56(2):350-9]

14. **a.** It is an acute inflammatory polyneuropathy. It is an acquired condition characterized by demyelination of the motor roots and the proximal segments of the peripheral nerves.
    Presentation consists of ascending paralysis associated with the lower back pain and radicular symptoms. Deep tendon reflexes are typically very depressed or lost. In very severe cases, respiratory muscle paralysis is seen and mechanical ventilation is required.
(Reference: James D, Steer PJ, Weiner CP, Gonik B, Robson SC. High Risk Pregnancy Management Options, 5th edition. Cambridge: Cambridge University Press; 2018)

15. **c.** Migraine describes periodic incapacitating neurological disorder characterized by episodic attacks of severe headache and autonomic nervous dysfunction. Migraine without aura is characterized by unilateral throbbing headache, nausea, vomiting, or photophobia.
[References: Headaches in Pregnancy and Postpartum: ACOG Clinical Practice Guideline No. 3. Obstet Gynecol. 2022;139(5):944-72.
Cunningham FG, Leveno KJ, Bloom SL, Spong CY, Dashe JS, Hoffman BL, et al. Williams Obstetrics, 24th edition. New York: McGraw Hill; 2014]

16. **c.** It is associated with sudden loss of consciousness with an uncontrolled fall without prior warning. It is also associated with a variable period of fetal hypoxia, with dramatic events with stiffening, then bilateral jerking, and a post-seizure state of confusion and sleepiness.
[Reference: Royal College of Obstetricians & Gynaecologists. (2016). Epilepsy in Pregnancy (Green-top Guideline No. 68). (online) Available from: https://

www.rcog.org.uk/media/rzldnacf/gtg68_epilepsy.pdf (Last accessed December, 2023)].

17. **b.** [Reference: Ajitkumar A, De Jesus O. Huntington Disease. In: StatPearls (Internet). Treasure Island (FL): StatPearls Publishing; 2023]

18. **a.** Multiple sclerosis is the demyelinating disease that affects central nervous system at different levels. Women are affected twice as often as men. Common symptoms include diplopia, gait instability, vertigo, bladder incontinence, loss of vision, and fatigue.
(Reference: James D, Steer PJ, Weiner CP, Gonik B, Robson SC. High Risk Pregnancy Management Options, 5th edition. Cambridge: Cambridge University Press; 2018)

19. **a.** Magnesium sulfate was compared with phenytoin for the prevention of eclampsia in four randomized controlled trials (RCTs) (2,343 women). Compared with phenytoin, magnesium sulfate significantly reduced the risk of eclampsia [three trials, 2,291 women; relative risk (RR) 0.08, 95% confidence interval (CI) 0.01–0.60].
[Reference: World Health Organization. (2011). WHO recommendations for prevention and treatment of pre-eclampsia and eclampsia. (online) Available from: https://iris.who.int/bitstream/handle/10665/44703/9789241548335_eng.pdf?sequence=1 (Last accessed December, 2023)]

20. **b.** Postpartum psychosis is characterized by abrupt onset of hallucinations, delusions, mixed affective symptoms (fluctuation between depressive and manic symptoms) disturbed or bizarre behavior and confusion or perplexity. A woman's risk of developing a postpartum psychosis is increased with a personal history of bipolar disorder and/or family history of bipolar disorder.
(Reference: James D, Steer PJ, Weiner CP, Gonik B, Robson SC. High Risk Pregnancy Management Options, 5th edition. Cambridge: Cambridge University Press; 2018)

21. **d.** Magnesium sulfate continues to be the mainstay of seizure prophylaxis for neuroprotection. Dosing recommendation is 4–6 g intravenous load given over 5–30 minutes followed by maintenance dose of 1–3 g/h intravenously. The serum levels of 4–8 mEq/L is considered optimal. It is continued for approximately for 24 hours into the postpartum period. Complications associated with the use of magnesium centers on its calcium antagonism at the neuromuscular junction which results in neuromuscular blockade.

At levels above 10 mEq/L deep tendon reflexes are lost. Levels 12–15 mEq/L result in respiratory paralysis. Higher levels can cause cardiac arrest.
(Reference: James D, Steer PJ, Weiner CP, Gonik B, Robson SC. High Risk Pregnancy Management Options, 5th edition. Cambridge: Cambridge University Press; 2018. p. 1276)

22. **c.** Magnesium sulfate administered parenterally is an effective anticonvulsant that is an effective anticonvulsant that avoids producing central nervous system depression. It is given intravenously by continuous infusion or intramuscularly by intermittent injection. Proposed mechanism of action include reduced presynaptic release of the neurotransmitter glutamate, blockade of glutaminergic N-methyl-D aspartate (NMDA) receptors, reduction in the cerebral vasospasm through calcium antagonism, and NMDA receptor channel blockade providing neuroprotection.

23. **c.** It is the neurological manifestation in preeclampsia. Preeclampsia is associated with intraendothelial cell leak which develops at blood pressure levels much lower than those that usually cause vasogenic edema and is coupled with loss of upper limit autoregulation. With imaging studies, these manifest as posterior reversible encephalopathy syndrome. The lesions of this syndrome principally involves posterior brain the occipital and parietal cortices.
(Reference: Cunningham FG, Leveno KJ, Bloom SL, Dashe JS, Hoffman BL, Casey BM, et al. Williams Obstetrics, 25th edition. United States: McGraw Hill; 2018)

24. **b.** Magnetic resonance imaging is used to study eclamptic women. Common findings are hyperintense T2 lesions like posterior reversible encephalopathy syndrome in the subcortical and cortical regions of the parietal and occipital lobes.
(Reference: Cunningham FG, Leveno KJ, Bloom SL, Dashe JS, Hoffman BL, Casey BM, et al. Williams Obstetrics, 25th edition. United States: McGraw Hill; 2018. p. 724)

25. **c.** Psychosis complicating the peripartum can occur as a part of a preexisting chronic psychotic illness such

as schizophrenia or with an abrupt onset in the early postpartum. It affects between 1 in 500 and 1 in 1,000 maternities. The condition is most strongly linked with personal or family history of bipolar disorders, especially with perinatal onset of an episode. The presentation of postpartum psychosis is usually within the first month postpartum.
(Reference: James D, Steer PJ, Weiner CP, Gonik B, Robson SC. High Risk Pregnancy Management Options, 5th edition. Cambridge: Cambridge University Press; 2018)

26. **b.** It is relatively rare manifestation of psychological disorder during puerperium with an incidence of 0.89-2.6 per 1000 women. Risk factors include previous history of postpartum psychosis, bipolar disorder, schizophrenia or schizoaffective disorder in self or in family, first pregnancy or discontinuation of antipsychotic medications during pregnancy)
[References: Renu Misra, Ion Donalds Practical Obstetric Problems, Eighth Edition, Wolter Kluwer (India) Pvt. Ltd., New Delhi, India.
James D, Steer PJ, Weiner CP, Gonik B, Robson SC. High Risk Pregnancy Management Options, 5th edition. Cambridge: Cambridge University Press; 2018]

27. **b.** Multiple sclerosis is a demyelinating disease that affects the central nervous system at different levels and at varying times. It is common among young adults peaking at the age of 30 years. Common symptoms include diplopia, vertigo, gait instability, bladder incontinence, loss of vision, and fatigue.
(Reference: James D, Steer PJ, Weiner CP, Gonik B, Robson SC. High Risk Pregnancy Management Options, 5th edition. Cambridge: Cambridge University Press; 2018)

28. **a.** The most common mechanism is external compression of the common peroneal nerve (formerly called common fibular nerve). This is caused by inappropriate leg positioning in stirrups, especially during prolonged second stage of labor.
(Reference: Cunningham FG, Leveno KJ, Bloom SL, Spong CY, Dashe JS, Hoffman BL, et al. Williams Obstetrics, 24th edition. New York: McGraw Hill; 2014)

29. **c.** Epidural analgesia is the most effective and titrable methods of labor and delivery analgesia.

    The epidural technique can be converted to surgical anesthesia for an instrumental or operative delivery, laceration repair, or postpartum tubal ligation by changing the dose or type of local anesthesia administered through catheter. The goal during labor and delivery is to provide lumbar and sacral sensory analgesia with minimal motor blockade. This should allow pregnant women to appreciate the sense of pressure, without pain, during contractions, while retaining the ability to move her lower extremities. Once the initial sensory blockade has been established epidural analgesia can be maintained by intermittent bolus injections, continuous infusions, or both simultaneously.
(Reference: James D, Steer PJ, Weiner CP, Gonik B, Robson SC. High Risk Pregnancy Management Options, 5th edition. Cambridge: Cambridge University Press; 2018. p. 1817)

Chapter 60: Disseminated Intravascular Coagulation in Pregnancy

Meenal S Sarmalkar, Honey M Gemavat

QUESTIONS

1. **Disseminated intravascular coagulation was first described as a fatal hemorrhagic diathesis following placental abruption by:**
   a. Edward Rigby
   b. Joseph DeLee
   c. Baudelocque
   d. Dieckmann

2. **The incidence of consumptive coagulopathy in gravidas varies and ranges from:**
   a. 0.03–0.35%
   b. 0.02–0.22%
   c. 0.03–0.38%
   d. 0.03–0.45%

3. **Disseminated intravascular coagulation (DIC) is characterized by:**
   a. Intravascular microcoagulation
   b. Fibrinolysis
   c. Consumption of coagulation factors and inhibitors
   d. End-organ damage
   e. All the above

4. **One of the principal initiators of disseminated intravascular coagulation (DIC) is:**
   a. A transmembrane glycoprotein called tissue factor (TF)
   b. Histamines
   c. Prostaglandins
   d. Cytokines

5. **Which of the following plasma protein is involved in coagulation of blood?**
   a. Albumin
   b. Globulin
   c. Fibrinogen
   d. Amylase

6. **All are true about the coagulation system in women with a normal pregnancy, *except*:**
   a. Excessive thrombin generation
   b. Increased platelet aggregation
   c. Increased fibrinogen concentrations
   d. Increased factor XIII and XI concentrations

7. **The most sensitive test for diagnosis of disseminated intravascular coagulation (DIC) is:**
   a. D-dimer test
   b. Fibrinogen test
   c. Antithrombin
   d. Protein C test

8. **All of the following conditions can trigger disseminated intravascular coagulation (DIC) in pregnancy, *except*:**
   a. Preeclampsia and HELLP (hemolysis, elevated liver enzymes, and low platelet count)
   b. Acute fatty liver of pregnancy
   c. Hypothyroidism
   d. Abruptio placenta

9. **In patients with amniotic fluid embolism (AFE), what is the approximate incidence of disseminated intravascular coagulation (DIC)?**
   a. 40% patients
   b. 60% patients
   c. 80% patients
   d. 100% patients

10. **In severe cases of disseminated intravascular coagulation (DIC), what is the potential risk for the fetus?**
    a. Fetal growth restriction
    b. Birth defects
    c. Neonatal jaundice
    d. Intrauterine fetal demise

11. **What is the primary cause of mortality in cases of disseminated intravascular coagulation (DIC) during pregnancy?**
    a. Maternal hemorrhage
    b. Maternal infection
    c. Fetal demise
    d. Multiorgan failure

12. **In severe cases of disseminated intravascular coagulation (DIC), the primary treatment objective is:**
    a. Stabilizing the mother's blood pressure
    b. Inducing labor and delivering the baby

c. Administering blood transfusions
d. Correction of the underlying cause of DIC

13. **Laboratory findings in disseminated intravascular coagulation (DIC) include:**
    a. Thrombocytopenia, prolonged prothrombin time (PT) and partial thromboplastin time (PTT), low fibrinogen, and raised D-dimers
    b. Thrombocytopenia, decreased prothrombin time (PT) and partial thromboplastin time (PTT), low fibrinogen, and decreased D-dimers
    c. Thrombocytopenia, prolonged prothrombin time (PT) and partial thromboplastin time (PTT), increased fibrinogen, and raised D-dimers
    d. Thrombocytopenia, prolonged prothrombin time (PT) and partial thromboplastin time (PTT), increased fibrinogen, and decreased D-dimers

14. **All are disseminated intravascular coagulation (DIC) scoring systems, *except*:**
    a. Japanese Ministry of Health and Welfare (JMHW) score
    b. The International Society on Thrombosis and Haemostasis (ISTH) score
    c. The Japanese Association for Acute Medicine (JAAM) score
    d. HAS-BLED (Hypertension, Abnormal renal/liver function, Stroke, Bleeding history or predisposition, Labile INR, Elderly, Drugs/alcohol concomitantly) score

15. **The International Society of Thrombosis and Hemostasis (ISTH) scoring system includes following investigations:**
    a. Platelet count, PT, fibrin marker, fibrinogen
    b. Platelet count, PT and fibrin marker
    c. Prothrombin time (PT) and fibrin marker
    d. Platelet count, fibrin marker, fibrinogen

16. **Japanese Association for Acute Medicine (JAAM) score includes all investigations, *except*:**
    a. Platelet count   b. Fibrin
    c. Prothrombin time   d. Fibrinogen

17. **The score for classifying overt disseminated intravascular coagulation (DIC) as per the International Society of Thrombosis and Hemostasis (ISTH) scoring system is:**
    a. >4   b. >5
    c. >6   d. >3

18. **A 32-year-old pregnant woman at 28 weeks of gestation presents to her obstetrician with complaints of sudden abdominal pain and vaginal bleeding. The obstetrician suspects the possibility of abruption and decides to use a pregnancy-specific disseminated intravascular coagulation (DIC) score to assess her condition. What parameters were included in the pregnancy-specific DIC score used by the obstetrician to assess her condition?**
    a. D-dimer, fibrinogen concentrations, and platelet count
    b. Fibrinogen concentrations, the PT difference, and platelet count
    c. Fibrinogen concentration, PT, and aPTT
    d. Fibrinogen concentration, fibrin/fibrinogen degradation products (FDP) and platelet count

19. **How does the pregnancy-specific disseminated intravascular coagulation (DIC) score perform in diagnosing DIC with a cutoff of ≥26 points?**
    a. 50% sensitivity, 90% specificity
    b. 88% sensitivity, 96% specificity
    c. 96% sensitivity, 88% specificity
    d. 75% sensitivity, 85% specificity

20. **Following is false about Japanese Association for Acute Medicine (JAAM) score:**
    a. It is specifically designed for the acute onset of "sepsis induced coagulopathy"
    b. It consists of a systemic inflammatory response syndrome criteria score (SIRS criteria) and three laboratory values (platelet count, PT, and fibrin marker)
    c. JAAM DIC score of 4 or more supports the diagnosis of DIC
    d. JAAM DIC score of 5 or more supports the diagnosis of DIC

21. **What is the recommended plasma fibrinogen level that should be maintained during ongoing postpartum hemorrhage (PPH)?**
    a. >1   b. >2
    c. >1.5   d. >2.5

22. **In major obstetric hemorrhage, fresh frozen plasma (FFP) is transfused at a dose of:**
    a. FFP at dose of 12–15 mL/kg administered every 6 units of RBCS with aim to maintain PT and APTT at <1.5 * normal
    b. FFP at dose of 15–20 mL/kg administered every 6 units of RBCS with aim to maintain PT and APTT at <1.5 * normal

c. FFP at dose of 12-15 mL/kg administered every 4 units of RBCS with aim to maintain PT and APTT at <1.5 * normal
d. FFP at dose of 15-20 mL/kg administered every 4 units of RBCS with aim to maintain PT and APTT at <1.5 * normal

23. What platelet count should trigger transfusion in acutely bleeding patient?
   a. 75,000
   b. 50,000
   c. 20,000
   d. 100,000

24. Which laboratory test is used to assess fibrin degradation products in disseminated intravascular coagulation (DIC)?
   a. D-dimer test
   b. Thrombin time
   c. International normalized ratio
   d. Antithrombin-2 assay

25. Most common cause of disseminated intravascular coagulation (DIC):
   a. Abruptio placentae
   b. Amniotic fluid embolism (AFE)
   c. Acute fatty liver of pregnancy (AFLP)
   d. Intrauterine fetal demise (IUFD)

26. If clotting time is <6 minutes, it indicates fibrinogen levels is more than:
   a. 100 mg percent
   b. 150 mg percent
   c. 200 mg percent
   d. 250 mg percent

27. Fresh frozen plasma contains:
   a. Fibrinogen, antithrombin III, clotting factors V and XI
   b. Fibrinogen, Protein S, clotting factors VIII, X, and XII
   c. Prothrombin, antithrombin III, clotting factors, V, XI, and XII
   d. Prothrombin, antithrombin III, clotting factors V, XI, and XII

28. Fresh frozen plasma (FFP) (250 mL) raises the fibrinogen levels by:
   a. 10–15 mg/dL
   b. 5–10 mg/dL
   c. 15–20 mg/dL
   d. 20–25 mg/dL

29. False about cryoprecipitate:
   a. It is obtained from thawed FFP
   b. It provides less volume (40 mL) compared to FFP (250 mL), so not useful for volume replacement
   c. It is rich in fibrinogen, factor VII, Von Willebrand's factor and factor XIII
   d. One unit increases fibrinogen levels by 5–10 mg/dL

30. What is false about role of antifibrinolytic agents?
   a. Inhibits plasminogen and plasmin
   b. Indicated in postpartum hemorrhage (PPH) following abruptio placenta
   c. Blood fibrinogen levels should be below 200 mg/dL
   d. Risk of thrombosis exists

31. In the case of a 30-year-old multigravida who developed massive postpartum hemorrhage with disseminated intravascular coagulation (DIC), and her serum fibrinogen levels are 150 mg/dL, what is the most appropriate product to elevate the fibrinogen level and manage the condition?
   a. Fresh frozen plasma (FFP)
   b. Packed red blood cells (PRBCs)
   c. Cryoprecipitate
   d. Platelet concentrate

32. Which of the following tests are considered viscoelastic tests used to assess hemostasis?
   a. Thromboelastography (TEG), thromboelastometry (ROTEM) and Sonoclot
   b. Prothrombin time (PT) and activated partial thromboplastin time (aPTT)
   c. Sonoclot and hemoglobin electrophoresis
   d. Thromboelastometry (ROTEM) and platelet count

33. In the context of major postpartum hemorrhage, when is fibrinogen replacement indicated to improve clinical hemostasis?
   a. When FIBTEM A5 is >7 mm
   b. When FIBTEM A5 is <7 mm, or <12 mm with ongoing bleeding
   c. When platelet count is <100,000/mm^3
   d. When activated partial thromboplastin time (aPTT) is prolonged

34. A FIBTEM A5 value of <15 in women with PPH can be correlated with which of the following fibrinogen concentrations?
   a. 1 g/L or 100 mg/dL
   b. 3 g/L or 300 mg/dL
   c. 5 g/L or 500 mg/dL
   d. 10 g/L or 1,000 mg/dL

35. Heparin is given in all case, *except:*
   a. Amniotic fluid embolism
   b. Venous thromboembolism
   c. Retained dead fetus
   d. Acute DIC with bleeding

36. A 28-year-old primigravida at 28 weeks of gestation presented to labor room with acute PV bleeding with severe pain in abdomen. Examination reveals clinical pallor with raised BP of 140/90 mm Hg, stony hard uterus with FHS 100 beats/min. PV reveals cervical os closed with active bleeding and hematuria in urinary catheter. Management includes:
   a. Expedite delivery in view of (i/v/o) abruptio placenta with DIC, antihypertensive treatment, laboratory investigations of CBC, LFT, KFT coagulation profile, FFP: RBC transfusion in ratio 1:1 to be given till reports of laboratory results are awaited
   b. Expedite delivery i/v/o abruptio placenta with DIC, antihypertensive treatment, laboratory investigations of CBC, LFT, KFT, coagulation profile, FFP: RBC transfusion in ratio 1:4 to be given till reports of laboratory results are awaited
   c. Expedite delivery i/v/o abruptio placenta with DIC, antihypertensive treatment, laboratory investigations of CBC, LFT, KFT, coagulation profile PRBC transfusion, FFP to be given only after reports of laboratory results available
   d. FFP: PRBC transfusion, anti-hypertensive treatment, injectable tranexamic acid, and conserve pregnancy

37. A 29-year-old G3P2L2 underwent Emergency Lower Segment Cesarean Section (LSCS) in view of fetal distress. Postoperatively patient had sudden onset of bleeding followed by collapse after 3 hours. Patient on examination was clinically pale, tachypnea, and tachycardia with hypotension uterus was flabby with passage of clots per vaginum. Blood investigations revealed Hb of 6 gms%, platelets of 40,000, coagulation profile was awaited. Management would include:
   a. Airway breathing circulation assessment, O_2, fluid resuscitation, uterotonics, PRBC transfusion, platelet transfusion, up to 4 units FFP and 10 units cryoprecipitate if ongoing bleeding
   b. Airway breathing circulation assessment, O_2, fluid resuscitation, uterotonics, PRBC transfusion, 4 units FFP and 10 units cryoprecipitate
   c. Airway breathing circulation assessment, O_2, fluid resuscitation, uterotonics, PRBC transfusion, platelet transfusion, 4 units FFP, and 10 units cryoprecipitate only if coagulation profile reports are deranged
   d. Airway breathing circulation assessment, O_2, fluid resuscitation, uterotonics, and PRBC transfusion only

ANSWERS

1. **b.** Edward Rigby, an English physician, in a classic essay in 1776, first defined and distinguished between the two main types of third trimester bleeding arising from either low-lying or normal implantation of the placenta. The hemorrhage attributed to a low implantation, or placenta previa, in which the placenta must separate for delivery to occur, was labeled "unavoidable," whereas premature separation of a normally implanted placenta was called "accidental."
   Baudelocque, in 1819, expanded this term to concealed accidental hemorrhage.
   DeLee, who, in 1892, described the condition as abruptio placentae because of the rupture of vascular elements, later attended a patient with uncontrollable uterine hemorrhage in association with placental abruption and postulated a hemophilia-like condition.
   Dieckmann, in 1936, first suggested a causal relationship between low fibrinogen levels and hemorrhage in premature separation of the placenta. *(References: 1. Yeo L, Ananth C, Vintzileos AM. Placental Abruption. Glob Libr Women's Med. 2008.*
   2. DeLee JB. A case of fatal haemorrhagic diathesis with premature detachment of placenta. Am J Obstet Dis Women Child. 1901;44:784-92)

2. **a.** *[Reference: Cunningham F, Leveno KJ, Bloom SL, Dashe JS, Hoffman BL, Casey BM, et al. (Eds). Williams Obstetrics, 25e. New York: McGraw Hill; 2018. p. 782]*

3. **e.** *[Reference: Donald I. Chapter 16: Antepartum Haemorrhage. In: Donald I (Ed). Practical Obstetric Problems, 7th edition. London: Lloyd-Luke (Medical Books); 2014. p. 331]*

4. **a.** Tissue factor—an integral membrane glycoprotein—serves as the principal initiator of coagulation (Levi, 2016). Tissue factor is found in highly vascularized organs such as the brain, lungs, and placenta; in amniotic fluid; and in certain other cells (Kuczyfiski, 2002; Østerud, 2006; Uszyfiski, 2001). Tissue factor forms complexes with factor VII/VIIa to activate factors IX and X and to initiate clotting.

[Reference: Cunningham F, Leveno KJ, Bloom SL, Dashe JS, Hoffman BL, Casey BM, et al. (Eds). Williams Obstetrics, 25th edition. Chapter 44. New York: McGraw Hill; 2018]

5. **c.** Fibrinogen is a high-molecular-weight protein (molecular weight = 340,000) that occurs in the plasma in quantities of 100–700 mg/dL. Fibrinogen is formed in the liver, and liver disease can decrease the concentration of circulating fibrinogen.

   Thrombin is a protein enzyme with weak proteolytic capabilities. It acts on fibrinogen to remove four low molecular-weight peptides from each molecule of fibrinogen, forming one molecule of fibrin monomer that has the automatic capability to polymerize with other fibrin monomer molecules to form fibrin fibers. Therefore, many fibrin monomer molecules polymerize within seconds into long fibrin fibers that constitute the reticulum of the blood clot.

   Albumin and globulin are also plasma proteins, but they are not directly involved in the coagulation process. The major function of albumin is to provide colloid osmotic pressure in the plasma which prevents plasma loss from the capillaries.

   Globulins perform a number of enzymatic functions in plasma and are principally responsible for body's both natural and acquired immunity against invading organisms.

   Amylase, on the other hand, is not a plasma protein involved in coagulation at all. It is an enzyme produced mainly by the pancreas and salivary glands, and it helps in the digestion of carbohydrates.
   [Reference: Hall JE. Unit VI, Chapter 37: Haemostasis and Blood Coagulation. In: Hall JE (Ed). Guyton and Hall Textbook of Medical Physiology, 13th edition. United States: WB Saunders; 2015. p. 483]

6. **d.** Women with a normal pregnancy have: (1) Excessive thrombin generation; (2) increased agonist derived platelets aggregation; (3) two- to threefold increase in fibrinogen concentrations; and (4) toward term they experience a 20–1,000% increase in factors VII, VIII, IX, X, and XII, as well as up to 400% increase in von Willebrand factor. By contrast, factors XIII and XI concentrations decrease during gestation and those of factors II and V unchanged.
   [Reference: Cunningham F, Leveno KJ, Bloom SL, Dashe JS, Hoffman BL, Casey BM, et al. (Eds). Williams Obstetrics, 25th edition. New York: McGraw Hill; 2018]

7. **a.** Normally D-dimer is not present in blood except when coagulation system is activated. Abnormal levels are seen in 94% cases of confirmed disseminated intravascular coagulation (DIC).
   [Reference: Donald I. Chapter 16: Antepartum Haemorrhage. In: Donald I (Ed). Practical Obstetric Problems, 7th edition. London: Lloyd-Luke (Medical Books); 2014. p. 333]

8. **c.** Disseminated intravascular coagulation (DIC) during pregnancy constitutes one of the leading causes for maternal mortality worldwide and its rate varies from 0.03 to 0.35%. This complication is often secondary to underlying maternal and/or fetal complications including placental abruption, postpartum hemorrhage, amniotic fluid embolism, acute fatty liver of pregnancy, preeclampsia and HELLP (hemolysis, elevated liver enzymes, and low platelet count), and retained stillbirth.

   The most frequent pregnancy complication associated with DIC according to Rattray et al. was placental abruption followed by PPH and preeclampsia. Similarly, Erez et al. reported that placental abruption was the leading underlying obstetrical disorder leading to DIC especially when it was accompanied by fetal death. Other groups reported preeclampsia and fetal death to be the leading obstetrical complications associated with DIC.
   [Reference: Erez O, Othman M, Rabinovich A, Leron E, Gotsch F, Thachil J. DIC in Pregnancy—Pathophysiology, Clinical Characteristics, Diagnostic Scores, and Treatments. J Blood Med. 2022;13:21-44]

9. **c.** Disseminated intravascular coagulation (DIC) occurs in approximately 80% of patients with amniotic fluid embolism (AFE). AFE is a rare but life-threatening obstetric emergency where amniotic fluid enters the maternal circulation, leading to various systemic complications, including DIC. DIC is a serious condition characterized by abnormal widespread activation of the clotting cascade, leading to both excessive clotting and bleeding. The high incidence of DIC in AFE highlights its significant association with this particular obstetric complication.
   [Reference: Haftel A, Chowdhury YS. Amniotic Fluid Embolism. In: StatPearls (Internet). Treasure Island (FL): StatPearls Publishing; 2023]

10. **d.** [Reference: Cunningham F, Leveno KJ, Bloom SL, Dashe JS, Hoffman BL, Casey BM, et al. (Eds). Williams Obstetrics, 25th edition. New York: McGraw Hill; 2018. p. 783]

11. **a.** At present time, obstetric bleeding remains to be the world's main cause of maternal mortality, early identification of factors leading to hemorrhage and early management of underlying pathological process is the key stone of the treatment. The most important pregnancy related condition leading to bleeding with high maternal mortality and morbidity rate is disseminated intravascular coagulation.
(Reference: Kadikar SK, Diwan FJ, Topiwala U, Agasiwala S. Study of Pregnancy with Disseminated Intravascular Coagulation. Int J Reprod Contracept Obstet Gynecol. 2021;10:4220-5)

12. **d.** Disseminated intravascular coagulation (DIC) does not occur as primary condition. Treatment of the underlying condition is the mainstay of treatment and at times may be sufficient to revert the process of DIC without instituting any specific therapy for coagulopathy.
[Reference: Donald I. Chapter 16: Antepartum Haemorrhage. In: Donald I (Ed). Practical Obstetric Problems, 7th edition. London: Lloyd-Luke (Medical Books); 2014. p. 333]

13. **a.** Disseminated intravascular coagulation (DIC) is a consequence of aberrant activation of coagulation cascade. The laboratory abnormalities reported in DIC are thrombocytopenia, elevated fibrin degradation products, prolonged PT, prolonged aPTT, and low fibrinogen levels, in order of frequency. Laboratory results should be interpreted with the understanding that normal range in nonpregnant women may differ from what is normal during pregnancy. Serial testing with clinical correlation is more useful than single time assessment.
[Reference: Donald I. Chapter 16: Antepartum Haemorrhage. In: Donald I (Ed). Practical Obstetric Problems, 7th edition. London: Lloyd-Luke (Medical Books); 2014. p. 332]

14. **d.** Disseminated intravascular coagulation (DIC) enhances the inflammatory response and causes the systemic inflammatory response syndrome (SIRS) and microvascular thrombosis, which result in multiple organ dysfunction syndrome. In this regard, several DIC scoring systems have been developed to predict the risk of mortality in critically ill patients. Of these, the Japanese Ministry of Health and Welfare (JMHW) score, the International Society on Thrombosis and Haemostasis (ISTH) score, the Japanese Association for Acute Medicine (JAAM) score, and the Korean Society on Thrombosis and Hemostasis (KSTH) score are commonly used to predict the risk of mortality in various diseases.

    HAS-BLED Score estimates risk of major bleeding for patients on anticoagulation to assess risk-benefit in atrial fibrillation care.
[References: 1. Lee DH, Lee BK, Jeung KW, Park JS, Lim YD, Jung YH, et al. Performance of 5 disseminated intravascular coagulation score systems in predicting mortality in patients with severe trauma. Medicine (Baltimore). 2018;97(33):e11912.
2. Zhu W, He W, Guo L, Wang X, Hong K. The HAS-BLED Score for Predicting Major Bleeding Risk in Anticoagulated Patients with Atrial Fibrillation: A Systematic Review and Meta-analysis. Clin Cardiol. 2015;38(9):555-61]

15. **a.** *[Reference: Iba T, Umemura Y, Watanabe E, Wada T, Hayashida K, Kushimoto S; Japanese Surviving Sepsis Campaign Guideline Working Group for disseminated intravascular coagulation. Diagnosis of sepsis-induced disseminated intravascular coagulation and coagulopathy. Acute Med Surg. 2019;6(3):223-32]*

16. **d.** *[Reference: Iba T, Umemura Y, Watanabe E, Wada T, Hayashida K, Kushimoto S; Japanese Surviving Sepsis Campaign Guideline Working Group for disseminated intravascular coagulation. Diagnosis of sepsis-induced disseminated intravascular coagulation and coagulopathy. Acute Med Surg. 2019;6(3):223-32]*

17. **a.** The International Society of Thrombosis and Hemostasis (ISTH) scoring system is a scoring system used only after a condition known to cause intravascular coagulation is identified and calculated using a combination of laboratory tests. The scoring is done based on the thrombocyte count, fibrin split products, D-dimer, prolonged aPTT, and fibrinogen levels. A score of 5 and higher is considered as overt DIC.
[Reference: Cunningham F, Leveno KJ, Bloom SL, Dashe JS, Hoffman BL, Casey BM, et al. (Eds). Williams Obstetrics, 25th edition. Chapter 44. New York: McGraw Hill; 2018. p. 785]

18. **b.** Diagnosis of DIC can be elusive during pregnancy and requires vigilance and knowledge of the physiologic changes during pregnancy. It can be facilitated by using a pregnancy specific DIC score including three components: 1) fibrinogen

concentrations; 2) the PT difference – relating to the difference in PT result between the patient's plasma and the laboratory control; and 3) platelet count.
(Reference: Erez O, Othman M, Rabinovich A, Leron E, Gotsch F, Thachil J. DIC in Pregnancy - Pathophysiology, Clinical Characteristics, Diagnostic Scores, and Treatments. J Blood Med. 2022;13:21-44. Published 2022 Jan 6. doi:10.2147/JBM.S273047)

19. **b.** At a cutoff of ≥26 points, the pregnancy specific DIC score has 88% sensitivity, 96% specificity, a positive likelihood ratio (LR) of 22, and a negative LR of 0.125.
(Reference: Erez O, Othman M, Rabinovich A, Leron E, Gotsch F, Thachil J. DIC in Pregnancy - Pathophysiology, Clinical Characteristics, Diagnostic Scores, and Treatments. J Blood Med. 2022;13:21-44. Published 2022 Jan 6. doi:10.2147/JBM.S273047)

20. **d.** *[Reference: Iba T, Umemura Y, Watanabe E, Wada T, Hayashida K, Kushimoto S; Japanese Surviving Sepsis Campaign Guideline Working Group for disseminated intravascular coagulation. Diagnosis of sepsis-induced disseminated intravascular coagulation and coagulopathy. Acute Med Surg. 2019;6(3):223-32]*

21. **b.** A plasma fibrinogen level of >2 g/L should be maintained during ongoing PPH. During ongoing postpartum hemorrhage, it is recommended to maintain a plasma fibrinogen level of >2 g/L. Fibrinogen plays a critical role in clot formation and stability, and maintaining adequate levels is essential for effective hemostasis in managing PPH. Keeping the fibrinogen concentration above 2 g/L helps to support clotting mechanisms and prevents excessive bleeding during this critical period after childbirth.
[Reference: Prevention and management of Postpartum hemorrhage, Green top guideline no.52, RCOG. BJOG. 2017;124(5):e106-e149]

22. **a.** FFP at a dose of 12–15 mL/kg should be administered for every 6 units of red cells during major obstetric hemorrhage. Subsequent FFP transfusion should be guided by results of clotting test if they are available in a timely manner, aiming to maintain prothrombin time (PT) and activated partial thromboplastin time (APTT) ratios at <1.5 times normal.
[Reference: RCOG. (2015). Blood transfusion in obstetrics; Green top guidelines no. 47. [online] Available from: https://www.rcog.org.uk/guidance/browse-all-guidance/green-top-guidelines/blood-transfusions-in-obstetrics-green-top-guideline-no-47/ (Last accessed December, 2023)].

23. **a.** Aim to maintain the platelet count above 50 × 10/L in the acutely bleeding patient as this represents the critical level for hemostasis. A platelet transfusion trigger of 75 × 10/L is recommended to provide a margin of safety. The platelets should ideally be group compatible. RhD-negative women should also receive RhD-negative platelets.
[Reference: RCOG. (2015). Blood transfusion in obstetrics; Green top guidelines no. 47. (online) Available from: https://www.rcog.org.uk/guidance/browse-all-guidance/green-top-guidelines/blood-transfusions-in-obstetrics-green-top-guideline-no-47/ (Last accessed December, 2023)].

24. **a.** Fibrin degradation products are blood components produced by degradation of blood clot or fibrinolysis. The fibrinolytic activity in DIC is enhanced which can be detected by measuring fibrin degradation products. However, FDP assays do not differentiate between degradation products of fibrin and fibrinogen, and may be raised in other conditions such as trauma, recent surgery, or thromboembolism. D-dimer is a fragment of fibrinogen which can be detected by assays using monoclonal antibody. D-dimers are not normally present in blood except when the coagulation system has been activated as in thrombosis or DIC. Of all tests, D-dimer assay has been found to be the most sensitive test for diagnosing DIC, abnormal levels reported in 94% of patients with DIC.
[Reference: Donald I. Practical Obstetric Problems, 7th edition. London: Lloyd-Luke (Medical Books); 2014]

25. **a.** The most frequent pregnancy complication associated with DIC according to Rattray et al. was placental abruption followed by PPH and preeclampsia. Similarly, Erez et al. reported that placental abruption was the leading underlying obstetrical disorder leading to DIC especially when it was accompanied by fetal death. Other groups reported preeclampsia and fetal death to be the leading obstetrical complications associated with DIC.
(Reference: Erez O, Othman M, Rabinovich A, Leron E, Gotsch F, Thachil J. DIC in Pregnancy—Pathophysiology, Clinical Characteristics, Diagnostic Scores, and Treatments. J Blood Med. 2022;13:21-44)

26. **b.** Clotting time: 5 mL of venous blood placed in 15 mL dry test tube at 37°C.

    Usually blood clot forms within 6–12 minutes. If the clotting time is <6 minutes, fibrinogen level is >150 mg%. If no clot forms within 30 minutes, the fibrinogen level is probably <100 mg%.
    [Reference: Begum F. Chapter 10: Coagulation Disorders in Pregnancy. In: Begum F (Ed). Textbook on High-Risk Pregnancy for Postgraduates, 1st Edition. New Delhi: Jaypee Brothers Medical Publishers (P) Ltd.; 2022. p. 121]

27. **a.** Fresh frozen plasma (FFP) is extracted from whole blood. It contains fibrinogen, antithrombin III, clotting factors II, V, VIII, IX, X, and XI.

    FFP transfusion provides both volume replacement and coagulation factors.
    [Reference: Begum F. Chapter 10: Coagulation Disorders in Pregnancy. In: Begum F (Ed). Textbook on High-Risk Pregnancy for Postgraduates, 1st Edition. New Delhi: Jaypee Brothers Medical Publishers (P) Ltd.; 2022. p. 121]

28. **b.** One unit of FFP (250 mL) raises the fibrinogen by 5–10 mg/dL.
    [Reference: Begum F. Chapter 10: Coagulation Disorders in Pregnancy. In: Begum F (Ed). Textbook on High-Risk Pregnancy for Postgraduates, 1st Edition. New Delhi: Jaypee Brothers Medical Publishers (P) Ltd.; 2022. p. 121]

29. **c.** Cryoprecipitate is obtained from thawed FFP. It is rich in fibrinogen, factor VIII, Von Willebrand's factor, and XIII. Cryoprecipitate provides less volume (40 mL) compared to FFP (250 mL). So, it should not be used for volume replacement. One unit of cryoprecipitate increases the fibrinogen level by 5–10 mg/dL.
    [Reference: Begum F. Chapter 10: Coagulation Disorders in Pregnancy. In: Begum F (Ed). Textbook on High-Risk Pregnancy for Postgraduates, 1st Edition. New Delhi: Jaypee Brothers Medical Publishers (P) Ltd.; 2022. p. 121]

30. **c.** Commonly available antifibrinolytic agents are— (1) EACA—inhibits plasminogen and plasmin (2) Trasylol—inhibits plasmin (3) Aprotinin—nonspecific enzyme inhibitor. Fibrinolytic inhibitors are mainly indicated in postpartum hemorrhage following abruptio placenta in spite of a firm and contracted uterus and when blood fibrinogen level is 200 mg% or more. However, these drugs can increase the risk of thrombosis.
    [Reference: Begum F. Chapter 10: Coagulation Disorders in Pregnancy. In: Begum F (Ed). Textbook on High-Risk Pregnancy for Postgraduates, 1st Edition. New Delhi: Jaypee Brothers Medical Publishers (P) Ltd.; 2022. p. 125]

31. **c.** The appropriate fibrinogen intervention trigger or target level is unknown. A pragmatic view based on available evidence is that, during continuing postpartum hemorrhage, cryoprecipitate or fibrinogen concentrate should be used to maintain a fibrinogen level of at least 2 g/L, even if PT or aPTT is normal.

    In this scenario, the most appropriate product to elevate the fibrinogen level is cryoprecipitate. Cryoprecipitate is a blood product derived from plasma and contains concentrated fibrinogen, along with other coagulation factors, von Willebrand factor, and fibronectin. Since the patient's serum fibrinogen level is 15 mg/dL, indicating low fibrinogen levels, cryoprecipitate is the ideal choice to rapidly replenish fibrinogen and support clot formation in cases of massive postpartum hemorrhage with DIC. Fresh frozen plasma (FFP) contains all coagulation factors, but cryoprecipitate is preferred in situations where fibrinogen deficiency is the primary concern due to its higher fibrinogen concentration. Packed red blood cells (PRBCs) and platelet concentrate are not appropriate for elevating fibrinogen levels as they do not contain significant amounts of fibrinogen.
    [References: 1. Prevention and management of Postpartum Haemorrhage, Green top guideline no. 52, RCOG. BJOG. 2017;124(5):e106-e149.
    2. Mavrides E, Allard S, Chandraharan E, Collins P, Green L, Hunt BJ, et al. Prevention and management of postpartum haemorrhage. BJOG. 2016;124:e106-49]

32. **a.** Viscoelastic tests, such as thromboelastography (TEG), rotational thromboelastometry (ROTEM) and Sonoclot, are used to assess the whole blood coagulation process, providing a dynamic assessment of clot formation and dissolution.

    While PT and aPTT are coagulation tests, they are not viscoelastic tests and measure specific aspects of the coagulation cascade rather than the overall

clotting process. Platelet count is a standard blood test to measure the number of platelets and not a viscoelastic test. Hemoglobin electrophoresis is used to detect abnormal hemoglobin types and is unrelated to coagulation assessment.
(Reference: Curry NS, Davenport R, Pavord S, Mallett SV, Kitchen D, Klein AA, et al. The use of viscoelastic haemostatic assays in the management of major bleeding. Br J Haematol. 2018;182:789806)

33. **b.** FIBTEM is a specific test in rotational thromboelastometry (ROTEM) used to assess the contribution of fibrinogen to clot formation. A5 refers to the amplitude of clot firmness at 5 minutes after the initiation of clotting. In the context of major postpartum hemorrhage, if FIBTEM A5 is <7 mm, or if it remains below 12 mm with ongoing bleeding, it suggests a deficiency in fibrinogen and indicates the need for fibrinogen replacement therapy to improve clinical hemostasis. Fibrinogen replacement helps to strengthen the clot and stabilize the hemostatic process during significant bleeding after childbirth.
[Reference: Curry NS, Davenport R, Pavord S, Mallett SV, Kitchen D, Klein AA, et al. The use of viscoelastic haemostatic assays in the management of major bleeding. Br J Haematol. 2018;182:789-806]

34. **b.** According to the given information, a FIBTEM A5 value of <15 in women with postpartum hemorrhage can be translated to a fibrinogen concentration of 3 grams per liter (g/L) or 300 milligrams per deciliter (mg/dL). This correlation helps to assess fibrinogen levels based on ROTEM results, guiding appropriate fibrinogen replacement therapy to support effective clot formation in managing postpartum hemorrhage.
(Reference: Erez O, Othman M, Rabinovich A, Leron E, Gotsch F, Thachil J. DIC in Pregnancy - Pathophysiology, Clinical Characteristics, Diagnostic Scores, and Treatments. J Blood Med. 2022;13:21-44)

35. **d.** Heparin should be used when the vascular compartment remains intact. In acute condition such as amniotic fluid embolism, intravenous heparin 5,000 units repeated 4–6 hours intervals are useful to stop DIC and may be lifesaving. In retained dead fetus, there is progressive but slow defibrination due to DIC. In such cases, the process can be arrested by intravenous heparin. In acute DIC, heparin may aggravate bleeding.
[Reference: Begum F. Chapter 10: Coagulation Disorders in Pregnancy. In: Begum F (Ed). Textbook on High-Risk Pregnancy for Postgraduates, 1st Edition. New Delhi: Jaypee Brothers Medical Publishers (P) Ltd.; 2022. p. 125]

36. **a.** Data regarding transfusion of blood products in APH is limited. In management of military trauma, a decrease in coagulopathy and improvement in survival is reported with a high fresh frozen plasma to packed red cell transfusion ratio of 1:1 to 1:1.4.

    In women who have experienced a massive blood loss or major abruption, the development of DIC should be considered. Clotting studies and platelet count should be urgently requested and advice from hematologist sought. Up to four units of FFP and 10 units of cryoprecipitate may be given while awaiting results.
[Reference: RCOG. (2011). RCOG Green top guidelines no. 63. (online) Available from: https://www.rcog.org.uk/guidance/browse-all-guidance/green-top-guidelines/antepartum-haemorrhage-green-top-guideline-no-63/(Last accessed December, 2023)]

37. **a.**
Fluid therapy and blood product transfusion:
- With continuing massive hemorrhage and awaiting coagulation studies, up to four units FFP and 10 units cryoprecipitate can be given if ongoing bleeding.
- Platelet concentrates can be given if platelet count is below 50,000 with aim to keep platelet count >75,000.

[Reference: RCOG. (2011). RCOG Green top guidelines no. 63: Antepartum haemorrhage, Appendix 2. (online) Available from https://www.rcog.org.uk/guidance/browse-all-guidance/green-top-guidelines/antepartum-haemorrhage-green-top-guideline-no-63/(Last accessed December, 2023)]

Chapter 61

Blood Transfusion

Kalyani Sai Dhandapani, Ruchika Garg

QUESTIONS

1. A P1L1 mother had severe PPH after a normal vaginal delivery crossmatching and was infused with 1,500 mL of crystalloids till the arrival of blood products. How much percentage of this fluid is expected to stay in the intravascular compartment after 1 hour?
   a. 10% b. 20%
   c. 30% d. 50%

2. Crossmatching before blood transfusion is:
   a. Maternal serum with standard reagent red cell
   b. Maternal serum with actual donor erythrocytes
   c. Standard reagent with donor erythrocytes
   d. Maternal RBC with donor erythrocytes

3. For a patient who had severe PPH, due to gestational thrombocytopenia, had massive blood transfusion protocol. Of the following, which blood products will help to improve platelet count?
   A. Whole blood
   B. Packed cell
   C. Single donor platelet
   D. Fresh frozen plasma (FFP)
   a. A and C   b. B and C
   c. C only   d. D and C

4. Hematocrit is maximum in which of the following blood products?
   a. Whole blood
   b. Packed red blood cell (PRBC)
   c. Cryoprecipitate
   d. Equal in whole blood and PRBC

5. In the woman with obstetrical hemorrhage, indications for blood product transfusion are all, *except*:
   a. Platelet count <50,000/μL
   b. A fibrinogen level <150 mg/dL
   c. A sufficiently prolonged PT or PTT in a woman with surgical bleeding
   d. Hematocrit <30%

6. One unit of whole blood transfusion raises the hematocrit by:
   a. 3-4 volume percent   b. 7-8 volume percent
   c. 10-12 volume percent d. 1-2 volume percent

7. Drawback of massive hemorrhage treatment with crystalloid solutions and packed red blood cells is depletion of platelets and clotting factors are:
   a. Dilutional coagulopathy
   b. Hypofibrinogenemia
   c. Thrombocytopenia
   d. Disseminated intravascular coagulation (DIC)

8. Each single donor-apheresis equivalent to six-unit bag raises the platelet count by approximately:
   a. 10,000/uL   b. 20,000/uL
   c. 30,000/uL   d. 15,000/uL

9. Minimum duration needed to thaw FFP.
   a. 30 minutes b. 45 minutes
   c. 60 minutes d. 15 minutes

10. This never frozen plasma, which is used as the best alternative to FFP is called:
    a. Cryoprecipitate
    b. Liquid plasma
    c. Fibrinogen concentrate
    d. PRBC

11. Which of the following is not found in cryoprecipitate?
    a. Factor V   b. Factor VIII
    c. Factor XIII d. Fibronectin

12. One unit raises the hematocrit by:
    a. 3 volume percent b. 5 volume percent
    c. 1 volume percent d. 10 volume percent

13. **False regarding recombinant activated factor VII (rFVIIa)**
    a. rFVIIa will not be effective if the plasma fibrinogen level is <50 mg/dL
    b. rFVIIa will not be effective if the platelet count is <30,000/μL
    c. rFVIIa is associated with arterial-and to a lesser degree-venous thrombosis
    d. rFVVIIa is transfused for volume replacement

14. **This is a picture of:**

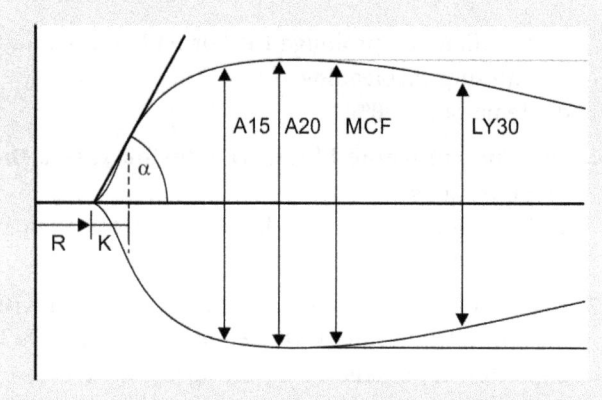

    a. Thromboelastography (TEG)
    b. Rotational thromboelastometry (ROTEM)
    c. Coagulation curve
    d. None of the above

15. **A 30-year-old primigravida at 36 weeks gestation with β-thalassemia trait had hemoglobin of 6 g/dL. She was transfused with PRBC and developed rash within 1 hour of transfusion. Which of the following should not be done?**
    a. Treating hypotension
    b. Treating hyperkalemia
    c. Preventing diuresis
    d. Alkalinizing the urine

16. **The most often implicated contaminants of red cells transfusion are:**
    a. *Yersinia*
    b. *Pseudomonas*
    c. *Serratia*
    d. *Staphylococcus*

17. **A 36-year-old multigravida with placenta previa was initiated on massive transfusion protocol during her intraoperative PPH. She developed septicemia of acinetobacter within 5 days of delivery. Which of the following blood products has the greatest probability of causing this septicemia?**
    a. Packed red blood cell (PRBC)
    b. Fresh frozen plasma (FFP)
    c. Cryoprecipitate
    d. Platelet

18. **Find the odd one out:**
    a. Consumptive coagulopathy
    b. Dilutional coagulopathy
    c. Defibrination syndrome
    d. Disseminated intravascular coagulation (DIC)

19. **False out of the following regarding pregnancy induced coagulation changes:**
    a. Elevated fibrinogen
    b. Elevated factor X
    c. Elevated plasminogen
    d. Low FDP

ANSWERS

1. **b.** 20%
   Serious hemorrhage demands prompt and adequate refilling of the intravascular compartment with crystalloid solutions. These rapidly equilibrate into the extravascular space, and only 20% of crystalloid remains intravascular in critically ill patients after 1 hour (Zuckerbraun, 2010). Because of this, initial fluid is infused in a volume two to three times the estimated blood loss.
   [Reference: Cunningham F, Leveno KJ, Dashe JS, Hoffman BL, Spong CY, Casey BM (Eds). Williams Obstetrics, 26th edition. New York: McGraw-Hill; 2022. p. 1977]

2. **b.** Screening involves mixing maternal serum with standard reagent red cells that carry antigens to which most of the common clinically significant antibodies react. Instead, crossmatching involves the use of actual donor erythrocytes rather than the standardized red cells. Importantly, administration of screened blood rarely results in adverse clinical sequelae.
   [Reference: Cunningham F, Leveno KJ, Dashe JS, Hoffman BL, Spong CY, Casey BM (Eds). Williams Obstetrics, 26th edition. New York: McGraw-hill; 2022. p. 1978]

3. **c.** C only
   [Reference: Cunningham F, Leveno KJ, Dashe JS, Hoffman BL, Spong CY, Casey BM (Eds). Management of obstetrical hemorrhage. Williams Obstetrics, 26th edition. New York: McGraw Hill; 2022. p. 1981]

4. **b.** Packed red blood cell (PRBC)
   Hematocrit in whole blood is 40% when compared to PRBC with 55–80%.

5. **d.** Hematocrit <30%
[Reference: Cunningham F, Leveno KJ, Dashe JS, Hoffman BL, Spong CY, Casey BM (Eds). Management of obstetrical hemorrhage. Williams Obstetrics, 26th edition. New York: McGraw Hill; 2022. p. 1980]

6. **a.** 3-4 volume percent
[Reference: Cunningham F, Leveno KJ, Dashe JS, Hoffman BL, Spong CY, Casey BM (Eds). Management of obstetrical hemorrhage. Williams Obstetrics, 26th edition. New York: McGraw Hill; 2022. p. 1981]

7. **d.** Disseminated intravascular coagulation (DIC)
[Reference: Cunningham F, Leveno KJ, Dashe JS, Hoffman BL, Spong CY, Casey BM (Eds). Management of obstetrical hemorrhage. Williams Obstetrics, 26th edition. New York: McGraw Hill; 2022. p. 1981]

8. **b.** 20,000/uL
[Reference: Cunningham F, Leveno KJ, Dashe JS, Hoffman BL, Spong CY, Casey BM (Eds). Management of obstetrical hemorrhage. Williams Obstetrics, 26th edition. New York: McGraw Hill; 2022. p. 1982]

9. **a.** 30 minutes
[Reference: Cunningham F, Leveno KJ, Dashe JS, Hoffman BL, Spong CY, Casey BM (Eds). Management of obstetrical hemorrhage. Williams Obstetrics, 26th edition. New York: McGraw Hill; 2022. p. 1982]

10. **b.** Liquid plasma
An alternative to frozen plasma is liquid plasma (LQP). This never frozen plasma is stored at 1–60°C for up to 40 days, and its use compares favorably with fresh-frozen plasma. Liquid plasma is not universally available in many centers
[Reference: Cunningham F, Leveno KJ, Dashe JS, Hoffman BL, Spong CY, Casey BM (Eds). Management of obstetrical hemorrhage. Williams Obstetrics, 26th edition. New York: McGraw Hill; 2022. p. 1982]

11. **a.** Fibronectin
[Reference: Cunningham F, Leveno KJ, Dashe JS, Hoffman BL, Spong CY, Casey BM (Eds). Management of obstetrical hemorrhage. Williams Obstetrics, 26th edition. New York: McGraw Hill; 2022. p. 1982]

12. **a.** 3 volume percent
Compatible whole blood is ideal for management of severe obstetrical hemorrhage. It has a shelf-life of 40 days, and 70% of the transfused red cells function for at least 24 hours following transfusion. One unit raises the hematocrit by 3-4 volume percent.
[Reference: Cunningham F, Leveno KJ, Dashe JS, Hoffman BL, Spong CY, Casey BM (Eds). Management of obstetrical hemorrhage. Williams Obstetrics, 26th edition. New York: McGraw Hill; 2022. p. 1981]

13. **d.** rFVVIIa is transfused for volume replacement.
Recombinant activated factor VII (rFVIIa) binds to exposed tissue factor at the injury site to generate thrombin that activates platelets and the coagulation cascade. Since its introduction, rFVIIa has been used to help control hemorrhage from surgery, trauma, and obstetrical causes.
[Reference: Cunningham F, Leveno KJ, Dashe JS, Hoffman BL, Spong CY, Casey BM (Eds). Management of obstetrical hemorrhage. Williams Obstetrics, 26th edition. New York: McGraw Hill; 2022. p. 1981]

14. **a.** Thromboelastography (TEG)

15. **c.** Preventing diuresis
A transfusion reaction is characterized by fever, hypotension, tachycardia, dyspnea, chest or back pain, flushing, severe anxiety, and hemoglobinuria. Immediate supportive measures include stopping the transfusion, treating hypotension and hyperkalemia, provoking diuresis, and alkalinizing the urine.

16. **d.** *Staphylococcus*
Bacterial infection from transfusion of a contaminated blood component is unusual because organism growth is discouraged by refrigeration. The most often implicated contaminants of red cells include *Yersinia, Pseudomonas, Serratia, Acinetobacter*, and *Escherichia* species.

17. **d.** Platelet
The most important risk is from bacterial contamination of platelets, which are stored at room temperature. Current estimates are that 1 in 1,000–2,000 platelet units are contaminated.

18. **b.** Dilutional coagulopathy

19. **d.** Low FDP

Chapter 62

Fetal Growth Restriction

Shobana Mahadevan, Ruchika Garg

QUESTIONS

1. **Primi at 28 weeks gestation has a scan at 28 weeks which shows abdominal circumference (AC) at 10th centile and estimated fetal weight (EFW) at 8th centile. Biparietal diameter (BPD) at 21st centile, head circumference (HC) at 18th centile, femur length (FL) at 20th centile. Doppler of umbilical artery, middle cerebral artery (MCA) and ductus venosus (DV) are within normal range. She is normotensive. Body mass index (BMI) is 23 kg/m^2. She has gestational diabetes managed with diet control. The appropriate next step will be:**
   a. As the EFW is at 8th centile, growth restriction is diagnosed and a Doppler study should be done after 1 week to rule out progression of the condition
   b. Daily fetal movement chart, twice weekly biophysical profile, cardiotocography (CTG) should be commenced for fetal surveillance
   c. This is a small for gestational age fetus and a scan should be scheduled 2–3 weeks later to determine the interval growth
   d. The next scan should be done at 36 weeks to determine the interval growth

2. **Choose the correct statement:**
   a. Aneuploidy fetuses are always symmetrically growth restricted
   b. All small for gestational age (SGA) fetuses are not growth restricted; most are likely to be constitutionally small
   c. The terms symmetrical and asymmetrical growth restriction are useful to understand the underlying etiology and prognosis
   d. All early onset growth restrictions are symmetrical and late onset ones are asymmetrical

3. **Regarding assignment of gestational age:**
   a. Gestational assessment between 6 and 7 weeks by crown-rump length (CRL) is the most accurate method
   b. If the first scan is done in the second trimester, AC is used to estimate the gestational age
   c. USG estimated date of delivery (EDD) should be preferred if the discrepancy between the menstrual dates and USG dates is >2 days in the first trimester
   d. If CRL exceeds 84 mm, HC should be used to estimate the gestational age

4. **A scan done at 34 weeks in a woman in her second pregnancy with no medical comorbidities shows AC at 20th centile and EFW at 15th centile. Umbilical artery pulsatility index (PI) and MCA Doppler are normal. CPR is 1.4. Amniotic fluid index (AFI) is 12. Her scan at 22 weeks showed EFW at 65th centile and AC at 48th centile. Uterine artery Doppler was not done. The most appropriate action will be:**
   a. As the EFW and AC are above the 10th centile, a repeat scan can be done after 4 weeks
   b. This is diagnostic of late onset of fetal growth restriction (FGR) and a repeat Doppler should be done in 2 weeks
   c. Corticosteroids should be given to the mother now for fetal lung maturity anticipating an early delivery
   d. No further scans are needed and expectant labor management until 40 weeks

5. **Small for gestational age (SGA) was diagnosed at 32 weeks by EFW 9th centile and BPD, HC, AC, and FL above the 10th centile. Uterine artery Doppler showed high resistance flow. Previous scan at 20 weeks showed all parameters above the 10th centile. Uterine artery Doppler was normal at**

20 and 32 weeks. All the following sentences are true, *except:*
a. Follow-up scan should be done after 3–4 weeks as this is SGA and not FGR
b. Uterine artery Doppler once assessed at 32 weeks need not be assessed at every scan visit later as it does not change
c. Growth should be assessed every 2 weeks to see if there is a crossover to FGR
d. In the case of SGA, induction should be considered at 37–38 weeks and not later than 39 weeks

6. Among the differences between early and late onset FGR, all are true, *except:*
   a. Late onset of FGR is more common
   b. Early onset of FGR is more difficult to diagnose while late onset of FGR is more difficult to manage
   c. Placental histopathology shows abnormal placental perfusion with early onset of FGR whereas it is a problem of diffusion in late onset of FGR
   d. There is usually abnormal Doppler flow in umbilical, middle cerebral arteries, and DV in early onset of FGR; in late onset of FGR, these indices may be abnormal but cerebroplacental ratio may show abnormality

7. At 19 weeks, the biometry shows growth restriction. Choose the correct statement.
   a. A positive immunoglobulin (Ig)M and IgG with high avidity for cytomegalovirus (CMV) is diagnostic of recent maternal infection
   b. A large placenta with normal liquor/polyhydramnios points to an infective cause
   c. Normal liquor rules out placental dysfunction
   d. Amniocentesis done before 20 weeks can detect fetal IgM antibodies to congenital infections

8. 29 weeks pregnancy with AC <10th centile and umbilical artery Doppler shows pulsatility index (PI) above 95th centile, normal ductus venosus (DV) Doppler. After 1 week, there is absence of umbilical artery diastolic flow. BP is normal. Liquor is normal. There is no reversal of flow in umbilical artery and DV is normal. What should be the management plan?
   a. Repeat Doppler after 1 week to confirm absent flow in umbilical artery
   b. Maternal corticosteroids and plan delivery by cesarean section now
   c. Induce labor by mechanical methods
   d. Repeat Doppler every 2–3 days to detect reversal of flow in umbilical artery till 32–34 weeks when delivery can be planned

9. Intrapartum fetal cardiotocography (CTG) abnormalities are most likely in:
   a. SGA with normal Dopplers and liquor at 39 weeks
   b. EFW at 10th centile with normal Doppler and liquor at 37–38 weeks
   c. EFW at 2nd centile with umbilical artery PI above the 95th centile with oligohydramnios
   d. EFW at 10th centile with umbilical artery Doppler at 95th centile

10. Regarding amniotic fluid measurement, the following are true, *except:*
    a. Using a measurement of single vertical deepest liquor pool <2 cm reduces overdiagnosis of oligohydramnios compared to a four-quadrant value cutoff below 5 cm
    b. An isolated finding of oligohydramnios is not associated with acidosis at birth
    c. Amniotic fluid measurement is a component of biophysical profile assessment
    d. EFW between 4 and 10th centile with AFI 6 cm is an indication for an elective cesarean section

11. The following conditions are at risk of fetal growth restriction, *except:*
    a. Hypertensive disorders of pregnancy
    b. Rh isoimmunization
    c. Type 2 diabetes mellitus
    d. Systemic lupus erythematosus (SLE)

12. A PAPP-A value less than the following value is a risk factor for SGA:
    a. 0.8 MOM   b. 0.6 MOM
    c. 0.5 MOM   d. 0.4 MOM

13. The following are recognized as risk factors for SGA, *except:*
    a. Cigarette smoking
    b. Previous SGA
    c. Cocaine use
    d. Subclinical hypothyroidism

14. In different customized growth charts, fetal growth and weight are adjusted for all the following variables, *except:*
    a. Maternal weight   b. Ethnicity
    c. Maternal comorbidities d. Fetal sex

15. In TRUFFLE study, the three timing-of-delivery arms that were compared did not include one of the following:
    a. Short-term variability in computerized CTG
    b. Reversal of umbilical artery end-diastolic flow
    c. High resistance flow in ductus venosus
    d. Reversal of flow in ductus venosus

16. The Doppler study of one of the following is useful both in the diagnosis and surveillance in FGR:
    a. Uterine artery pulsatility index (PI)
    b. Umbilical artery PI
    c. Middle cerebral artery (MCA) PI
    d. Ductus venosus (DV) PI

17. The following intervention improves neonatal outcome in preterm FGR fetuses:
    a. Bed rest
    b. Intravenous albumin infusion
    c. Maternal antenatal corticosteroids and $MgSO_4$
    d. Antithrombotic therapy of low-molecular-weight heparin (LMWH)

18. The most important predictor of intact neonatal survival in FGR fetuses before 28 weeks is:
    a. Uterine artery Doppler
    b. Gestational age
    c. Normal DV Doppler
    d. Normal umbilical artery Doppler

19. The TRUFFLE study was designed to assess:
    a. The differences in the outcomes between early onset and late onset FGR
    b. To compare the two surveillance methods namely umbilical artery Doppler and ductus venosus Doppler in early onset of FGR
    c. To assess whether changes in the fetal ductus venosus Doppler waveform or the short-term variation (STV) in computerized CTG should be the trigger for delivery in early onset FGR
    d. To compare the different methods of delivery in early onset FGR

20. One of the following is not typically associated with a small fetus:
    a. A small placenta
    b. Subchorionic fibrin deposition
    c. Low lying placenta
    d. Extensive placental calcification

21. Regarding MCA Doppler, all are true, *except:*
    a. There is a high interobserver variability
    b. In early onset of FGR, it is not useful in determining time of delivery
    c. Ratio of MCA-PI and umbilical artery PI is more sensitive in picking up fetal hypoxia than the individual values in late onset of FGR
    d. The vasodilatation of MCA with brain-sparing effect as a response to fetal hypoxia is represented by increasing PI

22. Choose the wrong statement:
    a. The most common cause of fetal growth restriction is deficient placental nutritional transfer due to abnormal invasion of fetal trophoblast
    b. Among the chromosomal abnormalities, trisomy-21 is the most common cause of FGR
    c. Maternal age, parity, ethnicity, and previous SGA are nonmodifiable causes of FGR
    d. Among the fetal infections, CMV and toxoplasmosis are the most common causes of FGR

23. A 25-year-old woman with a body mass index (BMI) 23 kg/m^2 with no medical comorbidities attends the clinic for preconception clinic. She is a smoker and has had the SGA baby at 10th centile in her first pregnancy. Which of the following will help in reducing the risk of having a growth restricted baby?
    a. Antiplatelet agents
    b. Smoking cessation
    c. Progesterone therapy in pregnancy
    d. All of the above

24. A 27-year-old gravida 3, para 2 had a growth scan at 32 weeks gestation. Her body mass index (BMI) is 25 kg/m^2. There are no medical comorbidities. She had one SGA baby born at term. Her umbilical artery pulsatility index (PI) is 0.73. Umbilical artery Doppler flow measurement has the following role:
    a. A low PI means the child should be delivered before 34 weeks
    b. It can predict growth restriction
    c. Management based on umbilical artery Doppler reduces perinatal mortality in growth restricted fetuses
    d. Reduces the incidence of SGA babies

25. The neonatal complications of growth-restricted neonates are all, *except:*
    a. Hypocalcemia   b. Hyperglycemia
    c. Hyperbilirubinemia   d. Polycythemia

26. The different screening methods to predict SGA are all, *except*:
    a. Symphysiofundal height plotted on a population-based or a customized chart
    b. Uterine artery Doppler PI at 20–22 weeks
    c. Ratio between soluble fms-like tyrosine kinase-1 (sFlt-1) and placental growth factor SFlt-1 to tyrosine kinase
    d. Risk factor-based prediction such as parity, BMI, smoking, and medical comorbidities

27. A 25-year-old woman in her second pregnancy attends antenatal clinic at 18 weeks. She delivered the previous growth restricted baby at 3rd centile at 37 weeks. What is the most appropriate plan of care for her pregnancy?
    a. Aspirin 150 mg, serial growth scans every 2–4 weeks from 28 weeks
    b. Aspirin 150 mg, uterine artery Doppler at anomaly scan, serial growth scans every 2–4 weeks from 28 weeks depending on uterine artery Doppler
    c. Aspirin 75 mg, serial growth scans every 2–4 weeks from 28 weeks
    d. Uterine artery Doppler at anomaly scan, serial growth scans every 2–4 weeks from 26 to 28 weeks depending on uterine artery Doppler

28. Elective induction of labor is a reasonable option in one of the following:
    a. EFW at 3rd centile with absent end-diastolic flow in the umbilical artery at 33 weeks
    b. Early-onset of FGR with spontaneous unprovoked deceleration at 29 weeks
    c. EFW at 10th centile at 37 weeks with umbilical artery PI above the 95th centile and normal MCA and DV Dopplers
    d. EFW at 2nd centile with normal Doppler at 32 weeks gestation with severe preeclampsia with imminent symptoms

29. A 36-year-old primi is seen in the routine antenatal clinic at 24 weeks of gestation. She has no significant past medical, family, or social history other than a BMI of 19.9 kg/m^2. A uterine artery Doppler performed at 20 weeks of gestation was normal. What is the most appropriate next step?
    a. Growth scans every 3 weeks from 28 weeks
    b. A single biometry scan at 34–36 weeks
    c. Serial symphysiofundal height assessment alone from 26–34 weeks
    d. Repeat uterine artery Doppler at 28 weeks

30. A 36-year-old woman at 35 weeks gestation has fetal weight plotted on the second centile. There is raised umbilical artery pulsatility index and absent end-diastolic flow is recorded in some loops of cord. What is the single best next plan?
    a. Induction of labor by mechanical method
    b. Corticosteroids and a cesarean section
    c. Induction of labor by prostaglandin pessary
    d. Administer corticosteroids and continue to monitor with daily Doppler and CTG

31. The following images denote:

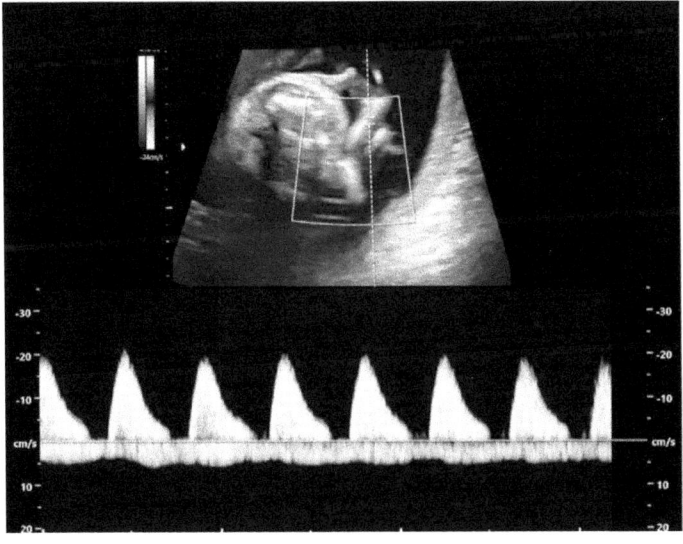
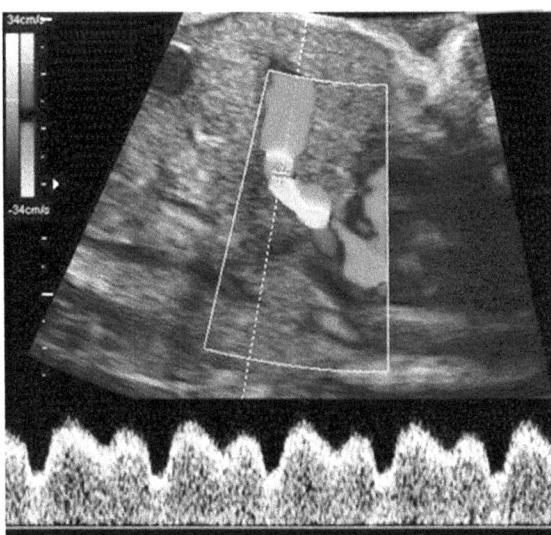

a. High resistance umbilical artery and normal MCA
b. Absent EDF in umbilical artery and normal ductus venosus
c. Absent end-diastolic flow in umbilical artery and abnormal DV waveform
d. Reversed end-diastolic flow in umbilical artery and normal DV waveform

ANSWERS

1. **c.** (ISUOG practice Guidelines. SGA is diagnosed when the AC or EFW are between 3rd and 10th centile with normal Dopplers-Delphi consensus. The follow-up scan is done for interval growth to ascertain there is no further drop in centiles when the diagnosis may have to be reassigned as FGR)

2. **b.** Though early onset FGRs are more likely to be symmetrical and late onset ones are asymmetrical, there can be considerable overlap. Classification based on the timing of growth restriction has more useful in understanding etiology and prognosis than the symmetry.

3. **d.** (Dating by crown-rump length (CRL) 8–14 weeks is the most reliable way to date the pregnancy. In the second trimester and when CRL exceeds 84 mm, HC should be used to assign gestational age. In the 1st trimester, USG-based gestational age should be assigned if the discrepancy between menstrual dates and USG is >5–7days. ISUOG Practice Guidelines, 2019)

4. **b.** (FGR is diagnosed as there is a drop of two quartiles-50: in centiles even though AC and EFWare above the 10th centile. Doppler is recommended in 2 weeks.)

5. **a.** (FIGO and RCOG)

6. **b.** (Stage-based management of FGR by Figueras and Gratacos)
   Early onset FGR is easy to diagnose but difficult to manage whereas with late onset FGR, the converse is true-Stage-based management of FGR by Figueras and Gratacos

7. **b.** (High avidity indicates distant past infection. Fetus produces IgM after 20 weeks.)

8. **d.** (Stage-based management of FGR by Figueras and Gratacos)

9. **c.** Intrapartum fetal distress is most likely with severe growth restriction < 3rd centile with abnormal umbilical artery Doppler.

10. **d.** (Isolated oligohydramnios without growth restriction is not associated with acidosis at birth. Induction can be considered for SGA with AFI 6 cm)

11. **b.** The risk of fetal growth restriction is extremely low in Rh isoimmunized pregnancies.

12. **d.**

13. **d.**

14. **c.** Maternal comorbidities are the commonest reason for FGR whereas the other responses cause inherent variation in fetal growth.

15. **b.**

16. **b.**

17. **c.** [None of the others have been proved to be useful. (RCOG and FIGO)]

18. **b.**

19. **c.**

20. **c.**

21. **d.** (Pulsatility index decreases in brain sparing.)

22. **b.** (Triploidy and trisomy-18 are the most common chromosomal causes of FGR.)

23. **b.**

24. **c.** (High Pi means high resistance flow. Umbilical artery Doppler is useful in the diagnosis and management of FGR. It is not useful in the prediction or prevention of FGR.)

25. **b.**

26. **c.** Soluble fms-like tyrosine kinase-1 (sFlt-1) to placental growth factor (PlGF) ratio has been validated as a short-term predictor to rule out preeclampsia in women in whom this condition is suspected clinically—Hypertension in pregnancy, NICE guideline 2019, updated 2022. It is not a routine screening test for FGR.

(Reference: NICE guideline on Antenatal Care 2021 and RCOG Greentop guideline 2013)

27. **d.** (RCOG, FIGO: 150 mg of aspirin is recommended from 16 weeks in high-risk women based on 1st trimester screening for preeclampsia. Benefit is more for preeclampsia than FGR. It may be considered

from 16 weeks in previous placental dysfunction related FGR in the absence of 1st trimester screening as prevention for FGR. However, there may not be any benefit if started after 16 weeks. Uterine artery Doppler is recommended at anomaly scan in high-risk pregnancy which includes previous FGR.)

28. **c.** (RCOG Greentop Guidelines, FIGO)
29. **b.** (RCOG Greentop Guideline: Three risk factors age, nulliparity, and low BMI. So, a biometry scan in 3rd trimester is indicated. Routine serial growth scans from 26 weeks are not needed. In low-risk pregnancies, routine third trimester scan is not recommended by FIGO/RCOG.)
30. **b.** (Stage-based management of FGR, RCOG)
31. **b.**

REFERENCES

1. The Royal College of Obstetricians and Gynecologists. (2013). Small-for-Gestational-Age Fetus, Investigation and Management (Green-top Guideline No. 31). Greentop guideline on The Investigation and Management of the Small-for-gestational-age Fetus 2013. [online] Available from https://www.rcog.org.uk/guidance/browse-all-guidance/green-top-guidelines/small-for-gestational-age-fetus-investigation-and-management-green-top-guideline-no-31/ [Last accessed December, 2023].
2. Melamed N, Baschat A, Yinon Y, Athanasiadis A, Mecacci F, Figueras, et al. FIGO (international Federation of Gynecology and obstetrics) initiative on fetal growth: Best practice advice for screening, diagnosis and management of fetal growth restriction. Int J Gynaecol Obstet. 2021;152(Suppl 1):3-57.
3. NICE Guidance on Hypertension in Pregnancy: diagnosis and management updated 2023.
4. Lees CC, Stampalija T, Baschat A, da Silva Costa F, Ferrazzi E, Figueras F, et al. ISUOG Practice Guidelines: diagnosis and management of small-for-gestational-age fetus and fetal growth restriction. Ultrasound Obstet Gynecol. 2020;56(2):298-312.
5. Salomon LJ, Alfirevic Z, Da Silva Costa F, Deter RL, Figueras F, Ghi T, et al. ISUOG Practice Guidelines: ultrasound assessment of fetal biometry and growth. Ultrasound Obstet Gynecol. 2019;53(6):715-23.
6. Francesc F, Gratacos E. Update on the Diagnosis and Classification of Fetal Growth Restriction and Proposal of a Stage-based Management Protocol. Fetal Diagn Ther. 2014;36(2):86-8.
7. Lees C, Marlow N, Arabin B, Bilardo CM, Brezinka C, Derks JB, et al. Perinatal morbidity and mortality in early-onset fetal growth restriction: cohort outcomes of the trial of randomized umbilical and fetal flow in Europe (TRUFFLE) C. Ultrasound Obstet Gynecol. 2013;42(4):400-8.

Chapter 63: Physiology of Pregnancy

Kalpana Kumari, Shilpi Srivastava

QUESTIONS

1. Which of the following cardiovascular changes is characteristic of pregnancy?
   a. Decreased cardiac output
   b. Increased peripheral vascular resistance
   c. Decreased blood volume
   d. Increased heart rate

2. What respiratory change occurs during pregnancy?
   a. Increased respiratory rate
   b. Decreased tidal volume
   c. Decreased oxygen consumption
   d. Decreased residual volume

3. Which of the following renal changes is seen in pregnancy?
   a. Decreased glomerular filtration rate (GFR)
   b. Decreased urinary output
   c. Increased tubular reabsorption of glucose
   d. Increased sensitivity to antidiuretic hormone (ADH)

4. What gastrointestinal change occurs during pregnancy?
   a. Decreased gastric motility
   b. Decreased gastric acid secretion
   c. Increased liver enzyme production
   d. Increased bile flow

5. What is the average increase in blood volume during pregnancy?
   a. 10-15%
   b. 20-25%
   c. 30-35%
   d. 40-45%

6. Which of the following changes occurs in the hematological system during pregnancy?
   a. Decreased red blood cell count
   b. Increased white blood cell count
   c. Decreased plasma volume
   d. Increased platelet count

7. What is the term used to describe the separation of the rectus abdominis muscles during pregnancy?
   a. Diastasis recti
   b. Ventral hernia
   c. Umbilical hernia
   d. Inguinal hernia

8. What is the hormone responsible for softening and relaxing the pelvic ligaments and joints during pregnancy?
   a. Relaxin
   b. Human chorionic gonadotropin (hCG)
   c. Oxytocin
   d. Progesterone

9. What is the hormone responsible for promoting uterine contractions during labor?
   a. Estrogen
   b. Progesterone
   c. Oxytocin
   d. Human chorionic gonadotropin

10. Which of the following changes occurs in the breasts during pregnancy?
    a. Decreased blood supply to the mammary glands
    b. Decreased size and firmness of the breasts
    c. Increased glandular tissue and vascularity
    d. Decreased production of colostrum

11. What is the hormone responsible for promoting uterine and breast development during pregnancy?
    a. Estrogen
    b. Progesterone
    c. Prolactin
    d. Oxytocin

12. What is the hormone responsible for softening the cervix and preparing it for labor?
    a. Estrogen
    b. Progesterone
    c. Oxytocin
    d. Relaxin

13. What is the term used to describe the stretching and thinning of the cervical canal during labor?
    a. Effacement
    b. Dilation
    c. Station
    d. Engagement

14. Which of the following changes occurs in the endocrine system during pregnancy?
    a. Decreased production of human chorionic gonadotropin
    b. Decreased insulin sensitivity
    c. Increased thyroid hormone production
    d. Increased adrenal gland activity

15. What is the term used to describe the enlargement of the uterus during pregnancy?
    a. Hyperplasia   b. Hypertrophy
    c. Hypoplasia   d. Hypotrophy

16. What is the hormone responsible for stimulating milk production after childbirth?
    a. Estrogen   b. Progesterone
    c. Prolactin   d. Oxytocin

17. Which of the following changes occurs in the integumentary system during pregnancy?
    a. Decreased hair growth
    b. Decreased oil production
    c. Increased nail strength
    d. Increased pigmentation of the skin

18. Which of these findings in heartbeat is abnormal during pregnancy?
    a. Ejection systolic murmur
    b. Diastolic murmur
    c. S3
    d. S4

19. Which hormone has the highest rise during pregnancy?
    a. hCG   b. hPL
    c. Relaxin   d. Oxytocin

20. Maximum levels of hCG is achieved at what gestation?
    a. 14 weeks   b. 10 weeks
    c. 36 weeks   d. 28 weeks

21. All of the following increases during pregnancy, *except:*
    a. Blood volume   b. Cardiac output
    c. Mean arterial pressure   d. Basal metabolic rate

22. During labor oxygen consumption increases to:
    a. 20-25%   b. 40-60%
    c. 25-30%   d. Remains unchanged

23. Which of the following decreases during pregnancy?
    a. Kidney size   b. GFR
    c. Renal plasma flow rate   d. Serum creatinine

24. Bluish coloration of the vaginal mucosa is called as_____
    a. Jaquemier's sign   b. Chadwick sign
    c. Kehr's sign   d. Goodell's sign

25. Montgomery's tubercles are:
    a. Sweat glands of the areola
    b. Sebaceous glands of the areola
    c. Sweat glands of the skin
    d. Sebaceous glands of the skin

26. In pregnancy all of the following increases, *except:*
    a. Blood volume   b. Plasma volume
    c. RBC mass   d. Hematocrit

27. Uterine blood flow near term is:
    a. ~750 mL/min   b. ~500 mL/min
    c. ~1,000 mL/min   d. ~1,500 mL/min

28. Basal metabolic rate in pregnancy increased to the extent of:
    a. 10%   b. 50%
    c. 30%   d. 60%

29. Which of the following is not true about lipid metabolism in pregnancy?
    a. HDL level increases by 15%
    b. LDL increased and utilized for placental steroid synthesis
    c. Activity of lipoprotein lipase is increased
    d. Hyperlipidemia of pregnancy is atherogenic

30. Which of the following are false in pregnancy?
    a. Motility of gastrointestinal tract decreased due to high progesterone level
    b. Cardiac sphincter is relaxed and may produce chemical esophagitis and hurtburn
    c. Risk of peptic ulcer disease is increased
    d. Atonicity of gut leads to constipation

ANSWERS

1. **d.** The heart rate rises on an average of 10 bpm during pregnancy but physiological increase always remains <100 bpm.
   (Reference: Williams Obstetrics, 25th Edition, Chapter 4, page 60)

2. **d.** During pregnancy RR remains unchanged, tidal volume and oxygen consumption increases and residual volume decreases by 20-25% or 200-400 mL.
   (Reference: Williams Obstetrics, 25th Edition, Chapter 4, page 64)

3. d. During pregnancy GFR increases by 25% by 2nd week of pregnancy and up to 50% by 2nd trimester of pregnancy. Along with this urine output also increases and reabsorption of glucose decrease from tubules. But ADH sensitivity increases.
(Reference: Williams Obstetrics, 25th Edition, Chapter 4, page 65)

4. a. During pregnancy the peristalsis wave has lower wave speed and lower amplitude thus gastric motility is decreased during pregnancy.
(Reference: Williams Obstetrics, 25th Edition, Chapter 4, page 68)

5. d. Hypervolemia associated with normal pregnancy averages 40–45% above nonpregnant blood volume after 32–34 weeks of gestation.
(Reference: Williams Obstetrics, 25th Edition, Chapter 4, page 57)

6. b. Normal leukocyte count during pregnancy can be higher than nonpregnant values, and upper values approach 15,000/μL.
(Reference: Williams Obstetrics, 25th Edition, Chapter 4, page 59)

7. a. Muscles of abdominal wall do not withstand the tension of expanding pregnancy. As a result, rectus muscle separates in midline creating diastasis recti of varying extent.
(Reference: Williams Obstetrics, 25th Edition, Chapter 4, page 53)

8. a. Relaxin has a role in extracellular matrix remodeling. Thus, it helps in softening and relaxing pelvic joints.
(Reference: Williams Obstetrics, 25th Edition, Chapter 5, page 102)

9. c. Oxytocin means quick birth. It acts as uterotonic during parturition and subsequent observations support this theory: (1) Near-term number of oxytocin receptors in decidua and myometrium. (2) Oxytocin acts on decidual tissue to promote prostaglandin release. (3) Oxytocin is synthesized directly in decidual and extraembryonic fetal tissues in placenta.
(Reference: Williams Obstetrics, 25th Edition, Chapter 21, page 417)

10. c. During pregnancy breast undergo increased in milk secreting glandular tissue and vascularity under the effect of prolactin, progesterone, and estrogen.
(References: Williams Obstetrics, 25th Edition, Chapter 4, page 53)

11. a. Uterine hypertrophy and breast enlargement are both stimulated by estrogen.
(Reference: Williams Obstetrics, 25th Edition, Chapter 4, page 49)

12. d. Relaxin plays a role in collagen and extracellular matrix remodeling, thus helps in softening of cervix.
(References: Williams Obstetrics, 25th Edition, Chapter 5, page 103)

13. a. Cervical effacement is obliteration or taking up of cervix. It is manifested by clinical shortening of cervix from a length of approximately 3 cm to merely a circular orifice.
(Reference: Williams Obstetrics, 25th Edition, Chapter 21, page 413)

14. d. During pregnancy maternal production of mineralocorticoid, deoxycortisone, and androgens increases.
(Reference: Williams Obstetrics, 25th Edition, Chapter 4, page 71)

15. b. During pregnancy, uterine enlargement involves stretching and marked hypertrophy of muscle cells, whereas production of new myocytes is limited.
(Reference: Williams Obstetrics, 25th Edition, Chapter 4, page 49)

16. c. With delivery, maternal serum levels of progesterone and estrogen decline abruptly and this drop removes the inhibitory influence of progesterone and this progesterone withdrawal allows prolactin to unopposed action in its stimulation of alpha lactoglobulin and milk production.
(Reference: Williams Obstetrics, 25th Edition, Chapter 36, page 656)

17. d. Hyperpigmentation develops in about 90% of patients and is more in dark-skinned people.
(Reference: Williams Obstetrics, 25th Edition, Chapter 4, page 53)

18. b. During pregnancy diastolic murmur are abnormal. Normal findings in heartbeat during pregnancy are: S3, S4, ejection systolic murmur, S1 split, bounding/collapsing pulse, relative sinus tachycardia, and few ectopic beats.

19. b. Human placental lactogen hormone has maximum levels during pregnancy. It is a polypeptide hormone directly proportional to placental size. It is a diabetogenic hormone.

Unlike hCG its levels keep increasing up to 36 weeks.

20. **b.** Maximum levels of β-hCG are achieved at 10 weeks of gestation after which level plateaus till 32 weeks after which it started declining.

21. **c.** Mean arterial pressure
    In pregnancy, MAP decreases by 5–10 mm Hg.

22. **b.** 40–60%
    Oxygen consumption increases by ~20% during pregnancy, and 10% higher in multifetal gestations. During labor, oxygen consumption increases ~40–60%.

23. **c.** Serum creatinine
    In pregnancy, kidney size increases ~1.5 cm, GFR and renal plasma flow increases, while serum creatinine levels decrease from a mean of 0.7 to 0.5 mg/dL.

24. **a.** *Jaquemier's sign:* Increased blood supply of the venous plexus surrounding the walls of vagina gives the bluish coloration of the vaginal mucosa.

25. **b.** Sebaceous glands of the areola
    Variable number of sebaceous glands remains invisible in the nonpregnant state in the areola, becomes hypertrophied, and is called Montgomery's tubercles.

26. **d.** Hematocrit
    The disproportionate increase in plasma and RBC volume produces state of hemodilution resulting in fall in hematocrit during pregnancy.

27. **a.** ~750 mL/min
    Uterine blood flow is increased from 50 mL/min in nonpregnant state to about 750 mL near term.

28. **c.** 30%
    Total metabolism is increased due to the needs of the growing fetus and the uterus. Basal metabolic rate is increased to the extent of 30% higher than that of the average for the nonpregnant women.

29. **d.** Hyperlipidemia of pregnancy is atherogenic.
    Hyperlipidemia of pregnancy is not atherogenic.

30. **c.** Risk of peptic ulcer disease is increased.
    Risk of peptic ulcer disease is reduced due to diminished gastric secretion and delayed gastric emptying.

Section 2

Gynecology

Chapter Outline

64. Ultrasound in Infertility
65. Ovarian Reserve
66. Laparoscopy in Infertility
67. Hysteroscopy in Infertility
68. Amenorrhea
69. Polycystic Ovary Syndrome
70. Endometriosis
71. Ovulation Induction
72. Tubal Factor Infertility
73. Female Genital Tuberculosis
74. Male Infertility
75. Intrauterine Insemination
76. In vitro Fertilization
77. Preimplantation Genetic Diagnosis
78. Mullerian Anomalies
79. Fibroid
80. Endocrinology of Reproduction
81. Menstruation
82. Abnormal Uterine Bleeding
83. Premenstrual Syndrome
84. Postmenopausal Bleeding
85. Vaginal Infection and Pelvic Inflammatory Diseases
86. Hyperprolactinemia
87. Prolapse Uterus: Part 1
88. Prolapse Uterus: Part II
89. Urogynecology
90. Contraception
91. Vulvodynia
92. Contraception Miscellaneous
93. Premature Ovarian Insufficiency
94. Myomectomy
95. Ovarian Hyperstimulation Syndrome: Part 1
96. Ovarian Hyperstimulation Syndrome: Part 2
97. Thyroid in Pregnancy
98. Cervical Cancer
99. Human Papillomavirus and Vaccination
100. Carcinoma of Ovary
101. Germ Cell Tumors
102. Menopause General: Part 1
103. Menopause General: Part 2
104. Vaginal Discharge

Chapter 64

Ultrasound in Infertility

Astha Lalwani, Shubhra Agarwal

QUESTIONS

1. **Normal ovary in ultrasound is the one with all, *except*:**
   a. 3–6 cc volume
   b. Antral follicle count (AFC) of 4–19/ovary
   c. Stromal resistance index (RI) of 0.6–0.7
   d. Echogenic stroma

2. **Baseline ovarian scan is done to:**
   a. Assess the ovarian volume
   b. Count the antral follicles
   c. Quantitative and qualitative assessment of stromal density
   d. Pulse Doppler is used to calculate intraovarian resistance index (RI) and peak systolic blood flow velocity (PSV)
   e. All the above

3. **Antral follicles can be counted by:**
   a. Two-dimensional (2D) USG, scrolling through the entire ovary and counting
   a. Specialized three-dimensional (3D) ultrasound software
   b. Sonoautomated volume count (AVC)
   c. (a) and (b)
   d. On day 10 of menstrual cycle

4. **A software called VOCAL (volume calculation by computer) is used to calculate the:**
   a. Ovarian volume   b. Endometrial volume
   c. Number of follicles d. Stromal blood flow

5. **USG features of preovulatory follicles are:**
   a. 16–18 mm
   b. Thin wall, no internal echos, halo
   c. Vascularity around three-fourths of the circumference
   d. All of these

6. **Peak systolic blood flow velocity (PSV) of the preovulatory follicle is:**
   a. >10 mm/sec   b. >15 mm/sec
   c. >5 mm/sec   d. >7 mm/sec

7. **USG features of preovulatory endometrium are all, *except*:**
   a. Thickness 8–10 mm
   b. Vascularity in zone 1–2
   c. Morphology grade A/B
   d. Resistance index (RI) <0.5

8. **Three-dimensional (3D) USG is better for:**
   a. Identifying intrafollicular cumulus to find the presence of fertilizable ovum.
   b. Follicular volume and size
   c. Uterine artery pulsatility index (PI)
   d. Vascularity of the ovum
   e. Both (a) and (b)

9. **Zones of vascularity in the endometrium are defined according to Applebaum as:**
   a. Zone 1 when vascularity on power Doppler is seen only at endometrium–myometrium junction
   b. Zone 2 when vessels penetrate through hyperechogenic endometrial edge
   c. Zone 3 is when these reach the intervening hypoechogenic zone
   d. Zone 4 is when these reach the endometrial cavity (central line)
   e. All are true

10. **All are true for correlation of ultrasound finding with progesterone, *except*:**
    a. The blurring of the outer margin of multilayered endometrium suggests initiation of progesterone
    b. Low resistance flow in corpus luteum with echogenic endometrium suggests normal luteal phase

c. High resistance flow in corpus luteum suggests corpus luteal inadequacy
d. High resistance flow in the endometrium suggests adequate progesterone receptors in the endometrium

11. **True about triple-line endometrium in late proliferative phase is all, *except*:**
    a. The outer bright line comprises nonfunctional zone of endometrium
    b. The inner predominantly dark (hypoechoic) zone is inner functional endometrium
    c. Innermost white line represents endometrial cavity
    d. In secretory phase, the functional zone starts decreasing echogenicity and becomes dark

12. **Question mark sign in ultrasound is seen in:**
    a. Fibroid uterus   b. Endometriosis
    c. Adenomyosis   d. Endometrial polyp

13. **Minimum endometrial thickness needed for PV to achieve pregnancy:**
    a. 7 mm   b. 10 mm
    c. 5 mm   d. 12 mm

14. **The dominant follicle grows at a rate of:**
    a. 0.5–2 mm/day   b. 2–3 mm/day
    c. 3–4 mm/day   d. 4–5 mm/day

15. **Features of ovarian hyperstimulation on ultrasound are all, *except*:**
    a. Large ovarian >10 cm
    b. Multiple follicles
    c. Stromal edema
    d. The features are severe if large follicles comprise the bulk

16. **Definite ultrasound features suggestive of ovulation are all, *except*:**
    a. Disappearance of the follicle or regress in size
    b. Follicle becoming echogenic with intrafollicular echos
    c. Irregular of extended margins of the follicle
    d. None

17. **"Water fall sign" seen in the ultrasound is suggestive of:**
    a. Fluid spillage from the tubal end adjacent to the ovaries
    b. Increase stromal flow in the ovaries
    c. Ovarian hyperstimulation syndrome (OHSS)
    d. Polycystic ovarian syndrome (PCOS)

18. **As per the European Society of Human Reproduction and Embryology (ESHRE)/the American Society for Reproductive Medicine (ASRM) 2018, ultrasound criteria to define polycystic ovarian syndrome (PCOS) are all, *except*:**
    a. Volume > 10 cc of either of the ovary
    b. >20 antral follicles
    c. Each follicle 2–9 mm in diameter
    d. Increased stromal echogenicity

19. **Three-dimensional HyCosy, a recently evolved procedure, has the following advantages over the routine—**
    HyCosy:
    a. Lesser amount of contrast is needed
    b. The accuracy to identify the free spillage from the tube is improved
    c. Uterine cavity and the whole length of the tube can be seen together
    d. All of the above

20. **Three-dimensional (3D) ultrasound is better than conventional B-mode in the following conditions:**
    a. Uterine lesions can be demonstrated better such as polyp, fibroid, and synechiae
    b. Better delineation of endomyometrial junctions in diagnosis of adenomyosis
    c. In tubal patency assessment by HyCosy
    d. For volume assessment of the follicles and the endometrium
    e. All of the above

21. **"Red Indian Head sign" in B mode of USG is suggestive of:**
    a. Bowel endometriosis
    b. Ureteric endometriosis
    c. Uterosacral endometriosis
    d. Ovarian endometriomas

22. **All ultrasound features are suggestive of ovarian endometriosis, *except*:**
    a. Birds nest sign on 3D power Doppler
    b. Ground glass appearance with the internal echogenicity in the ovarian cyst
    c. Vertical fluid—fluid level
    d. Rokitansky tubercle

23. **Ultrasound features of adenomyosis are all, *except*:**
    a. Venetian blind or rain in forest (Fan shadows of myometrium)
    b. Irregular junctional zone

c. Salt and pepper appearance of the myometrium due to hyper- and hypoechoic areas
d. Well-encapsulated mass with peripheral vascularity

24. **Chronic endometritis can be suspected in ultrasound on the following features:**
    a. Persistently thin endometrium with synechiae or narrow endometrial cavity
    b. Endometrial, subendometrial, and myometrial calcifications
    c. Fluid in the endometrial cavity in the mid-proliferative phase with hyperechoic endometrial lining
    d. Vertical orientation of the interstitial part of the tube
    e. All of the above

25. **Volume ultrasound [three-dimensional (3D)] has following features to diagnose bicornuate uterus, *except*:**
    a. Fundus of a uterus has a dimple
    b. If a straight line is drawn joining the top of the endometrial cavities, the fundus dimple is <5 mm above than this line
    c. Thick myometrial layers/tissue can be seen dipping in between the endometrial cavities
    d. Angle between the two cavities is <90°

26. **3D ultrasound is conclusive to diagnose the Müllerian anomalies, which is best done in the:**
    a. Menstrual phase
    b. Early proliferative phase
    c. Late proliferative phase
    d. Secretory phase or preovulatory phase

27. **Ultrasound features of septate/subseptate uterus are all, *except*:**
    a. No/minimal indentation on the uterus
    b. At least 5 mm of uterine wall can be seen above the line joining tips of two endometrial cavities
    c. The distance between this line and the deepest point between endometrial cavities is >10 mm
    d. Angle between cavities is >90°

28. **Arcuate uterus can be diagnosed by all, *except*:**
    a. Endometrial cavity is concave at fundus
    b. Distance between line touching the tips of endometrial cavities and the deepest point between the endometrial cavities is <10 mm
    c. Angle between the cavities is >90°
    d. External fundal shows dipping

29. **Acute endometritis is seen in ultrasound as:**
    a. Thick isoechoic endometrium with disruption of junctional zone
    b. Minimal fluid in endometrial cavity
    c. Increased vascularity even in early follicular phase
    d. All of the above

30. **Luteinized unruptured follicle can be seen and diagnosed by following features:**
    a. Persistent follicle with thick walls and progressive loss of cystic appearance difficult to differentiate from corpus luteum
    b. Endometrium is thick echogenic with flow
    c. 3. No free fluid in pouch of Douglas (POD)
    d. 4. On Doppler perifollicular RI is 0.51–0.59 which is higher than normal and remains steady till the end
    e. All of the above

31. **True about endometrial grading on 2D USG is:**
    a. Grade A endometrium is multilayered endometrium with intervening area more echogenic than myometrium
    b. Grade B endometrium is multilayered with intervening area hypoechoic to myometrium
    c. Grade C endometrium is homogenous isoechoic to endometrium
    d. All of the above

ANSWERS

1. **d.** Normal ovaries have the largest diameter of 2–3 cm, ovarian volume of 3–6.6 cc, antral follicle count (AFC) per ovary 4–19, isoechoic stroma, stromal peak systolic blood flow velocity (PSV) of 5–10 cm/s. They are normal because they respond to standard stimulation protocols.

2. **e.** Baseline ovarian scan is done for assessing ovarian volume, counting antral follicles, quantitative and qualitative assessment of stromal density. Pulse doppler is used to calculate intraovarian resistance index (RI) and peak systolic blood flow velocity (PSV).

3. **c.** Antral follicles are counted by two-dimensional (2D) USG and 3D with inversion mode rendering and sonoautomated volume count (AVC).

4. **a.** VOCAL (volume calculation by computer) is used to calculate ovarian volume. It calculates the ovarian volume. VOCAL calculates the volume by rotating it 180°. A step of rotation of 6–30° can be selected. A circumference is drawn around the structure of

interest at every step of rotation and at the end of 180° total volume is calculated.

5. **a.** A preovulatory follicle is 16-18 mm size, thin isoechoic walls, regular round shape, thin hypoechoic rim surrounding follicle, at least two-thirds to three-fourths vascularity in follicular circumference.

6. **a.** Peak systolic blood flow velocity (PSV) of preovulatory follicle >10 cm/sec

7. **c.** On color Doppler, the endometrium which is mature shows vascularity in zone 3 or 4 or may be called subendometrial and endometrial layers.

8. **e.** Three-dimensional (3D) USG is better for identifying intrafollicular cumulus to find presence of fertilizable ovum. Also, it calculates the longest orthogonal diameters, mean diameter, and volume of individual follicle. This information helps to decide the time of trigger and to decide the type of trigger.

9. **e.** Zones of vascularity are defined according to Applebaum as:
    - *Zone 1:* Vascularity seen only at endometrium-myometrial junction
    - *Zone 2:* When vessels penetrate through hyperechogenic endometrial edge.
    - *Zone 3:* When these reach intervening hypoechogenic zone.
    - *Zone 4:* When these reach the endometrial cavity (central line).

10. **d.** High-resistance endometrial flow in the mid-luteal phase suggests either inadequate progesterone levels or inadequate progesterone receptors in the endometrium.

11. **d.** In secretory phase, the functional zone is echogenic and brighter.

12. **c.** Question mark sign is seen in adenomyosis, there is abnormal curvature of fundal endometrial cavity in the direction opposite to the normal curvature of uterus.

13. **a.** An endometrial thickness of a minimum of 6 mm is required on the day of ovulation trigger, but 8-10 mm is optimum.

14. **b.** A dominant follicle grows at the rate of 2-3 mm/day.

15. **d.** The syndrome is severe if small follicles comprise the bulk and mild when majority of follicles are intermediate size. Small (<9 mm), intermediate (<9-15 mm), and large (>15 mm).

16. **d.** USG findings suggestive of ovulation: Follicle suddenly disappears or regresses in size, irregular margins, intrafollicular echoes.

17. **a.** Waterfall sign is seen in ultrasound and is suggestive of fluid spillage from tubal end adjacent to ovaries.

18. **d.** The European Society of Human Reproduction and Embryology (ESHRE)/the American Society for Reproductive Medicine (ASRM) ultrasound criteria to define polycystic ovarian syndrome (PCOS) PCOS are ovary >10 cc in volume or has >20 antral follicles of 2-9 mm in diameter.

19. **d.** Three-dimensional (3D) HyCosy shows whole uterine cavity and tubes together, condition of lumen and fimbriae can be studied, it shortens procedure time and patient discomfort, less amount of contrast is required, storage of volumes allows reassessment and reviews, spill is better appreciated, it is more accurate.

20. **e.** Three-dimensional (3D) ultrasound is better than conventional B mode as uterine lesions such as polyp, fibroid, or synechiae. Better delineation of endomyometrial junctions in diagnosis of adenomyosis, for volume assessment of the follicles and the endometrium, in tubal patency assessment by HyCosy.

21. **a.** In rectosigmoid deep penetrating endometriosis when the submucosa is involved, fibrotic retraction of the lesion in submucosa leads to a typical Red Indian head appearance. A negative sliding organ sign between the uterus and bowel may be an additional sign.

22. **d.** Three-dimensional (3D)-PD shows the multiple short coursed regularly separated pericystic vessels giving it typical bird nest appearance. 3D-PD shows the multiple short course regularly separated pericystic vessels giving it typical bird nest appearance.

23. **d.** There is marked increase in vascularity with vascular dilation which is penetrating type and intralesional.

24. **e.** Chronic endometritis can be suspected in ultrasound based on persistently thin endometrium with synechiae or narrow endometrial cavity Endometrial, subendometrial, and myometrial

calcification Fluid in the endometrial cavity in the midproliferative phase with hyperechoic endometrial lining

Vertical orientation of the interstitial part of the tube

25. **d.** in a bicornuate uterus, the angle between the two cavities is >90°
26. **d.** Three-dimensional (3D) ultrasound is conclusive to diagnose Müllerian anomalies which is best done in the secretory or preovulatory phase.
27. **d.** In a septate or subseptate uterus the angle is <90°.
28. **d.** The external fundal contour is flat or convex.
29. **d.** Acute endometritis is seen in ultrasound as thick isoechoic endometrium with disruption of junctional zone. There is minimal fluid in endometrial cavity, increased vascularity even in early follicular phase.
30. **e.** Luteinized unruptured follicle can be seen and diagnosed by following:
Persistent follicle with thick walls and progressive loss of cystic appearance difficult to differentiate from corpus luteum, endometrium is thick echogenic with flow, no free-fluid in pouch of Douglas (POD), on Doppler perifollicular resistance index (RI) is 0.51–0.59 which is higher than normal and remains steady till the end, rising peak systolic blood flow velocity (PSV) with steady low resistance index (RI) suggests follicle is close to rupture. Steady or decrease PSV with rising RI suggests that follicle is proceeding toward LUI-LUF- Luteinized Unruptured Follicle.
31. **d.** Endometrial grading on two-dimensional (2D) USG is:
    - *Grade A endometrium:* Multilayered endometrium with intervening area more echogenic than myometrium.
    - *Grade B endometrium:* Multilayered endometrium with intervening area hypoechoic to myometrium
    - *Grade C endometrium:* Homogenous isoechoic to endometrium

REFERENCES

1. Nagori C, Panchal S (Eds). Practical guide to Infertility Management & IVF. New Delhi: Jaypee Brothers Medical Publishers (P) Ltd.; 2021.
2. Berek JS. Berek & Novak's Gynecology, 16th edition. Gurugram (Haryana), India: Wolters Kluwer India (P) Ltd.; 2019.
3. Tutorial notes by Dr. Randhawa institute of Ultrasound training, Delhi by Dr JS Randhawa and Dr Sonal Randhawa.
4. Rao KA. Principles and Practice of Assisted Reproductive Technology,-Volume 1: Infertility. New Delhi: Jaypee Brothers Medical Publishers (P) Ltd.; 2018.
5. Nagori C, Panchal S. Handbook of Infertility and Ultrasound for practicing Gynecologists. New Delhi: Jaypee Brothers Medical Publishers (P) Ltd.; 2021.

Chapter 65: Ovarian Reserve

Astha Lalwani, Shubhra Agarwal

QUESTIONS

1. Ovarian reserve testing can be justified for women with any of the following criteria:
   i. Age over 35
   ii. Unexplained infertility to identify unexpected loss of ovarian reserve
   iii. Family history of early menopause
   iv. Previous ovarian surgery/ovarian cystectomy, drilling, chemotherapy or radiation
   v. Smoking
   vi. Demonstrated poor response to exogenous gonadotropin stimulation

   a. i, ii
   b. i, iii, iv
   c. i, iv, v, vi
   d. All

2. Which is not true for the ovarian reserve?
   a. Ovarian reserve test always should be interpreted with caution
   b. An abnormal test result does not preclude the possibility of pregnancy
   c. Ovarian reserve test (ORT) should be easy to perform, easily reproducible, and noninvasive
   d. None of the above

3. Following is/are the biochemical ovarian reserve tests (ORTs):
   a. Baseline serum follicle-stimulating hormone (FSH) and serum estradiol
   b. Serum inhibin B
   c. Anti-Müllerian hormone (AMH)
   d. All of the above

4. Following are the biophysical, ultrasonological evaluation ovarian reserve test (ORT), except:
   a. Antral follicle count (AFC)
   b. Ovarian volume
   c. Ovarian Doppler
   d. Clomiphene citrate challenge (CCT)

5. All are true, except:
   a. Exhibits high intra- and intercycle variability and hence has to be measured on second day of menstrual cycle
   b. It is the earliest marker to show decline in ovarian reserve
   c. Serum anti-Müllerian hormone (AMH) levels strongly correlate with antral follicle count (AFC) by transvaginal ultrasound scan (TVS)
   d. Levels below 1.26 ng/mL indicate poor ovarian response to ovarian stimulation

6. The dynamic test for ovarian reserve are all, except:
   a. Clomifene citrate challenge test (CCCT)
   b. Exogenous FSH ORT (EFORT)
   c. GAST (Gonadotropin-releasing hormone agonist stimulation test)
   d. Anti-Müllerian hormone (AMH)

7. The best predictive value for ovarian reserve (OR) is for the following test:
   a. Antral follicle count (AFC)
   b. AMH
   c. Both 1 and 2
   d. Ovarian biopsy

8. True statements about AFC are all, except:
   a. AFC are small follicles seen in the ovary mainly 2–10 mm in diameter
   b. AFC is measured in the early follicular phase, day 2–4
   c. The follicles of each ovary is considered separately for AFC
   d. AFC of 8–16 is considered to have normal over ovarian response in in vitro fertilization (IVF)

9. Other uses of anti-Müllerian hormone (AMH) are:
   a. To know the residual ovarian reserve in young cancer survivors who have received gonadotropin therapy previously

b. At levels 0.5–1.26 ng/mL, AMH indicates menopausal within 3–5 years
c. Sensitive marker to predict hyper-response as well; hence in vitro fertilization (IVF) protocols can be individualized
d. Helps to assume ovarian reserve in women who wish to delay the childbearing to plan their future childbearing accordingly
e. All of the above

10. **False statement about ovarian reserve (OR) is:**
    a. Biological age is the best measure of oocyte quality and single reliable factor
    b. All ovarian reserve tests are considered screening tests and abnormal test results should be confirmed by another test
    c. The short follicular phase indicates the diminishing OR
    d. AMH can surely predict non pregnancy

11. **Bologna criteria [(ESHRE) European Society of Human Reproduction and Embryology] says that out of 3 any 2 criteria should be present to define poor ovarian reserve. Those criteria are all,** *except***:**
    a. Maternal age >40 years or other risk factors for poor ovarian reserve
    b. Previous history of <3 oocytes with a conventional stimulation protocol
    c. Abnormal ovarian reserve test, i.e., antral follicle count (AFC) <5–7, anti-Müllerian hormone (AMH) <0.5–1.1 ng/mL
    d. Serum (FSH follicle-stimulating hormone) >20

12. **Facts about ovarian reserve test (ORT) as in ASRM (American Society for Reproductive Medicine) practice committee are all,** *except***:**
    a. ORT does not predict pregnancy and live birth rates and there are many other variables that play important roles
    b. ORT predicts the reproductive potential among women with unproven infertility
    c. ORT predicts the success after controlled ovarian hyperstimulation and intrauterine insemination
    d. In vitro fertilization (IVF) can be refused on the basis of low ORT

13. **Favorable results are all,** *except***:**
    a. Age <35, follicle-stimulating hormone (FSH) <10, inhibin B >45
    b. Age <35, FSH <20, inhibin > 45
    c. Age <30, FSH <10, inhibin >45
    d. Age <35, FSH <10, inhibin <45

14. **Decreased ovarian reserve (DOR) is indicated by all,** *except***:**
    a. Day 2–3 FSH >12–15
    b. Day 2 estradiol (E2) >80 pg/mL
    c. The follicle-stimulating hormone (FSH)/ luteinizing hormone (LH) ratio, if high
    d. Inhibin B >45 pg/mL

15. **Ovarian response predictive index (ORPI) is calculated as:**
    a. AMH × AFC/Patient's age
    b. AMH/AFC × Patient's age
    c. AMH × AFC Patient's age
    d. Patient's age × AFC/AMH

16. **Incorrect statement about antral follicular count (AFC) is:**
    a. AFC can predict poor response and also hyperstimulation after gonadotropin stimulation
    b. AFC has low intercycle and interobserver variability, though it is more significant in young women when AFC is high
    c. Three dimensional ultrasonography (USG) is extremely useful for counting antral fluid
    d. Sono automated volume calculate (AVC) is very convenient and accurate
    e. AFC is better predictor than anti-Müllerian hormone (AMH)

17. **Ovarian 3D power Doppler (PD) flow indices are:**
    a. Total ovarian vascularization index (VI)
    b. Vascularization flow index (VFI)
    c. Ovarian stromal flow index (FI)
    d. All the three

18. **Higher dose of gonadotropin is needed in following conditions,** *except***:**
    a. Age >35 years
    b. Body mass index (BMI) <20 kg/m^2
    c. Antral follicle count (AFC) <3 [(FNPO) follicle number per ovary]
    d. Ovarian volume <3 cc

19. **Lower dose of gonadotropin is needed in following condition,** *except***:**
    a. Age <25 years
    b. Body mass index (BMI) >28 kg/m^2
    c. Amniotic fluid index (AFI) >12 [(FNOP) follicle number per ovary]
    d. Ovarian volume >10 cc

20. **Three-dimensional power Doppler (PD) indices in ovaries in polycystic ovary syndrome (PCOS) are:**
    a. Vascularization index (VI) = 5, 10; vascularization flow index (VFI) = 2–3
    b. VI = 2–5; VFI = 1–2
    c. VI <2; VFI = <0.5
    d. VI ≥5; VFI ≥3

21. **Three-dimensional PD indices in normal-responding ovaries are:**
    a. VI = 2–5; VFI = 1–2
    b. VI = 5–10; VFI = 2–3
    c. VI ≤2; VFI ≤0.5
    d. VI >5; VFI >3

22. **Three-dimensional PD indices in poor response ovaries:**
    a. VI = 5–10; VFI = 2–3
    b. VI = 2–5; VFI = 1–2
    c. VI ≤2; VFI ≤0.5
    d. VI >5; VFI >3

23. **Following correlation of FSH level and response to ovulation induction drug is correct:**
    a. FSH <8 min/mL—reassurance
    b. FSH 8–12 min/mL—average reserve
    c. FSH 12–17 min/mL—demand ovarian reserve
    d. FSH >17 min/mL—extremely poor pregnancy rates
    e. All are true

24. **Day 2 serum estradiol (E2) is a static ovarian reserve test (ORT). TRUE are all, *except*:**
    a. A high E2 level on day 2 or 3 of menstrual cycle indicates early follicular recruitment
    b. Cycle cancellation is higher in IVF if E2 >80 pg/mL or more on day 2
    c. Cycle cancellation is high if day 2 E2 is <20 pg/mL or less on day 2
    d. E2 alone can be used as a sole marker for ovarian reserve

25. **Follicle-stimulating hormone/luteinizing hormone (FSH/LH) ratio is static OR test. TRUE are all, *except*:**
    a. Day 2/day 3, low FSH/LH ratio indicates poor OR
    b. The FSH/LH ratio is an early indicator of ovarian aging
    c. FSH rises earlier than LH
    d. Frequent menstruation with short cycles may diagnose the risk earlier

26. **Inhibin B is a static ovarian reserve test (ORT), false statement is**
    a. It is secreted from small antral follicles and inhibits FSH release
    b. It is not used as a routine ORT
    c. Decrease in inhibin B occurs earlier than rise in FSH with decreasing ovarian reserve
    d. A level more than 45 pg/mL on day 2–3 is indicative of normal response

27. **True option about AMH:**
    a. It is produced by antral follicles, dominant follicle, and corpus luteum
    b. AMH is considered to be reflective of FSH-dependent follicular growth
    c. AMH is produced by granulosa cells of primordial, preantral, and small antral follicles
    d. It inhibits the later stages of follicular development

28. **Chances of hyperstimulation are when:**
    a. AMH >5
    b. AMH >15
    c. AMH >10
    d. AMH >12

29. **Clinical uses of AMH:**
    a. To confirm the presence of testicular tissue in children
    b. Differential diagnosis of patients with intersex
    c. For diagnosis of polycystic ovary syndrome (PCOS)
    d. All are correct

30. **Clomiphene citrate challenge (CCT) test is a dynamic test; false statement is:**
    a. The basal level of FSH is measured on day 3 and repeated on day 10 after CCT stimulation
    b. A higher value of FSH (>10 mIU/mL) either on day 3 or 10 indicates diminished ovarian reserve
    c. Normally luteinizing hormone (LH) rises more than FSH after clomiphene but in patients with low reserve, FSH rises more than LH
    d. This test has a high prognostic value and is routinely used

31. **True statement about OR is:**
    a. The ovarian reserve depends on only the quality of the ovarian antral follicles
    b. The OR depends on only the quantity of the ovarian antral follicles
    c. The OR depends on the quality and quantity of the antral follicles
    d. The OR depends on the quality and quantity of preantral and antral follicles

32. **True options about the number of ova available are all, *except*:**
    a. At birth 2 million
    b. At puberty 3–4 lakh
    c. After 40 years—25,000
    d. At menopause—<1,000

CHAPTER 65: Ovarian Reserve

33. **POSEIDON criteria are used to identify the women with poor ovarian reserve and to decide upon the best stimulation protocol. It depends upon the following markers,** *except:*
    a. Age
    b. Ovarian biomarkers (AFC and/or AMH)
    c. Number of oocytes retrieved in previous Ovarian stimulation cycle
    d. FSH

ANSWERS

1. **d.** Ovarian reserve (OR) needs to be assessed in females >35 years of age, females with unexplained infertility and in females who have had a previous cycle of ovulation induction with gonadotropins and had a poor response, females who have a history of ovarian surgery in the past, smokers, and females who have maternal relations with early menopause.

2. **d.** The ovarian reserve tests are considered screening tests and abnormal tests should be confirmed by another test. They should be easy to perform, reproducible, and noninvasive.

3. **d.** Biochemical tests for ovarian reserve are serum follicle-stimulating hormone (FSH), luteinizing hormone (LH), serum estradiol, serum inhibin B, serum anti-Müllerian hormone (AMH), and inhibin B

4. **d.** Biophysical or ultrasound markers of ovarian reserve are ovarian volume, ovarian blood flow (ovarian doppler), antral follicle count (AFC).

5. **a.** Serum anti-Müllerian hormone (AMH) is constant throughout the menstrual cycle, except that has lower thresholds in late luteal phase.

6. **d.** Dynamic tests for ovarian reserve are clomifene citrate challenge test (CCCT), exogenous FSH ovarian reserve test (EFORT), gonadotrophin releasing hormone analog stimulation test (GAST)
   [Chapter 3 - Practical Guide to Infertility Management and IVF- Chaitanya Nagori, Sonal Panchal][2]

7. **c.** Receiver operating characteristics curves showed high accuracy for anti-Müllerian hormone (AMH) and antral follicle count (AFC) for the prediction of poor ovarian reserve.
   [Chapter 3 - Practical Guide to Infertility Management and IVF- Chaitanya Nagori, Sonal Panchal][3]

8. **c.** Antral follicle count is defined as total number of follicles seen in both the ovaries up to 9 mm in early follicular phase.
   [Chapter 3 - Practical Guide to Infertility Management and IVF- Chaitanya Nagori, Sonal Panchal][3]

9. **e.** Anti-Müllerian hormone (AMH) is used to know residual ovarian reserve in young cancer survivors who have received gonadotrophin therapy previously, AMH of 0.5–1.26 ng/mL indicates menopause within 3–5 years, AMH is a sensitive marker to predict hyper response hence in vitro fertilization (IVF) protocols can be individualized. It helps to assume ovarian reserve in women who wish to delay childbearing to plan their future childbearing accordingly.
   [Chapter 3 - Practical Guide to Infertility Management and IVF- Chaitanya Nagori, Sonal Panchal][4]

10. **d.** Anti-Müllerian hormone (AMH) cannot surely predict nonpregnancy
    [Chapter 3 - Practical Guide to Infertility Management and IVF- Chaitanya Nagori, Sonal Panchal][1]

11. **d.** Bologna criteria [(ESHRE) European Society of Human Reproduction and Embryology] says 2 out of 3 should be present to define poor ovarian reserve. Those criteria are:
    - Maternal age >40 years or other risk factors for poor ovarian reserve (genetic or acquired conditions)
    - Previous history of <3 oocytes with a conventional stimulation protocol
    - Abnormal ovarian reserve test, i.e., antral follicle count (AFC) <5–7 or anti-Müllerian hormone (AMH) <0.5–1.1 ng/mL
    [Chapter 3 - Practical Guide to Infertility Management and IVF- Chaitanya Nagori, Sonal Panchal][3]

12. **d.** ASRM (American Society for Reproductive Medicine) practice committee opinion gives the following facts:
    - Ovarian reserve markers do not predict the reproduction potential in women with unproven or proven fertility.
    - Markers of ovarian reserve test (ORT) do not predict likelihood of success following ovarian stimulation and intrauterine insemination.
    - Low AMH is for counseling the women regarding suboptimal response and yield of oocytes but should not be used to refuse treatment.
    - Ovarian reserve tests do not predict pregnancy and live birth rates.
    - AFC and AMH give the same information about ovarian reserve and dose of gonadotrophins required for IVF.

[Chapter 3 - Practical Guide to Infertility Management and IVF- Chaitanya Nagori, Sonal Panchal]²

13. **a.** Age <35 years, FSH <10, inhibin B >45
[Chapter 3 - Practical Guide to Infertility Management and IVF- Chaitanya Nagori, Sonal Panchal]¹

14. **d.** Diminishing ovarian reserve is indicated by:
Day 2–3 FSH >12–15
Day 2 E2 >80 pg/mL
FSH/LH ratio, if high indicates decreased ovarian reserve (DOR)
Inhibin B >45 pg/mL indicates good reserve
[Chapter 3 - Practical Guide to Infertility Management and IVF- Chaitanya Nagori, Sonal Panchal]²

15. **a.** Ovarian response predictive index (ORPI) is calculated as AMH × AFC/Patient's age
[Chapter 3 - Practical Guide to Infertility Management and IVF- Chaitanya Nagori, Sonal Panchal]¹

16. **e.** Antral follicle count is found to be as effective as AMH in determining ovarian response.
[Chapter 3 - Practical Guide to Infertility Management and IVF- Chaitanya Nagori, Sonal Panchal]⁴

17. **d.** The ovarian volume, AFC and VI (vascularization index), FI (ovarian stromal flow index), and VFI (vascularization flow index) determined.
[Chapter 3 - Practical Guide to Infertility Management and IVF- Chaitanya Nagori, Sonal Panchal]²

18. **b.** Higher dose gonadotrophin is needed for age >35 years, body mass index (BMI) >28 kg/m², AFC <3, ovarian volume <3 cc
[Chapter 3- Practical Guide to Infertility Management and IVF- Chaitanya Nagori, Sonal Panchal]³

19. **b.** Lower dose of gonadotrophin are needed if age <25 years, BMI <20 kg/m², AFC >12, ovarian volume >10 cc
[Chapter 3- Practical Guide to Infertility Management and IVF- Chaitanya Nagori, Sonal Panchal]²

20. **a.** In polycystic ovary syndrome (PCOS) 3D-PD-VI: 5–10, VFI: 2–3.
[Chapter 3- Practical Guide to Infertility Management and IVF- Chaitanya Nagori, Sonal Panchal]³

21. **a.** Normally responding ovaries—3D-PD VI: 2–5, VFI: 1–2
[Chapter 3- Practical Guide to Infertility Management and IVF- Chaitanya Nagori, Sonal Panchal]¹

22. **c.** Poor responding ovaries: 3D-PD VI <2, VFI <0.5
[Chapter 3- Practical Guide to Infertility Management and IVF- Chaitanya Nagori, Sonal Panchal]²

23. **e.** *FSH levels:*
- <8 mIU/mL: Reassure
- 8–12 mIU/mL: Average reserve
- 12–17 mIU/mL: Decreased ovarian reserve (DOR)
- >17 mIU/mL: Extremely poor pregnancy rates

[Chapter 3- Practical Guide to Infertility Management and IVF- Chaitanya Nagori, Sonal Panchal]³

24. **d.** Estradiol (E2) level on day 2 is high because of cumulative E2 produced from granulosa cells of multiple small follicles. E2 level alone, therefore, is never used as a sole marker for ovarian reserve. It has to be always used along with serum FSH; if both are high, it reflects poor ovarian reserve. As high E2 can mask an abnormal FSH in lower ovarian reserve patient due to negative feedback mechanism.
[Chapter 3- Practical Guide to Infertility Management and IVF- Chaitanya Nagori, Sonal Panchal]⁴

25. **a.** High FSH/LH ratio indicates poor ovarian reserve. FSH/LH ratio is an early indicator of ovarian aging and a rising FSH/LH ratio could be the first marker of ovarian aging and decreased ovarian reserve (DOR).
[Chapter 3- Practical Guide to Infertility Management and IVF- Chaitanya Nagori, Sonal Panchal]²

26. **d.** A level >45 pg/mL on day 2–3 is indicative of hyper-response to ovulation induction.
[Chapter 3- Practical Guide to Infertility Management and IVF- Chaitanya Nagori, Sonal Panchal]³

27. **c.** AMH inhibits the early stages of follicular development till 6-mm size, then the follicle grows under the effect of FSH.
[Chapter 3- Practical Guide to Infertility Management and IVF- Chaitanya Nagori, Sonal Panchal]⁴

28. **b.** *AMH levels*:
- Less than 1: Cycle cancellation or ovum donation
- 1–5: Poor response
- 5–15: Adequate response
- More than 15: Chances of OHSS

[Chapter 3- Practical Guide to Infertility Management and IVF- Chaitanya Nagori, Sonal Panchal]²

29. **d.** AMH is increased in polycystic ovary syndrome (PCOS) due to hyperandrogenemia and hyperinsulinemia. But in new Rotterdam's criteria July 2018, AMH cannot be used as only criteria to diagnose PCOS.

[Chapter 3- Practical Guide to Infertility Management and IVF- Chaitanya Nagori, Sonal Panchal][2]

30. **d.** There is no standard definition of abnormal test, hence not used routinely, as better tests like AFC and AMH are available. Smaller follicles produce less inhibin B and less E2 resulting in less negative feedback to FSH that is released due to clomifene stimulation.
[Chapter 3- Practical Guide to Infertility Management and IVF- Chaitanya Nagori, Sonal Panchal][4]

31. **d.** The ovarian reserve is the capacity of the ovaries to produce fertilizable ova. This depends on the quality and quantity of ovarian antral and preantral follicles.
[Chapter 3- Practical Guide to Infertility Management and IVF- Chaitanya Nagori, Sonal Panchal][3]

32. **d.** *Number of ova:*
    - At 20 weeks: 6–7 million
    - At birth 2 million
    - At puberty 3–4 lakh
    - After 30 years, 25,000
    - After 40 years, 8,000
    - At menopause <1,000

[Chapter 3- Practical Guide to Infertility Management and IVF- Chaitanya Nagori, Sonal Panchal][1]

33. **d.** Young old
Age <35; age >35
And AFC >5 AFC >5
OR AMH >1.2 ng/mL AMH >1.2 Group 1 Group 2
Poor; age >35 age >35 OR; AFC <5 AFC <5 AMH <1.2 AMH <1.2 Group 3 Group 4

REFERENCES

1. Natarajan P, Pandiyan R, Thanikachalam P. Speroff's Clinical Gynecologic Endocrinology and Infertility, 1st South Asia edition. New Delhi: Wolters Kluwer India Pvt. Ltd.; 2023.
2. Berek JS. Berek and Novak's Gynecology, 16th edition. Philadephia: Lippincott Williams & Wilkins; 2019.
3. Rao K A, Krishna D, Jaffar M, Ashraf C M. Principles and Practice of Assisted Reproductive Technology. volume 1 Infertility, 2nd edition. New Delhi: Jaypee Brothers Medical Publishers; 2019.
4. Nagori C, Panchal S. Handbook of Infertility & Ultrasound for Practicing Gynecologists, 2nd edition. New Delhi: Jaypee Brothers Medical Publishers; 2021.

Chapter 66: Laparoscopy in Infertility

Astha Lalwani, Shubhra Agarwal

QUESTIONS

1. **In a lady with infertility with bilateral tubal block at cornua, the best method of next management is:**
   a. Laparoscopy and hysteroscopy
   b. Hydrotubation
   c. In vitro fertilization (IVF)
   d. Tuboplasty

2. **The best management of endometrioma through laparoscopy is:**
   a. Drainage of endometrioma
   b. Cystectomy
   c. Aspiration
   d. CO_2 laser excision

3. **Indications of diagnostic laparoscopy in infertility are all, *except*:**
   a. Unexplained infertility
   b. Previous history of any pelvic surgery, severe dysmenorrhea, chronic pelvic pain
   c. Hysterosalpingogram (HSG) symptomatic of suggestive of bilateral tubal block
   d. Decrease ovarian reserve
   Before taking the patient for laparoscopic tubal reconstructive surgery following things are considered.
   1. Age of the patient
   2. Ovarian reserve
   3. Site and extent of tubal disease

4. **Before taking the patient for laparoscopic tubal reconstructive surgery, following things are considered.**
   1. Age of the patient
   2. Ovarian reserve
   3. Site and extent of tubal disease
   4. Semen analysis
   a. 1,3   b. 1,2
   c. 1,2,3   d. All

5. **Proximal tubal block, can be due to the following conditions, *except*:**
   a. Obstruction resulting from plugs of mucus and debris
   b. Spasm of the uterotubal ostium
   c. Occlusion from fibrosis due to salpingitis isthmica nodosa (SIN), pelvic inflammatory disease (PID) or endometriosis
   d. Fimbrial phimosis

6. **Success rate of opening of proximal tubal block after surgery is around:**
   a. 10–15%   b. 50%
   c. 80%–85%   d. 100%

7. **Distal tubal disease with hydrosalphinges and fimbrial phimosis usually has bad prognosis, hence the options of management are:**
   a. Laparoscopic tubal clipping
   b. Hysteroscopic occlusion of ostia
   c. Salpingectomy followed by in vitro fertilization (IVF)
   d. Any of the above

8. **Prognosis is better and the patient can be offered benefit of salpingostomy in distal block in the following conditions:**
   a. No more than limited filmsy adnexal adhesions
   b. Mildly dilated (<3 cm) tubes with thin and walls
   c. A lush endosalphinx with presentation of mucosal folds
   d. All of the above

9. **True about salpingoscopy is all, *except*:**
   a. Salpingoscopy is very easily practiced during fertiloscopy by the use of a small telescope
   b. The telescope is pushed gently in the fimbriae and then extended in ampulla

c. It is necessary to irrigate the tube
d. Intratubal pathologies like flattened mucosal folds and intra-ampullary adhesions can be identified
e. None of the above

10. **An attempt to create new ostia when there is hydrosalpinx or complete obstruction and original fimbria have completely disappeared is called:**
    a. Neosalpingostomy   b. Fimbrioplasty
    c. Salpingoscopy   d. Falloposcopy

11. **Reconstruction of fimbriae in a partially or completely occluded oviduct is called:**
    a. Neosalpingostomy   b. Fimbrioplasty
    c. Salpingoscopy   d. Falloposcopy

12. **Thing to be kept in mind during ovarian drilling:**
    a. The ovary has to be mobile and can fall freely on/off
    b. We can overcook the ovaries as it will not cause any harm
    c. Cooling the ovaries by thorough suction, irrigation, and lavage is a must
    d. Hydroflotation at the end of the procedure is not necessary to prevent adhesion formation

13. **Contraindications to minimal access surgeries are all, except:**
    a. Severe chronic obstructive pulmonary disease
    b. Stage 3 and stage 4 shock
    c. Coagulopathy
    d. Previous history of surgeries

14. **Azimuth angle is:**
    a. Angle between instrument and optical axis of endoscope
    b. Angle between endoscope and body of patient
    c. Angle between instrument and horizontal plane
    d. Angle between two tips of operating instruments

15. **Manipulation angle is:**
    a. Angle between instrument and optical axis of endoscope
    b. Angle between instrument and horizontal plane
    c. Angle between two tips of two operating instruments
    d. Angle between endoscope and body of patients

16. **The elevation angle is:**
    a. Between two tips of operating instruments
    b. Angle between instrument and optical axis of endoscope
    c. Angle between endoscope and body of patient
    d. Angle between instrument and horizontal plane

17. **True about Strassman metroplasty is all, except:**
    a. It is the unification surgery of two uterine cavities in bicornuate or uterine didelphys
    b. It is indicated in patients with recurrent pregnancy loss (RPL) or midtrimester miscarriages
    c. Broad rectovesical fold of peritoneum has to be resected hence cannot be performed hysteroscopically due to risk of uterine rupture
    d. The surgery is indicated in asymptomatic patients also irrespective of the obstetric outcome

18. **Which of the following is correct regarding endometrioma excision?**
    a. Endometrioma excision before in vitro fertilization (IVF) increases the live birth rate
    b. Endometrioma excision before IVF can increase the number of embryo yield but does not affect the quality of embryos and fertilization rates
    c. Endometrioma excision is needed in those patients when there is severe pelvic pain, ovulation is affected or oocytes cannot be retrieved during IVF
    d. Endometrioma excision should be done in all patients presenting with infertility irrespective of their anti-Müllerian hormone (AMH) levels

19. **The correct statement regarding management of an infertile patient, with history and examination suggestive of pelvic endometriosis is all, except:**
    a. Diagnostic laparoscopy with proper staging of disease and simultaneous fulguration of endometriotic deposits should be planned with see and treat approach
    b. Mild to minimal endometriosis can be offered ovulation induction with intrauterine insemination (IUI) and moderate to severe endometriosis can be given an option of in vitro fertilization (IVF)
    c. There is a definite role of adjuvant pre- and post-operative gonadotropin-releasing hormone (GnRh) analogs in such patients who are anxious to conceive
    d. The best time to conceive is within 6 months of the surgery

20. **Mechanism of electrothermal injuries include:**
    a. Defective insulation
    b. Alternative site burns
    c. Lateral thermal spread
    d. All of the above

21. Regarding mechanism of ultrasonic devices like harmonic, which is correct?
    i. Acts through tissue by heating
    ii. Acts through tissue by vibrating
    iii. Range of 20,000–60,000 Hz
    iv. Seals by using protein denaturation
    v. Converts the applied electric energy to thermal energy then converted mechanical vibration
    a. i, ii
    b. ii, iii, iv
    c. i, v
    d. ii, iii, iv, v

22. In case of suspected intra-abdominal adhesions Veress needle can be inserted through:
    a. Palmer's point
    b. Lee-huang point
    c. Jain point
    d. Umbilicus

23. Confirmation for the correct intraperitoneal placement of Veress needle is done by:
    i. Double click test
    ii. Hanging drop test
    iii. Aspiration test
    iv. Intraperitoneal pressure test
    a. i, iii
    b. ii, iv
    c. iii, iv
    d. All of the above

24. Carbon dioxide is used to create pneumoperitoneum because it is:
    i. Noncombustible
    ii. Inert and colorless
    iii. Highly soluble in blood so risk of embolism is less
    iv. Easily available and inexpensive
    a. i, ii, iii
    b. ii, iii
    c. iii, iv
    d. All of the above

25. The decision about whether to operate for ovarian endometrioma or pursue assisted reproduction depends upon following factor/factors:
    a. Size of endometrioma
    b. Ovarian reserve
    c. History of previous surgery
    d. Associated pelvic pain
    e. Ovarian access for in vitro fertilization (IVF) (anatomical distortion)
    f. All of the above

26. Decision to operate in adenomyosis (AD) depends upon all, *except:*
    a. Diffuse or focal adenoma with size
    b. Severity of symptoms (pain, bleeding)
    c. Distance from the endometrial cavity
    d. Ovarian reserve

27. Laparoscopic myomectomy is different from laparoscopic adenomyomectomy in the following way/ways, *except:*
    a. No proper capsule in adenoma hence plane of cleavage is not well maintained
    b. In myomectomy, complete myoma can be excised but in adenectomy the end point of the surgery is not satisfactorily achieved and part of myometrium is also excised
    c. In myomectomy hydrodissection and intracapsular vasopressin have a significant role to prevent blood loss, unlike in adenectomy
    d. The healing of the defect is better in adenoma excision as compared to myoma excision

28. True about laparoscopic transabdominal cerclage (TAC) is all, *except:*
    a. Indicated in patients with history of previous failed vaginal cerclage
    b. Better performed in patients with short, irregular cervix or with history of conization
    c. Success rate is better than transcervical route
    d. Has to always be done in the interpregnancy period, and never during pregnancy

29. A 25-year-old presented with primary infertility with ultrasound suggestive of bilateral tubo-ovarian abscess not responding to intravenous (IV) antibiotics. Next line of management should be:
    a. Hysterosalpingogram (HSG)
    b. Diagnostic laparoscopy with drainage and collection of pus for CBNAAT (cartridge-based nucleic acid amplification test)
    c. Hysteroscopy
    d. Ovulation induction followed by intrauterine insemination (IUI)

30. A 35-year-old patient presented with infertility with reduced ovarian reserve and planned for intra-ovarian platelet rich plasma. True is:
    a. Can be done laparoscopically
    b. Can be done transvaginally
    c. Repeat anti-Müllerian hormone (AMH) should be done after 6 weeks
    d. All of the above

31. **ACUM (Accessory and cavitated uterine mass) is a rare entity, often misdiagnosed leading to refractory dysmenorrhea. The diagnosis is based on following surgicopathological criteria,** *except:*
    a. An isolated accessory cavitated mass usually located under the round ligament
    b. Normal uterus fallopian tubes and ovaries are not identified
    c. Chocolate brown-colored fluid content
    d. An accessory cavity lined by endometrial epithelium with glands and stroma

ANSWERS

1. **a.** Laparoscopic surgery is the best method of management for bilateral tubal block as consequently Assisted reproductive technologies such as in vitro fertilization and embryo transfer[3]

2. **b.** Laparoscopic endometriotic cystectomy of ovary when performed with accurate surgical technique leads to no significant ovarian tissue removal and thus does not result in reduction of ovarian reserve.[1]

3. **d.** Diagnostic laparoscopy has no effect on decreasing or increasing ovarian reserve.[2]

4. **d.** Before taking the patient for laparoscopic tubal reconstructive surgery following things are considered. 1. Age of the patient 2. Ovarian reserve 3. Site and extent of tubal disease 4. Semen analysis.[1]

5. **d.** It is distal tubal disease

6. **c.** Success rate of opening of proximal tubal block after surgery is around 80–85%.[3]

7. **d.** Tuboplasty is not appropriate for women with severe disease or with both proximal and distal occlusions, as success rate is not good. Further it can lead to life-threatening ectopic pregnancies.

8. **d.** Prognosis is better and the patient can be offered benefit of salpingostomy in distal block in the following conditions: a. No more than limited flimsy adnexal adhesions b. Mildly dilated (<3 cm) tubes with thin and walls c. A lush endosalphinx with presentation of mucosal folds.[2]

9. **e.** All options provided for salpingoscopy are true.[2]

10. **a.** An attempt to create new ostia when there is hydrosalpinx or complete obstruction and original fimbria have completely disappeared is called Neosalpingostomy.[3]

11. **b.** Reconstruction of fimbriae in a partially or completely occluded oviduct is called Fimbrioplasty.[3]

12. **c.** During ovarian drilling, Cooling the ovaries by thorough suction, irrigation, and lavage is a must to prevent damage to ovarian reserve.[2]

13. **d.** Minimal access surgeries can be performed with history of previous surgeries.[1]

14. **a.** Azimuth angle is the angle between instrument and optical axis of endoscope.[3]

15. **c.** Manipulation angle is the angle between two tips of two operating instruments.[3]

16. **d.** The elevation angle is the angle between instrument and horizontal plane.[3]

17. **d.** The surgery is indicated only if there is midtrimester loss or recurrent pregnancy loss (RPL).

18. **c.** Clinicians should not routinely perform surgery for ovarian endometrioma prior to assisted reproductive technology (ART) to improve live birth rates, as the current evidence shows no benefit and surgery is likely to have a negative impact on ovarian reserve.

19. **c.** Management of an infertile patient, with history and examination suggestive of pelvic endometriosis there is no definite role of pre and post operative GnRh analogues.[1]

20. **d.** Mechanism of electrothermal injuries include: Defective insulation, alternative site burns, lateral thermal spread.[2]

21. **b.** Ultrasonic device like harmonic acts by vibrating on a range of 20,000–80,000Hz and seals by using protein denaturation.[3]

22. **a.** In case of suspected intra-abdominal adhesions veress needle can be inserted through Palmer's point.[3]

23. **d.** Confirmation for the correct intraperitoneal placement of Veress needle is done by: i. Double click test ii. Hanging drop test iii. Aspiration test iv. Intraperitoneal pressure test.[4]

24. **d.** Carbon dioxide is used to create pneumoperitoneum because it is: i. Noncombustible ii. Inert and colorless iii. Highly soluble in blood so risk of embolism is less iv. Easily available and inexpensive.[4]

25. **d.** Overall patients with focal adenomyosis (AD) have higher pregnancy rates after conservative surgery as compared to diffuse AD, and higher risk of uterine

rupture is also found in patients with diffuse AD excision. In diffuse AD, the decision for surgery to improve pregnancy rates also depends upon the distance of AD from the endometrial cavity, severity of other symptoms like pelvic pain, heavy menstrual bleeding, with history of recurrent pregnancy loss (RPL), implantation failure, or failed medical management.

26. **d.** The myometrium is inadvertently excised in adenoma excision as there is no well-developed capsule, it can lead to risk of uterine rupture in the consequent pregnancy. Minimum 9–15 mm of optimal uterine wall thickness is needed for conception and preventing uterine rupture.

27. **d.** It can be successfully performed in antenatal patients before 12 weeks under general anesthesia.

28. **b.** Diagnostic laparoscopy should be preferred, followed by tissue sampling for timely intervention in the form of antitubercular treatment (ATT). In case histopathologically proven diagnosis is not made, as the genital tuberculosis (TB) is paucibacillary, empirical treatment can be started. The tubal damage is irreversible if ATT not started timely but the uterine cavity can still be functional for the need of future possible in vitro fertilization (IVF).

29. **d.** Primary infertility with ultrasound suggestive of bilateral tuboovarian abscess not responding to intravenous (IV) antibiotics. Next line of management is ovulation induction followed by intrauterine insemination.[4]

30. **d.** Infertility with reduced ovarian reserve and planned for intra-ovarian platelet rich plasma. It can be done laparoscopically, can be done transvaginally and repeat anti-Müllerian hormone (AMH) should be done after 6 weeks.[4]

31. **b.** Accessory and cavitated uterine mass (ACUM) is lateralized to right or left of the uterine cavity, with regular borders, located under the insertion of round ligament. Uterine cavity and adnexa is usually normal which could be differentiated from unicornuate uterus by Magnetic resonance imaging (MRI). Laparoscopic excision is usually preferred as it is mostly found as progressive dysmenorrhea in young women <30 years of age.

REFERENCES

1. Rao KA, Chen C. Endoscopy in Infertility, 1st edition. New Delhi: Jaypee Brothers Medical Publishers; 2007.
2. Tandulwadkar SR, Nizari Mangeshikar N. Practical Endoscopy Tips by Experts, 2nd edition. New Delhi: Jaypee Brothers Medical Publishers; 2015.
3. Berek JS. Berek and Novak's Gynecology, 16th edition. Philadephia: Lippincott Williams & Wilkins; 2019.
4. Mishra RK. Textbook of Laparoscopy for Surgeons and Gynecologists, 4th edition. New Delhi: Jaypee Brothers Medical Publishers; 2021.

Chapter 67: Hysteroscopy in Infertility

Shubhra Agarwal, Astha Lalwani

QUESTIONS

1. Indication of hysteroscopy in infertility:
   a. Abnormal hysterosalpingogram (HSG) or transvaginal sonography (TVS)
   b. Unexplained infertility
   c. Routine assessment prior to embryo transfer
   d. All of above

2. Low viscosity fluids are:
   i. 1.5% glycine
   ii. Dextran
   iii. 3% sorbitol
   iv. 5% Mannitol

   Which is correct?
   a. i and ii
   b. i, iii, and iv
   c. ii, iii, and iv
   d. i, ii, and iii

3. Complications related to low viscosity media:
   a. Pulmonary edema
   b. Hyponatremia
   c. Cerebral edema
   d. All of above

4. Pressure required to distend endometrial cavity to visualize tubal ostia:
   a. 85 mm Hg
   b. 80 mm Hg
   c. 45 mm Hg
   d. 60 mm Hg

5. Management of recurrent pregnancy loss (RPL) with r-AFS class V or CONUTA U2:
   a. Observe
   b. Abdominal metroplasty
   c. Division of septum
   d. None of above

6. Distension media are all, *except:*
   a. CO_2 gas
   b. N_2O gas
   c. 0.9% normal saline
   d. 3% Mannitol

7. What degree of telescope is the best for diagnostic procedures?
   a. 0°
   b. 15°
   c. 30°
   d. 45°

8. What is the endpoint of septal resection in hysteroscopy?
   a. Attainment of two out of three criteria (Pain, bleeding, visualization of myometrial fibers)
   b. Attainment of visualization of myometrial fibers
   c. Attainment of all three criteria
   d. None of above

9. How much maximum fluid deficit allowed when normal saline is used?
   a. 1.5 L
   b. 2.5 L
   c. 2.0 L
   d. 1.0 L

10. Which degree of telescope is the best for hysteroscopic tubal cannulation/sterilization?
    a. 0°
    b. 15–25°
    c. 25–30°
    d. 45–60°

11. Indication of hysteroscopy myomectomy in infertility is all, *except:*
    a. Symptoms related to presence or fibroid
    b. Subfertility due to fibroid
    c. Submucous fibroid < 5 cm
    d. FIGO grade 7

12. Techniques of tubal cannulation are all, *except:*
    a. Selective salpingography
    b. Under sonographic guidance
    c. Hysteroscopy
    d. Hysterosalpingography

13. What is the indications of metroplasty in septate uterus?
    i. Recurrent pregnancy loss (RPL)
    ii. Preterm birth
    iii. Menorrhagia
    a. i and ii
    b. i and iii
    c. i, ii, and iii
    d. ii and iii

14. **In case of wide uterine septum second phase of surgery is performed:**
    a. After 1 month
    b. Not before 2 months
    c. Not before 6 months
    d. After next menses

15. **True about local injury to endometrium is all, *except*:**
    a. Implantation rate increases after injury to endometrium
    b. Rapid growth of endometrial cells
    c. Secretion of CK and GF increases wound healing
    d. Asherman's syndrome is more common

16. **What is the most sensitive imaging techniques for deciding hysteroscopic resection of fibroid?**
    a. USG
    b. MRI
    c. HSG
    d. CT

17. **Complication of hysteroscopy is all, *except*:**
    a. Perforation
    b. Bleeding
    c. Fluid overload
    d. Pneumothorax

18. **Hysteroscopic polypectomy is debatable if polyp is:**
    a. <2 cm
    b. 2–3 cm
    c. <4 cm
    d. Size has no value

19. **Hysteroscopic septal resection can be done by?**
    a. Scissors
    b. Collins knife
    c. Monopolar cautery
    d. All of above

20. **What is true for hysteroscopy in women for first IVF treatment?**
    a. Should routinely be offered hysteroscopy
    b. Offered hysteroscopy and laparoscopic chromopertubation
    c. Should not be offered hysteroscopy if TVS is normal
    d. Routine hysteroscopy improves fertility outcome

21. **Infertility with polyp management is:**
    a. Medical treatment
    b. Saline infusion sonography
    c. Hysteroscopy polypectomy
    d. Endometrial ablation

22. **Vaginoscopy in infertile patient:**
    i. Decreases pain
    ii. Decreases time
    iii. Decreases complications
    a. ii and iii
    b. i, ii, and iii
    c. i and iii
    d. i and ii

23. **Chronic endometritis in hysteroscopy is characterized by all, *except*:**
    a. Micropolyps
    b. Localized hyperemia
    c. Stippling
    d. Localized edema

24. **Endometrial polyp causes infertility by:**
    a. Release of glycodelin
    b. Reduced levels of HOXA-10 and -11
    c. Increased level of inflammatory markers
    d. All of above

25. **Hysteroscopic adhesiolysis aims at all, *except*:**
    a. Restore size and shape of cavity
    b. Leave a spur of 1 cm
    c. Prevent recurrence by amnion graft, catheter, estradiol valerate
    d. Promote regeneration of destroyed endometrium

26. **Classification used for selection of cases for hysteroscopic myomectomy:**
    a. STEP-W classification
    b. Sim's classification
    c. The American Society for Reproductive Medicine (ASRM) classification
    d. The European Society of Human Reproduction and Embryology (ESHRE) classification

27. **Hysteroscopy test to confirm tubal patency is:**
    a. Micropellet test
    b. Bubble test
    c. Methylene blue dye best
    d. Essure test

28. **All are true regarding fluid overload in hysteroscopy, *except*?**
    a. Fluid deficit > 1,000 mL in hypotonic solution
    b. 2.5 L in 0.9% normal saline (NS)
    c. 750 mL in cardiovascular impairment
    d. >3.0 L in glycine media

29. **All are true regarding intrauterine pressure, *except*:**
    a. For short procedures, intrauterine pressure (IUP) around 40 mm Hg is feasible
    b. The higher the IUP the lesser is the fluid absorption
    c. Significant absorption can occur if IUP exceeds mean arterial pressure (MAP)
    d. Pressure in venous sinuses in myometrium is 10–15 mm Hg

30. **Office hysteroscopy is defined as:**
    i. 2.7 mm scope
    ii. No need of OT
    iii. Outer sheath of 5–5.5 mm

    Which is correct?
    a. i, ii, and iii
    b. i and ii
    c. i and iii
    d. ii and iii

ANSWERS

1. **d.** Unexplained infertility cases, abnormal hysterosalpingogram (HSG), and assessment prior to ET are indications for hysteroscopy.

2. **b.** 1.5% glycine, 3% sorbitol, and 5% mannitol are low viscosity fluids and can be used with monopolar surgical instruments as they are electrolyte free.

3. **d.** Low viscosity media can cause pulmonary edema, hyponatremia, heart failure, cerebral edema, and death.

4. **c.** The main aim is to stay below mean arterial pressure and keep pressure as low as possible to minimize extravasation.

5. **c.** Hysteroscopic division of septum improves reproductive outcome at a rate comparable to abdominal metroplasty with reduced morbidity and cost.

6. **b.** Various types of liquid media available and used for hysteroscopy like mannitol, normal saline, nitrous oxide gas.

7. **a.** 0-degree telescope provides a panoramic view and is the best for diagnostic procedures whereas 25–30° angles are often used for cannulation.

8. **a.** Office method of "see and treat" where dissection is continued until attaining 2 of the three criteria (pain, bleeding, visualization of myometrial fibres).

9. **c.** When using electrolyte free media deficit of >1 L requires repeat measurement of serum electrolyte level and furosemide. The maximum deficit allowed with normal saline is 2.5 L.

10. **c.** Rigid endoscopes require an angled lens to provide a field of view useful for operative hysteroscopy. In addition to 0-degree versions, they are commonly used in 12–15°, and 25–30° models.

11. **d.** Indications of hysteroscopic myomectomy are as follows:
    - Symptoms, which are considered to be related to the presence of submucous fibroids.
    - Subfertility due to submucous fibroids when they interfere with the uniformity of the uterine cavity and implantation.
    - Submucous fibroids < 5 cm in diameter at the time of surgery.

12. **d.** Techniques of cannulation:
    - Selective salpingography
    - Under sonographic guidance
    - Hysteroscopic cannulation

13. **a.** Indications of metroplasty in uterine septa:
    - Recurrent pregnancy loss (RPL)
    - Primary and secondary infertility
    - Preterm births
    - Dysmenorrhea (therapy resistant)
    - In few cases before IVF (as a preventive measure)

14. **b.** *Follow-up:* Estrogen therapy is administered for 2 months following which diagnostic hysteroscopy will be performed.

15. **d.** Not a local injury but a curettage that erodes the basal endometrial layer leaving it exposed which in turn heals by fibrous tissue formation known as Asherman syndrome.

16. **b.** Most sensitive imaging techniques for deciding hysteroscopic resection of fibroid is MRI to determine the number, size, location, degree of intramural extension of submucous myomas as well as the distance between the myoma and the serosa.

17. **d.** Complication of hysteroscopy:
    - Perforation is reported in up to 6% of attempted procedures. It is left to heal on its own.
    - Infection (rare)
    - Bleeding
    - Fluid overload

18. **a.** Hysteroscopic polypectomy is debatable if polyp is <2 cm as it can removed by using neodymium-doped yttrium aluminum garnet (Nd:YAG) laser.

19. **d.** Hysteroscopic septal resection can be done by:
    - Monopolar or bipolar system
    - Collins knife
    - Scissors

20. **c.** Hysteroscopy in women for first IVF treatment should not be performed if the transvaginal sonography (TVS) is normal as it will undue instrumentation.

21. **c.** Infertility with polyp management is hysteroscopic polypectomy as it is the definitive treatment and will aid in fertility.

22. **b.** Vaginoscopy in infertile patients decreases time, pain, and complications.

23. **c.** Chronic endometritis in hysteroscopy is characterized by micropolyps, localized hyperemia, and edema.

24. **d.** Endometrial polyp causes infertility by release of glycodelin, reduced levels of HOXA-10 and -11, increased level of inflammatory markers.

25. **b.** Hysteroscopic adhesiolysis aims at restoring the size and shape of cavity, prevents recurrence and promotes regeneration of destroyed endometrium.

26. **a.** STEP-W classification that considers size, topography, extent, penetration, and location on wall of uterus is used to decide for hysteroscopic myomectomy.

27. **b.** Bubble test is the test performed to visualize the patency of tubes via hysteroscopy.

28. **d.** Fluid deficit of 1 L is acceptable for hypotonic solution in normal individuals, 750 mL in cardiac patient, and 2.5 L with normal saline.

29. **b.** The main aim in hysteroscopy is to keep intrauterine pressure below the mean arterial pressure. More the intrauterine pressure more is the fluid absorption.

30. **b.** Office hysteroscopy is usually performed in OPD with a 2.7-mm scope and outer sheath of 3.5–4.0 mm.

REFERENCES

1. Falcone T, Ridgeway B. Gynaecologic Endoscopy. In: Berek JS (Ed). Berek and Novac's Gynaecology, 16th edition. Philadelphia: Wolters Kluwer; 2020. pp. 1286-406.
2. Jain N, singh TG, Jain V, Srivastava K. Endoscopy in infertility: Hysteroscopy in infertility. In: Rao KA (Ed). Principles and practice of Assisted Reproductive Technology, 2nd edition, vol. 1. New Delhi: The health Science publisher (Jaypee Brothers Medical Publishers (Pvt. Ltd.); 2018. pp. 559-69.

Chapter 68

Amenorrhea

Vejainty Chauhan, Shefali Singh

QUESTIONS

1. **Patient fulfilling any of the following criteria should be evaluated for amenorrhea:**
   a. No menses by age of 14 years in the absence of growth or development of secondary sexual characteristics
   b. No menses by age of 15 years regardless of the presence of normal growth and development of secondary sexual characteristics
   c. In women who have menstruated previously, no menses for an interval of time equivalent to a total of at least three previous cycles or no menses over a 12-month period
   d. All of the above

2. **Which of the following is true regarding sequence of Tanner staging of breast and pubic hair in a normal individual?**
   a. Breast development is a reliable indicator of endogenous estrogen production or exposure to exogenous estrogens and within 2 years pubarche is noted
   b. The presence of pubic hair growth reliably reflects androgen production or exposure and noted before thelarche
   c. Breast development and growth of pubic hair typically progress in a symmetrical manner, their Tanner stages should be consistent in normal individual
   d. All of the above

3. **Which of the following is not correct?**
   a. Compartment I involves the uterus, cevix, and vagina
   b. Compartment II involves the disorders of the ovary
   c. Compartment III involves the disorders of the posterior pituitary
   d. Compartment IV involves the disorders of the hypothalamus or central nervous system (CNS)

4. **Which compartment disorder is the most common overall cause of primary and secondary amenorrhea?**
   a. Ovary
   b. Outflow tract
   c. Hypothalamo-pituitary outflow
   d. Uterus

5. **Which of the following is the most common form of hypergonadotropic hypogonadism in women with absent secondary sexual characters and primary amenorrhea?**
   a. Turner syndrome
   b. Kallmann syndrome
   c. Swayer syndrome
   d. Galactosemia

6. **Second most common hypothalamic cause of primary amenorrhea with hypogonadotropic hypogonadism is:**
   a. Turner syndrome
   b. Kallmann syndrome
   c. Swayer syndrome
   d. Cushing syndrome

7. **Transverse vaginal septum and imperforate hymen have all common, *except*:**
   a. Cyclical pelvic or abdominal pain with amenorrhea
   b. Secondary sexual characters are present
   c. On physical examination, Valsalva maneuver causes distention of bulge
   d. Laboratory investigations are not required, imaging—abdominal/pelvic magnetic resonance imaging (MRI) differentiates the two

8. Mutation of the variant of *GALT* gene is seen associated with:
   a. Müllerian agenesis
   b. Classical galactosemia
   c. Kallmann syndrome
   d. None of the above

9. Patient with primary amenorrhea with normal, symmetrical breast and pubic hair development, no visible vagina, and have no symptoms or signs of cryptomenorrhea.
   Has few urologic anomalies on ultrasonologic findings. Which of the diagnosis can be considered?
   a. Turner syndrome
   b. Type A Müllerian agenesis
   c. Type B Müllerian agenesis
   d. True hermaphrodite

10. A 20-year-old female with primary amenorrhea came to gynecology OPD. On examination, it was noticed that she had well-developed breast but Tanner 2 stage pubic hairs and short blind vagina. Pelvic ultrasound reveals no uterus, no cervix. Her 16 years old younger sister did not attained menarche yet. Which of the following is incorrect for this?
    a. She had normal male karyotype (46,XY), testes as gonads producing testosterone and AMH
    b. An inactivating mutation in the gene encoding the intracellular androgen receptor (AR) (located on the long arm of the X chromosome, Xq)
    c. Gonads show evidence of spermatogenesis
    d. Other family members such as sister or maternal aunt are often affected

11. How is the third most common cause of amenorrhea is differentiated from the second most common cause of amenorrhea?
    a. The absence of pubic and axillary hair
    b. Serum testosterone and serum LH levels
    c. Karyotyping
    d. All of the above

12. The management of patients with complete AIS has two major components:
    1. Creating functional vagina to allow attainment and optimization of potential for sexual relations
    2. Can bear own offsprings with surrogacy
    3. Risk for developing malignancy in the cryptorchid testes
    4. Gonadectomy done at the time of diagnosis
    a. 1 and 2 are correct
    b. 2 and 4 are correct
    c. 3 and 2 are correct
    d. 1 and 3 are correct

13. Gonadectomy is recommended by approximately at age of 16–18 years in:
    a. Swayer syndrome
    b. Complete AIS
    c. Incomplete AIS
    d. All of the above

14. A 34-year-old woman presents to OPD with the complaints of hypomenorrhea and secondary infertility. She had history of previous two abortions (4 years back) followed by suction and evacuation and curettage thereafter. She did not resume her normal menses for 4 years, while her hormonal profile is normal. Which of the following is not true regarding this condition?
    a. Amenorrhea traumatic—the most common cause is curettage done for postpartum hemorrhage
    b. Asherman syndrome is an uncommon but recognized complication of cesarean section, abdominal, or hysteroscopic myomectomy or metroplasty, and uterine artery embolization
    c. Asherman syndrome from any cause results only in amenorrhea and so most women with intrauterine adhesions present with infertility, or recurrent pregnancy loss
    d. End-organ endometrial damage and intrauterine adhesions also may result from intrauterine infections such as tuberculosis and schistosomiasis

15. Which of the following statement is false?
    a. The diagnosis of Asherman syndrome is based primarily on a high index of suspicion, based on history
    b. In women with Asherman syndrome, scant or no withdrawal bleeding after sequential treatment with exogenous estrogen and progestin occurs
    c. Saline infusion sonogram (SIS) or hysterosalpingography (HSG) provides a definitive diagnosis of Asherman syndrome
    d. Operative hysteroscopy is the primary method for treatment of intrauterine adhesions

16. The American Fertility Society classifies the severity of Asherman syndrome in three stages as follows. Which is false?
    a. Mild disease: Few flimsy adhesions involving less than a third of the uterine cavity with normal menses or hypomenorrhea
    b. Moderate disease: Flimsy and dense adhesions, the involvement of one-third to two-thirds of the cavity, and hypomenorrhea
    c. Severe disease: Dense adhesions involving more than two-thirds of the cavity with amenorrhea

d. Severe disease: Dense adhesions involving whole of the cavity with amenorrhea

17. Which of the following leads to Asherman syndrome?
    a. Elective endometrial ablation
    b. Schistosomiasis
    c. Cesarean section
    d. All of the above

18. Females with Turner syndrome is associated with increased risk cancers, *except:*
    a. Endometrial cancer
    b. Bladder cancer
    c. Breast cancer
    d. Central nervous system tumors

19. Women with Turner syndrome is strongly discouraged for pregnancy as:
    a. The risk of death during pregnancy is increased as much as 100-fold, primarily due to complications of aortic dissection or rupture
    b. Preimplantation genetic screening technology can be utilized to minimize the risk of aneuploidy in the progeny
    c. Turner syndrome generally should be regarded as a relative contraindication to pregnancy
    d. All are true

20. A short statured 13 years old female with absent axillary and pubic hairs, deafness, shielded chest with widely spaced nipples came to OPD. Which of the following is true?
    a. Treatment with GH should be delayed till treatment with estrogen therapy is effective
    b. Combined Estrogen-progesterone therapy should be given in high dose as soon as the diagnosis is confirmed
    c. Fluorescence in situ hybridization (FISH) analysis is most clearly indicated for those exhibiting any evidence of virilization or having a chromosomal fragment of uncertain origin
    d. Risk for developing gonadoblastoma is <5%

21. Which of the following is not required for initial evaluation of primary ovarian insufficiency?
    a. Menstrual history
    b. Follicle-stimulating hormone (FSH) and estradiol levels
    c. Pelvic ultrasound—antral follicle count
    d. Prolactin and thyroid function test

22. After the diagnosis of POI is confirmed, which of the testing is done?
    a. Karyotype and pelvic ultrasonography
    b. FMR1 premutation
    c. 21-hydroxylase (CYP21) by immunoprecipitation or indirect immunofluorescence
    d. All of the above

23. Maximum risk of premature ovarian failure seen in:
    a. Numerical and structural chromosomal abnormalities
    b. Hypothyroidism
    c. Fragile X premutation
    d. Autoimmune disease

24. Which of the following is true regarding fragile X syndrome?
    a. POF associated with premutation may reflect *FMR1* mRNA loss-of-function toxicity
    b. Least common inherited cause of mental retardation and autism
    c. Results from abnormal expansion of an unstable trinuclcotide (CGC) repeat sequence in the *FMR1* gene
    d. Women with POF should be offered testing for *FMR1* premutation

25. Functional ovarian failure resulting from disorder of follicular development with hypergonadotropic hypogonadism is known as:
    a. Swayer syndrome
    b. Simmond syndrome
    c. Sheehan syndrome
    d. Savage syndrome

26. Low gonadal toxicity is shown by which chemotherapeutic drugs?
    a. Cyclophosphamide
    b. Adriamycin
    c. Nitrogen mustard
    d. Bleomycin

27. BPES—a rare autosomal dominant disease characterized by:
    a. The blepharophimosis/ptosis/epicanthus inversus
    b. Premature ovarian failure
    c. caused by a variety of mutations in the gene encoding a forkhead box transcription factor (FOXL2) required for normal granulosa cell function
    d. All of the above

28. A 30-year-old woman presents with secondary amenorrhea since her last childbirth. Pregnancy test is negative. She gives history of severe PPH in last pregnancy for which she received five units of blood transfusion. She was not able to breastfeed her child as milk formation was not enough. Which one of the following statements is not correct for this situation?
    a. Acute infarction and ischemic necrosis of posterior pituitary gland
    b. Most common cause is hypovolemic hypotension from postpartum hemorrhage
    c. Failed lactation after delivery is the classical presenting symptom
    d. Skull X-ray shows partially or completely empty Sella

29. Which of the following is not true for secondary amenorrhea?
    a. Infiltrative pituitary lesions act by damaging the gonadotrophs and cause hypogonadotropic hypogonadism
    b. Excessive absorption of dietary iron leading iron overload and subsequently damage the gonadotrophs in pituitary in hereditary hemochromatosis
    c. Hereditary hemochromatosis is a common cause of hypogonadotropic hypogonadism, iron studies must be performed in all patients with hypopituitarism and normal imaging
    d. In lymphocytic hypophysitis, patients are treated by transsphenoidal surgery, dopamine agonists, anti-inflammatory or immunosuppressive drugs, or pituitary radiotherapy

30. Diseases associated with the amenorrhea are:
    a. Granulomatous infiltrative processes of sarcoidosis
    b. Tuberculous meningitis
    c. Intrasellar tuberculoma
    d. All of the above

31. The critical level of body fat required for the onset and regularity of menstrual function corresponds to:
    a. 17% for menarche, and at 22% for regular menstruation
    b. 27% for menarche, and at 22% for regular menstruation
    c. 22% for menarche, and at 17% for regular menstruation
    d. 17% for menarche, and at 27% for regular menstruation

32. Perimenopausal transition is associated with:
    a. High FSH, high LH
    b. Low FSH, high LH
    c. High FSH, normal LH
    d. Normal FSH, normal LH

33. All are true for Kallmann syndrome, *except:*
    a. It is a congenital gonadotropin-releasing hormone (GnRH) deficiency is associated with anosmia or hyposmia (an absent or grossly impaired sense of smell)
    b. Patients with the disorder also may have a family history of delayed puberty and other abnormalities, including cleft lip/palate, urogenital tract anomalies, or syndactyly
    c. Always inherited in an autosomal recessive fashion
    d. Associated with inactivating mutation in the gene encoding the fibroblast growth factor-1 receptor (FGFR1)

34. All are true in congenital gonadotropin-releasing hormone deficiency, *except:*
    a. Patients with the disorder also may have a family history of delayed puberty and other abnormalities, including cleft lip/palate, urogenital tract anomalies, or syndactyly
    b. At puberty, both males and females with Kallmann syndrome usually present with delayed growth and sexual development
    c. The diagnosis of congenital GnRH deficiency can be inferred by demonstrating a complete lack of pulsatile LH secretion and little or no LH secretion in response to exogenous pulsatile GnRH treatment
    d. Congenital GnRH deficiency is more common in females than in males (5:1)

35. All are true regarding empty Sella syndrome, *except:*
    a. Most commonly idiopathic, associated with pituitary insufficiency
    b. A less common mechanism for an empty Sella is of pituitary infarction
    c. In women presenting with amenorrhea and galactorrhea, the prevalence of empty Sella is between 4 and 15%
    d. Patients with hyperprolactinemia and an empty sella should undergo annual surveillance (prolactin assay and imaging)

36. Which is not true about corticotroph adenomas causing amenorrhea?
    a. Causes the Cushing disease associated with excessive circulating glucocorticoids
    b. Most common cause of Cushing syndrome is inhaled glucocorticoids
    c. Moon face and buffalo hump are characteristics of Cushing disease
    d. Menstrual abnormalities are common, affecting 80% women and one-third develop amenorrhea

ANSWERS

1. **a.**
   - No menses by age of 14 years in the absence of growth or development of secondary sexual characteristics.
   - No menses by age of 16 years regardless of the presence of normal growth and development of secondary sexual characteristics.
   - In women who have menstruated previously, no menses for an interval of time equivalent to a total of at least three previous cycles or no menses over a 6-month period.

   [Reference: Taylor HS, Pal L, Seli E (Eds). Speroff's Clinical Gynecologic Endocrinology and Infertility, 9th edition. Gurugram: Wolters Kluwer Pvt. Ltd.; 2019. p. 822]

2. **c.** Breast development is a reliable indicator of endogenous estrogen production or exposure to exogenous estrogens. The Tanner stage of breast development should be noted. A secondary arrest of breast development suggests a disruption of the HPO axis. When menarche has not followed breast development at the expected time (ideally, within 2 years of thelarche), a developmental anomaly of the reproductive tract as a mechanism for primary amenorrhea should be high in the list of differential diagnoses.

   The presence of pubic hair growth reliably reflects androgen production or exposure. Because breast development and growth of pubic hair typically progress in a symmetrical manner, their Tanner stages should be consistent. Absent or scant growth of sexual hair can be expected in otherwise sexually infantile girls, but also is a classical sign of androgen insensitivity syndrome (AIS) when breast development may be asymmetrically advanced.

   [Reference: Taylor HS, Pal L, Seli E (Eds). Speroff's Clinical Gynecologic Endocrinology and Infertility, 9th edition. Gurugram: Wolters Kluwer Pvt. Ltd.; 2019. p. 831]

3. **c.** Compartment I: Disorders of the genital outflow tract and uterus
   Compartment II: Disorders of the ovary
   Compartment III: Disorders of the anterior pituitary
   Compartment IV: Disorders of the hypothalamus or central nervous system

   [Reference: Taylor HS, Pal L, Seli E (Eds). Speroff's Clinical Gynecologic Endocrinology and Infertility, 9th edition. Gurugram: Wolters Kluwer Pvt. Ltd.; 2019. p. 826]

4. **a.** Abnormalities of ovarian function are the most common overall cause of amenorrhea (primary and secondary) and include a wide variety of disorders ranging from simple chronic anovulation as in women with polycystic ovarian syndrome (PCOS) to ovulatory dysfunction associated with obesity, thyroid disorders, and hyperprolactinemia, to ovarian failure or POI. Several conditions are associated with POI including genetic abnormalities [these can be chromosomal abnormalities or single gene disorders such as fragile X (FMR1) permutation or genetically inherited metabolic disorders such as galactosemia] or, autoimmune disease, or following exposure to radiation or chemotherapy.

   [Reference: Taylor HS, Pal L, Seli E (Eds). Speroff's Clinical Gynecologic Endocrinology and Infertility, 9th edition. Gurugram: Wolters Kluwer Pvt. Ltd.; 2019. p. 834]

5. **a.** Turner syndrome
   Turner syndrome (45,X) and its variants represent the most common form of hypergonadotropic hypogonadism in women with primary amenorrhea. Here, gonadotropin levels are elevated because of the lack of negative estrogen feedback on the hypothalamic–pituitary axis. Most patients with these conditions have primary amenorrhea and lack secondary sexual characteristics.

   Turner syndrome (45,X) is the most common karyotypic abnormality causing gonadal failure and primary amenorrhea. It appears that patients with Turner syndrome initially have normal ovarian development in utero. Amenorrhea is the result of accelerated atresia of the follicles. The fibrotic ovaries are called streak ovaries.

   In addition to gonadal failure, there are associated stigmata with Turner syndrome that include short stature, webbed neck, shield chest, cubitus valgus (increased carrying angle of the arms), low hair line, high arched palate, multiple pigmented nevi, and short fourth metacarpals. X inactivation is a process that inactivates most of the genes on one X chromosome.

   Of the genes on the X chromosome, 20% escape X inactivation, and it is believed that loss of the second copy of these genes in a 45,X patient causes the stigmata associated with Turner syndrome. After the diagnosis of Turner syndrome is confirmed by karyotype, studies should be performed to ensure that cardiac (30% have coarctation of the aorta), renal (especially horseshoe kidney), and autoimmune (thyroiditis) abnormalities are diagnosed and treated.

Cardiac magnetic resonance imaging should be used in addition to echocardiography. Evaluation should be performed in childhood to identify potential attention-deficit or nonverbal learning disorders. Women with Turner syndrome should be screened for diabetes mellitus, aortic enlargement, hypertension, and hearing loss throughout their lives.

In girls, galactosemia often is associated with ovarian failure, but this condition usually is detected by newborn screening programs. A galactose-1 phosphate uridyltransferase level can be measured to assess the patient for galactosemia or carrier status.
[Reference: Berek JS (Ed). Berek & Novak's Gynecology, 16th edition. United States: Lippincott (Wolters Kluwer); 2019. p. 867]

6. **b.** Kallmann syndrome
The second most common hypothalamic cause of primary amenorrhea associated with hypogonadotropic hypogonadism is insufficient pulsatile secretion of GnRH (Kallmann syndrome), which has varied modes of genetic transmission. Insufficient pulsatile secretion of GnRH leads to deficiencies in FSH and LH. Kallmann syndrome is often associated with anosmia (inability to perceive odors), although a woman may not be aware of her impaired sense of smell. The hypogonadism and anosmia arise because of failure of proper neuronal migration during fetal development. *Physiologic or constitutional delay of puberty is the most common* manifestation of hypogonadotropic hypogonadism. Amenorrhea may result from the lack of physical development caused by delayed reactivation of the GnRH pulse generator. Levels of GnRH are functionally deficient in relation to chronologic age but normal in terms of physiologic development.
[Reference: Berek JS (Ed). Berek & Novak's Gynecology, 16th edition. United States: Lippincott (Wolters Kluwer); 2019. p. 872]

7. **c.** A transverse vaginal septum results when the vaginal plate, formed from the fused sinovaginal bulbs, fails to break down or canalize during embryogenesis. As could be expected, girls with a transverse vaginal septum or cervical atresia, like those with an imperforate hymen, generally present at or soon after the age of expected menarche with primary amenorrhea and complaints of cyclic pelvic or abdominal pain due to obstructed menses and exhibit symmetrical, and age-appropriate secondary sexual development. Physical examination reveals a *normal vaginal orifice, a shortened vagina of varying length, no visible cervix, and a palpable hematocolpos in the proximal vaginal segment above the obstruction and/or a pelvic mass resulting from hematometra and hematosalpinges. A Valsalva maneuver will cause distention at the introitus in those with an imperforate hymen, but not in those with a transverse vaginal septum or cervical atresia, and can help to distinguish the two.* Imaging is necessary to define the anatomy of the disorder, but laboratory investigation generally is not required. Pelvic ultrasonography can reveal the level and extent of the hematocolpos and any associated hematometra or hematosalpinges.
[Reference: Taylor HS, Pal L, Seli E (Eds). Speroff's Clinical Gynecologic Endocrinology and Infertility, 9th edition. Gurugram: Wolters Kluwer Pvt. Ltd.; 2019. p. 857]

8. **a.** The prevalence of a mutation in the galactose-1-phosphate uridyltransferase (*GALT*) gene (different from that associated with classical galactosemia) is increased in daughters with Müllerian agenesis and their mothers. This observation suggests that errors in fetal or maternal galactose metabolism resulting in increased intrauterine galactose exposure may have adverse effects on Müllerian development and is consistent with studies in rodents wherein a high galactose diet during pregnancy delayed vaginal opening in the female offspring. Given the relationship between classical galactosemia and POI (discussed later in this chapter), patients with Müllerian agenesis who carry such a variant *GALT* gene mutation may be at increased risk for the same.

Galactosemia is an autosomal recessive disorder of galactose metabolism caused by a deficiency of the enzyme GALT and is another, albeit very rare, cause of POF. Affected women have fewer primordial follicles, presumably due to the cumulative toxicity of galactose metabolites on germ cell migration and survival. Diagnosis usually is made in the first few days of life after feeding with breast or cows' milk-based formulas begin, causing jaundice, vomiting, and failure to thrive.

[Reference: Taylor HS, Pal L, Seli E (Eds). Speroff's Clinical Gynecologic Endocrinology and Infertility, 9th edition. Gurugram: Wolters Kluwer Pvt. Ltd.; 2019. p. 859]

9. **c.** Patients with Müllerian agenesis typically present in late adolescence or as young adults, well after menarche was expected, with primary amenorrhea as their only complaint. They exhibit normal, symmetrical breast and pubic hair development, have no visible vagina, and have no symptoms or signs of cryptomenorrhea because the rudimentary uteri contain no functional endometrium. Two forms of the disorder have been described.

(1) Type A is characterized by symmetrical, muscular, rudimentary uteri and normal fallopian tubes and (2) type B by asymmetrical rudimentary uteri and absent or hypoplastic fallopian tubes.

In the great majority of patients with Müllerian agenesis, the ovaries are entirely normal histologically and functionally.

Urologic anomalies are relatively common (15–40%), particularly in type B Müllerian agenesis, and include unilateral renal agenesis, ectopic or horseshoe kidney, and duplication of the collecting system(s).

Because patients with Müllerian agenesis can exhibit characteristics similar to those observed in some types of male pseudohermaphroditism, a karyotype is justified and definitive.

In the absence of a karyotype, serum testosterone concentration in the normal female range effectively excludes AIS.

[Reference: Taylor HS, Pal L, Seli E (Eds). Speroff's Clinical Gynecologic Endocrinology and Infertility, 9th edition. Gurugram: Wolters Kluwer Pvt. Ltd.; 2019. p. 859]

10. **c.** Complete AIS (testicular feminization) has gonadal sex (male) and the contrasting phenotype (female). the third most common cause of primary amenorrhea, after gonadal dysgenesis and Müllerian agenesis.

AMH signaling is intact in AIS, the internal genitalia follow the male pattern of differentiation with regression of the Müllerian structures; individuals with AIS are phenotypic females with absent cervix and uterus (due to normal AMH action); the vagina is short and ends blindly (derived only from the urogenital sinus). The breasts may become relatively large and have subtle abnormalities; lacking the actions of progesterone, they have little glandular tissue, small nipples, and pale areolae. The labia minora usually are underdeveloped and the vagina is short and ends blindly. Pubic and axillary hair do not develop due to the absence of androgen action. The gonads are testes, and their location may be intra-abdominal, but often are partially descended into the inguinal canal; more than half of patients with complete AIS have an inguinal hernia, and the testes are frequently palpable in the inguinal canals, most commonly at the level of the external inguinal ring. Histologically, the gonads generally resemble any cryptorchid testes but may be nodular. After puberty, the testes contain immature seminiferous tubules lined by immature germ cells and Sertoli cells with no evidence of spermatogenesis.

[Reference: Taylor HS, Pal L, Seli E (Eds). Speroff's Clinical Gynecologic Endocrinology and Infertility, 9th edition. Gurugram: Wolters Kluwer Pvt. Ltd.; 2019. p. 863]

11. **d.** Patients with complete AIS generally are easily distinguished from those with Müllerian agenesis by the absence of pubic and axillary hair.

Serum testosterone concentration easily distinguishes patients with AIS from those with Müllerian agenesis because levels are normal or modestly elevated well above the normal range for females and often above the range observed in normal males. Serum LH levels also are elevated, reflecting androgen insensitivity at the hypothalamo-pituitary level. A karyotype (46,XY) firmly establishes the diagnosis.

[Reference: Taylor HS, Pal L, Seli E (Eds). Speroff's Clinical Gynecologic Endocrinology and Infertility, 9th edition. Gurugram: Wolters Kluwer Pvt. Ltd.; 2019. p. 863]

12. **a.** The management of patients with complete AIS has two major components, one focusing on creation of a functional vagina to allow attainment and optimization of potential for sexual relations and another relating to the risk for developing malignancy in the cryptorchid testes. In patients with AIS, the options for creation of a neovagina are the same as discussed earlier for those with Müllerian agenesis—progressive vaginal dilation and vaginoplasty. The short but distinct vagina observed in most patients with AIS speeds the progress of efforts at vaginal dilation. Good results also can be expected with surgical treatment, when necessary. Gonadectomy

is indicated because the incidence of neoplasia in cryptorchid testes is relatively high. In one early series of 50 cases, 11 malignancies, 15 adenomas, and 10 benign cysts were observed: a 22% incidence of malignancy and a 52% overall incidence of neoplasia. More recent series suggest a lower 5–10% overall incidence of gonadal tumors.
[Reference: Taylor HS, Pal L, Seli E (Eds). Speroff's Clinical Gynecologic Endocrinology and Infertility, 9th edition. Gurugram: Wolters Kluwer Pvt. Ltd.; 2019. p. 863]

13. **b.** Gonadectomy is recommended at the time of diagnosis in other intersex states such as XY gonadal dysgenesis (Swyer's syndrome), it is better delayed in those with AIS, for two reasons. First, the smooth pubertal development that results from endogenous gonadal hormone production is difficult to achieve with exogenous hormone treatment, and second, gonadal tumors develop less often in patients with AIS and rarely before puberty. Therefore, gonadectomy and hormone therapy (physiologic estrogen treatment) generally are best postponed until after pubertal development is complete, by approximately age of 16–18 years. Complete AIS is the only exception to the rule that gonads with a Y chromosome should be removed as soon as the diagnosis is made. Gonadectomy usually can be accomplished endoscopically with relative ease when the testes reside within the abdomen and via inguinal incisions when they are partially descended. In patients with the incomplete form of AIS, surgery should not be postponed because prompt gonadectomy will prevent further unwanted virilization that can occur at puberty.
[Reference: Taylor HS, Pal L, Seli E (Eds). Speroff's Clinical Gynecologic Endocrinology and Infertility, 9th edition. Gurugram: Wolters Kluwer Pvt. Ltd.; 2019. p. 863]

14. **c.** Disruption of the full thickness of the endometrium including the zona basalis, commonly resulting from instrumentation of the uterine cavity, is the most common mechanism for intrauterine scarring. Risk for developing intrauterine adhesions is increased by inflammation, as may result from endometritis or retained products of conception, and when the endometrium is relatively thin and inactive, as it is during the early postpartum period.

Asherman syndrome is an uncommon but recognized complication of cesarean section, abdominal, or hysteroscopic myomectomy, or metroplasty, and uterine artery embolization. Elective endometrial ablation procedures that utilize various modalities to achieve endometrial damage such as electrocautery, laser, thermal ablation, or cryoablation for the management of menorrhagia frequently result in amenorrhea, by intent.

End-organ endometrial damage and intrauterine adhesions also may result from intrauterine infections such as tuberculosis and schistosomiasis, which are rare in the United States but not in other regions of the world.

Although Asherman syndrome from any cause may result in amenorrhea, most women with intrauterine adhesions present with *dysmenorrhea, hypomenorrhea, infertility, or recurrent pregnancy loss, rather than absence of menses*. The diagnosis of Asherman syndrome is based primarily on a high index of suspicion, based on history.
[Reference: Taylor HS, Pal L, Seli E (Eds). Speroff's Clinical Gynecologic Endocrinology and Infertility, 9th edition. Gurugram: Wolters Kluwer Pvt. Ltd.; 2019. p. 865]

15. **c.** In women whose history suggests this possibility, scant or no withdrawal bleeding after sequential treatment with exogenous estrogen (e.g., conjugated equine estrogens 1.25 mg daily for 21 days) and progestin (e.g., MPA 10 mg daily for the last 5–7 days of estrogen dosing) reflects end-organ endometrial failure and corroborates the clinical suspicion. The clinical impression is further strengthened by ultrasound evidence of a thin, hyperechoic, and often irregular endometrial echo. Saline infusion sonogram (SIS) or hysterosalpingography (HSG) provides more specific information regarding the location and extent of intrauterine adhesions that partially or completely obliterate or obstruct the endometrial cavity or the cervical canal. Hysteroscopy provides a definitive diagnosis. Operative hysteroscopy is the primary method for treatment of intrauterine adhesions.
[Reference: Taylor HS, Pal L, Seli E (Eds). Speroff's Clinical Gynecologic Endocrinology and Infertility, 9th edition. Gurugram: Wolters Kluwer Pvt. Ltd.; 2019. p. 865]

16. **d.** The American Fertility Society classifies the severity of Asherman syndrome in three stages as follows:
    1. *Mild disease:* Few flimsy adhesions involving less than a third of the uterine cavity with normal menses or hypomenorrhea.

2. *Moderate disease:* Flimsy and dense adhesions, the involvement of one-third to two-thirds of the cavity, and hypomenorrhea.
3. *Severe disease:* Dense adhesions involving more than two-thirds of the cavity with amenorrhea.

[Reference: Smikle C, Yarrarapu SNS, Khetarpal S. Asherman syndrome. In: StatPearls (Internet). Treasure Island (FL): StatPearls Publishing; 2023]

17. **d.** Risk for developing intrauterine adhesions is increased by inflammation, as may result from endometritis or retained products of conception, and when the endometrium is relatively thin and inactive, as it is during the early postpartum period.

    Consequently, most cases arise in close temporal proximity to a pregnancy and are associated with surgical trauma, primarily curettage. Asherman syndrome is an uncommon but recognized complication of cesarean section, abdominal or hysteroscopic myomectomy or metroplasty, and uterine artery embolization.

    Elective endometrial ablation procedures that utilize various modalities to achieve endometrial damage such as electrocautery, laser, thermal ablation, or cryoablation for the management of menorrhagia frequently result in amenorrhea, by intent.

    End-organ endometrial damage and intrauterine adhesions also may result from intrauterine infections such as tuberculosis and schistosomiasis.

    [Reference: Taylor HS, Pal L, Seli E (Eds). Speroff's Clinical Gynecologic Endocrinology and Infertility, 9th edition. Gurugram: Wolters Kluwer Pvt. Ltd.; 2019. p. 865]

18. **c.** Overall cancer risks in women with Turner syndrome are similar to those in the general population, but the incidence of central nervous system tumors, bladder cancer, and endometrial cancer may be increased, the risk of breast cancer is decreased compared to the general population and may be attributable to the early deprivation of ovarian hormones.

    [Reference: Taylor HS, Pal L, Seli E (Eds). Speroff's Clinical Gynecologic Endocrinology and Infertility, 9th edition. Gurugram: Wolters Kluwer Pvt. Ltd.; 2019. p. 869]

19. **d.** This mortality risk is greatest for those with preexisting cardiac abnormalities such as a bicuspid aortic valve or a dilated aortic root, but even those without obvious cardiac abnormalities remain at risk. Turner syndrome generally should be regarded as a relative contraindication to pregnancy.

    Those expressing serious interest in oocyte donation must receive thorough evaluation and counseling, and those with evidence of any significant cardiac abnormality must be strongly discouraged.

    Advances in the field of fertility preservation, such as oocyte or ovarian tissue cryopreservation, now can offer a realistic possibility for preservation of fertility potential for a subset of girls and women with Turner syndrome who demonstrate evidence of residual ovarian function.

    Eggs and embryos of these patients are at a higher risk for sex chromosome aneuploidy, and preimplantation genetic screening technology can be utilized to minimize the risk of aneuploidy in the progeny.

    [Reference: Taylor HS, Pal L, Seli E (Eds). Speroff's Clinical Gynecologic Endocrinology and Infertility, 9th edition. Gurugram: Wolters Kluwer Pvt. Ltd.; 2019. p. 870]

20. **c.** Treatment with GH generally should begin as soon as growth curve falls below the fifth percentile of normal female growth, and the regimen must be individualized, according to response.

    Treatment with estrogen must be timed carefully with the goals of minimizing its adverse effects on growth and adult height and inducing puberty at an approximately normal age. Ideally, estrogen therapy should begin no later than age of 15 years and not before the age of 12 years when growth is a priority, unless height already has been maximized.

    Estrogen therapy should begin at a low dose (e.g., 0.25–0.5 mg micronized estradiol or its equivalent), increasing gradually at intervals of 3–6 months according to response (Tanner stage, bone age), with the goal of completing sexual maturation over a period of 2–3 years. When vaginal bleeding first occurs, or after 12–24 months of estrogen therapy, a progestin (e.g., MPA) should be added to the treatment regimen to prevent dysfunctional bleeding, to achieve differentiation of breast tissue, and to protect the endometrium from long-term adverse effects of unopposed estrogen.

    A karyotype is definitive, and specifically indicated, in part because it may reveal a cell line containing a Y chromosome otherwise not suspected or identified (e.g., 45,X/46,XY); approximately 5% of women with Turner syndrome have a karyotype containing all or part of a Y chromosome. Further analysis with fluorescence in situ hybridization using one or more probes specific for segments of the Y chromosome will identify another 5% having occult Y chromosome material.

It is important to identify a Y chromosome because affected individuals are at significant increased risk for developing gonadoblastoma (20–30%), that risk appears lower (5–10%) in women with Turner syndrome and limited to those having detectable Y chromosome on karyotype.

[Reference: Taylor HS, Pal L, Seli E (Eds). Speroff's Clinical Gynecologic Endocrinology and Infertility, 9th edition. Gurugram: Wolters Kluwer Pvt. Ltd.; 2019. p. 870]

21. **c.**
    - Diagnosis of primary ovarian insufficiency
    - Menstrual irregularity for at least 3 consecutive months
    - Follicle-stimulating hormone and estradiol levels (two random tests at least 1 month apart). If gonadotropins are elevated into the menopausal range (typically, basal FSH levels will be >30–40 mIU/mL, depending on the laboratory used), a repeat FSH measurement is indicated in 1 month. If the result indicates that FSH is elevated, a diagnosis of primary ovarian insufficiency can be established. Estradiol levels of <50 pg/mL indicate hypoestrogenism.
    - Prolactin and thyroid function test.

    (Reference: Data from Nelson LM. Clinical practice. Primary ovarian insufficiency. N Engl J Med. 2009;360: 606-14)

22. **d.** If diagnosis is confirmed:
    - Karyotype
    - *FMR1* premutation
    - Adrenal antibodies
        - 21-hydroxylase (CYP21) by immunoprecipitation
        - Indirect immunofluorescence
        - Pelvic ultrasonography

    (Reference: Data from Nelson LM. Clinical practice. Primary ovarian insufficiency. N Engl J Med. 2009;360: 606-14)

23. **a.** Numerical and structural chromosomal abnormalities such as translocations, deletions, and mosaicism run high risk of premature ovarian failure.

    Convincing evidence has demonstrated an association between premature ovarian failure (POF) and fragile X "permutations".

    Ovarian failure sometimes may be the consequence of autoimmune disease.

    [Reference: Taylor HS, Pal L, Seli E (Eds). Speroff's Clinical Gynecologic Endocrinology and Infertility, 9th edition. Gurugram: Wolters Kluwer Pvt. Ltd.; 2019. p. 873]

24. **d.** A dynamic trinucleotide (CGG) repeats sequence mutation in the X-linked *FMR1* gene, located near the terminal end of the long arm of the X chromosome (Xq27.3). The normal *FMR1* gene contains approximately 30 repeats. The fully expanded form of the mutation, characterized by *200 or more CGG repeats, results in FXS, the most common known genetic cause of mental retardation and autism*. The full mutation silences the *FMR1* gene, resulting in little or no production of the corresponding mRNA or gene product (fragile X mental retardation protein FMRP), the POF associated with permutations may reflect *FMR1* mRNA *gain-of-function toxicity.*

    Guidelines issued by the American College of Medical Genetics, the American College of Obstetricians and Gynecologists, and the American Society for Reproductive Medicine all recommend *FMR1* testing for women with unexplained POF. There is consensus that testing should be offered to those having a family history of POF, FXS, or FXTAS or having relatives with unexplained mental retardation or autism. Additionally, screening merits consideration in women demonstrating evidence of diminished ovarian reserve.

    Prevalence of permutations:
    - *Familial POF:* 14%
    - *Sporadic cases of POF:* 1–7%

    [Reference: Taylor HS, Pal L, Seli E (Eds). Speroff's Clinical Gynecologic Endocrinology and Infertility, 9th edition. Gurugram: Wolters Kluwer Pvt. Ltd.; 2019. p. 874]

25. **d.** *Savage syndrome or resistant ovary syndrome* results from intrinsic defects in follicular development. Whereas accelerated follicular depletion is the underlying mechanism for the most common causes

of POI, a variety of rare genetic disorders causing impaired or abnormal follicular development may result in a functional ovarian failure. *Examples include disorders of intraovarian regulation, steroidogenic enzyme defects, and abnormalities in gonadotropins and their receptors.* In 1969, Jones and de Moraes Ruehsen described three patients with amenorrhea and hypergonadotropic hypogonadism who also *were resistant to high doses of exogenous gonadotropins, although their ovaries contained numerous follicles.*
[Reference: Taylor HS, Pal L, Seli E (Eds). Speroff's Clinical Gynecologic Endocrinology and Infertility, 9th edition. Gurugram: Wolters Kluwer Pvt. Ltd.; 2019. p. 884]

26. **d.** Bleomycin
Chemotherapy causes depletion of the primordial follicular pool in a drug- and dose-dependent manner and is a relatively common cause of POI.
Chemotherapeutic drugs vary in potential for gonadotoxicity:
- *High gonadal toxicity:* Cyclophosphamide, chlorambucil, melphalan, busulfan, nitrogen mustard, procarbazine
- *Moderate gonadal toxicity:* Cisplatin and adriamycin
- *Low gonadal toxicity:* Bleomycin, actinomycin-D, vincristine, methotrexate, 5-flurouracil, taxanes.

[Reference: Taylor HS, Pal L, Seli E (Eds). Speroff's Clinical Gynecologic Endocrinology and Infertility, 9th edition. Gurugram: Wolters Kluwer Pvt. Ltd.; 2019. p. 882]

27. **d.** All of the above
The blepharophimosis/ptosis/epicanthus inversus syndrome (BPES) is a rare autosomal dominant disease characterized by eyelid malformations and POF, caused by a variety of mutations in the gene encoding a forkhead box transcription factor (*FOXL2*) required for normal granulosa cell function.
[Reference: Taylor HS, Pal L, Seli E (Eds). Speroff's Clinical Gynecologic Endocrinology and Infertility, 9th edition. Gurugram: Wolters Kluwer Pvt. Ltd.; 2019. p. 885]

28. **a.** Acute infarction and ischemic necrosis of posterior pituitary gland.
Acute infarction and ischemic necrosis of the pituitary gland resulting from postpartum hemorrhage and consequent hypovolemic hypotension are known as "Sheehan syndrome".

One of the most common causes of hypopituitarism in the underdeveloped or developing countries.
Anterior pituitary is most commonly involved.
Failed lactation after delivery is the classical and earliest presenting symptom.
The rest of the clinical picture varies with the severity of the pituitary insult, ranging from severe hypopituitarism soon after delivery, manifesting as lethargy, anorexia, and weight loss, to secondary amenorrhea, loss of sexual hair, and less severe symptoms of fatigue that emerge weeks and months later.
Deficiencies in GH, prolactin, and gonadotropins are most common, although the majority also exhibit adrenocorticotropic hormone (ACTH) and thyroid-stimulating hormone (TSH) deficiencies.
A partially or completely empty Sella is a common later finding.
Any ACTH stimulation test that may be performed to detect a *secondary adrenal insufficiency should be postponed until approximately 6 weeks after delivery.*
[Reference: Taylor HS, Pal L, Seli E (Eds). Speroff's Clinical Gynecologic Endocrinology and Infertility, 9th edition. Gurugram: Wolters Kluwer Pvt. Ltd.; 2019. p. 904]

29. **c.** Hereditary hemochromatosis is a common cause of hypogonadotropic hypogonadism, iron studies must be performed in all patients with hypopituitarism and normal imaging.
The best screening test for hereditary hemochromatosis is a fasting transferrin saturation (a ratio of serum iron to total iron binding capacity, expressed as a percentage); values >45% are an indication for proceeding with HFE genotyping to establish the diagnosis. Early diagnosis and treatment (periodic phlebotomy, chelation therapy) help to prevent serious multisystem end-organ damage relating to excess iron deposition; organs particularly susceptible to iron toxicity are the liver, pancreas, anterior pituitary, and heart. *Hereditary hemochromatosis is an uncommon cause of hypogonadotropic hypogonadism, some have suggested that iron studies should be performed in all patients with hypopituitarism and normal imaging.*
Lymphocytic hypophysitis is a rare autoimmune disorder causing enlargement of the pituitary that mimics a pituitary tumor, most often occurring during pregnancy or in the first 6 months postpartum.

The chronic inflammatory process results in focal or diffuse adenohypophysial destruction of varying severity and subsequent fibrosis. In the initial phase of hypophysitis, hyperprolactinemia is common, followed by progressive hypopituitarism.

The disorder should be considered in women with Sellar enlargement soon after pregnancy and in those with hypogonadism and a coexisting autoimmune disorder.

Patients with symptoms and signs of pituitary enlargement and suprasellar extension can be treated by transsphenoidal surgery, dopamine agonists, anti-inflammatory or immunosuppressive drugs, or pituitary radiotherapy.

[Reference: Taylor HS, Pal L, Seli E (Eds). Speroff's Clinical Gynecologic Endocrinology and Infertility, 9th edition. Gurugram: Wolters Kluwer Pvt. Ltd.; 2019. p. 905]

30. **d.** Granulomatous infiltrative processes of sarcoidosis involving the hypothalamus and/or the pituitary gland and presenting as amenorrhea have been reported. Similarly, cases of tuberculous meningitis and intrasellar tuberculoma resulting in amenorrhea have also been described.

    [Reference: Taylor HS, Pal L, Seli E (Eds). Speroff's Clinical Gynecologic Endocrinology and Infertility, 9th edition. Gurugram: Wolters Kluwer Pvt. Ltd.; 2019. p. 905]

31. **a.** The critical weight hypothesis holds that the onset and regularity of menstrual function require that weight remains above a critical threshold level, with a corresponding critical level of body fat, which is estimated at *17% for menarche and at 22% for regular menstruation*. This level enables extra ovarian aromatization of androgens to estrogen.

    According to this hypothesis, excessive exercise or malnutrition may decrease the amount of body fat to below threshold values, resulting in delayed menarche in adolescents and in amenorrhea in postpubertal women.

    Logically, those at or near their critical thresholds of weight and body fat content would be at the greatest risk for loss of menstrual function.

    Fat appears to be critical to a normally functioning hypothalamic-pituitary-gonadal axis.

    [Reference: Taylor HS, Pal L, Seli E (Eds). Speroff's Clinical Gynecologic Endocrinology and Infertility, 9th edition. Gurugram: Wolters Kluwer Pvt. Ltd.; 2019. p. 913]

32. **c.** During perimenopausal period it is normal for FSH levels to begin to rise even before bleeding has ceased. This is true whether the perimenopausal period is premature at age of 25–35 years or at the usual time.

    This increase in FSH is associated with a decrease in inhibin production by less competent ovarian follicles. Period of elevated levels of FSH can be followed by a pregnancy.

    The value of measuring both FSH and LH is again emphasized because this special perimenopausal condition is associated with a high follicle stimulating hormone but a normal LH.

    [Reference: Matthews ML. Chapter 4: Menstrual Disorders during the Reproductive Years. In: Marshburn PB, Hurst BS (Eds). Disorders of Menstruation. United States: Blackwell Publishing Ltd.; 2011. p. 47]

33. **c.** It is a congenital GnRH deficiency is associated with anosmia or hyposmia (an absent or grossly impaired sense of smell), the disorder is known as Kallmann syndrome.

    The classical X-linked form of the disorder is caused by a variety of genetic mutations in the *KAL* gene (located on the short arm of the X chromosome, Xp22.3) encoding anosmin-1, a neural adhesion molecule that promotes migration of GnRH neurons, and olfactory neurons, from the olfactory placode into the hypothalamus during embryonic development.

    Kallmann syndrome also can be *inherited in an autosomal dominant or recessive fashion*. The autosomal dominant form has been linked to an inactivating mutation in the gene encoding the fibroblast growth factor-1 receptor (FGFR1).

    At puberty, both males and females with Kallmann syndrome usually present with delayed growth and sexual development.

    The presence of pubic hair, reflecting a normal adrenarche, helps to distinguish them from those with a constitutional delay of puberty in whom adrenarche typically also is delayed.

    However, the most distinguishing feature of Kallmann syndrome is the inability to perceive odors, such as coffee or perfume.

    Patients with the disorder also may have a family history of delayed puberty and other abnormalities, including cleft lip/palate, urogenital tract anomalies, or syndactyly.

    [Reference: Taylor HS, Pal L, Seli E (Eds). Speroff's Clinical Gynecologic Endocrinology and Infertility, 9th edition. Gurugram: Wolters Kluwer Pvt. Ltd.; 2019. p. 917]

34. d. In rare individuals, hypothalamic amenorrhea results from a congenital GnRH deficiency relating to specific genetic mutations that prevent normal GnRH neuronal migration during embryogenesis or to mutations in the pituitary GnRH receptor.

Although seldom necessary, the diagnosis of congenital GnRH deficiency can be inferred by demonstrating a complete lack of pulsatile LH secretion and little or no LH secretion in response to exogenous pulsatile GnRH treatment.

Congenital GnRH deficiency is more common in males than in females (5:1).

[Reference: Taylor HS, Pal L, Seli E (Eds). Speroff's Clinical Gynecologic Endocrinology and Infertility, 9th edition. Gurugram: Wolters Kluwer Pvt. Ltd.; 2019. p. 917]

35. a. The "empty Sella syndrome" is a misnomer because the Sella turcica is not, in fact, empty.

It is most commonly iatrogenic, consequent to previous removal or destruction of a pituitary adenoma by surgery or radiation.

A less common mechanism for an empty Sella is of pituitary infarction.

Alternatively, an empty Sella may result from a congenital defect in the sellar diaphragm (primary empty Sella).

In autopsy studies, the prevalence of an empty Sella is approximately 5%, with the prevalence being disproportionately higher in women (nearly 85% of affected individuals are women).

In women presenting with amenorrhea and galactorrhea, the prevalence of empty Sella is between 4 and 15%.

Not surprisingly, the syndrome may coexist with an adenoma and, less commonly, with deficiencies in pituitary hormone secretion that can be severe.

However, the condition usually is quite benign and does not progress to pituitary failure. *There is no convincing evidence to indicate that a primary empty Sella causes pituitary insufficiency.*

Because of the possibility of a coexisting adenoma, patients with hyperprolactinemia and an empty Sella should undergo annual surveillance (prolactin assay and imaging) for a few years to detect any evidence of tumor growth.

Treatment for the condition is dictated by the associated symptoms and disturbances in pituitary hormone secretion.

[Reference: Taylor HS, Pal L, Seli E (Eds). Speroff's Clinical Gynecologic Endocrinology and Infertility, 9th edition. Gurugram: Wolters Kluwer Pvt. Ltd.; 2019. p. 903]

36. b. *Corticotroph adenomas*

Functional ACTH-secreting corticotroph adenomas are the specific cause of Cushing disease and one cause of the more general disorder, Cushing syndrome, which results from an excess of circulating glucocorticoids.

The most common cause of Cushing syndrome is *the ingestion of prescribed glucocorticoids* (e.g., prednisone), although oral, injected, topical, and inhaled glucocorticoids also may cause the disorder.

The most common features are progressive central obesity, features resulting from excess fat accumulation in the buccal (moon face) and nuchal (buffalo hump) fat pads, those caused by atrophy of the skin and subcutaneous tissue (such as easy bruising and purple striae on the abdomen and flanks), and hyperpigmentation (caused by excess ACTH), which is most noticeable in areas exposed to light (the face, neck, and back of the hands) or at skin sites exposed to chronic mild trauma, friction, or pressure (the elbows, knees, knuckles, and shoulders); hyperpigmentation of Cushing disease may additionally involve mucosal surfaces such as the inner lip.

Menstrual abnormalities are common, affecting up to 80% of women, with one-third developing amenorrhea.

[Reference: Taylor HS, Pal L, Seli E (Eds). Speroff's Clinical Gynecologic Endocrinology and Infertility, 9th edition. Gurugram: Wolters Kluwer Pvt. Ltd.; 2019. p. 896]

Chapter 69: Polycystic Ovary Syndrome

Mona Asnani, Meher Narain

QUESTIONS

1. During the evaluation of secondary amenorrhea in a 24-year-old woman, hyperprolactinemia is diagnosed. Which of the following conditions could cause increased circulating prolactin concentration and amenorrhea in this patient?
   a. Anorexia nervosa
   b. Stress
   c. Primary hyperthyroidism
   d. Polycystic ovarian disease
   e. Congenital adrenal hyperplasia (CAH)

2. Mrs X brings her 14-year-old daughter to your outpatient department (OPD) for consultation. She is concerned that her daughter is shorter than her friends at school and should have started her period by now. On physical examination, the girl is 4 ft 9 inch tall. Evidence of breast development is consistent with Tanner stage 2. She has no axillary or pubic hair. You reassure the mother that her daughter seems to be developing normally. What is your best advice regarding educating the mother and daughter?
   a. The daughter is likely to start her period when her breasts reach Tanner stage 5
   b. The daughter's growth spurt will be followed by pubic hair development, heralding the onset of menstruation
   c. The daughter's period is likely to start by the age of 18 years, but if she has not had her period by then, she should come back for further evaluation
   d. The daughter's period should start within 1–2 years since her breast buds have just started developing
   e. The daughter is likely to start her period, and then have her growth spurt

Questions 3 and 4

A 26-year-old P0 comes to your OPD with the chief complaint of being "too hairy." She reports that her menses began at the age of 13 years and have always been very irregular and infrequent, occurring every 2–6 months. She also complains of acne but reports no other medical problems. Her only surgery was an appendectomy at the age of 8 years. Her height is 5 ft 5 inch, weight is 82 kg, and blood pressure is 100/60 mm Hg. On physical examination, there are a few coarse, dark hairs around the nipples, chin, and upper lip. No galactorrhea, thyromegaly, or temporal balding is noted. Pelvic examination is normal and there is no evidence of clitoromegaly.

3. Which of the following is the most likely explanation for this patient's problem?
   a. Late-onset CAH
   b. Idiopathic hirsutism
   c. Adrenal tumor
   d. Polycystic ovarian syndrome (PCOS)
   e. Sertoli–Leydig cell tumor of the ovary

4. Which of the following blood tests has no role in the evaluation of this patient?
   a. Estrone
   b. Total testosterone
   c. 17α-hydroxyprogesterone
   d. Dehydroepiandrosterone sulfate (DHEA-S)
   e. Thyroid-stimulating hormone (TSH)

5. A 26-year-old P0 with PCOS presents to the emergency department with the chief complaint of prolonged and heavy vaginal bleeding for 8 days. She had been taking oral contraceptives to regulate her periods until 4 months ago when she stopped taking them since she and her spouse decided to try and get pregnant. She thought she might be

pregnant because she had not had her period since her last one 4 months ago. Her bleeding has been very heavy, requiring her to double up on her sanitary napkins and change them five to six times daily since the bleeding began. In the emergency department, the patient has a supine blood pressure of 100/62 mm Hg with a pulse of 96 beats/min. Upon standing, the patient feels light headed. Her blood pressure while standing is 106/68 mm Hg with an increase in her pulse to 126 beats/min. While waiting for laboratory work to come back, you order intravenous hydration. After 2 hours, she is no longer orthostatic. Her pregnancy test is negative, and her hematocrit (Hct) is 31%. A transvaginal ultrasound showed an atrophic-appearing endometrial stripe. Which of the following is the best next step in the management of this patient?

a. Send her home with a prescription for iron therapy
b. Perform a dilation and curettage (D&C)
c. Start blood transfusion to treat her severe anemia
d. Administer antiprostaglandins
e. Administer high-dose estrogen therapy

Questions 6 and 7
A 23-year-old woman presents with the chief complaint of 7 months of amenorrhea. She has no other major medical problems. Examination reveals bilateral galactorrhea and normal breast and pelvic examinations. Her pregnancy test is negative. Serum prolactin is ordered, and the result is 47 ng/mL.

6. Which of the following is the next step in management?
   a. Reassure the patient and keep on regular follow-up
   b. Refer her to a breast surgeon
   c. Order a magnetic resonance imaging (MRI) of the brain
   d. Check glycated hemoglobin (HbA1c)
   e. Repeat the serum prolactin in 1 month

7. Which of the following classes of medication is also a possible cause of galactorrhea?
   a. Phenothiazines
   b. Antiestrogens
   c. Gonadotropin hormone-releasing hormone (GnRH) analogs
   d. Gonadotropins
   e. Prostaglandins

Questions 8 and 9
A 22-year-old woman consults you for the treatment of hirsutism. Physical examination demonstrates facial acne as well as dark, coarse hair on her upper lip, chin, and midsternum. She has a body mass index (BMI) of 35 kg/m^2. Serum luteinizing hormone (LH) level is 35 mIU/mL and follicle-stimulating hormone (FSH) is 9 mIU/mL. Androstenedione and testosterone levels are mildly elevated, whereas serum DHEA-S is normal. The patient does not wish to conceive at this time.

8. Which of the following single agents is the most appropriate treatment for her condition?
   a. GnRH agonists
   b. Oral contraceptives
   c. Corticosteroids
   d. Spironolactone
   e. Metformin

9. The patient returns 3 years later. She discontinued her medication 1 year ago as she and her husband wanted to get pregnant. Since then, her periods have been very unpredictable and infrequent, usually occurring every 3-6 months. She now wants your advice regarding the best way to conceive. Which of the following is the most appropriate first-line therapy to help her conceive?
   a. Metformin
   b. Intrauterine insemination
   c. Laparoscopic ovarian drilling
   d. In vitro fertilization
   e. Letrozole

10. Which of the following pubertal events in girls is not estrogen dependent?
    a. Hair growth
    b. Menses
    c. Production of cervical mucus
    d. Vaginal cornification
    e. Reaching adult height

11. All the following statements are true about liver disorders in women with PCOS, *except:*
    a. Prevalence of nonalcoholic fatty liver disease (NAFLD) in women with PCOS is 27-60%
    b. Insulin resistance is the primary cause of NAFLD in PCOS
    c. Obesity is the most important driver for the development of NAFLD in PCOS
    d. Androgens independently predict NAFLD in women with PCOS
    e. Diet, exercise, and metformin have been demonstrated to improve NAFLD

12. All the following are true about biochemical hyperandrogenism, *except*:
    a. Testosterone levels are elevated in most, but not all, women with PCOS
    b. Testosterone is the most important androgen produced by the ovary
    c. Direct radioimmunoassay (RIA) for free testosterone measurement is the most accurate
    d. Free testosterone level is more sensitive for the diagnosis of hyperandrogenic disorders
    e. The AE-PCOS (Androgen Excess and Polycystic Ovary Syndrome) Society regards elevated serum DHEA-S levels as sufficient evidence of hyperandrogenism to support the diagnosis of PCOS

13. All the following are true about clinical hyperandrogenism, *except*:
    a. Ludwig visual score is preferred for assessing the degree and distribution of acne
    b. Clinical manifestations of hyperandrogenism include hirsutism, acne, and androgenic alopecia, all of which relate to the effects of androgens on the pilosebaceous unit
    c. The modified Ferriman–Gallwey score is the accepted standard for assessing the severity of hirsutism in clinical investigations
    d. Androgenic alopecia is a recognized but relatively uncommon feature of PCOS
    e. The pattern of hair loss in women with PCOS follows the well-recognized "female hair loss" phenotype wherein hair thinning is most apparent at the caput while the frontal hairline remains well preserved

14. All the following are true regarding the management of clinical hyperandrogenism, *except*:
    a. Mild focal hirsutism can be managed effectively with cosmetic measures such as shaving, plucking, waxing, electrolysis, or laser hair removal
    b. *Combined oral contraceptives* (COCs) are an effective treatment for hirsutism
    c. Antiandrogens are effective for the treatment of hirsutism
    d. Eflornithine hydrochloride is available as an oral treatment which is effective in slowing the growth of unwanted facial hair
    e. Topical minoxidil in concentrations recommended for men (5%) offers some benefit with minimal side effects and should be offered to women with alopecia

15. Which of the following is a requirement in the Rotterdam criteria for the diagnosis of PCOS?
    a. Elevated low-density lipoprotein (LDL)
    b. Insulin resistance
    c. Metabolic syndrome
    d. Hypothyroidism
    e. Ovarian volume >10 mL^3 and/or >12 follicles between 2 and 9 mm in size in at least one ovary.

16. All the following are true regarding ethnic variations affecting the prevalence of PCOS, *except*:
    a. More severe hirsutism is noted in Middle Eastern, Hispanic, and Mediterranean women
    b. Increased central adiposity and insulin resistance in Southeast Asian women
    c. Lower BMI in East Asians
    d. Utilizing the Rotterdam criteria reduces the number of women diagnosed with PCOS
    e. Milder hirsutism in East Asians

17. All the following are true regarding ultrasound assessment of ovarian morphology for diagnosis of PCOS, *except*:
    a. Ovarian volume >10 mL^3
    b. Total number of small follicles measuring between 2 and 9 mm in size ≥ 12 is a prerequisite of the National Institutes of Health (NIH) 1990 criteria
    c. Presence of any one of the two morphologic ultrasonographic findings (volume >10 mL^3 and number >12) in a single ovary serves as meeting the Rotterdam criteria for polycystic ovary (PCO)
    d. PCO is commonly observed during normal pubertal development and even in women with hypothalamic amenorrhea and hyperprolactinemia
    e. The AE-PCOS Society has recommended increasing the minimal number of small follicles from a threshold of 12 to a minimum of 25

18. Which of the following sonographic parameters is included in the ultrasound diagnosis of PCOS?
    a. Follicle number per ovary
    b. Ovary length
    c. Stromal echogenicity
    d. Stromal volume
    e. Stromal blood flow

19. Which of the following statements is suggested by AE-PCOS criteria regarding the diagnosis of PCOS?
    a. Add follicular distribution as an adjunctive marker
    b. Follicle size to be increased to >9 mm

c. Increase the threshold of follicle number per ovary to 25
d. Increase the threshold of ovarian volume to >15 mL³
e. Include stromal blood flow as diagnostic criteria.

20. All the following are the components for the diagnosis of metabolic syndrome, *except:*
    a. Increased blood pressure
    b. Increased waist circumference
    c. Increased triglycerides
    d. Increased fasting insulin
    e. Decreased high-density lipoproteins (HDL)

21. All the following are true regarding lifestyle intervention in PCOS, *except:*
    a. Weight loss of >15% is needed to improve metabolic and reproductive outcomes
    b. Weight reduction is a first-line management strategy for overweight and obese women
    c. Metformin should not be used primarily for weight reduction
    d. A significant overall decrease in net calorie intake is the most important dietary strategy for weight reduction
    e. Exercise helps improve diabetes and cardiovascular health

22. Which of the following is not an indication for the use of metformin in PCOS?
    a. Women with indices of dysglycemia (impaired fasting glucose and elevated hbA1c)
    b. Women with acanthosis nigricans
    c. Women with peripheral obesity
    d. Women with NAFLD
    e. Women with hypertension

23. All are true about antimüllerian hormone (AMH), *except:*
    a. Expression of AMH is greatest in the granulosa cells of follicles measuring <4 mm (preantral and antral follicles)
    b. Serum AMH is significantly higher in women with PCOS
    c. High serum AMH concentrations in PCOS are due to increased concentration of antral follicles
    d. AMH is significantly higher in the ovulatory phenotype of PCOS
    e. A positive correlation has been noted between androgen levels and AMH

24. Which of the following is the single most sensitive marker for biochemical hyperandrogenism?
    a. Free testosterone
    b. Total testosterone
    c. DHEA
    d. DHEA-S
    e. Androstenedione

25. All of the following conditions masquerade as PCOS, *except:*
    a. Late-onset CAH
    b. Cushing syndrome
    c. Hyperprolactinemia
    d. Hyperthyroidism
    e. Androgen-secreting tumors

26. A patient has just had a pelvic ultrasound which showed bilateral polycystic ovaries; however, she has normal menstrual cycles as well as normal androgen levels. The patient asks, "So does this mean I have PCOS?" What would be the most appropriate response?
    a. Only women who are postmenopausal can have PCOS
    b. Since the ultrasound shows cysts in the ovaries, it should be diagnosed as PCOS
    c. In order to be diagnosed with PCOS, irregular menstrual cycles and/or elevated androgen levels along with cysts on your ovaries are required
    d. The patient must have low androgen levels to be diagnosed with PCOS
    e. The patient must have elevated AMH levels to be diagnosed as PCOS

27. Which of the following hormone level patterns is consistent with PCOS?
    a. Decreased testosterone and decreased prolactin
    b. Decreased testosterone and decreased estrone
    c. Decreased LH and increased FSH
    d. Increased testosterone and LH and decreased FSH
    e. Decreased LH and increased testosterone

28. A patient with PCOS came to the OPD and asked if her weight gain of 10 kg will affect her PCOS symptoms. How will you respond?
    a. Weight gain will not affect PCOS symptoms
    b. Weight gain usually exacerbates symptoms of PCOS; hence, patients with PCOS are encouraged to exercise and maintain a balanced diet
    c. PCOS patients tend to lose weight, not gain
    d. Increase in weight is a marker of improvement of PCOS symptoms
    e. None of the above

29. Which of the following conditions is at an increased risk due to elevated estrogen levels in PCOS?
    a. Hirsutism
    b. Metabolic syndrome
    c. Obstructive sleep apnea
    d. Endometrial cancer
    e. Dyslipidemia

30. All of the following are true regarding infertility management in PCOS, *except*:
    a. Letrozole should be considered a first-line pharmacological treatment for ovulation induction
    b. Clomiphene citrate can be used alone in women with PCOS with anovulatory infertility
    c. For women with PCOS who fail to achieve successful pregnancy despite multiple successful ovulation with the use of either clomiphene or letrozole, consideration should be given to proceeding directly to in vitro fertilization
    d. Induction of ovulation with exogenous gonadotropins is highly effective but requires careful monitoring to avoid the intrinsic risks of multiple pregnancy and ovarian hyperstimulation syndrome (OHSS)
    e. All the above are true

ANSWERS

1. **b.** Physical or psychological stress may result in an increase in prolactin. Prolactin is under the control of prolactin-inhibiting factor (PIF), which is produced in the hypothalamus. Many drugs (e.g., phenothiazines), stress, hypothalamic lesions, stalk lesions, and stalk compression decrease PIF. In anorexia nervosa, prolactin, TSH, and thyroxine levels are normal; FSH and LH levels are low; and cortisol levels are elevated. In hypothyroidism, elevated thyrotropin-releasing hormone (TRH) acts as a prolactin-releasing hormone to cause the release of prolactin from the pituitary; hyperthyroidism is not associated with hyperprolactinemia. There are many other conditions, such as acromegaly and pregnancy, which are associated with elevated prolactin levels. Hyperandrogenic conditions such as CAH or polycystic ovarian disease are not typically associated with hyperprolactinemia.
   (*Reference: Taylor HS, Pal L, Seli E. Abnormal uterine bleeding. Speroff's Clinical Gynecologic Endocrinology and Infertility, 9th edition. Philadelphia: Lippincott Williams & Wilkins; 2019. pp. 545-6.*)

2. **d.** Significant emotional concerns develop when puberty is delayed. Delayed puberty is defined as absent or incomplete sexual maturation by the age at which 95% of children of same sex have started pubertal development. Breast development, the usual first sign, begins by the age of 12 years in >95% of girls. Menarche usually follows about 2.6 years after the beginning of puberty and after the peak of growth has passed. On average, the pubertal sequence of accelerated growth, thelarche, pubarche, and menarche, requires a period of 4.5 years. Appropriate laboratory tests include circulating pituitary and steroid hormone levels, karyotypic analysis, and central nervous system (CNS) imaging when indicated. Hypergonadotropic hypogonadism is seen in girls with gonadal dysgenesis, such as with Turner syndrome.
   (*Reference: Taylor HS, Pal L, Seli E. Normal and abnormal sexual development. Speroff's Clinical Gynecologic Endocrinology and Infertility, 9th edition. Philadelphia: Lippincott Williams & Wilkins; 2019. pp. 312, 324-6.*)

3. **d.**

4. **a.** Polycystic ovarian syndrome is the most common cause of androgen excess and hirsutism. Women with this syndrome often have irregular menstrual cycles due to anovulation. Given the history and physical examination of this patient, PCOS is the most likely diagnosis. Women with late-onset CAH are hirsute due to an increase in adrenal androgen production caused by a deficiency in 21-hydroxylase. In order to rule out CAH caused by a deficiency in 21-hydroxylase, a follicular phase morning serum 17α-hydroxyprogesterone level should be drawn, although specific testing can safely be reserved for those having early onset hirsutism, women with a family history of the disorder, or those in high-risk ethnic groups.

   Women with idiopathic hirsutism have greater activity of 5α-reductase. It is defined as hirsutism accompanied by normal ovulatory and menstrual function and with normal circulating androgen levels. By definition, a diagnosis of idiopathic hirsutism requires measurement of serum androgen levels, which otherwise is not necessary for those with mild hirsutism. It is generally assumed that idiopathic hirsutism results from increased peripheral

5α-reductase activity, which amplifies the action of normal circulating testosterone concentrations via increased intracellular conversion to the more potent androgen, dihydrotestosterone (DHT).

Androgen-secreting tumors almost always are accompanied by severe or rapidly progressive hirsutism or symptoms or signs of virilization (deepening of the voice, temporal or male pattern balding, breast atrophy, increased muscle mass, and clitoromegaly). *The possibility of a tumor is excluded primarily by the clinical history and physical examination. A serum total testosterone concentration >150 ng/dL identifies almost all women with a potential androgen-producing tumor.* However, a tumor should still be suspected and excluded in women with rapidly progressive hirsutism or signs or symptoms of virilization, even when the serum testosterone concentration is below the threshold value.

Elevated levels of DHEA-S would be consistent with PCOS. There is no role for ordering an isolated estrone level in the workup and evaluation of hirsutism. Thyroid dysfunction and hyperprolactinemia can both be associated with hirsutism, and therefore it is important to check levels of TSH and prolactin.
(Reference: Taylor HS, Pal L, Seli E. Amenorrhea. Speroff's Clinical Gynecologic Endocrinology and Infertility, 9th edition. Philadelphia: Lippincott Williams & Wilkins; 2019. p. 418.)

5. **e.** This patient has bleeding due to ovulatory dysfunction related to PCOS. The transvaginal ultrasound helps direct the next step in the care of this patient. Her endometrial stripe is thin, suggesting that she has shed her endometrium to its basalis layer. Women who have experienced acute heavy bleeding and have an atrophic endometrium should be treated with 25 mg of conjugated estrogen every 4 hours until the bleeding subsides. Estrogen will help stop the bleeding by rebuilding the endometrium and stimulating clotting at the capillary level. Since this patient's bleeding is due to an atrophic endometrium, estrogen therapy is the preferred treatment. Had the transvaginal ultrasound shown a thickened endometrial stripe, hysteroscopy and D&C would be options to stop the bleeding more rapidly than medical treatment. In older women, D&C might be helpful in obtaining tissue for pathology to rule out endometrial hyperplasia or cancer. In this young patient who is resuscitated and stabilized with intravenous fluids, there is no indication for a blood transfusion as long as the bleeding abates. Iron therapy alone would not be adequate for this patient; the bleeding must be stopped first. Antiprostaglandins have no role in curtailing hemorrhage in a woman bleeding due to anovulation. They have been used with some success in ovulatory women who have heavy cycles or in women with menorrhagia caused by the use of the intrauterine contraceptive device (IUD). It is thought that prostaglandin synthetase inhibitors reduce the amount of bleeding by promoting vasoconstriction and platelet aggregation.
(Reference: Taylor HS, Pal L, Seli E. Menstrual disorders. Speroff's Clinical Gynecologic Endocrinology and Infertility, 9th edition. Philadelphia: Lippincott Williams & Wilkins; 2019. p. 522.)

6. **e.** A modest increase in serum prolactin should be reevaluated at least once prior to ordering an imaging study because prolactin can be transiently increased by many factors such as stress, breast stimulation, or eating. If it is persistently elevated, she should undergo an MRI of the pituitary. It is also important to check a TSH to rule out thyroid disease and an FSH to rule out ovarian failure (as a cause of amenorrhea). There is no indication to refer her to a breast surgeon or to check her HbA1c.
(Reference: Taylor HS, Pal L, Seli E. Normal and abnormal growth and pubertal development. Speroff's Clinical Gynecologic Endocrinology and Infertility, 9th edition. Philadelphia: Lippincott Williams & Wilkins; 2019. p. 351.)

7. **a.** Amenorrhea and galactorrhea may be seen when something causes an increase in prolactin secretion or action. The differential diagnosis involves several possible causes. Excessive estrogens, such as birth control pills, can reduce PIF, thus raising serum prolactin levels. Similarly, intensive suckling during lactation can activate the reflex arc that results in hyperprolactinemia. Many antipsychotic medications, especially phenothiazines, are also known to have mammotropic properties. Hypothyroidism appears to cause galactorrhea secondary to TRH stimulation of prolactin release. When prolactin levels are persistently elevated without an obvious cause (e.g., in breastfeeding), evaluation for pituitary adenoma becomes necessary.

(Reference: Taylor HS, Pal L, Seli E. Abnormal uterine bleeding. Speroff's Clinical Gynecologic Endocrinology and Infertility, 9th edition. Philadelphia: Lippincott Williams & Wilkins; 2019. p. 545.)

8. **b.** This patient has PCOS, diagnosed by the clinical picture and laboratory values, including abnormally high LH to FSH ratio (which should normally be approximately 1:1), elevated androgens, and normal DHEA-S. DHEA-S is a marker of adrenal androgen production; when normal, it essentially excludes adrenal sources of hyperandrogenism. Several medications have been used to treat hirsutism associated with PCOS. Oral contraceptives are the most frequently used agents to treat hirsutism in a patient who does not desire pregnancy. They act by increasing sex hormone-binding globulin (SHBG) and suppressing LH-driven ovarian androgen production, thereby reducing levels of free circulating androgen. GnRH agonists suppress ovarian steroid production, but they are expensive, cause bone demineralization, and result in menopausal symptoms by causing medical menopause. Metformin may be used to treat women with PCOS who want to conceive, as it has been shown to improve ovulation rates in women with a high BMI; however, it has not been shown to improve hirsutism. Spironolactone is an antiandrogen that may be used to treat hirsutism; however, it is rarely selected as a first-line therapy due to the possibility of adverse effects on a developing male fetus in utero.
(Reference: Taylor HS, Pal L, Seli E. Amenorrhea. Speroff's Clinical Gynecologic Endocrinology and Infertility, 9th edition. Philadelphia: Lippincott Williams & Wilkins; 2019. p. 420.)

9. **e.** Letrozole is a first-line therapy for anovulatory women, including women with PCOS. Most women with PCOS will ovulate with clomiphene citrate, and approximately 50% will conceive. Intrauterine insemination is not an ideal treatment in a setting where ovulation is unpredictable. Metformin may improve ovulation and is sometimes used in combination with clomiphene citrate. Laparoscopic ovarian drilling is not used as much anymore since there are so many other pharmacologic options to induce ovulation. In vitro fertilization would be considered in patients who failed medical therapy.
(Reference: Taylor HS, Pal L, Seli E. Amenorrhea. Speroff's Clinical Gynecologic Endocrinology and Infertility, 9th edition. Philadelphia: Lippincott Williams & Wilkins; 2019. pp. 422-3.)

10. **a.** The presence of estrogen in a pubertal girl stimulates the formation of secondary sex characteristics, including development of breasts, production of cervical mucus, and vaginal cornification. As estrogen levels increase, menses begin and ovulation is maintained for several decades. Ovarian estrogen production late in puberty is at least in part responsible for the termination of the pubertal growth spurt, thereby determining adult height. Decreasing levels of estrogen are associated with a lower frequency of ovulation, eventually leading to menopause. Hair growth during puberty is caused by androgens from the adrenal gland and, later, the ovary.
(Reference: Taylor HS, Pal L, Seli E. Normal and abnormal sexual development. Speroff's Clinical Gynecologic Endocrinology and Infertility, 9th edition. Philadelphia: Lippincott Williams & Wilkins; 2019. p. 314.)

11. **c.** Insulin resistance appears to be the primary driver, as even in the absence of obesity, women with insulin resistance have an independent risk of developing NAFLD.
(Reference: Taylor HS, Pal L, Seli E. Amenorrhea. Speroff's Clinical Gynecologic Endocrinology and Infertility, 9th edition. Philadelphia: Lippincott Williams & Wilkins; 2019. p. 427.)

12. **c.** Radioimmunoassay for free testosterone is highly inaccurate. More sophisticated and accurate methods (equilibrium dialysis, gas, or liquid chromatography-mass spectrometry) are technically complex and costly.
(Reference: Taylor HS, Pal L, Seli E. Amenorrhea. Speroff's Clinical Gynecologic Endocrinology and Infertility, 9th edition. Philadelphia: Lippincott Williams & Wilkins; 2019. p. 411.)

13. **a.** Ludwig visual score is preferred for assessing the degree and distribution of alopecia. There are no universally accepted visual assessments for the evaluation of acne.
[Reference: Monash University. (2018). International evidence-based guideline for assessment and management of polycystic ovarian syndrome 2018. (online) Available from: https://www.monash.edu/data/assets/pdf_file/0004/1412644/PCOS_Evidence-Based-Guidelines_20181009.pdf (Last accessed December, 2023).]

14. **d.** Eflornithine hydrochloride is available as a topical treatment which is effective in slowing the growth of unwanted facial hair. COCs are an effective treatment for hirsutism primarily because they suppress LH-dependent ovarian androgen production and stimulate hepatic SHBG production. Antiandrogens, although are effective for the treatment of hirsutism, must be used in combination with a highly reliable contraceptive method because of their potential to adversely affect sexual development in a male fetus if the patient were to conceive unexpectedly.
(Reference: Taylor HS, Pal L, Seli E. Amenorrhea. Speroff's Clinical Gynecologic Endocrinology and Infertility, 9th edition. Philadelphia: Lippincott Williams & Wilkins; 2019. p. 422.)

15. **e.** Rotterdam criteria state that diagnosis of PCOS should be based on at least two of the three major criteria: (1) Oligoanovulation, (2) clinical or biochemical signs of hyperandrogenism, and (3) polycystic-appearing ovary(ies) assessed by ultrasonography described as an ovarian volume of >10 mL^3 and/or >12 follicles measuring between 2 and 9 mm in size in at least one ovary, also excluding other endocrinopathies having a similar clinical presentation.
(Reference: Taylor HS, Pal L, Seli E. Amenorrhea. Speroff's Clinical Gynecologic Endocrinology and Infertility, 9th edition. Philadelphia: Lippincott Williams & Wilkins; 2019. p. 401.)

16. **d.** Health professionals should consider ethnic variation in the presentation and manifestations of PCOS, including:
    - A relatively mild phenotype in Caucasians
    - Higher BMI in Caucasian women, especially in North America and Australia
    - More severe hirsutism in Middle Eastern, Hispanic, and Mediterranean women
    - Increased central adiposity, insulin resistance, diabetes, metabolic risks and acanthosis nigricans in Southeast Asians and Indigenous Australians
    - Lower BMI and milder hirsutism in East Asians
    - Higher BMI and metabolic features in Africans

    The overall prevalence of PCOS among different populations (accounting for the three different diagnostic criteria) is relatively similar (NIH 6%, Rotterdam and AE-PCOS 10%).

    [Reference: Monash University. (2018). International evidence-based guideline for assessment and management of polycystic ovarian syndrome 2018. [online] Available from: https://www.monash.edu/data/assets/pdf_file/0004/1412644/PCOS_Evidence-Based-Guidelines_20181009.pdf (Last accessed December, 2023).]

17. **b.** Polycystic ovarian morphology was not a part of the diagnostic criteria of NIH criteria 1990. NIH 1990 criteria specify that the presence of clinical/biochemical hyperandrogenemia and menstrual irregularities is required for the diagnosis of PCOS.
(Reference: Taylor HS, Pal L, Seli E. Amenorrhea. Speroff's Clinical Gynecologic Endocrinology and Infertility, 9th edition. Philadelphia: Lippincott Williams & Wilkins; 2019. p. 401.)

18. **a.** The Rotterdam consensus criterion for an ovary to be considered polycystic weighs equally on the ovarian volume (>10 mL^3) and the total number of small follicles measuring between 2 and 9 mm in size (≥12); the presence of any one of these two morphologic ultrasonographic findings in a single ovary serves as meeting the Rotterdam criteria for polycystic ovary.
(Reference: Taylor HS, Pal L, Seli E. Amenorrhea. Speroff's Clinical Gynecologic Endocrinology and Infertility, 9th edition. Philadelphia: Lippincott Williams & Wilkins; 2019. p. 401.

19. **c.** The AE-PCOS Society has recommended that in order to characterize ovarian appearance as PCO, the minimal number of small follicles should be increased from a threshold of 12, as is specified by Rotterdam criteria, to a minimum of 25.
(Reference: Taylor HS, Pal L, Seli E. Amenorrhea. Speroff's Clinical Gynecologic Endocrinology and Infertility, 9th edition. Philadelphia: Lippincott Williams & Wilkins; 2019. p. 401.)

20. **d.** As defined by the National Heart, Lung, and Blood Institute and the American Heart Association, a diagnosis of metabolic syndrome requires the presence of any three of the following five clinical characteristics:
    1. Increased waist circumference (population specific, >88 cm in women in the United States)
    2. Increased blood pressure (≥130 mm Hg systolic; ≥85 mm Hg diastolic) or receiving medication for hypertension

3. Increased triglycerides (≥150 mg/dL) or receiving medication for hypertriglyceridemia
4. Decreased HDL cholesterol (<50 mg/dL) or receiving medication for reduced HDL
5. Increased fasting glucose (≥100 mg/dL) or receiving medication for hyperglycemia

(Reference: Taylor HS, Pal L, Seli E. Amenorrhea. Speroff's Clinical Gynecologic Endocrinology and Infertility, 9th edition. Philadelphia: Lippincott Williams & Wilkins; 2019. p. 425.)

21. **a.** At least 50% of women with PCOS are obese. It is important to stress that even a small reduction in weight (2–5%) can result in significant improvements in metabolic and reproductive function.

(Reference: Taylor HS, Pal L, Seli E. Amenorrhea. Speroff's Clinical Gynecologic Endocrinology and Infertility, 9th edition. Philadelphia: Lippincott Williams & Wilkins; 2019. p. 421.)

22. **c.** Metformin is indicated in women with central obesity. The most logical candidates for treatment with metformin (aimed at preventing or slowing progression to type 2 diabetes and at reducing longer-term risks for cardiovascular disease) are women with indices of dysglycemia including impaired fasting glucose, impaired glucose tolerance, abnormally elevated HbA1c levels, or diabetes; those with obvious evidence of severe insulin resistance (acanthosis nigricans); and women having other features of the metabolic syndrome, such as *central obesity*, hypertension, and dyslipidemia. All women with PCOS should be screened with an oral glucose tolerance test (OGTT) at the time of presentation and at least every 2 years thereafter (or sooner if the clinical picture worsens); those with impaired glucose tolerance warrant annual screening. Evaluation must include assessment of blood pressure and should include measuring waist circumference and assessing lipid profile, to help quantify their metabolic risk by identifying those with features of the metabolic syndrome.

(Reference: Taylor HS, Pal L, Seli E. Amenorrhea. Speroff's Clinical Gynecologic Endocrinology and Infertility, 9th edition. Philadelphia: Lippincott Williams & Wilkins; 2019. pp. 427-8.)

23. **d.** Recently, AMH has been implicated as another potential marker to PCOS. AMH is produced by granulosa cells, and expression is greatest in the granulosa cells of follicles measuring <4 mm (preantral and antral follicles). In women with PCOS, there is an excessive amount of AMH, which is likely explained by increased follicles in the antral and preantral stages, which produce the greatest amounts of AMH. While the mechanism of increased production is not known, evidence supports a role for androgens, as there is a positive correlation between androgen and AMH levels. AMH also decreases FSH receptor and ovarian aromatase expression. In doing so, it prevents the continued follicular growth and development needed to reach maturity, resulting ultimately in follicular arrest, with no dominant follicle selected. Hence, AMH has been proposed as an inclusion criterion for the diagnosis of PCOS, likely replacing (or serving as a surrogate for) PCO morphology, as studies have demonstrated that an AMH of 5 ng/mL has a high specificity (97%) and greater sensitivity than the current criteria for PCO morphology. However, given no standardization/validation across populations as of yet, exercising caution is recommended before replacing PCO-appearing ovaries on US with AMH level; rather, a threshold of AMH ≥ 5 ng/mL may be used as a further suggestion of PCOS.

(Reference: Taylor HS, Pal L, Seli E. Amenorrhea. Speroff's Clinical Gynecologic Endocrinology and Infertility, 9th edition. Philadelphia: Lippincott Williams & Wilkins; 2019. p. 402.)

24. **a.** Testosterone levels are elevated in most, but not all, women with PCOS. The free testosterone level is more sensitive for diagnosis of hyperandrogenic disorders.

(Reference: Taylor HS, Pal L, Seli E. Amenorrhea. Speroff's Clinical Gynecologic Endocrinology and Infertility, 9th edition. Philadelphia: Lippincott Williams & Wilkins; 2019. p. 411.)

25. **d.** Hypothyroidism masquerades as PCO and not hyperthyroidism.

(Reference: Taylor HS, Pal L, Seli E. Amenorrhea. Speroff's Clinical Gynecologic Endocrinology and Infertility, 9th edition. Philadelphia: Lippincott Williams & Wilkins; 2019. p. 418.)

26. **c.** *(Reference: Taylor HS, Pal L, Seli E. Amenorrhea. Speroff's Clinical Gynecologic Endocrinology and Infertility, 9th edition. Philadelphia: Lippincott Williams & Wilkins; 2019. p. 401.)*

CHAPTER 69: Polycystic Ovary Syndrome

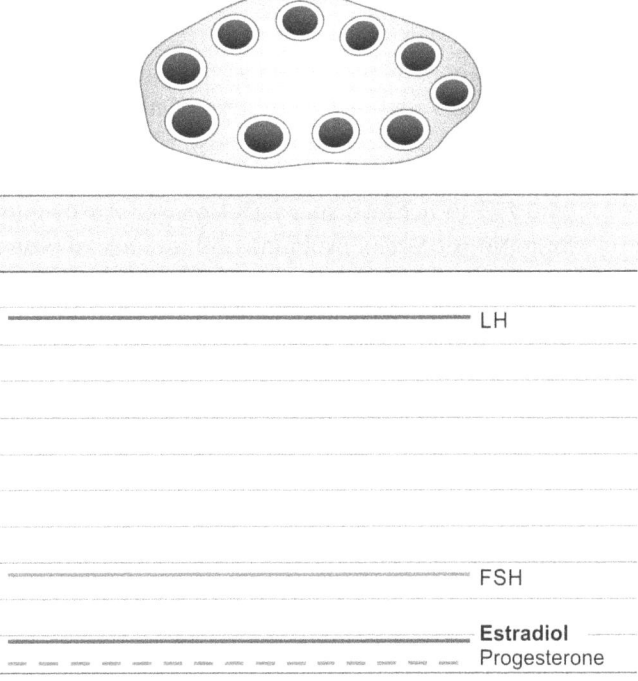

Criteria	National Institute of Health (NIH) Criteria 1990	Rotterdam criteria 2003	Androgen Excess and Polycystic Ovarian Syndrome (AE-PCOS) Society criteria 2006

• Irregular periods[†]
• Elevated serum androgens or hyperandrogenism
  – Hirsutism
  – Acne
  – Androgenetic alopecia
• Polycystic ovarian morphology (PCOM) or polycystic ovary (PCO)[‡]
	1 and 2[*]	Any 2 of 3[*]	1 and 2[*] or 2 and 3[*]

[*]Differential diagnoses that can mimic clinical presentation must be excluded.
[†]Eight or fewer menses per year.
[‡]Ovarian volume >10 mL^3 and/or >12 follicles between 2 and 9 mm in size in at least one ovary.

27. **d.** The average daily production of both androgens and estrogens is increased in women with PCOS. Serum estrone concentrations are modestly elevated, due to peripheral conversion of increased amounts of androstenedione. In contrast, serum estradiol levels in women with PCOS fluctuate but generally remain within the range typically observed in the early follicular phase, reflecting continued low-level production from limited follicular development. An altered pattern of GnRH release that leads to an increased LH pulse frequency offers a unifying mechanism for both ovarian androgen excess (due to LH-mediated stimulation of androgen production by ovarian stroma) and impaired follicle development that results in chronic anovulation (due to the relatively low FSH levels that occur secondary to altered GnRH release pattern).
(Reference: Taylor HS, Pal L, Seli E. Amenorrhea. Speroff's Clinical Gynecologic Endocrinology and Infertility, 9th edition. Philadelphia: Lippincott Williams & Wilkins; 2019. p. 402.)

28. **b.** Weight reduction is the first-line management strategy for overweight and obese women with PCOS. Weight loss increases SHBG concentrations, thereby reducing free androgen levels and decreasing androgen stimulation of the hair and skin. Weight loss also improves ovulatory function, thereby increasing conception rates and also possibly decreasing the risk for miscarriage.
(Reference: Taylor HS, Pal L, Seli E. Amenorrhea. Speroff's Clinical Gynecologic Endocrinology and Infertility, 9th edition. Philadelphia: Lippincott Williams & Wilkins; 2019. p. 421.)

29. **d.** Chronic anovulation, obesity, and hyperinsulinemia provide an environment that is conducive to risk for proliferative endometrial pathologies such as endometrial hyperplasia and even endometrial cancer in women with PCOS. The risk for endometrial cancer may be as high as threefold greater in anovulatory women with PCOS compared to women with normal reproductive physiology.
(Reference: Taylor HS, Pal L, Seli E. Amenorrhea. Speroff's Clinical Gynecologic Endocrinology and

Infertility, 9th edition. Philadelphia: Lippincott Williams & Wilkins; 2019. p. 417.)

30. **e.** Based on existing evidence, letrozole should be considered a first-line agent for ovulation induction in women with PCOS and in those with a history of resistance to clomiphene. For women with PCOS who fail to achieve successful pregnancy despite multiple successful ovulation with the use of either clomiphene or letrozole, consideration should be given to proceeding directly to in vitro fertilization with single-embryo transfer as a strategy that maximizes the likelihood of achieving pregnancy while minimizing the risks of OHSS and multiple pregnancies that women with PCOS are particularly susceptible to with the use of gonadotropins to achieve ovulation induction.

(Reference: Taylor HS, Pal L, Seli E. Amenorrhea. Speroff's Clinical Gynecologic Endocrinology and Infertility, 9th edition. Philadelphia: Lippincott Williams & Wilkins; 2019. p. 423.)

Chapter 70

Endometriosis

Ganesh Dangal, Nishma Bajracharya

QUESTIONS

1. Which of the following is a more favored theory to explain the development of endometriosis?
   a. Lymphatic spread
   b. Coelomic metaplasia
   c. Retrograde menstruation
   d. Abnormal differentiation of Müllerian remnants

2. An enzyme important in creating a unique estrogenic environment within endometriotic implants includes which of the following?
   a. Aromatase
   b. 17α-hydroxylase
   c. 17β-hydroxylase
   d. 17β-hydroxysteroid dehydrogenase type 2

3. Which of the following is the focus of the classification system by the American Society of Reproductive Medicine (ASRM)?
   a. Pelvic pain severity
   b. Degree of infertility
   c. Anatomic extent of endometriosis
   d. All of the above

4. Which of the following is the most likely etiology for infertility in a woman with endometriosis?
   a. Tubal obstruction
   b. Implantation defect
   c. Ovulatory dysfunction
   d. Poor embryo development

5. A 24-year-old woman with endometriosis diagnosed laparoscopically during late adolescence complains of worsening dysmenorrhea, dyspareunia, dysuria, and urinary urgency. The urinalysis and urine cultures have been negative for infection. Which of the following would be the least suitable to further evaluate this patient?
   a. Cystoscopy
   b. Computed tomography (CT)
   c. Transvaginal sonography (TVS)
   d. Magnetic resonance imaging (MRI)

6. A 35-year-old woman presents with a large, firm, and fixed mass along a prior Pfannenstiel incision. It usually becomes more painful and tender during menses. Which of the following is NOT true regarding the typical management of such abdominal wall masses?
   a. Mesh may be needed to close the large fascial defect
   b. Excision is offered to provide a diagnosis and symptom relief
   c. Such masses are typically managed conservatively with hormonal suppression
   d. CT scan delineates involvement of the mass with the anterior rectus sheath or with the rectus abdominis muscle

7. Which of the following is true regarding laboratory testing during the evaluation of suspected endometriosis?
   a. It should rarely be performed
   b. It identifies most cases of endometriosis
   c. It is used mainly to exclude other conditions.
   d. Elevated cancer antigen-125 (CA 125) levels are pathognomic for endometriosis

8. Sonographically, endometriomas are typically described by which of the following?
   a. Solid with intracystic blood flow
   b. Solid with diffuse internal low-level echoes
   c. Cystic with focal hyperechoic internal echoes
   d. Cystic with diffuse internal low-level echoes

9. Endometriomas have often an appearance similar to which of the following?
   a. Tubo-ovarian abscess
   b. Pedunculated myoma

c. Mature cystic teratoma
d. Hemorrhagic corpus luteal cyst

10. A 22-year-old nulligravida undergoes diagnostic laparoscopy for dysmenorrhea and chronic pelvic pain (CPP). The endometriotic implants are ablated. She is not currently planning for conception; however, she desires future fertility. Which is the most appropriate postoperative treatment for her?
    a. Androgens
    b. Aromatase inhibitors
    c. Combination of oral contraceptive pills (OCPs)
    d. Gonadotropin-releasing hormone (GnRH) antagonist

11. A 25-year-old nulligravida was treated with GnRH agonist 1 month ago. However, she now complains of decreased sleep, decreased libido, and dyspareunia due to vaginal dryness. Which of the following agents taken orally might be least effective for this patient?
    a. Fluoxetine
    b. Norethindrone
    c. Norethindrone plus conjugated equine estrogen
    d. Medroxyprogesterone acetate plus transdermal estradiol

12. Which of the following is a suitable time to begin add-back therapy during the course of GnRH agonist treatment?
    a. At 1 month   b. At 6 months
    c. At initiation of therapy   d. Each one is suitable

13. All of the following are side effects of aromatase inhibitors, *except:*
    a. Hyperglycemia   b. Vaginal atrophy
    c. Vasomotor symptoms   d. Ovarian cyst formation

14. With deep infiltrating endometriosis, which of the following surgical approaches may most likely benefit the patient?
    a. Laser ablation
    b. Radical excision
    c. Bipolar electrosurgical ablation
    d. Monopolar electrosurgical ablation

15. For the surgical treatment of endometriomas, which of the following approaches is superior in lowering the recurrence rates?
    a. Drainage   b. Cystectomy
    c. Cyst wall ablation   d. None

16. Which of the following statements is true regarding presacral neurectomy (PSN)?
    a. It effectively treats lateral adnexal pain.
    b. It is a procedure that excises the uterosacral ligaments
    c. Postoperative side effects may include constipation and voiding dysfunction
    d. It should be recommended to most women undergoing endometriosis surgery

17. Which of the following is appropriate for diagnosing rectal endometriosis?
    a. Laparoscopy
    b. Transvaginal ultrasound
    c. Transrectal ultrasound
    d. MRI

18. Which of the following pharmacological agents has been proven to be more effective than others for the prevention of adhesion formation post surgery for endometriosis?
    a. Oxidized regenerated cellulose
    b. Polytetrafluoroethylene surgical membrane
    c. Icodextrin 4%
    d. All are equally effective

19. Which of the following procedures are effective for achieving spontaneous pregnancy in women with endometriosis-associated infertility?
    a. In infertile women with the American Fertility Society (AFS)/ASRM stage I/II endometriosis, CO_2 laser vaporization of endometriosis, instead of monopolar electrocoagulation
    b. In infertile women with ovarian endometrioma undergoing surgery, excision of the endometrioma capsule, instead of drainage and electrocoagulation of the endometrioma wall
    c. In infertile women with AFS/ASRM stage III/IV endometriosis, operative laparoscopy, instead of expectant management
    d. All of the above are effective

20. What is the effectiveness of medically assisted reproduction in women with endometriosis-associated infertility?
    a. Intrauterine insemination (IUI) with controlled ovarian stimulation, instead of expectant management, does not increase live birth rates
    b. IUI with controlled ovarian stimulation has similar results compared with IUI along with increasing pregnancy rates

c. Use of assisted reproductive technologies for infertility associated with endometriosis is recommended, especially if tubal function is compromised or if there is male factor infertility, and/or other treatments have failed
d. None are true

21. Which of the following is the most common site of extrapelvic endometriosis?
    a. Broad ligament
    b. Rectum
    c. Sigmoid colon
    d. Ovary

22. A 40-year-old infertile woman suspected to be suffering from endometriosis is subjected to diagnostic laparoscopy. Findings include a normal uterus, but both ovaries show the presence of chocolate cysts. Endometriotic deposits are seen on the round ligament, both fallopian tubes and pouch of Douglas (POD), and moderately dense adhesions are present. The treatment of choice in this case is:
    a. Total hysterectomy with bilateral salpingo-oophorectomy
    b. Danazol therapy
    c. Progesterone therapy
    d. Fulguration of endometriotic deposits

23. A 30-year-old female complains of dysmenorrhea, dyspareunia, and infertility. TVS shows a thin-walled cyst 4 × 5 cm in diameter with echogenic fluid and no solid areas in the left ovary. She wishes to conceive soon. What is the best treatment option?
    a. Perform laparoscopic cystectomy
    b. Treat with continuous OCP
    c. Treat with GnRH
    d. Treat with injection of medroxyprogesterone acetate

24. The organ not involved in endometriosis is:
    a. Liver
    b. Lymph nodes
    c. Brain
    d. Spleen

25. Pain in endometriosis correlates with:
    a. Depth of invasion
    b. Multiple sites
    c. CA 125
    d. Stage of disease

26. Which of the following does not attribute to the pain associated with endometriosis?
    a. Actions of inflammatory cytokines in the peritoneal cavity
    b. Direct and indirect effects of focal bleeding from endometriotic implants
    c. Irritation or direct infiltration of nerves in the pelvic floor
    d. Hormonal milieu has no influence in pain perception

27. Which of the following is false regarding the medical treatment of endometriosis?
    a. Danazol has androgenic side effects that limit its clinical utility
    b. OCPs are generally well tolerated; episodic breakthrough bleeding is more common with continuous than with cyclic treatment
    c. Treatment with GnRH agonists results in a hypogonadal state with associated symptoms of hot flushes, genitourinary atrophy, and bone mineral depletion
    d. The medical treatment of endometriosis improves fertility

28. Risk factors for persistent or recurrent disease and pain include:
    a. Ovarian preservation
    b. Incomplete excision of disease
    c. Postoperative unopposed estrogen therapy in women with extensive or residual disease
    d. All of the above

29. Which of the following is not true regarding the use of progesterone for medical management of endometriosis?
    a. It suppresses serum estrogen levels and causes decidualization and atrophy of endometrial cells
    b. It reduces inflammation and inhibition of matrix metalloproteinases (MMPs) and has antiangiogenic and immune modulatory action
    c. Commonly used progesterone preparations are dienogest, antiangiogenic, dydrogesterone, microscopic polyangiitis (MPA), and norethindrone
    d. Dienogest cannot be safely used in adolescent girls for long term

30. All the following are true regarding endometriosis in postmenopausal women, *except*:
    a. Medical management still should be the first line of treatment
    b. Patients refractory to initial medical management and who have completed the family can go for radical surgical treatments

c. Retaining ovaries increases the incidence of recurrence from 6 to 18%
d. Postoperative suppression with GnRH agonist and dienogest has no role in patients with postmenopausal endometriosis

ANSWERS

1. **c.** Retrograde menstruation
   The most favored theory describes retrograde menstruation through the fallopian tubes. These refluxed endometrial fragments invade the peritoneal mesothelium and develop a blood supply for implant survival and growth. In correlation, women with outflow tract obstruction also have a high incidence of endometriosis, which often resolves following obstruction relief.
   [Reference: Hoffman BL, Schorge JO, Schaffer JI, Bradshaw KD, Halvorson LM, Corton MM (Eds). Endometriosis. Williams Gynecology, 3rd edition. New York: McGraw Hill; 2020. pp. 230-48]

2. **a.** Aromatase
   Estrogen plays a causative role in endometriosis formation and is derived from multiple sources. Most estrogen in women is produced directly by the ovaries. Second, peripheral tissues also produce estrogens through the conversion of ovarian and adrenal androgens by the enzyme aromatase. Endometriotic implants express aromatase and 17β-hydroxysteroid dehydrogenase type 1, which are the enzymes responsible for the conversion of androstenedione to estrone and of estrone to estradiol, respectively. Implants, however, are deficient in 17β-hydroxysteroid dehydrogenase type 2, which inactivates estrogen. This enzymatic combination ensures that implants create an estrogenic environment.
   [Reference: Hoffman BL, Schorge JO, Schaffer JI, Bradshaw KD, Halvorson LM, Corton MM (Eds). Endometriosis. Williams Gynecology, 3rd edition. New York: McGraw Hill; 2020. pp. 230-48]

3. **c.** Anatomic extent of endometriosis
   The primary method of endometriosis diagnosis is the visualization of endometriotic lesions by laparoscopy, with or without biopsy for histologic confirmation. The extent of endometriosis can vary widely between individuals, and thus, one classification by ASRM (1997) allows the disease to be quantified. With this, endometriosis on the peritoneum, ovaries, fallopian tubes, and cul-de-sac is scored at surgery. At these sites, points are assigned for disease surface area, degree of invasion, morphology, and extent of associated adhesions. Also, endometriotic lesions are morphologically categorized as white, red, or black. In this system, endometriosis is classified as stage I (minimal), stage II (mild), stage III (moderate), and stage IV (severe).
   [Reference: Hoffman BL, Schorge JO, Schaffer JI, Bradshaw KD, Halvorson LM, Corton MM (Eds). Endometriosis. Williams Gynecology, 3rd edition. New York: McGraw Hill; 2020. pp. 230-48]

4. **a.** Tubal obstruction
   Adhesions are one intuitive explanation for endometriosis-related infertility. These may impair normal oocyte pickup and transport by the fallopian tube.
   [Reference: Hoffman BL, Schorge JO, Schaffer JI, Bradshaw KD, Halvorson LM, Corton MM (Eds). Endometriosis. Williams Gynecology, 3rd edition. New York: McGraw Hill; 2020. pp. 230-48.]

5. **b.** Computed tomography
   Endometriosis should be considered if urinary tract symptoms persist despite negative urine culture results. Symptoms, if present, are more common with bladder disease. These include dysuria, suprapubic pain, urinary frequency, and urgency. TVS has suitable accuracy for bladder endometriosis but is less sensitive for ureteral disease. In unclear cases, MRI can add additional anatomic information. Cystoscopy with biopsy can also help clarify the diagnosis.
   [Reference: Hoffman BL, Schorge JO, Schaffer JI, Bradshaw KD, Halvorson LM, Corton MM (Eds). Endometriosis. Williams Gynecology, 3rd edition. New York: McGraw Hill; 2020. pp. 230-48]

6. **c.** Such masses are typically managed conservatively with hormonal suppression.
   Some individuals with abdominal pain can have anterior abdominal wall endometriomas. Most of these lesions develop in the abdominal scar after uterine surgery or cesarean delivery. Implants usually are found within the subcutaneous layer, are palpable, and may involve the adjacent fascia. Less often, the rectus abdominis muscle is infiltrated. Abdominal wall sonography, CT, MRI, and fine-needle aspiration are options for diagnosis. In most instances, implants

are surgically excised for pain relief and diagnosis. For small implants, preoperative imaging may not be needed. But with larger implants and concerns for fascial or rectus abdominis muscle involvement, CT or MRI can aid surgery planning. Large fascial defects following excision may require mesh to close the defect.
[Reference: Hoffman BL, Schorge JO, Schaffer JI, Bradshaw KD, Halvorson LM, Corton MM (Eds). Endometriosis. Williams Gynecology, 3rd edition. New York: McGraw Hill; 2020. pp. 230-48]

7. **c.** It is used mainly to exclude other conditions.
Laboratory investigations are often undertaken to exclude other causes of pelvic pain. Initially, a complete blood count (CBC), human chorionic gonadotropin assay, urinalysis and urine cultures, vaginal cultures, and cervical swabs may be collected to exclude infections or pregnancy complications. CA 125 is a glycoprotein that is found in the fallopian tube epithelium, endometrium, endocervix, pleura, and peritoneum. This marker is used in ovarian cancer evaluation and surveillance. Recognized by monoclonal antibody assays, elevated CA 125 levels positively correlate with endometriosis severity. Unfortunately, the assay has poor sensitivity in detecting mild endometriosis and appears to be a better diagnostic test for stage III or IV endometriosis.
[Reference: Hoffman BL, Schorge JO, Schaffer JI, Bradshaw KD, Halvorson LM, Corton MM (Eds). Endometriosis. Williams Gynecology, 3rd edition. New York: McGraw Hill; 2020. pp. 230-48]

8. **d.** Cystic with diffuse internal low-level echoes
The sensitivity and specificity of TVS to diagnose endometriomas range from 64 to 90% and from 22 to 100%, respectively. An endometrioma classically is cystic with homogeneous, low-level internal echoes, often described as "ground glass" echogenicity. There is normal surrounding ovarian tissue.
[Reference: Hoffman BL, Schorge JO, Schaffer JI, Bradshaw KD, Halvorson LM, Corton MM (Eds). Endometriosis. Williams Gynecology, 3rd edition. New York: McGraw Hill; 2020. pp. 230-48]

9. **d.** Hemorrhagic corpus luteal cyst
An endometrioma classically is cystic with homogeneous, low-level internal echoes, often described as "ground glass" echogenicity. There is normal surrounding ovarian tissue. As such, these may have an identical appearance to hemorrhagic corpus luteum cysts. Although endometriomas are most often unilocular, one to four thin septations can be found. Less typically, these cysts can display thick septations or walls.
[Reference: Hoffman BL, Schorge JO, Schaffer JI, Bradshaw KD, Halvorson LM, Corton MM (Eds). Endometriosis. Williams Gynecology, 3rd edition. New York: McGraw Hill; 2020. pp. 230-48]

10. **c.** Combination oral contraceptive pills
Therapy for endometriosis depends on a woman's specific complaints, symptom severity, location of endometriotic lesions, goals for treatment, and desire to conserve future fertility. Whether a patient is seeking treatment for infertility or pain is essential, as therapy for these two is different. If pain is prominent and conception is not currently desired, medical therapy is typically selected. Treatment strives to atrophy ectopic endometrium and diminishes disease-associated inflammation. Available agents include nonsteroidal anti-inflammatory drugs (NSAIDs), sex steroid hormones, GnRH agents, and aromatase inhibitors. In general, suitable starting regimens are NSAIDs alone or combined with OCPs or with progestin. These agents may be initiated if endometriosis is suspected in a woman with CPP or maybe started following diagnostic laparoscopy. If initial therapy fails to control pain following laparoscopy, then the use of a different medication is reasonable. If initial empiric therapy is ineffective, then either diagnostic laparoscopy or medication change is suitable.
[Reference: Hoffman BL, Schorge JO, Schaffer JI, Bradshaw KD, Halvorson LM, Corton MM (Eds). Endometriosis. Williams Gynecology, 3rd edition. New York: McGraw Hill; 2020. pp. 230-48]

11. **a.** Fluoxetine
Concerns regarding the effects of prolonged hypoestrogenism such as hot flushes, insomnia, reduced libido, vaginal dryness, and headaches preclude extended treatment with GnRH agonists. Moreover, both spine and hip bone mineral density decrease at 3 and 6 months of GnRH agonist therapy, with only partial recovery at 12-15 months after treatment. Because of the increased osteoporosis risk, therapy is usually limited to the shortest possible

duration—usually not >6 months. Estrogen may be added to GnRH agonist therapy to counteract bone loss and is termed add-back therapy. With the addition of such hormonal add-back therapy, a GnRH agonist may occasionally be used longer than 6 months. The goal of add-back therapy is to supply enough estrogen to minimize GnRH agonist side effects while still maintaining a hypoestrogenic state sufficient to suppress endometriosis.
[Reference: Hoffman BL, Schorge JO, Schaffer JI, Bradshaw KD, Halvorson LM, Corton MM (Eds). Endometriosis. Williams Gynecology, 3rd edition. New York: McGraw Hill; 2020. pp. 230-48]

12. **d.** Each one is suitable.
Add-back therapy can be initiated either immediately with the GnRH agonist or after 3-6 months of agonist therapy.
[Reference: Hoffman BL, Schorge JO, Schaffer JI, Bradshaw KD, Halvorson LM, Corton MM (Eds). Endometriosis. Williams Gynecology, 3rd edition. New York: McGraw Hill; 2020. pp. 230-48]

13. **a.** Hyperglycemia
The aromatase inhibitors block aromatase action and estradiol production in both the ovary and extraovarian sites. As a result, estrogen levels are dramatically suppressed and have hypoestrogenic side effect profiles similar to those of GnRH agonists. In addition to hypoestrogenic side effects, a second concern is ovarian cyst formation by blocking the conversion of androgens to estrogens in ovarian granulosa cells; they reduce the negative feedback at the pituitary–hypothalamus level. This leads to increased GnRH secretion. Resulting elevations in luteinizing hormone (LH) and follicle-stimulating hormone promote increased ovarian follicular development.
[Reference: Hoffman BL, Schorge JO, Schaffer JI, Bradshaw KD, Halvorson LM, Corton MM (Eds). Endometriosis. Williams Gynecology, 3rd edition. New York: McGraw Hill; 2020. pp. 230-48]

14. **b.** Radical excision
The optimal method to address endometriotic implants for maximal symptom relief is controversial. First, laser ablation does not appear to be more effective than conventional electrosurgical ablation of endometriosis. Second, ablation and excision both appear to perform suitably. For deeply infiltrative endometriosis, some have advocated radical surgical excision, although well-designed trials are lacking.
[Reference: Hoffman BL, Schorge JO, Schaffer JI, Bradshaw KD, Halvorson LM, Corton MM (Eds). Endometriosis. Williams Gynecology, 3rd edition. New York: McGraw Hill; 2020. pp. 230-48]

15. **b.** Cystectomy
Endometriomas are typically treated surgically. To determine the best technique, total ovarian cystectomy compared against aspiration coupled with cyst wall ablation has been studied. Findings note that cystectomy lowers endometrioma recurrence rates and pain symptoms and improves subsequent spontaneous pregnancy rates. During surgery, ideally, normal ovarian tissue is preserved. Toward this goal, electrosurgical coagulation of bleeding sites should be limited.
[Reference: Hoffman BL, Schorge JO, Schaffer JI, Bradshaw KD, Halvorson LM, Corton MM (Eds). Endometriosis. Williams Gynecology, 3rd edition. New York: McGraw Hill; 2020. pp. 230-48]

16. **c.** Postoperative side effects may include constipation and voiding dysfunction.
For some women, the transection of presacral nerves lying within the presacral space may provide relief of CPP. Results from a randomized trial revealed significantly greater pain relief at 12 months postoperatively in women treated with PSN and endometriotic excision compared with that from endometriotic excision alone (86% vs. 57%). However, all of these women had midline pain. Neurectomy may be performed laparoscopically, but it is technically challenging. Due to involved nerve disruption, postoperative constipation and voiding dysfunction are common. For these reasons, PSN is used in a limited manner and not recommended routinely for the management of endometriosis-related pain.
[Reference: Hoffman BL, Schorge JO, Schaffer JI, Bradshaw KD, Halvorson LM, Corton MM (Eds). Endometriosis. Williams Gynecology, 3rd edition. New York: McGraw Hill; 2020. pp. 230-48]

17. **b.** Transvaginal ultrasound
In cases where there is a strong suspicion of endometriosis, especially in deep infiltrating disease, studies have been performed to evaluate the accuracy of TVS in diagnosing rectal endometriosis.

[Reference: Dunselman GA, Vermeulen N, Becker C, Calhaz-Jorge C, D'Hooghe T, De Bie, et al; European Society of Human Reproduction and Embryology. ESHRE guideline: Management of Women with Endometriosis: Hum Reprod. 2014;29(3):400-12]

18. **a.** Oxidized regenerated cellulose
The use of oxidized regenerated cellulose in the prevention of adhesion formation after laparoscopic surgery for endometriosis can be more effective than polytetrafluoroethylene surgical membrane (Gore-Tex®), fibrin sheet, sodium hyaluronate and carboxymethylcellulose combination, polyethylene oxide and carboxymethylcellulose gel, steroids, dextran, icodextrin 4%, hyaluronic acid products, and polyethylene glycol hydrogel. The others have been studied and proven effective for adhesion prevention in the context of pelvic surgery, although not specifically in women with endometriosis.
[Reference: Dunselman GA, Vermeulen N, Becker C, Calhaz-Jorge C, D'Hooghe T, De Bie, et al.; European Society of Human Reproduction and Embryology. ESHRE guideline: Management of Women with Endometriosis. Hum Reprod. 2014;29(3):400-12]

19. **d.** All of the above are effective.
[Reference: Dunselman GA, Vermeulen N, Becker C, Calhaz-Jorge C, D'Hooghe T, De Bie, et al.; European Society of Human Reproduction and Embryology. ESHRE guideline: Management of Women with Endometriosis. Hum Reprod. 2014;29(3):400-12]

20. **c.** The use of assisted reproductive technologies for infertility associated with endometriosis is recommended, especially if tubal function is compromised or if there is male factor infertility and/or other treatments have failed.
   In women with minimal to mild endometriosis, IUI with controlled ovarian stimulation may be effective in increasing the live birth rate, compared with expectant management. Furthermore, IUI with controlled ovarian stimulation may be more effective in increasing pregnancy rate than IUI alone and may be as effective in women with minimal or mild endometriosis within 6 months of surgical treatment as in women with unexplained infertility.
[Reference: Dunselman GA, Vermeulen N, Becker C, Calhaz-Jorge C, D'Hooghe T, De Bie, et al.; European Society of Human Reproduction and Embryology. ESHRE guideline: Management of Women with Endometriosis. Hum Reprod. 2014;29(3):400-12]

21. **c.** Sigmoid colon
[Reference: Dunselman GA, Vermeulen N, Becker C, Calhaz-Jorge C, D'Hooghe T, De Bie B, et al.; European Society of Human Reproduction and Embryology. ESHRE guideline: Management of Women with Endometriosis, Guideline of the European Society of Hum Reprod. 2014;29(3):400-12]

22. **d.** Fulguration of endometriotic deposits.
[Reference: Dunselman GA, Vermeulen N, Becker C, Calhaz-Jorge C, D'Hooghe T, De Bie B, et al.; European Society of Human Reproduction and Embryology. ESHRE guideline: Management of Women with Endometriosis. Hum Reprod. 2014;29(3):400-12]

23. **a.** Perform laparoscopic cystectomy
In infertile women with AFS/ASRM stage III/IV endometriosis, operative laparoscopy, instead of expectant management.
[Reference: Dunselman GA, Vermeulen N, Becker C, Calhaz-Jorge C, D'Hooghe T, De Bie B, et al.; European Society of Human Reproduction and Embryology. ESHRE guideline: Management of Women with Endometriosis. Hum Reprod. 2014;29(3):400-12]

24. **d.** Spleen
(Reference: Speroff L, Marc FA. Endometriosis. Clinical Gynecologic Endocrinology & Infertility, 7th edition. Philadelphia: Lippincott Williams & Wilkins; 2005)

25. **a.** Depth of invasion
The intensity of pain associated with deep infiltrating endometriosis relates to the depth of the penetration and to the proximity or direct invasion of nerves. However, there is no relationship between stage, site of the morphological characteristics of pelvic endometriosis, and pain.
(Reference: Speroff L, Mar FA. Endometriosis. Clinical Gynecologic Endocrinology & Infertility, 7th edition. Philadelphia: Lippincott Williams & Wilkins; 2005)

26. **d.** Hormonal milieu has no influence in pain perception.
   Numerous studies have examined measures of pain perception across the menstrual cycle. A meta-analysis including 16 such studies concluded that somatic sensory pain thresholds and tolerance are near their lowest levels just prior to and during menses.
(Reference: Speroff L, Marc FA. Endometriosis. Clinical Gynecologic Endocrinology & Infertility, 7th edition. Philadelphia: Lippincott Williams & Wilkins; 2005)

27. **d.** The medical treatment of endometriosis improves fertility.

    Established medical treatment options for women with pain associated with endometriosis include danazol, progestins, cyclic or continuous oral contraceptives, GnRH agonists, and gestrinone. All available evidence indicates that they are equally effective and that no one treatment is considered best; pain relief, subsequent pregnancy rates, and recurrence rates are similar for all forms of medical treatment. One form of therapy can prove effective in relieving pain when another has failed. Consequently, the choice of therapy should be determined on the basis of cost and side effects. There is no substantial evidence that medical treatment of endometriosis improves fertility.
    (Reference: Speroff L, Marc FA. Endometriosis. Clinical Gynecologic Endocrinology & Infertility, 7th edition. Philadelphia: Lippincott Williams & Wilkins; 2005)

28. **d.** All of the above
    Risk factors for persistent or recurrent disease and pain include ovarian preservation, incomplete excision of disease, and postoperative unopposed estrogen therapy in women with extensive or residual disease. However, when all visible endometriosis is removed, the risk for recurrent pain in women who receive immediate or delayed hormone treatment is similar. Ovarian remnant syndrome involves persistent or recurrent disease and pain associated with residual functional ovarian tissue. The syndrome is not altogether rare and occurs most frequently when the ovaries are enlarged or densely adherent to the pelvic sidewalls and dissection is technically difficult.
    (Reference: Speroff L, Marc FA. Endometriosis. Clinical Gynecologic Endocrinology & Infertility, 7th edition. Philadelphia: Lippincott Williams & Wilkins; 2005)

29. **d.** Dienogest cannot be safely used in adolescent girls for long term.
    Dienogest can be used in a dose of 2 mg/day and has a very good safety profile, efficacy, and minimal side effects. It is well tolerated and improves symptoms and the overall quality of life. It can safely be used in adolescent girls for the long term which reduces the size of lesions. Postoperative use of dienogest and GnRH agonists reduces the incidence of recurrence.
    (Reference: Arora M, Pai H, Kumari SS. Evidence-based Practices in Obstetrics and Gynecology, 1st edition. New Delhi: Evangel Publishing; 2023)

30. **d.** Postoperative suppression with GnRH agonist and dienogest has no role in patients with postmenopausal endometriosis.
    (Reference: Arora M, Pai H, Kumari SS. Evidence-based Practices in Obstetrics and Gynecology, 1st edition. New Delhi: Evangel Publishing. 2023)

Chapter 71

Ovulation Induction

Anuja Bhalerao

QUESTIONS

1. **Progesterone levels above _____ indicates ovulation.**
   a. 4 ng/mL
   b. 2 ng/mL
   c. 3 ng/mL
   d. 1 ng/mL

2. **Maximum dose of clomifene citrate that can be administered for ovulation induction is:**
   a. 150 mg/day
   b. 100 mg/day
   c. 250 mg/day
   d. 50 mg/day

3. **Ovulation induction should be initiated on day 2/3 only if:**
   a. E2 < 50 pg/mL
   b. E2 > 50 pg/mL
   c. E2 < 75 pg/mL
   d. E2 > 75 pg/mL

4. **Normal response to gonadotropins stimulation in IVF is indicated by:**
   a. 4–14 oocytes at OPU
   b. 20–25 oocytes at OPU
   c. 2–3 oocytes at OPU
   d. 15–20 oocytes at OPU

5. **In case of anovulatory infertility, diagnostic hormonal levels for hyperprolactinemia will be:**
   a. ↑follicle-stimulating hormone (FSH), ↑luteinizing hormone (LH), ↑E2
   b. ↓FSH, ↓LH, ↓E2
   c. ↑FSH, ↑LH, ↓E2
   d. ↓FSH, ↓LH, ↑E2

6. **Half-life of corifollitropin alfa is:**
   a. 65 hours
   b. 24 hours
   c. 48 hours
   d. 36 hours

7. **All are included in WHO classification of ovulatory disorders as end-organ failure, *except*:**
   a. Primary ovarian failure
   b. Fragile X syndrome
   c. Turner syndrome
   d. Polycystic ovarian syndrome (PCOS)

8. **DNA fragmentation studies needed in all, *expect*:**
   a. Unexplained infertility
   b. Recurrent pregnancy loss
   c. Varicocele associated infertility
   d. Routine husband/male partner evaluation

9. **A failed cycle is when:**
   a. You go through infertility treatment and it does not end in pregnancy.
   b. You go through infertility treatment and it does not end in ovulation.
   c. You go through infertility treatment and does not end completely.
   d. You go through infertility treatment and it is withdrawn.

10. **Cumulus like shadow is seen on USG _____ hours prior to ovulation.**
    a. 24 hours
    b. 36 hours
    c. 48 hours
    d. 72 hours

11. **Anti-Müllerian hormone (AMH) inhibits the recruitment of:**
    a. Primordial follicle
    b. Primary follicle
    c. Secondary follicle
    d. Antral follicle

12. **In polycystic ovarian syndrome (PCOS), if required ovarian drilling can be done by:**
    a. Electrocautery
    b. Laser
    c. (a) and (b)
    d. None

13. **Clomifene citrate failure means:**
    a. Failure to ovulate
    b. Failure to conceive
    c. All of the above
    d. None of the above

14. **Kisspeptin triggers oocyte maturation by:**
    a. Blocks action of vascular endothelial growth factor (VEGF)
    b. Stimulates gonadotropin-releasing hormone (GnRH) release thus increase follicle-stimulating hormone (FSH), and luteinizing hormone (LH)
    c. Inhibits vasopressin
    d. None of the above

15. **Drug of choice for hyperprolactemic women with ovulatory dysfunction is:**
    a. Gonadotropin-releasing hormone (GnRH)
    b. Dopamine agonist
    c. Selective estrogen receptor modulator (SERM)
    d. Aromatase inhibitor

16. **Most effective dose of exogenous GnRH treatment is:**
    a. 2.5–5 µg/pulse at constant interval of 60–90 mL
    b. 5–7.5 ug/pulse at constant interval of 60–90 mL
    c. 1.5–2.5 ug/pulse at constant interval of 60–90 mL
    d. 2.5–5.0 ug/pulse at constant interval of 60–90 mL

17. **Side effects of dopamine agonist minimized with:**
    a. Starting with low dose then gradually increasing
    b. Giving pulsatile dose of dopamine
    c. Giving high dose of dopamine
    d. Giving low dose of dopamine

18. **Ovarian hyperstimulation syndrome (OHSS) is reported with all, *except:***
    a. Clomifene citrate
    b. Exogenous gonadotropins
    c. Letrozole
    d. Both (a) and (b)

19. **With gonadotropin stimulation regimen best results are obtained when estradiol concentration peaks at:**
    a. 500–1,500 pg/mL
    b. <100 pg/mL
    c. >1,500 pg/mL
    d. 200–500 pg/mL

20. **Monitoring of gonadotropin therapy is done with:**
    a. Serial serum estradiol and transvaginal ultrasound scan (TVS)
    b. Serial serum estrone and TVS
    c. Serial serum estriol and TVS
    d. Serial serum estrone and transabdominal ultrasonography (TAS)

21. **All of the following risks are associated with gonadotropin therapy, *except:***
    a. Ovarian hyperstimulation syndrome (OHSS)
    b. Multifetal pregnancy
    c. Liver malignancy
    d. Breast cancer

22. **In following which is the most common treatment of luteal phase defect?**
    a. Progesterone therapy
    b. Estrogen therapy
    c. Clomifene
    d. Dexamethasone

23. **With pulsatile GnRH therapy, risk of which of the following can be eliminated?**
    a. Ovarian hyperstimulation syndrome (OHSS)
    b. Multiple gestation
    c. Liver cancer
    d. All of the above

24. **Reliable evidence that ovulation has occurred:**
    a. Progesterone > 3 ng/mL
    b. Progesterone > 10 ng/mL
    c. Progesterone > 13 ng/mL
    d. Progesterone > 16 ng/mL

25. **After treatment with dopamine agonist, menses restored within:**
    a. 6–8 weeks
    b. 8–10 weeks
    c. 10–12 weeks
    d. 12–14 weeks

26. **To support normal luteal function, dose of hCG required is:**
    a. 2,000–2,500 IU every 3–4 days
    b. 2,500–3,000 IU every 3–4 days
    c. 3,000–3,500 IU every 3–4 days
    d. 3,500–4,000 IU every 3–4 days

27. **Aromatase inhibitors act:**
    a. Block estrogen production centrally as well as periphery
    b. Block estrogen production centrally only
    c. Estrogen production periphery only
    d. None of the above

28. **Follicle-stimulating hormone (FSH) levels_____ have high specificity for predicting poor response to stimulation.**
    a. >10 IU/L
    b. >15 IU/L
    c. >20 IU/L
    d. >30 IU/L

29. A 26-year-old infertile PCOS patient treated with clomifene citrate presents with sudden onset of abdominal pain and distention after 20 days of starting treatment. What is the probable cause?
    a. Uterine rupture
    b. Ectopic pregnancy
    c. Multifetal pregnancy
    d. Ovarian hyperstimulation syndrome (OHSS)

30. Drug of choice for ovulation induction in anovulatory women is:
    a. Dopamine
    b. Letrozole
    c. Clomifene
    d. Gonadotropin-releasing hormone (GnRH)

31. In a woman with hypogonadotropins hypogonadism, regimen for ovulation induction contains:
    a. Follicle-stimulating hormone (FSH)
    b. Luteinizing hormone (LH)
    c. Both FSH and LH
    d. Follicle-stimulating hormone and estrogen

32. Most common side effect of letrozole is:
    a. Hot flushes
    b. Headache and cramps
    c. Breast tenderness
    d. Fatigue

33. In step-up treatment regimen in hypogonadotrophic hypogonadism, dose of gonadotropin to induce ovulation is:
    a. 75 IU
    b. 37.5 IU
    c. 100 IU
    d. 225 IU

ANSWERS

1. c.	2. a.	3. a.	4. a.
5. b.	6. a.	7. d.	8. d.
9. a.	10. b.	11. a.	12. b.
13. a.	14. b.	15. b.	16. a.
17. a.	18. c.	19. a.	20. a.
21. a.	22. a.	23. a.	24. a.
25. a.	26. a.	27. a.	28. a.
29. d.	30. b.	31. c.	32. b.
33. a.			

Chapter 72

Tubal Factor Infertility

Archana Kumari, Ruchika Garg

QUESTIONS

1. Which of the following is false regarding hydrosalpinx simplex?
    a. Plicae are few and widely separated
    b. Excessive distension and thinning of the wall of the uterine tube
    c. Lumen is broken up into compartments
    d. It is the end stage of tubal infection

2. Which of the following is not true regarding pregnancy outcome in women with hydrosalpinx?
    a. Risk of spontaneous abortion is doubled
    b. Clinical pregnancy rate is reduced by half
    c. There is an increased risk of ectopic pregnancy
    d. Bilateral hydrosalpinx is associated with a lower pregnancy rate compared to unilateral hydrosalpinx

3. The risk of ectopic pregnancy is increased:
    a. 2–3 fold after pelvic infection
    b. 4–5 fold after pelvic infection
    c. 5–6 fold after pelvic infection
    d. 6–7 fold after pelvic infection

4. Which of the following is incorrect regarding tubal obstruction?
    a. Proximal tubal obstruction is an all-or-none phenomenon
    b. Distal tubal occlusion exhibits a spectrum ranging from fimbrial agglutination to complete obstruction
    c. Inflammatory damage to internal tubal mucosal architecture can be easily detected
    d. Hysterosalpingography (HSG) and laparoscopy are two complementary methods to assess tubal patency

5. Which of the following is not used for tubal patency testing?
    a. Saline
    b. Hydroxyethyl cellulose
    c. Oxygen gas
    d. Sodium hexafluoride

6. Which of the following is false regarding HSG?
    a. When HSG reveals blocked tubes, there is a high probability that tube is open
    b. When HSG reveals patent tubes, there is little chance that tube is actually occluded
    c. A false-positive HSG may occur when contrast enters a widely dilated hydrosalpinx
    d. The positive predictive value (PPV) of HSG for tubal occlusion is 38%

7. Which dye is preferred for chromopertubation?
    a. Methylene blue   b. Indigo carmine
    c. Toulidene blue   d. Saline

8. Which of the following is the most important prognostic factor for achieving a live birth after microsurgical sterilization reversal?
    a. Type of procedure
    b. Location of procedure
    c. Age of the patient
    d. Final length of the repaired fallopian tube

9. Which of the following regarding distal tubal obstruction is incorrect?
    a. Fimbriolysis is the separation of adherent fimbria
    b. Fimbrioplasty is the correction of phimotic but patent fimbria
    c. Neosalpingostomy involves reopening of a completely obstructed tube
    d. In young women with a severe distal tubal obstructive disease, laparoscopic surgery may be viewed as an alternative to in vitro fertilization (IVF)

10. Which of the following is incorrect with respect to pregnancy rates in women with hydrosalpinges?
    a. Laparoscopic salpingectomy affects the ovarian reserve
    b. Laparoscopic salpingectomy improves the IVF pregnancy rates in women with hydrosalpinges
    c. Ultrasound-guided aspiration of hydrosalpingeal fluid at the time of oocyte aspiration does not fare better than laparoscopic salpingectomy
    d. Ultrasound-guided aspiration of hydrosalpingeal fluid can be reserved for women likely to have severe intra-abdominal adhesions

11. Which of the following is not an infectious cause of proximal tubal blockage?
    a. Tuberculosis
    b. Salpingitis isthmica nodosa
    c. Pelvic inflammatory disease
    d. Intratubal endometriosis

12. Fertiloscopy is:
    a. Hysteroscopy with falloscopy
    b. Hysteroscopy with salpingoscopy
    c. Hysteroscopy with falloscopy with salpingoscopy
    d. Hysteroscopy with falloscopy, salpingoscopy, and transvaginal hydrolaparoscopy

13. Jacobson and Westrom criteria is:
    a. Laparoscopic criteria for diagnosis and grading of salpingitis
    b. Laparoscopic criteria for diagnosis and grading of endometriosis
    c. Hysteroscopic criteria for diagnosis and grading of endometritis
    d. Hysteroscopic criteria for diagnosis and grading of Asherman syndrome

14. Which of the following is correct about salpingitis isthmica nodosa?
    a. It involves endosalpingeal compartments of the fallopian tube
    b. It is the most common cause of distal tubal disease
    c. It can be treated by tubal catheterization using Novy's system
    d. It is associated with peritubal adhesions

15. Which of the following endometrial receptivity markers is decreased in hydrosalpinx?
    a. HOXA10
    b. Cyclin E
    c. P27
    d. Leukemia inhibitory factor

ANSWERS

1. **c.** Lumen is broken up into compartments.

   Hydrosalpinx simplex is the end stage of tubal infection with excessive distension and thinning of the wall of the uterine tube with plicae being few and widely separated. However, hydrosalpinx follicularis describes a tube without a central cystic cavity with lumen being broken up into compartments due to fusion of the tubal plicae.

   [Reference: Gardner DK, Weissman A, Howles CM, Zeev S (Eds). Textbook of Assisted Reproductive Techniques, Volume 2: Clinical Perspectives, 5th edition. Boca Raton: CRC Press; 2017. p. 773]

2. **c.** There is an increased risk of ectopic pregnancy.

   Patients with tubal infertility have an increased risk of ectopic pregnancy after IVF compared to those with other indications, but it has not been possible to establish that patients with hydrosalpinges have an increased risk of ectopic pregnancy compared with patients suffering from other types of tubal infertility.

   [Reference: Gardner DK, Weissman A, Howles CM, Zeev S (Eds). Textbook of Assisted Reproductive Techniques, Volume 2: Clinical Perspectives, 5th edition. Boca Raton: CRC Press; 2017. pp. 773, 774]

3. **d.** 6-7 fold after pelvic infection

   (Reference: Taylor HS, Fritz MA, Pal L, Emre S. Speroff's Clinical Gynecologic Endocrinology and Infertility, 9th edition. Philadelphia: Wolters Kluwer; 2020. p. 1002)

4. **c.** Inflammatory damage to internal tubal mucosal architecture can be easily detected.

   (Reference: Taylor HS, Fritz MA, Pal L, Emre S. Speroff's Clinical Gynecologic Endocrinology and Infertility, 9th edition. Philadelphia: Wolters Kluwer, 2020. p. 1003)

5. **c.** Oxygen is a gas not being used for Tubal patency.

6. **a.** When HSG reveals blocked tubes, there is a high probability that tube is open.

   The clinical implications are that when HSG reveals obstruction, there is still a relatively high probability (approximately 60%) that the tube is open, but when HSG demonstrates patency, there is little chance that the tube is actually occluded (approximately 5%).

   (Reference: Taylor HS, Fritz MA, Pal L, Emre S. Speroff's Clinical Gynecologic Endocrinology and Infertility, 9th edition. Philadelphia: Wolters Kluwer, 2020. p. 1004)

7. **b.** Indigo carmine
   Indigo carmine is preferred over methylene blue which may rarely cause acute methemoglobinemia, particularly in patients with glucose-6-phosphate dehydrogenase (G6PDH) deficiency.
   (Reference: Taylor HS, Fritz MA, Pal L, Emre S. Speroff's Clinical Gynecologic Endocrinology and Infertility, 9th edition. Philadelphia: Wolters Kluwer, 2020. p. 1004)

8. **c.** Age of the patient
   The most important prognostic factor for achieving a live birth after microsurgical sterilization reversal is age. The type and location of procedure and the final length of the repaired fallopian tube are also considered to play a role.
   (Reference: Taylor HS, Fritz MA, Pal L, Emre S. Speroff's Clinical Gynecologic Endocrinology and Infertility, 9th edition. Philadelphia: Wolters Kluwer; 2020. p. 1006)

9. **d.** In young women with a severe distal tubal obstructive disease, laparoscopic surgery may be viewed as an alternative to in vitro fertilization (IVF).
   For younger women with mild distal tubal occlusive disease, laparoscopic surgery may be viewed as an alternative to IVF, but when disease is severe or pregnancy does not occur during first postoperative year, IVF is the logical choice.
   (Reference: Taylor HS, Fritz MA, Pal L, Emre S. Speroff's Clinical Gynecologic Endocrinology and Infertility, 9th edition. Philadelphia: Wolters Kluwer; 2020. pp. 1006-7)

10. **a.** Laparoscopic salpingectomy affects the ovarian reserve.
    (Reference: Taylor HS, Fritz MA, Pal L, Emre S. Speroff's Clinical Gynecologic Endocrinology and Infertility, 9th edition. Philadelphia: Wolters Kluwer; 2020. p. 1007)

11. **d.** Intratubal endometriosis
    (Reference: Taylor HS, Fritz MA, Pal L, Emre S. Speroff's Clinical Gynecologic Endocrinology and Infertility, 9th edition. Philadelphia: Wolters Kluwer; 2020. p. 1007)

12. **d.** Hysteroscopy with falloscopy, salpingoscopy, and transvaginal hydrolaparoscopy
    [Reference: Rao KA, Carp HJA, Fischer R (Eds). Principles and Practice of Assisted Reproductive Technology. Vol 1, 2nd edition. New Delhi: Jaypee Brothers Medical Publishers (P) Ltd; 2014. p. 400]

13. **a.** Laparoscopic criteria for diagnosis and grading of salpingitis
    [Reference: Rao KA, Carp HJA, Fischer R (Eds). Principles and Practice of Assisted Reproductive Technology. Vol 1, 2nd edition. New Delhi: Jaypee Brothers Medical Publishers (P) Ltd; 2014. P. 399]

14. **d.** It is associated with peritubal adhesions.

15. **a.** HOXA10

Chapter 73

Female Genital Tuberculosis

Sippy Agarwal, Prabhat Agrawal

QUESTIONS

1. What is the likelihood of fallopian tubes getting involved in female genital tuberculosis?
   a. Almost 100%
   b. 50%
   c. 75%
   d. 90%

2. What causes menstrual irregularities in cases of pulmonary tuberculosis with no demonstrable pathology in genital tract?
   a. The steroidogenic effect of *Mycobacterium tuberculosis*
   b. The antigonadotrophic effect of *Mycobacterium tuberculosis*
   c. The immune response of the body
   d. The spread of tuberculosis to the genital tract from the lungs occurs too fast before demonstrable lesions can be detected

3. Which of the following tests is most specific to diagnose genital tuberculosis?
   a. Mantoux test
   b. Erythrocyte sedimentation rate (ESR)
   c. Pelvic ultrasound
   d. Histopathological evidence in biopsy of premenstrual endometrial tissue

4. Which time of the menstrual cycle is the most ideal for histopathological detection of genital tuberculosis?
   a. 2-3 days postmenstrually
   b. 2-3 days premenstrually
   c. 9-10 days postmenstrually
   d. 9-10 days premenstrually

5. Which portion of the endometrium is most likely to show tubercles in genital tuberculosis?
   a. Fundus
   b. Anterior wall
   c. Cornu
   d. Posterior wall

6. Which of the following findings can be present in the hysterosalpingography of a patient suffering from genital tuberculosis?
   a. Rigid pipe stem appearance
   b. Hydrosalpinx
   c. Irregular calcified adnexa
   d. All of the above

7. What is the minimum numbers of bacterias present to call a culture positive while diagnosing genital tuberculosis on culturing upon Lowenstein-Jensen medium?
   a. 1,000/mL
   b. 10/mL
   c. 10,000/mL
   d. 100/mL

8. What does the BACTEC radiometric culture detect in order to diagnose growing *Mycobacterium tuberculosis*?
   a. Nitrogen
   b. Carbon dioxide
   c. Oxygen
   d. None of the above

9. Which amongst the following is the fastest diagnostic modality for genital tuberculosis?
   a. Culture in Lowenstein-Jensen media
   b. BACTEC radiometric assay
   c. Polymerase chain reaction assay
   d. All the modalities take equal time

10. What is the approximate time taken for a polymerase chain reaction (PCR) assay to diagnose genital tuberculosis?
    a. 1-2 weeks
    b. 1-2 days
    c. 3-4 days
    d. 5-6 days

11. Which of the following is a close mimic of tubo-ovarian mass of genital tuberculosis?
    a. Tubo-ovarian mass of pyogenic origin
    b. Pelvic endometriosis
    c. Both a and b
    d. Neither a nor b

12. Which of the following antitubercular drugs is a known enzyme inducer?
    a. Rifampicin   b. Isoniazid
    c. Ethambutol   d. Pyrazinamide

13. What is the likelihood of a female getting pregnant who has clinical features of genital tuberculosis after treatment is given?
    a. 5–10%   b. 20–30%
    c. Almost 100%   d. 40–50%

14. Which among the following is an indication for surgical management of genital tuberculosis?
    a. Persistence of pelvic mass
    b. Recurrence of pain or bleeding after 9 months of treatment
    c. On patient demand
    d. Both a and b

15. What is the minimum duration of having started a patient on antitubercular treatment before initiation of surgical management?
    a. 6 weeks   b. 8 weeks
    c. 4 weeks   d. 12 weeks

16. Which is the best modality for conception in a female who has had a history of genital tuberculosis?
    a. Spontaneous conception
    b. In vitro fertilization
    c. In utero insemination
    d. Adhesiolysis

17. Which is the most common mode of spread in female genital tuberculosis?
    a. Lymphatic spread
    b. Ascending infection
    c. Direct spread
    d. Hematogenous route

18. Which among the following is a differential diagnosis for tuberculosis of cervix?
    a. Carcinoma of cervix
    b. Cervical polyp
    c. Presence of nabothian cysts
    d. None of the above

19. What is the minimum number of bacilli to be present in a sample in order to be detected by PCR assay?
    a. 10 microorganisms
    b. 100 microorganisms
    c. 1 microorganism
    d. 100,000 microorganisms

20. Which of the following abnormalities can occur in a patient with genital tuberculosis?
    a. Hypomenorrhea
    b. Amenorrhea
    c. Postmenopausal bleeding
    d. All of the above

21. Which of the following conventional stains is used for the identification of *M. tuberculosis*?
    a. Ziehl-Neelsen stain   b. Malachite green stain
    c. Giemsa stain   d. Acridine orange stain

22. Which age group does genital tuberculosis mostly affect?
    a. Childhood
    b. Postmenopausal women
    c. Reproductive age group
    d. All of the above

23. What is the presence of dense adhesions of the liver capsule on the anterior abdominal wall called?
    a. Cushing's syndrome
    b. Fitz-Hugh-Curtis syndrome
    c. Blueberry syndrome
    d. Down's syndrome

24. By which of the following routes can tuberculosis be transmitted to a newborn of a mother infected with genital tuberculosis?
    a. Transplacental route
    b. Swallowing of amniotic fluid perinatally
    c. None of the above
    d. Both a and b

25. Which of the following parameters are assessed to monitor response to antitubercular treatment in genital tuberculosis?
    a. Improvement in constitutional symptoms
    b. Change in the size of pelvic mass and amount of ascitic fluid with the help of clinical examination and ultrasound.
    c. Changes in ESR
    d. All of the above

26. Which of the following conditions is an indication for surgical intervention in genital tuberculosis?
    a. Drainage of large residual pelvic abscess, pyosalpinx
    b. Persistence of fever, pain, ascites after medical management
    c. Fertility evaluation after treatment
    d. All of the above

27. Which of the following antitubercular drugs is known to cause optic neuritis?
    a. Ethambutol   b. Streptomycin
    c. Isoniazid   d. Rifampicin
28. Abnormalities of which of the following sites cannot be detected by hysteroscopy in female genital tuberculosis?
    a. Cervix   b. Endometrium
    c. Fallopian tubes d. Ostia
29. Which of the following signs can be found in the pelvis during per vaginal examination in a patient suffering from genital tuberculosis?
    a. Restricted mobility of uterus
    b. Tenderness on movement of cervix
    c. Enlarged uterus due to pyometra
    d. All of the above
30. Which among the following is not a second-line drug for the management of genital tuberculosis?
    a. Levofloxacin   b. Rifampicin
    c. Kanamycin   d. Capreomycin

ANSWERS

1. **a.** [Reference: Kumar P, Malhotra N. Jeffcoate's Principles of Gynaecology, 7th edition. New Delhi: Jaypee Brothers Medical Publishers (P) Ltd; 2008. p. 361]
2. **b.** [Reference: Kumar P, Malhotra N. Jeffcoate's Principles of Gynaecology, 7th edition. New Delhi: Jaypee Brothers Medical Publishers (P) Ltd; 2008. p. 361]
3. **d.** [Reference: Kumar P, Malhotra N. Jeffcoate's Principles of Gynaecology, 7th edition. New Delhi: Jaypee Brothers Medical Publishers (P) Ltd; 2008. p. 362]
4. **b.** [Reference: Kumar P, Malhotra N. Jeffcoate's Principles of Gynaecology, 7th edition. New Delhi: Jaypee Brothers Medical Publishers (P) Ltd; 2008. p. 362]
5. **c.** [Reference: Kumar P, Malhotra N. Jeffcoate's Principles of Gynaecology, 7th edition. New Delhi: Jaypee Brothers Medical Publishers (P) Ltd; 2008. p. 362]
6. **d.** [Reference: Kumar P, Malhotra N. Jeffcoate's Principles of Gynaecology, 7th edition. New Delhi: Jaypee Brothers Medical Publishers (P) Ltd; 2008. p. 362]
7. **d.** [Reference: Kumar P, Malhotra N. Jeffcoate's Principles of Gynaecology, 7th edition. New Delhi: Jaypee Brothers Medical Publishers (P) Ltd; 2008. p. 362]
8. **b.** [Reference: Kumar P, Malhotra N. Jeffcoate's Principles of Gynaecology, 7th edition. New Delhi: Jaypee Brothers Medical Publishers (P) Ltd; 2008. p. 362]
9. **c.** [Reference: Kumar P, Malhotra N. Jeffcoate's Principles of Gynaecology, 7th edition. New Delhi: Jaypee Brothers Medical Publishers (P) Ltd; 2008. p. 362]
10. **b.** [Reference: Kumar P, Malhotra N. Jeffcoate's Principles of Gynaecology, 7th edition. New Delhi: Jaypee Brothers Medical Publishers (P) Ltd; 2008. p. 362]
11. **c.** [Reference: Kumar P, Malhotra N. Jeffcoate's Principles of Gynaecology, 7th edition. New Delhi: Jaypee Brothers Medical Publishers (P) Ltd; 2008. p. 363]
12. **a.** [Reference: Kumar P, Malhotra N. Jeffcoate's Principles of Gynaecology, 7th edition. New Delhi: Jaypee Brothers Medical Publishers (P) Ltd; 2008. p. 363]
13. **b.** [Reference: Kumar P, Malhotra N. Jeffcoate's Principles of Gynaecology, 7th edition. New Delhi: Jaypee Brothers Medical Publishers (P) Ltd; 2008. p. 362]
14. **a.** [Reference: Kumar P, Malhotra N. Jeffcoate's Principles of Gynaecology, 7th edition. New Delhi: Jaypee Brothers Medical Publishers (P) Ltd; 2008. p. 363]
15. **a.** [Reference: Kumar P, Malhotra N. Jeffcoate's Principle of Gynaecology, 7th edition. New Delhi: Jaypee Brothers Medical Publishers (P) Ltd; 2008. p. 363]
16. **b.** [Reference: Kumar P, Malhotra N. Jeffcoate's Principles of Gynaecology, 7th edition. New Delhi: Jaypee Brothers Medical Publishers (P) Ltd; 2008. p. 363]
17. **d.** [Reference: Kumar P, Malhotra N. Jeffcoate's Principles of Gynaecology, 7th edition. New Delhi: Jaypee Brothers Medical Publishers (P) Ltd; 2008. p. 361]

18. **a.** *[Reference: Kumar P, Malhotra N. Jeffcoate's Principles of Gynaecology, 7th edition. New Delhi: Jaypee Brothers Medical Publishers (P) Ltd; 2008. p. 415]*

19. **a.** *[Reference: Kumar P, Malhotra N. Jeffcoate's Principles of Gynaecology, 7th edition. New Delhi: Jaypee Brothers Medical Publishers (P) Ltd; 2008. p. 362]*

20. **d.** *[Reference: Bangalore Society of Obstetrics and Gynaecology Focus. (2017). Female genital tuberculosis. (online) Available from: https://www.bsog.in/bsog-focus-v8-single-pages.pdf (Last accessed December 2023)].*

21. **a.** *[Reference: Kumar P, Malhotra N. Jeffcoate's Principles of Gynaecology, 7th edition. New Delhi: Jaypee Brothers Medical Publishers (P) Ltd; 2008. p. 361]*

22. **c.** *[Reference: Kumar P, Malhotra N. Jeffcoate's Principles of Gynaecology, 7th edition. New Delhi: Jaypee Brothers Medical Publishers (P) Ltd; 2008. p. 361]*

23. **d.** *[Reference: Bangalore Society of Obstetrics and Gynaecology Focus. (2017). Female genital tuberculosis. (online) Available from: https://www.bsog.in/bsog-focus-v8-single-pages.pdf (Last accessed December 2023)].*

24. **d.** *[Reference: Bangalore Society of Obstetrics and Gynaecology Focus. (2017). Female genital tuberculosis. (online) Available from: https://www.bsog.in/bsog-focus-v8-single-pages.pdf (Last accessed December 2023)].*

25. **d.** *[Reference: Bangalore Society of Obstetrics and Gynaecology Focus. (2017). Female genital tuberculosis. (online) Available from: https://www.bsog.in/bsog-focus-v8-single-pages.pdf (Last accessed December 2023)].*

26. **d.** *[Reference: Bangalore Society of Obstetrics and Gynaecology Focus. (2017). Female genital tuberculosis. (online) Available from: https://www.bsog.in/bsog-focus-v8-single-pages.pdf (Last accessed December 2023)].*

27. **a.** *[Reference: Bangalore Society of Obstetrics and Gynaecology Focus. (2017). Female genital tuberculosis. (online) Available from: https://www.bsog.in/bsog-focus-v8-single-pages.pdf (Last accessed December 2023)].*

28. **c.** *[Reference: Bangalore Society of Obstetrics and Gynaecology Focus. (2017). Female genital tuberculosis. (online) Available from: https://www.bsog.in/bsog-focus-v8-single-pages.pdf (Last accessed December 2023)].*

29. **d.** *[Reference: Bangalore Society of Obstetrics and Gynaecology Focus. (2017). Female genital tuberculosis. (online) Available from: https://www.bsog.in/bsog-focus-v8-single-pages.pdf (Last accessed December 2023)].*

30. **b.** *[Reference: Kumar P, Malhotra N. Jeffcoate's Principles of Gynaecology, 7th edition. New Delhi: Jaypee Brothers Medical Publishers (P) Ltd; 2008. p. 362]*

Chapter 74

Male Infertility

Divya Pandey, Shivam Yadav

QUESTIONS

1. What does not hold true as per WHO Semen Analysis Manual (6th edition, 2021)?
   a. Vitality—54%
   b. Total motility—30%
   c. Progressive motility—30%
   d. Total motility—42%

2. Which of the following tests has been discarded as per the new edition (6th edition) of WHO Semen Analysis 2021?
   a. Computer-assisted semen analysis (CASA)
   b. CatSper channels
   c. Hamster egg penetration test
   d. Sperm chromatin structure and stability

3. The main components of the 6th edition of WHO Semen Analysis Manual (2021) are all, *except*:
   a. Semen examination
   b. Semen preparation and cryopreservation
   c. Quality assessment and quality control
   d. Stains and plates for morphology

4. If A = Sperm concentration × Volume of semen × Motility percentage, what is the correct term for "A"?
   a. Total sperm count (TSC)
   b. Total motile sperm count (TMSC)
   c. Total sperm concentration
   d. Motile sperm count

5. Which of the following is true regarding sperm motility as per the WHO Semen Analysis Manual, 6th edition?
   a. Four-pointer system—rapidly progressive, slow progressive, nonprogressive, immotile
   b. Three-pointer system—forward progressive, nonprogressive, immotile
   c. Lower reference value for total motility = 30%
   d. Lower reference value for progressive motility = 42%

6. As per the 6th edition of WHO Semen Analysis Manual (2021), normal vitality is:
   a. 58
   b. 48
   c. 45
   d. 54

7. The semen reference parameters that have not changed from 5th to 6th edition of WHO Semen Analysis Manual are:
   a. Total motility and progressive motility
   b. Sperm concentration and total sperm number
   c. Volume and total sperm number
   d. Total sperm number and morphology

8. What are the indications for sperm DNA fragmentation (SDF) testing?
   a. Unexplained male infertility
   b. Recurrent pregnancy loss
   c. Intrauterine insemination (IUI) failure
   d. All of the above

9. Males with high DNA fragmentation in semen can be prescribed all, *except*:
   a. Vitamin C and E
   b. Selenium and zinc
   c. Coenzyme Q-10 and N-acetyl cysteine (NAC)
   d. L-carnitine and oxalic acid

10. Which of the following sperm selection techniques is based on morphology?
    a. Swim-up
    b. Magnetic-activated cell sorting (MACS)
    c. Motile sperm organelle morphology examination (MSOME)
    d. Microelectrophoresis

11. Which of the following methods can be used to differentiate viable nonmotile sperms from dead sperms when no motile sperms are observed?
    a. Supravital dye staining
    b. Hypo-osmotic sperm swelling test
    c. Both a and b
    d. Neither a nor b

12. A 35-year-old male presents with infertility and is found to have elevated serum follicle-stimulating hormone (FSH) levels. Which of the following conditions is the most likely cause?
    a. Klinefelter syndrome   b. Varicocele
    c. Testicular trauma   d. Prostate infection

13. A 38-year-old male presents with infertility and a history of mumps infection during adolescence. Which of the following conditions is the most likely cause of his infertility?
    a. Testicular torsion   b. Varicocele
    c. Epididymitis   d. Orchitis

14. A semen analysis reveals a low semen volume, acidic pH, and absence of fructose. Which of the following conditions is most likely responsible for these findings?
    a. Obstruction of the ejaculatory ducts
    b. Varicocele
    c. Cryptorchidism
    d. Prostate infection

15. A 42-year-old male with infertility is found to have bilateral testicular atrophy. Which of the following hormone levels is most likely to be elevated in this patient?
    a. Follicle stimulating hormone (FSH)
    b. Luteinizing hormone (LH)
    c. Testosterone
    d. Prolactin

16. At what doses of radiation do spermatogenesis suppression and permanent azoospermia/infertility generally occur?
    a. Spermatogenesis suppression at 0.015 Gy (15 rad) and permanent azoospermia at 6 Gy
    b. Spermatogenesis suppression at 0.015 Gy (15 rad) and permanent azoospermia at 0.06 Gy (60 rad)
    c. Spermatogenesis suppression at 0.15 Gy (150 rad) and permanent azoospermia at 6 Gy
    d. Spermatogenesis suppression at 0.15 Gy (150 rad) and permanent azoospermia at 0.6 Gy (600 rad)

17. A semen analysis reveals low semen volume, low sperm count, and normal sperm motility and morphology. Which of the following conditions is most likely responsible for these findings?
    a. Obstruction of the ejaculatory ducts
    b. Varicocele
    c. Testicular failure
    d. Retrograde ejaculation

18. In the initial evaluation for male factor infertility, when should another semen analysis be obtained, if the first one shows abnormal results?
    a. After at least 1 week
    b. After at least 2 weeks
    c. After at least 3 weeks
    d. After at least 4 weeks

19. When performing a routine semen analysis, which of the following situations warrants additional studies to differentiate between leukocytes and immature sperm (round spermatids, spermatocytes) and identify true leukocytospermia (>1 million leukocytes/mL) requiring further evaluation for genital tract infection or inflammation?
    a. Round cell count exceeding 1 million/mL
    b. Round cell count exceeding 5 million/mL
    c. Round cell count exceeding 10 million/mL
    d. Round cell count exceeding 20 million/mL

20. Which gene mutation has been implicated as a potential cause of male infertility due to its involvement in regulating the synapse between homologous chromosomes during meiosis?
    a. *DAZL*
    b. *PRM1* and *PRM2*
    c. *SYCP3*
    d. *SYCP1*

21. Which of the following accurately describes the genetic basis and association of 46,XX males?
    a. 46,XX males have an extra X chromosome, resulting in Klinefelter syndrome
    b. 46,XX males have a translocation of the testis-determining gene (SRY) to an X chromosome, leading to Klinefelter syndrome
    c. 46,XX males have a deletion of the testis-determining gene (SRY) from an X chromosome, causing Klinefelter syndrome
    d. 46,XX males have a mutation in the androgen receptor gene, resulting in Klinefelter syndrome

22. Which of the following best describes the contribution of seminal vesicle secretions to the ejaculate in men with congenital bilateral absence of the vas deferens (CBAVD)?
    a. High-volume alkaline ejaculate with abundant fructose
    b. Low-volume acidic ejaculate with little or no fructose
    c. High-volume acidic ejaculate with abundant fructose
    d. Low-volume alkaline ejaculate with little or no fructose

23. The primary marker of sperm apoptosis is:
    a. Externalization of annexin V
    b. Externalization of phosphatidylserine
    c. Reduction in the sperm Zeta potential
    d. All of the above

24. Surgical sperm retrieval procedures based on aspiration technique are usually reserved for:
    a. Varicocele
    b. Obstructive azoospermia
    c. Nonobstructive azoospermia
    d. Normozoospermia

25. At what temperature and for what duration the semen sample after collection should be incubated?
    a. 20 minutes, 27°C
    b. 30 minutes, 27°C
    c. 20 minutes, 37°C
    d. 30 minutes, 37°C

26. The WHO lab manual for human semen examination has been revised for how many times?
    a. 5 times
    b. 6 times
    c. 4 times
    d. 7 times

27. Which of the following is the method of assessing sperm chromatin abnormalities?
    a. Acidic aniline blue (AAB) stain
    b. CMA3 assay
    c. TUNEL assay
    d. COMET assay
    e. All of the above

28. Which of the following is the strategy to reduce sperm DNA damage?
    a. Electrophoretic separation of sperm
    b. Antioxidant treatment
    c. Magnetic cell separation
    d. All of the above

29. All of the following are risk factors for SDF, *except*:
    a. Varicocele
    b. Obesity
    c. Scrotal hypothermia
    d. Radiation exposure

30. All of the following are precautions taken during semen preparation to reduce sperm DNA damage, *except*:
    a. Slow dilution of samples, especially cryopreserved samples
    b. Gradual changes in temperature and tests performed at 37°C
    c. Mandatory use of centrifugation at high speed to segregate sperms
    d. Controlled exposure to potential toxic material

ANSWERS

1. **b. Table 1** shows the comparison between WHO Semen Analysis in 5th and 6th editions.
   The lower fifth percentile (with a 95% confidence interval) of semen parameters is mentioned from men in couples having a pregnancy within a year of unprotected sexual intercourse leading to a natural conception.

TABLE 1: WHO 2010 (5th Edition) versus WHO 2021 (6th Edition).

Semen parameters	WHO 2010	WHO 2021
Semen volume (mL)	1.5 (1.4–1.7)	1.4 (1.3–1.5)
Total sperm number (10^6 per ejaculate)	39 (33–46)	39 (35–40)
Total motility (%)	40 (38–42)	42 (40–43)
Progressive motility (%)	32 (31–34)	30 (29–31)
Nonprogressive motility (%)	1	1 (1–1)
Immotile sperm (%)	22	20 (19–20)
Vitality (%)	58 (55–63)	54 (50–56)
Normal forms (%)	4 (3–4)	4 (3.9–4)

(Reference: World Health Organization. *WHO Laboratory Manual for the Examination and Processing of Human Semen, 6th edition.* Geneva: World Health Organization; 2021)

2. **c.** As per the 6th edition, the following tests, which were described in the 5th edition, have been discarded:
   • Sperm cervical penetration test
   • Hamster egg penetration test

3. **d.**
   (Reference: World Health Organization. WHO Laboratory Manual for the Examination and Processing of Human Semen, 6th edition. Geneva: World Health Organization; 2021)

4. **b.** Sperm concentration × Volume of semen = Total sperm count
   Total sperm count × motility percentage (motile sperms/mL) = Total motile sperm count

5. **a.** (Reference: World Health Organization. WHO Laboratory Manual for the Examination and Processing of Human Semen, 6th edition. Geneva: World Health Organization; 2021)

6. **d.** 54
   (Reference: World Health Organization. WHO Laboratory Manual for the Examination and Processing of Human Semen, 6th edition. Geneva: World Health Organization; 2021)

7. **d.** (Reference: World Health Organization. WHO Laboratory Manual for the Examination and Processing of Human Semen, 6th edition. Geneva: World Health Organization; 2021)

Semen parameters	WHO 2010	WHO 2021
Semen volume (mL)	1.5 (1.4–1.7)	1.4 (1.3–1.5)
Total sperm number (10^6 per ejaculate)	39 (33–46)	39 (35–40)
Total motility (%)	40 (38–42)	42 (40–43)
Progressive motility (%)	32 (31–34)	30 (29–31)
Nonprogressive motility (%)	1	1 (1–1)
Immotile sperm (%)	22	20 (19–20)
Vitality (%)	58 (55–63)	54 (50–56)
Normal forms (%)	4 (3–4)	4 (3.9–4)

8. **d.** Routine SDF testing is not recommended and is indicated in specific indications such as unexplained male infertility, recurrent pregnancy loss, varicocele, and IUI and in vitro fertilization (IVF) failure. SDF testing may be indicated before IVF, and in case of high SDF, intracytoplasmic sperm injection (ICSI) should be considered.

9. **d.** Antioxidant therapy can reduce the SDF and the effect of oxidative stress on sperms. The antioxidants with positive effects that can be prescribed are vitamin C, selenium, zinc, coenzyme Q10, N-acetyl cysteine (NAC), and L-carnitine.

10. **c.** *Swim-up technique* in sperm is based on intrinsic motility.
    Magnetic-activated cell sorting is a sperm selection technique based on the separation of apoptotic from nonapoptotic sperms using annexin V conjugated supramagnetic microbeads.
    Externalization of phospatidylserine (PS) is a marker of apoptotic sperms. These microbeads bind to PS in apoptotic sperms selectively and separate it from the nonapoptotic sperms.
    Motile sperm organelle morphology examination-based selection of sperm is based on morphology. Under high magnification, MSOME allows assessment of sperm head, middle piece, and tail region.
    Micro-electrophoresis is based on the fact that the plasma membrane of physiologically normal and mature sperms contains a rich amount of sialoglycoproteins. This induces a negative charge on the sperm of the range –16 to –20 mV, which prevents self-agglutination and unnecessary binding of sperm to the genital tract. This is called *Zeta potential*. Microelectrophoresis selects normal mature sperms from immature and abnormal sperms based on the difference in this charge.
    Microfluidics is another method of sperm selection based on normal sperm morphology and motility. The microfluidic platform uses chemotactic and thermotactic gradients for selection.

11. **c.** When no motile sperms are observed, a sperm vitality test can differentiate viable nonmotile sperms from dead sperms. One method involves mixing fresh semen with a *supravital dye (eosin Y or trypan blue)*; sperms with intact membrane function do not take up the stain. Another method, the *hypo-osmotic sperm swelling* test, involves incubation of sperms in a hypo-osmotic solution; the tails of sperms with normal membrane function swell and coil as fluid is transported across the membrane. In men with few or no motile sperms, the hypo-osmotic swelling test can be used to identify living nonmotile sperms for ICSI.
    [Reference: Taylor HS, Pal L, Seli E. Speroff's Clinical Gynecologic Endocrinology and Infertility, 9th edition. Philadelphia: Lippincott Williams & Wilkins (LWW); 2019. p. 2709]

12. **a.** Klinefelter syndrome is characterized by an extra X chromosome (47,XXY) and is a common cause of male infertility. Elevated FSH levels can result from the impaired spermatogenesis seen in this condition.

(Reference: Taylor HS, Pal L, Seli E. Speroff's Clinical Gynecologic Endocrinology and Infertility, 9th edition. Philadelphia: Lippincott Williams & Wilkins; 2019. p. 2694)

13. **d.** Orchitis refers to inflammation of the testes, commonly caused by viral infections such as mumps. It can lead to impaired sperm production and subsequent infertility.
(Reference: Taylor HS, Pal L, Seli E. Speroff's Clinical Gynecologic Endocrinology and Infertility, 9th edition. Philadelphia: Lippincott Williams & Wilkins; 2019. p. 2701)

14. **a.** Obstruction of the ejaculatory ducts can result in a low semen volume due to reduced seminal fluid contribution from the seminal vesicles and absent fructose, which is mainly produced by the seminal vesicles. The acidic pH may be due to increased prostatic secretions in the absence of seminal fluid.
(Reference: Taylor HS, Pal L, Seli E. Speroff's Clinical Gynecologic Endocrinology and Infertility, 9th edition. Philadelphia: Lippincott Williams & Wilkins; 2019. p. 2707)

15. **a.** Bilateral testicular atrophy suggests testicular failure. In response, the pituitary gland increases FSH production in an attempt to stimulate spermatogenesis. Therefore, elevated FSH levels are commonly observed in patients with testicular failure.
(Reference: Taylor HS, Pal L, Seli E. Speroff's Clinical Gynecologic Endocrinology and Infertility, 9th edition. Philadelphia: Lippincott Williams & Wilkins; 2019. p. 2717)

16. **a.** Doses of radiation as low as 0.015 Gy (15 rad) can suppress spermatogenesis, and doses above 6 Gy generally cause permanent azoospermia and infertility.
(Reference: Taylor HS, Pal L, Seli E. Speroff's Clinical Gynecologic Endocrinology and Infertility, 9th edition. Philadelphia: Lippincott Williams & Wilkins; 2019. p. 2697)

17. **d.** Retrograde ejaculation occurs when semen enters the bladder instead of being expelled through the urethra during ejaculation. This can result in low semen volume and low sperm count, while sperm motility and morphology remain unaffected.
(Reference: Taylor HS, Pal L, Seli E. Speroff's Clinical Gynecologic Endocrinology and Infertility, 9th edition. Philadelphia: Lippincott Williams & Wilkins; 2019. p. 2707)

18. **d.** The initial evaluation for male factor infertility should include at least one properly performed semen analysis. If abnormal, another semen analysis should be obtained after at least 4 weeks.
(Reference: Taylor HS, Pal L, Seli E. Speroff's Clinical Gynecologic Endocrinology and Infertility, 9th edition. Philadelphia: Lippincott Williams & Wilkins; 2019. p. 2702)

19. **b.** In the given fact, it is stated that when the round cell count exceeds 5 million/mL during a routine semen analysis, additional studies should be performed to differentiate between leukocytes and immature sperm and to identify true leukocytospermia (>1 million leukocytes/mL) requiring further evaluation for genital tract infection or inflammation.
(Reference: Taylor HS, Pal L, Seli E. Speroff's Clinical Gynecologic Endocrinology and Infertility, 9th edition. Philadelphia: Lippincott Williams & Wilkins; 2019. p. 2711)

20. **c.** Several autosomal and X-linked genes have been identified as important regulators of spermatogenesis. Mutations in the *SYCP3* gene (involved in the regulation of the synapse between homologous chromosomes during meiosis) have been implicated as a potential cause of male infertility. Others include polymorphisms of *DAZL* (an autosomal homolog of the *DAZ*, deleted in azoospermia, gene), *PRM1* and *PRM2* (protamines involved in chromatin compaction), *Tnp1* and *Tnp2* (transition nuclear proteins), and *USP26* (deubiquitinating enzyme family).
(Reference: Taylor HS, Pal L, Seli E. Speroff's Clinical Gynecologic Endocrinology and Infertility, 9th edition. Philadelphia: Lippincott Williams & Wilkins; 2019. p. 2696)

21. **b.** 46,XX males, resulting from translocation of the testis-determining gene (SRY) to an X chromosome, also have Klinefelter syndrome. The phenotype varies with the number of extra X chromosomes and possibly also with the number of trinucleotide CAG repeats on the androgen receptor gene (a polymorphism); as the length of the repeat sequence increases, receptor activity decreases. A longer CAG repeat sequence has been associated with taller stature, lower bone

mineral density, gynecomastia, and decreased penile length.
(Reference: Taylor HS, Pal L, Seli E. Speroff's Clinical Gynecologic Endocrinology and Infertility, 9th edition. Philadelphia: Lippincott Williams & Wilkins; 2019. p. 2694)

22. **b.** In men with CBAVD, the seminal vesicles are often hypoplastic or absent. This leads to a low-volume ejaculate that is acidic (pH < 7.2) and lacks fructose, reflecting the diminished contribution of alkaline seminal vesicle secretions.
(Reference: Taylor HS, Pal L, Seli E. Speroff's Clinical Gynecologic Endocrinology and Infertility, 9th edition. Philadelphia: Lippincott Williams & Wilkins; 2019. p. 2706)

23. **b.** *Magnetic activated cell sorting* is a sperm selection technique based on separation of apoptotic from nonapoptotic sperms using annexin V conjugated supramagenetic microbeads. *Externalization of phospatidyl serine* (PS) is a marker of apoptotic sperms. These microbeads bind to PS in apoptotic sperms selectively and separates it from the nonapoptotic sperms.

24. **b.**

25. **d.**

26. **b.** The latest edition is the 6th edition, which was released in 2021.

27. **e.** *Various methods of assessing sperm chromatin abnormalities are:*
    - Acidic aniline blue (AAB) staining
    - Modified AAB assay with eosin-Y
    - Toluidine Blue (TB) staining
    - CMA3 assay (CA3 is a guanine-cytosine-specific fluorochrome, which can reveal poorly packaged chromatin in spermatozoa. It is the indirect measure of protamine deficiency in sperm DNA.)
    - DBD-FISH assay (This can detect DNA breaks in specific DNA sequences as well as whole genome in a single cell)

28. **d.**
[Reference: Gardner DK, Weissman A, Howles CM, Shoham Z (Eds). Sperm chromatin assessment. Textbook of Assisted Reproductive Techniques, Vol 1: Clinical Perspectives, 5th edition. Boca Raton: CRC Press; 2018. pp. 65-78]

29. **c.**

30. **c.** Most common methods like density gradient centrifugation, swim-up, and glass wool filtration method yield sperm with better DNA integrity than native semen. Precautions taken during semen preparation to reduce sperm DNA damage are:
    - Slow dilution of samples, especially cryopreserved sample
    - Gradual changes in temperature and tests are performed at 37°C.
    - Minimal use of centrifugation at high speed to segregate sperm
    - Controlled exposure of semen to potential toxic materials

[Reference: Gardner DK, Weissman A, Howles CM, Shoham Z (Eds). sperm chromatin assessment. Textbook of Assisted Reproductive Techniques, Vol 1: Clinical Perspectives, 5th edition. Boca Raton: CRC Press; 2018. pp. 65-78]

Chapter 75: Intrauterine Insemination

Kanchan Rani, Divya Suman

QUESTIONS

1. Which of the following is not an indication of intrauterine insemination (IUI)?
   a. Unexplained genital tract bleeding
   b. Unexplained infertility with a total motile sperm count more than 10 million
   c. Allergy to seminal plasma
   d. Mild/moderate endometriosis

2. A couple with unexplained infertility is visiting your clinic. Human sperm assay (IISA) shows that total motile sperm count is more than 10 million and prognosis of pregnancy is <30% within a year. What will you suggest?
   a. Spontaneous method with fertility cycle explanation for six cycles
   b. Spontaneous method with fertility cycle explanation for three cycles
   c. IUI with spontaneous ovulation
   d. IUI with ovulation induction

3. What is the minimum number of consecutive IUI cycles per couple/woman in which pregnancy rates still increase significantly?
   a. 3
   b. More than 3
   c. 6
   d. More than 6

4. Which of the following is not true for IUI?
   a. Chances of success are better after mild ovarian stimulation and the maturation of a maximum of two or three follicles
   b. The cycle must be monitored by ultrasound and hormonal analysis
   c. To cancel an IUI cycle, the limit of maximum mature follicles [on ultrasonography (USG)] is more than 6
   d. IUI in a natural (not ovarian stimulated) cycle should be performed 1 day after luteinizing hormone (LH) rise

5. Hunault scoring is valid for:
   a. Female <40 years
   b. Where there is no tubal pathology or azoospermia
   c. None of the above
   d. Both a and b

6. Which of the following is not true for Hunault model?
   a. It is a prediction model for natural conception
   b. It uses only five predictors
   c. The only male factor predictor is sperm motility
   d. Tubal pathology is one of the predictors

7. Which of the following is not a contraindication for IUI?
   a. Severe endometriosis
   b. Genetic abnormality in male partner
   c. Unexplained genital tract bleeding
   d. Vaginismus

8. Which of the following is true for sperm collection for IUI?
   a. Abstinence right in the beginning of the IUI in order to produce concentrated specimen on the day of IUI
   b. Abstinence of 2 days produces the highest number of live pregnancies
   c. Prolonged period of abstinence results in lesser reactive oxygen species (ROS) in specimen
   d. Prolonged period of abstinence results in increased motility of sperms

9. Which of the following is not a semen preparation technique for IUI?
   a. Wash and centrifugation
   b. Swim-up
   c. Gradient
   d. Migration sedimentation technique

10. **Which of the following is true for swim-up method of semen preparation?**
    a. The direct swim-up is used for semen with normal parameters. It is not used for viscous samples
    b. The pellet swim-up method is used for normal or marginally abnormal semen samples. It is the method of choice for viscous samples
    c. None of the above
    d. Both a and b

11. **Which among the following is not true for density gradient method?**
    a. It cannot be used for normal semen samples
    b. The density gradient method is effective for abnormal sperm
    c. It removes not only the abnormal sperm but also microbes, debris, and other cell contaminates from the sample
    d. It is also used in processing semen samples prior to freezing them, and for processing nonprocessed frozen semen samples

12. **Which of the following is not true for sperm viability test?**
    a. Absence of motility indicates that the sperm may or may not be viable
    b. Viability can be decided by hypo-osmotic swelling test (HOST)
    c. If more than 58% of the sperm tail coil and swell in HOST, it indicates that the sample has sperms with functional and intact plasma membrane
    d. These samples after the test are used for IUI, in vitro fertilization (IVF), or intracytoplasmic sperm injection (ICSI)

13. **Which of the following is not true for deoxyribonucleic acid fragmentation index (DFI)?**
    a. It indicates the cutoff value of extent of nuclear fragmentation
    b. The cutoff value is estimated to be 60%
    c. Below the cutoff of DFI value, pregnancy even with ICSI is not possible
    d. None of the above

14. **To prevent transfer of infectious diseases, a batch of donor sperm should be cryopreserved and kept in quarantine for at least:**
    a. 1 month
    b. 2 months
    c. 3 months
    d. 6 months

15. **Which of the following is not a criterion for donor sperm that can be used in IUI with donor sperm?**
    a. Volume >4 mL
    b. Normal morphology >4%
    c. Motility >50%
    d. Count >50 million/mL

16. **Anovulatory women with polycystic ovary syndrome (PCOS) and body mass index (BMI) >25 kg/m^2, who have not responded to clomiphene citrate (CC) alone, may be offered metformin in addition.**
    a. True
    b. False

17. **In order to improve the quality and outcome of IUI procedures, there is a need for simple, inexpensive, reliable, and safe sperm preparation techniques. Hence, which statement is not true for sperm preparation?**
    a. Seminal fluid acts as a transport medium for sperm, prostaglandins, ions and antioxidants
    b. Reactive oxygen species can be detrimental for the fertilizing potential of the spermatozoa
    c. Donor sperm is mainly cryopreserved and kept in quarantine for at least 6 months to prevent the transfer of infectious diseases
    d. Thawed sperm is mostly not used for IUI as compared to intracervical insemination

18. **Which of the following is an indication of use of gonadotrophins for ovarian stimulation in IUI?**
    a. Resistant to antiestrogenic therapy
    b. Hypothalamic failure or dysfunction
    c. Both a and b
    d. None of the above

19. **When an ovulation disorder is present, we should:**
    a. Give CC as first line of medical treatment up to 6 months
    b. Give CC as first line of medical treatment up to 12 months
    c. Give low dose of gonadotrophin or CC as first line of medical treatment
    d. Give CC with metformin

20. **Which of the following is not an indication of gonadotrophin therapy (GT)?**
    a. Clomiphene/Letrozole failure
    b. Ovarian cyst
    c. Persistent hypersecretion of LH
    d. Hypothalamic dysfunction

21. Which of the following is not true for human immunodeficiency virus (HIV)-discordant couple (when a male is HIV positive)?
    a. IUI should be offered to them
    b. IVF is the correct choice for them
    c. Donor sperm is not required if there is no abnormality other than HIV infection
    d. Semen wash is safe and prevents HIV infection transmission to a noninfected female partner

22. Which of the following is an indication of IUI in special cases?
    a. If a couple is unable to have vaginal sex due to a physical disability or psychosexual problem
    b. If a couple is serodiscordant and husband is HIV positive
    c. None of the above
    d. Both a and b

23. Which of the following statements is true for double IUI?
    a. In both unexplained and male infertility, there is insufficient evidence that a double IUI within the same cycle will lead to better pregnancy rates than a single IUI within a cycle
    b. In unexplained infertility, a double IUI within the same cycle will lead to better pregnancy rates than a single IUI within a cycle
    c. In male infertility, a double IUI within the same cycle will lead to better pregnancy rates than a single IUI within a cycle
    d. In any factor of infertility, a double IUI within the same cycle will lead to better pregnancy rates than a single IUI within a cycle

24. After an insemination, women undergoing IUI should have a bed rest of:
    a. 10–15 minutes
    b. 15–30 minutes
    c. 30–45 minutes
    d. 45–60 minutes

25. Which of the following is not true for the optimal method of timing in natural or stimulated IUI cycles?
    IUI in a natural (not ovarian stimulated) cycle should be performed 1 day after LH rise
    a. If a human chorionic gonadotropin (hCG) injection is used, single IUI can be performed any time between 24 and 40 hours after hCG injection
    b. Monitoring follicle growth by ultrasound combined with hCG injection is better than LH testing for determining the timing of IUI in a natural cycle
    c. Providers can determine the method of timing in IUI in natural cycles [no ovarian stimulation (OS)] as there is no evidence to recommend for or against a method

26. How can you prevent multiple pregnancies in an IUI program?
    a. IUI should be withheld when more than two dominant follicles >20 mm or more than five follicles >15 mm are present at the time of hCG injection or LH surge
    b. IUI should be withheld when more than two dominant follicles >20 mm or more than five follicles >10 mm are present at the time of hCG injection or LH surge
    c. IUI should be withheld when more than two dominant follicles >15 mm or more than five follicles >10 mm are present at the time of hCG injection or LH surge
    d. IUI should be withheld when more than two dominant follicles >15 mm or more than five follicles >8 mm are present at the time of hCG injection or LH surge

27. The most common risk factor associated with OS with gonadotrophin is:
    a. Multiple pregnancy
    b. Birth defects
    c. Gestational diabetes mellitus (GDM)
    d. Ovarian hyperstimulation syndrome (OHSS)

28. As an alternative to cycle cancellation, aspiration of excess follicles at the time of hCG injection or LH surge might be additional options for reducing the risk of multiple pregnancies in IUI OS.
    a. True   b. False

29. Which of the following is not an indication for IUI with donor sperm?
    a. Repeated failure at IVF/ICSI
    b. Azoospermia
    c. Hereditary disease in male partner
    d. Severe hypospadias

30. What are the indications of using husband's frozen semen?
    a. Vasectomy
    b. Post antineoplastic treatment
    c. Absentee husband
    d. All of the above

ANSWERS

1. **a.** In couples with unexplained infertility and men with a total motile sperm count (TMSC) above 10 million, IUI should be combined with OS to improve live birth rates. In case of allergy to seminal plasma, IUI should be the choice as the prepared semen sample is free of plasma. In mild-to-moderate endometriosis, there is a 7–8% chance of pregnancy with IUI.
   [Reference: Cohlen B, Bijkerk A, Van der Poel S, Ombelet W. IUI: Review and systematic assessment of the evidence that supports global recommendations. Hum Reprod Update. 2018;24(3):300-19]

2. **d.** In couples with unexplained infertility with a prognosis of becoming pregnant without assistance within the next 12 months (estimate >30%), IUI could be postponed for at least 6 months. In couples with unexplained infertility and men with a TMSC >10 million and a prognosis of spontaneous pregnancy <30% within a year, it is recommended that IUI plus OS is the treatment of first choice.
   [Reference: Cohlen B, Bijkerk A, Van der Poel S, Ombelet W. IUI: Review and systematic assessment of the evidence that supports global recommendations. Hum Reprod Update. 2018;24(3):300-19]

3. **a.** In couples with an indication for IUI, at least three consecutive IUI cycles should be performed. There is insufficient evidence to recommend the maximum number of IUI treatment cycles. The majority of pregnancies occur within the first six cycles.
   [Reference: Cohlen B, Bijkerk A, Van der Poel S, Ombelet W. IUI: Review and systematic assessment of the evidence that supports global recommendations. Hum Reprod Update. 2018;24(3):300-19]

4. **c.** In order to prevent high rates of multiple gestation pregnancies in IUI OS, IUI should be withheld when more than two dominant follicles >15 mm or more than five follicles >10 mm at the time of hCG injection or LH surge are present. There is a general agreement in the literature that chances of success are better after mild ovarian stimulation and the maturation of a maximum of two or three follicles. However, the cycle must be monitored by ultrasound and hormonal analysis.
   [Reference: Cohlen B, Bijkerk A, Van der Poel S, Ombelet W. IUI: Review and systematic assessment of the evidence that supports global recommendations. Hum Reprod Update. 2018;24(3):300-19]

5. **d.** The established standard prediction model for natural conception is the Hunault model, also known as the synthesis model, which was based on the original data collected in three cohorts of subfertile couples between 1974 and 1995. It is the one with the best calibration and has been externally validated of all the prediction models for natural conception. Data used for construction of the model was restricted to a subfertile population in whom female age was <40 years and in whom any tubal pathology and azoospermia had been excluded.
   [Reference: Hunault CC, Habbema JD, Eijkemans MJ, Collins JA, Evers JL, te Velde ER. Two new prediction rules for spontaneous pregnancy leading to live birth among subfertile couples, based on the synthesis of three previous models. Hum Reprod. 2004;19(9):2019-26]

6. **d.** This model is not valid for a female with tubal pathology. The synthesis of Hunault model encompasses five predictors: Female age, duration of subfertility, whether female subfertility is primary or secondary, sperm motility, and referral status.
   [Reference: Hunault CC, Habbema JD, Eijkemans MJ, Collins JA, Evers JL, te Velde ER. Two new prediction rules for spontaneous pregnancy leading to live birth among subfertile couples, based on the synthesis of three previous models. Hum Reprod. 2004;19(9):2019-26]

7. **d.**

8. **b.** Prolonged period of abstinence leads to increased ROS in the sample, thereby increasing DNA fragmentation, dead sperms, and debris. Recently, studies have shown that abstinence of 2 days produced the highest pregnancy rate. This higher conception rate occurred despite a decrease in the total number of motile sperms.
   [Reference: Sanchez-Martín P, Sánchez-Martin F, González-Martínez M, Gosálvez J. Increased pregnancy after reduced male abstinence. Syst Biol Reprod Med. 2013;59(5):256-60]

9. **d.** Swim-up, gradient, wash and centrifugation are the three different semen preparation techniques for IUI.
   [Reference: Cohlen B, Bijkerk A, Van der Poel S, Ombelet W. IUI: Review and systematic assessment of the evidence that supports global recommendations. Hum Reprod Update. 2018;24(3):300-19]

10. **d.** The direct swim-up method is used for semen with normal parameters. It is not used for viscous samples.

The pellet swim-up method is used for normal or marginally abnormal semen samples. It is the method of choice for viscous samples.
[Reference: Palshetkar N (Ed). (2011). FOGSI Focus Advanced Infertility Management. (online) Available from: https://www.fogsi.org/wp-content/uploads/fogsi-focus/advances_infertility.pdf (Last accessed December 2023)]

11. **a.** It can be used for normal semen sample also.
[Reference: Palshetkar N (Ed). (2011). FOGSI Focus Advanced Infertility Management. (online) Available from: https://www.fogsi.org/wp-content/uploads/fogsi-focus/advances_infertility.pdf (Last accessed December 2023)]

12. **d.** These samples after the test cannot be used for fertilization as they are placed in hypo-osmotic saline solution.
(Reference: World Health Organization. WHO Laboratory Manual for the Examination and Processing of Human Semen, 5th edition. Geneva: World Health Organization; 2010)

13. **b.** The cutoff value is estimated to be 60%
The cutoff value is 15–20%. The good results comes with 15% or less of that DNA sperm fragmentations.

14. **d.** *(Reference: World Health Organization. WHO Laboratory Manual for the Examination and Processing of Human Semen, 5th edition. Geneva: World Health Organization; 2010)*

15. **a.** The criterion used for donor sperm in IUI with donor is that the volume should be >2 mL.
[Reference: Sharma RS, Bhargava PM, Chandhiok N, Saxena NC (Eds). Code of practice, ethical considerations and legal issues. National Guidelines for Accreditation, Supervision and Regulation of ART Clinics in India. New Delhi: Indian Council of Medical Research; 2005]

16. **a.** Clomiphene citrate remains the first-line medical treatment and can be given for up to 12 months. Anovulatory women with PCOS and BMI >25 kg/m^2, who have not responded to clomiphene alone, may be offered metformin in addition.
[Reference: European Society of Human Reproduction and Embryology. (2008). Good Clinical Treatment in Assisted Reproduction-An ESHRE position paper. (online) Available from: https://www.eshre.eu/-/media/sitecore-files/Guidelines/Guidelines/Position-Papers/GCT-in-ART.pdf (Last accessed December 2023)]

17. **d.** The seminal plasma also contains decapitation factor(s) that needs to be removed for complete capacitation of the spermatozoa. This process of capacitation is essential for both fertilizations, in vivo or in vitro; hence, spermatozoa to be used in IUI must be separated from the seminal plasma and its decapacitating factors. Preparation of human semen samples should also result in the removal of nonviable spermatozoa, leukocytes and/or bacteria, and other sources of contamination. Thawed sperm is mostly used for IUI as compared to intracervical insemination, as supported by older evidence.
[References: Cohlen B, Bijkerk A, Van der Poel S, Ombelet W. IUI: Review and systematic assessment of the evidence that supports global recommendations. Hum Reprod Update. 2018;24(3):300-19.
Besselink MG, Van Santvoort HC, Buskens E, Boermeester MA, van Goor H, Timmerman HM, et al. Probiotic prophylaxis in predicted severe acute pancreatitis: a randomised, double-blind, placebo-controlled trial. Lancet. 2008;371(9613):651-9]

18. **c.** Gonadotrophin therapy is appropriate for women who fail to ovulate or conceive with antiestrogen therapy (CC) or have hypothalamic failure or dysfunction.
[Reference: European Society of Human Reproduction and Embryology. (2008). Good Clinical Treatment in Assisted Reproduction-An ESHRE position paper. (online) Available from: https://www.eshre.eu/-/media/sitecore-files/Guidelines/Guidelines/Position-Papers/GCT-in-ART.pdf (Last accessed December 2023)].

19. **b.** Clomiphene citrate remains the first-line medical treatment and can be given for up to 12 months. Anovulatory women with PCOS and BMI >25 kg/m^2, who have not responded to clomiphene alone, may be offered metformin in addition. GT is appropriate for women who fail to ovulate or conceive with antiestrogen therapy (clomiphene citrate) or have hypothalamic failure or dysfunction.
[Reference: European Society of Human Reproduction and Embryology. (2008). Good Clinical Treatment in Assisted Reproduction-An ESHRE position paper. (online) Available from: https://www.eshre.eu/-/media/sitecore-files/Guidelines/Guidelines/

Position-Papers/GCT-in-ART.pdf (Last accessed December 2023)].

20. **b.** *[Reference: Palshetkar N (Ed). (2011). FOGSI Focus Advanced Infertility Management. (online) Available from: https://www.fogsi.org/wp-content/uploads/fogsi-focus/advances_infertility.pdf (Last accessed December 2023)]*

21. **b.** *[Reference: Carvalho WAP, Catafesta E, Rodart IF, Takata S, Estevam DL, Barbosa CP. Prevention of HIV transmission with sperm washing within fertile serodiscordant couples undergoing non-stimulated intrauterine insemination. AIDS Care. 2021;33(4):478-85. doi: 10.1080/09540121.2020. 1739201. Epub 2020 Mar 16. PMID: 32178530]*

22. **d.** *[Reference: NHS UK. (2020). Accessing IUI on the NHS. (online) Available from: https://www.nhs.uk/conditions/artificial-insemination/#:~:text= Accessing%20IUI%20on%20the%20NHS,need%20 specific%20help%20to%20conceive. (Last accessed December 2023)].*

23. **a.** Women undergoing IUI should be offered a single insemination per cycle. In both unexplained and male infertility there is insufficient evidence that the intervention, a double IUI, within the same cycle will lead to better pregnancy rates than a single IUI within a cycle.
[Reference: Cohlen B, Bijkerk A, Van der Poel S, Ombelet W. IUI: Review and systematic assessment of the evidence that supports global recommendations. Hum Reprod Update. 2018;24(3):300-19]

24. **a.** Women undergoing IUI, should have 10–15 minutes of bed rest after an insemination.
[Reference: Cohlen B, Bijkerk A, Van der Poel S, Ombelet W. IUI: Review and systematic assessment of the evidence that supports global recommendations. Hum Reprod Update. 2018;24(3):300-19]

25. **c.** There is no such evidence available that one of these methods is better than another.
[Reference: Cohlen B, Bijkerk A, Van der Poel S, Ombelet W. IUI: Review and systematic assessment of the evidence that supports global recommendations. Hum Reprod Update. 2018;24(3):300-19]

26. **c.** In order to prevent high rates of multiple gestation pregnancies in IUI OS, IUI should be withheld when more than two dominant follicles >15 mm or more than five follicles >10 mm at the time of hCG injection or LH surge are present.
[Reference: Cohlen B, Bijkerk A, Van der Poel S, Ombelet W. IUI: Review and systematic assessment of the evidence that supports global recommendations. Hum Reprod Update. 2018;24(3):300-19]

27. **a.** The most common side effects of IUI in cycles with OS are multiple pregnancies and OHSS. However, OHSS is very rare in IUI OS treatment because the aim of the stimulation protocol should be two to three dominant follicles. Regular ultrasound monitoring should identify any hyper-response early, such that HCG to induce ovulation can be withheld to avoid OHSS. With an adequate program to prevent multiple pregnancies, OHSS should be rarely encountered.
[References: Cohlen B, Bijkerk A, Van der Poel S, Ombelet W. IUI: Review and systematic assessment of the evidence that supports global recommendations. Hum Reprod Update. 2018;24(3):300-19.
Van Rumste MM, Custers IM, Van der Veen F, Van Wely M, Evers JL, Mol BW. The influence of the number of follicles on pregnancy rates in intrauterine insemination with ovarian stimulation: a meta-analysis. Hum Reprod Update. 2008;14(6):563-70]

28. **a.** It is a good practice point to aspirate excess follicles at the time of hCG injection or LH surge as an alternative to cycle cancelation for reducing the risk of multiple pregnancy in IUI OS.
[References: Cohlen B, Bijkerk A, Van der Poel S, Ombelet W. IUI: Review and systematic assessment of the evidence that supports global recommendations. Hum Reprod Update. 2018;24(3):300-19]

29. **d.** *(Reference: Taylor HS, Pal L, Seli E. Speroff's Clinical Gynecologic Endocrinology and Infertility. 9th edition. Philadelphia: Lippincott Williams & Wilkins; 2019)*

30. **d.** *(Reference: Taylor HS, Pal L, Seli E. Speroff's Clinical Gynecologic Endocrinology and Infertility. 9th edition. Philadelphia: Lippincott Williams & Wilkins; 2019)*

Chapter 76

In vitro Fertilization

Shreedevi Tanksale, Tejal Poddar

QUESTIONS

1. All of the following can be used as predictors of ovarian response to controlled ovarian stimulation (COS), *except:*
   a. Serum anti-müllerian hormone (AMH) and antral follicle count (AFC)
   b. Basal follicle-stimulating hormone (FSH) levels
   c. Duration of infertility
   d. Previous in vitro fertilization (IVF) response

2. Gonadotrophin-releasing hormone (GnRH) antagonist protocol is associated with:
   a. Increased number of retrieved oocytes as compared to GnRh agonist
   b. Longer duration of stimulation as compared to agonist protocol
   c. Lower incidence of ovarian hyperstimulation syndrome (OHSS)
   d. Increased chances of cycle cancellation

3. Bologna criteria for poor ovarian responders include all of the following, *except:*
   a. Advanced age >40 years
   b. Serum AMH value <0.5–1.1 ng/mL
   c. Day 5 estradiol level <100 pg/mL
   d. In previous COS cycles, using conventional stimulation protocols, three or less oocytes were retrieved.

4. Two cell–two-gonadotrophin theory suggests that steroidogenesis is a result of the action of gonadotrophins. FSH and luteinizing hormone (LH) act on the granulosa and theca cells through receptors to promote production of estradiol. LH stimulated conversion of ____ to ____ in ____ cells.
   a. Dehydroepiandrosterone (DHEA), testosterone, theca
   b. Androgen, estradiol, theca
   c. Cholesterol, androstenedione, theca
   d. Androstenedione, estradiol, granulosa

5. All of the following statements are true about GnRH antagonists, *except:*
   a. Antagonists have a direct inhibitory, reversible suppression on gonadotrophin secretion
   b. Initial flare-up effect followed by suppression of FSH and LH hormones
   c. As compared to agonist analogs, a higher dose of antagonists is required for effective pituitary suppression
   d. A constant supply of antagonists is required for effective pituitary suppression

6. The endometrial pattern and thickness are noted during ovarian stimulation in IVF. Endometrial pattern is considered a key factor in implantation and successful pregnancy outcomes following assisted reproductive technology (ART). Which of the following best describes a type A endometrium?
   a. Isoechoic endometrium with less defined outer myometrium and central echogenic line
   b. Hyperechoic endometrium with subendometrial linear striations
   c. Multilayered endometrium with hyperechogenic two outer and one central lines with hypoechoic endometrium in between
   d. Homogenous endometrium

7. Hormonal changes occur during the menstrual cycle. Which of the following events occurs during the periovulatory phase of menstrual cycle?
   a. Estradiol (E2) levels start to increase
   b. Dominant follicle gets selected
   c. FSH declines
   d. First meiotic division of oocyte is completed

8. The figure shows the protocol for frozen embryo transfer (FET). Identify the protocol used for FET.

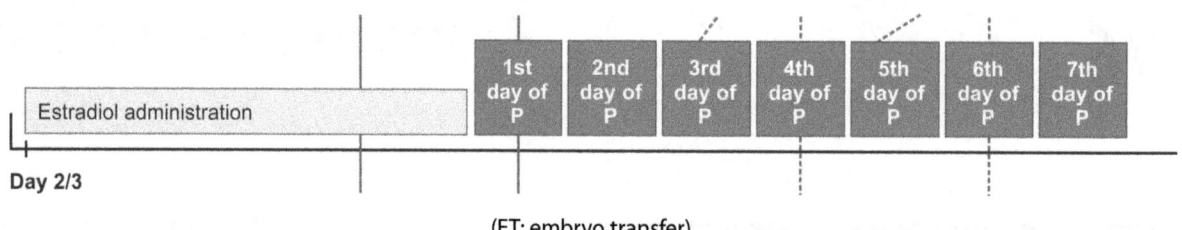

(ET: embryo transfer)

   a. Modified natural cycle
   b. Hormone replacement therapy (HRT)
   c. Downregulated FET
   d. Stimulated FET

9. Y chromosome microdeletion is the second most common genetic etiology in male factor infertility. Which of the following statements is true about Y chromosome microdeletion?
   a. Microdeletions are more commonly seen in the long arm of Y chromosome
   b. There is no risk of transmission from father to son
   c. There is complete absence of Y chromosome
   d. Y chromosome microdeletions are mapped to four regions

10. Which of the following events occurs during the implantation of an embryo?
    a. After fertilization, in the ampullary region, the embryo moves in the tubal lumen due to rhythmic contractions and ciliary movement in the cornual-ampullary direction
    b. Blastocyst rolls for 2 days in the uterine cavity before the onset of hatching
    c. Embryo implantation events occur in the sequence of penetration, apposition, and adhesion
    d. Interleukins play an important role in adhesion of embryo

11. The European Society of Human Reproduction and Embryology (ESHRE) Preimplantation Genetic Diagnosis (PGD) consortium described recurrent implantation failure (RIF) as failure to achieve objective evidence of pregnancy after:
    a. Transfer of 3 top-quality embryos (TQEs)
    b. Transfer of ≥10 embryos in multiple transfers
    c. Transfer of ≥2 embryos by a senior fertility specialist
    d. Both a and b

12. A 28-year-old female comes to your clinic. She is married for 2 years and trying to conceive for the last 12 months. After taking history and physical examination, which of the following tests would you recommend?
    a. Hysterosalpingography (HSG)
    b. Hormonal profile and husband's semen analysis
    c. Hysterolaparoscopy
    d. Hormonal, ultrasonography, HSG, and karyotyping of only female partner

13. As per American Society for Reproductive Medicine (ASRM)–Society for Assisted Reproductive Technology (SART) guidelines, how many euploid embryos in the blastocyst stage can be transferred in a woman aged 40 years and more?
    a. 2
    b. 1
    c. 2–3
    d. 4

14. Which of the following conditions is an indication for cryopreservation of embryos and FET, *except*?
    a. On the day of pickup, progesterone level >1.5 ng
    b. Agonist trigger given for oocyte retrieval
    c. Excess endometrial contractions with fluid in the endometrial cavity and delayed growth potential in embryos
    d. Endometrial grading on Applebaum criteria shows endometrial blood flow in zone 4

15. Identify the embryo in the figure.

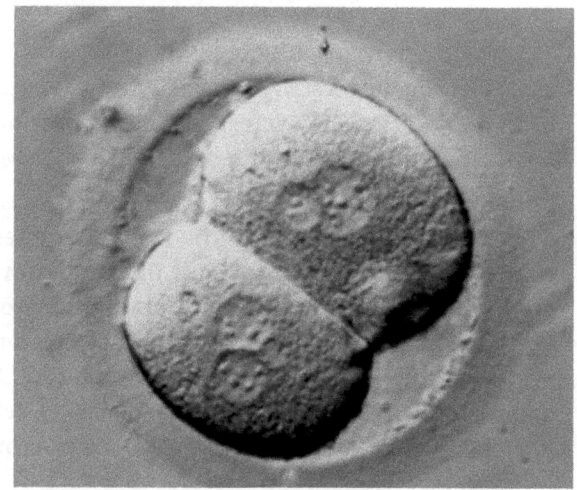

a. Triploid embryo
b. Premature chromosomal condensation
c. Euploid embryo
d. Binucleated embryo

16. **With regards to conceiving using ART in women with advanced-stage endometriosis, which of the following statements is true?**
    a. Ovulation induction alone is a valid treatment option
    b. IVF-embryo transfer (ET) is considered as first-line treatment with good success rates
    c. Medical therapy prior to assisted reproduction increases success rates
    d. Surrogacy is the option for such couples

17. **As per the WHO 2021, Which of the following parameters is correct value for the fifth percentile (with 95% confidence interval) of semen parameters from men in couples starting a pregnancy within one year of unprotected sexual intercourse leading to a natural conception?**
    a. Total motility—42%
    b. Immotile sperm—68%
    c. Semen volume—1.1 mL
    d. Abnormal forms—6%

18. **Identify the part marked by arrow in the figure.**

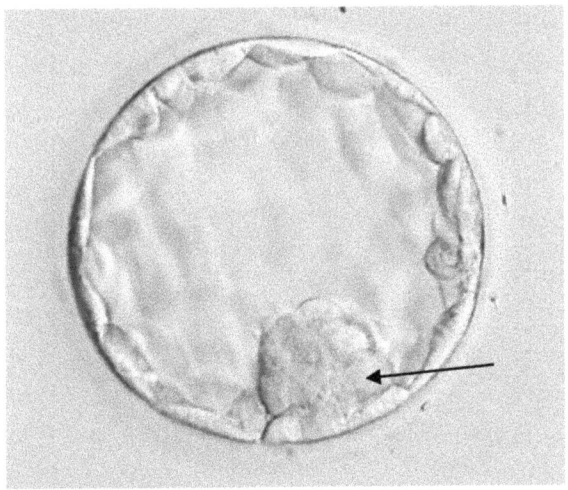

    a. Trophectoderm   b. Zona pellucida
    c. Inner cell mass d. Blastocoel

19. **Which of the following statements is true regarding female gametogenesis, *except*?**
    a. During prefertilization, there is completion of meiosis I and release of first polar body
    b. After ovulation, the oocyte is arrested in prophase of meiosis II until fertilization
    c. At fertilization, the secondary oocyte completes meiosis II to form a mature oocyte (23,1N) and a second polar body
    d. All primary oocytes are formed by the fifth month of fetal life and remain dormant in prophase of meiosis I until puberty

20. **A 28-year-old female with previous two miscarriages comes to you with a 3D ultrasound report. The image is as shown the figure. What would be your next line of management considering all her other parameters are within normal range?**

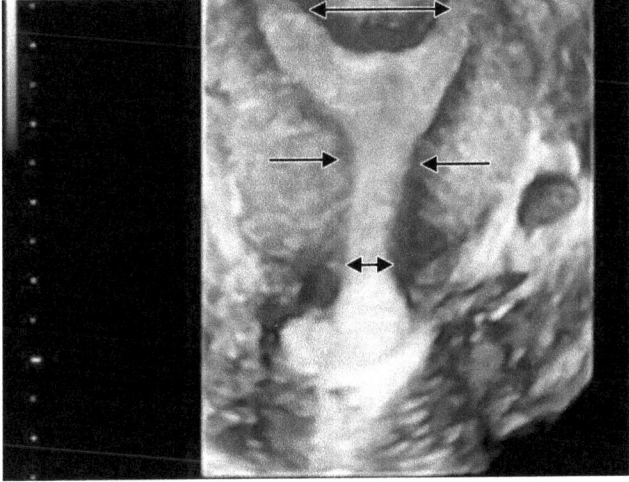

    a. IVF-ET using antagonist protocol
    b. Surrogacy
    c. Ovulation induction with gonadotrophins and intrauterine insemination (IUI)
    d. Hysteroscopy

21. **As per the 2023 meta-analysis and guidelines, which of the following is the first line of oral ovulogen for anovulatory polycystic ovary syndrome (PCOS) patients?**
    a. Letrozole
    b. Clomiphene citrate
    c. Clomiphene citrate + metformin
    d. Gonadotrophins

22. **Assessment of embryo quality is an important step in the success of ART procedure. Identify which is the correct assessment.**
    a. Day 2 at 42 hours post insemination with two-cell stage
    b. Day 3 at 68 hours post insemination with eight-cell stage

c. Day 4 at 84 hours post insemination with morula stage
d. Day 5 at 120 hours insemination with compacted stage

23. In hyperresponders, what is the preferred choice of IVF protocol?
    a. Long agonist
    b. Antagonist protocol with agonist trigger
    c. Short protocol
    d. Ultrashort protocol

24. These are the steps of afterloading ET procedure. Arrange them as per actual order of events.
    1. Introduction of speculum
    2. Loading of inner catheter
    3. Introducing the outer catheter
    4. Identification of the patient and confirmation of embryos

    a. 2, 3, 1, 4   b. 4, 1, 3, 2
    c. 1, 2, 3, 4   d. 4, 3, 2, 1

25. Which protocol is described in the following figure?

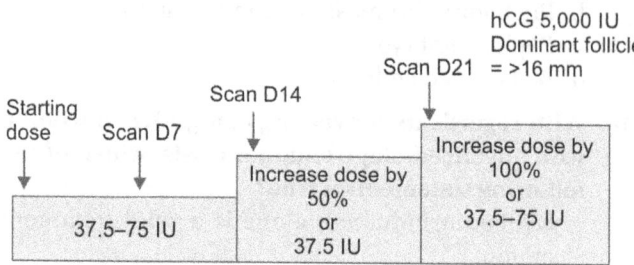

Treatment cycles long –28–35 days
Multiple folliculogenesis and OHSS less
(hCG: human chorionic gonadotropin; OHSS: ovarian hyperstimulation syndrome)

    a. Chronic low-dose step-up protocol
    b. Step-down protocol
    c. Conventional step-up protocol
    d. Sequential regimen

26. All of the following drugs are GnRH agonists, *except:*
    a. Triptorelin   b. Cetrorelix
    c. Leuprolide   d. Buserelin

27. Identify the correct hormone in the box marked the following figure.

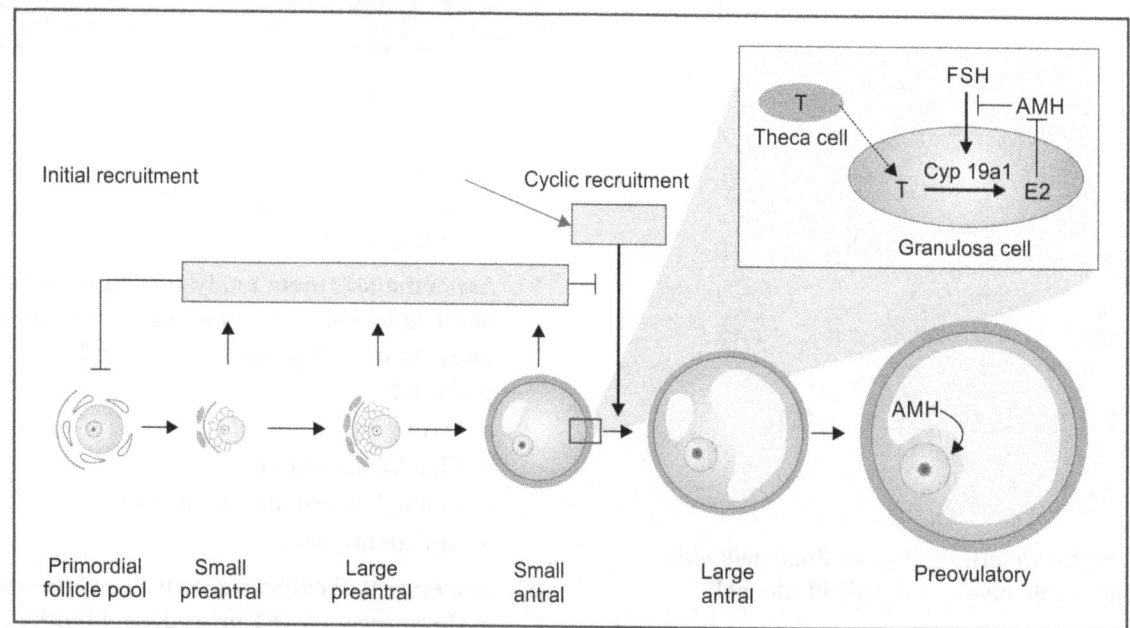

(AMH: anti-müllerian hormone; FSH: follicle stimulating hormone)

    a. FSH
    b. LH
    c. Estradiol
    d. Anti-müllerian hormone (AMH)

28. **Which of the following is the basic principle of oocyte pickup, *except*?**
    a. The ovary should be lined up to the most accessible position on the screen
    b. It is advisable to keep the needle at the edge of the aspirating follicle
    c. Identify the echogenic tip of the needle at all times
    d. Aspiration of follicular fluid is done using a suction pump

29. **As per the Government of India ART Rules 2022, which of the following is not a responsibility of the gynecologist at ART clinic?**
    a. Interviewing of the infertile couple initially, history taking, and physical examination of the female
    b. Recommending appropriate tests to be carried out, interpreting them, and treating medical disorders (such as infections and endocrine anomalies)
    c. Carrying out gynecological endoscopy and ultrasonographic intervention for diagnosis and therapy of infertility
    d. Providing adequate anesthesia comfort and pain relief to the patients during oocyte retrieval and embryo transfer procedures

30. **As per the ART Rules 2022, which of the following is not needed in a level 1 ART clinic?**
    a. Centrifuge machine
    b. Ultrasound machine
    c. Laminar air flow
    d. Micromanipulator

ANSWERS

1. **c.** Treatment individualization in IVF depends on predicting individual response to COS. AMH, basal FSH, and basal estradiol are the blood markers, while AFC and the ovarian volume are the ultrasound markers.

2. **c.** Gonadotrophin-releasing hormone antagonist protocols are associated with a reduction in OHSS, reduction in cycle cancellation, lesser duration of stimulation as compared to agonist cycle, and also slightly reduced number of retrieved oocytes as compared to agonist protocol.

3. **c.** The Bologna criteria were released to standardize the definition of poor ovarian response (POR) and pave the way for the formulation of evidence-based, efficient modalities of treatment for women undergoing IVF-ET. An agreement was reached on the minimal criteria needed to define POR. At least two of the following three criteria had to be present to establish the definition:
    - Advanced maternal age (>40 years) or any other risk factor for POR
    - A previous POR (≤3 oocytes with a conventional stimulation protocol)
    - An abnormal ovarian reserve test (i.e., AFC less than 5–7 follicles or AMH <0.5–1.1 ng/mL).

4. **c.** According to the two-cell-two-gonadotrophin theory, LH stimulates thecal cells to produce androgens, and FSH stimulates granulosa cells to produce estrogens from androgens. LH stimulates conversion of cholesterol to androstenedione in theca cells. Androstenedione diffuses into the granulosa cells, where under the influence of FSH, it is aromatized to estrogens. The classic *two-cell–two-gonadotrophin model* of estrogen synthesis was first proposed by Armstrong et al. in 1979.

5. **b.** Suppression achieved by GnRH antagonists is immediate, having no flare-up effect. There is no receptor loss, so a constant supply of antagonists is needed to keep receptors occupied. Consequently, as compared to dot agonist, a higher dose of antagonists is needed to maintain effective pituitary suppression.

6. **c.** Synchronized endometrial maturation and embryo development is the key to successful pregnancy. Type A pattern is a triple-line endometrium with hyperechoic outer lines and a prominent central line. Hyperechoic endometrium with subendometrial linear striations is usually associated with adenomyosis.

7. **d.** Periovulatory events consist of completion of the first meiotic division of oocyte, luteinization of granulosa cells, LH surge, and ovulation. Rest of the events described occur in early and mid-follicular phases.

8. **b.** Hormone replacement therapy cycles for FET were first introduced by Lutjen et al. in 1984. HRT involves supplementing with estrogen in the follicular phase in incremental doses. Starting estrogen prior to day 4 of cycle prevents selection of dominant follicle. HRT is a one of the most frequently used protocols for FET.

9. **a.** Y chromosome microdeletion is described as the absence of DNA segments or genes from functionally active Y chromosome. These occur mostly in the long

arm of Y chromosome and in three regions, namely AZFa, AZFb, and AZFc. There is a genetic risk of transmitting these microdeletions to the sons.

10. **b.** After fertilization, the embryo moves by contraction in the ampullary–cornual direction. It rolls in the uterine cavity to find a favorable place for implantation. Implantation occurs as apposition, adhesion, penetration, and invasion. Interleukins are responsible for apposition of embryo to endometrium.

11. **d.** The ESHRE guidelines define RIF as failure to achieve objective evidence of pregnancy after transfer of three TQEs or transfer of ≥10 embryos in multiple transfers.

12. **b.** Since the couple is trying for 1 year, basic hormonal workup of the female partner and semen analysis of the male are the basic investigations recommended. Evaluation of tubal patency is not to be considered at the first visit unless indicated by history.

13. **b.** In an effort to promote singleton gestations, reduce twin gestations, and eliminate high-order multiple gestations, the ASRM and SART have developed guidance to assist ART programs and patients in determining the appropriate number of cleavage-stage embryos or blastocysts to transfer. The guidelines recommend transferring a single euploid day 5 embryo in a woman aged 40 years and above.

14. **d.** Cryopreservation and FET are increasingly being used for multiple indications including elevated progesterone on the day of pickup, agonist trigger, and excess uterine contractility. Applebaum criteria showing endometrial blood flow till zone 4 is a receptive endometrium and does not indicate cryopreservation by itself.

15. **d.** This is an image of a binucleated embryo. Multinucleation in one or more blastomeres at the earliest stages of development would seem to be an unambiguous indicator of incompetence and pending demise because this defect should be, and generally is, associated with errors in chromosomal replication and segregation.

16. **b.** Ovulation induction alone, in the presence of tubal disease, is associated with a high risk of ectopic pregnancy. If a patient does not want to undergo surgery, IVF-ET is the ideal treatment of choice. Medical therapy is only of benefit in alleviating symptoms.

17. **a.** Total motility—42%

	WHO 2010	WHO 2021
Semen volume (mL)	1.5 (1.4–1.7)	1.4 (1.3–1.5)
Total sperm number (10^6 per ejaculate)	39 (33–46)	39 (35–40)
Total motility (%)	40 (38–42)	42 (40–43)
Progressive motility (%)	32 (31–34)	30 (29–31)
Nonprogressive motility (%)	1	1 (1–1)
Immotile sperm (%)	22	20 (19–20)
Vitality (%)	58 (55–63)	54 (50–56)
Normal forms (%)	4 (3–4)	4 (3.9–4)

18. **c.** The blastocyst possesses an inner cell mass (ICM), or embryoblast, which subsequently forms the embryo, and an outer layer of cells, or trophoblast, which later forms the placenta.

19. **b.** After *ovulation*, the oocyte is arrested in *metaphase of meiosis II* until fertilization. Rest all statements are true about oogenesis.

20. **d.** The 3D ultrasound image shows a T-shaped uterus. Considering her history of previous miscarriages, the next step should be correction with hysteroscopic lateral metroplasty.

21. **a.** Meta-analysis showed that letrozole was superior for ovulation rate (per patient and per cycle), pregnancy rate, clinical pregnancy rate, and live birth rate per patient. Certainty, the evidence is high for live birth rate and moderate for pregnancy rate, clinical pregnancy rate, and ovulation rate.
(Reference: Teede H, Tay CT, Laven J, Dokras A, Moran L, Piltonen T, et al. International Evidence-based Guideline for the assessment and management of polycystic ovary syndrome. Melbourne: Monash University; 2023)

22. **b.** A day 2 embryo is examined at 44 hours for four-cell stage. A day 3 embryo is examined 68 hours after insemination for eight-cell stage. A day 4 embryo is assessed at 92 hours for morula stage. A blastocyst is examined at 116 hours for a day 5 embryo.

23. **b.** The use of low-dose gonadotrophins with antagonist protocol and the use of GnRH agonist trigger is the most preferred protocols for hyperresponders to prevent OHSS.

24. **b.** In afterloading technique, after correctly identifying the patient, a speculum is inserted and an outer

catheter is introduced; later, a loaded inner catheter is introduced.

25. **a.** The principle behind this regimen is to find the *threshold* level of FSH which will lead to the development of a single preovulatory follicle. This regimen was proposed mainly by the ESHRE and ASRM Thessaloniki group joint consensus to prevent the OHSS. The key feature of this regimen is the low-starting dose (37.5–75 units/day) of drug and a stepwise increase in subsequent doses, if necessary, with the aim of achieving the development of a single dominant follicle rather than the development of many large follicles, so as to avoid the complications of OHSS and multiple pregnancies.

26. **b.** Cetrorelix is a GnRH antagonist. Rest all are GnRH agonists.

27. **a.** FSH is responsible for recruitment of follicles from antral stage to preovulatory phase.

28. **b.** It is advisable to keep the needle at the center of the follicle being aspirated. Rest all are standard guidelines for oocyte pickup.

29. **d.** The last option is the primary duty of anesthetist during oocyte retrieval.

30. **d.** Micromanipulator is used for intracytoplasmic sperm injection (ICSI), an essential requirement for a level 2 ART clinic.

Chapter 77: Preimplantation Genetic Diagnosis

Athulya Shajan

QUESTIONS

1. **What are the units involved in a preimplantation genetic diagnosis (PGD) program?**
   a. Clinical genetics unit only
   b. IVF unit only
   c. Diagnostic testing laboratories only
   d. All of the above

2. **What is the recommended method for insemination during polymerase chain reaction (PCR)-based diagnostic tests on single embryonic cells?**
   a. Conventional insemination
   b. In vitro fertilization (IVF)
   c. Intracytoplasmic sperm injection (ICSI)
   d. Fluorescence in situ hybridization (FISH)

3. **How should counseling be conducted in PGD/PGS programs, according to the guidelines?**
   a. By nonphysician healthcare providers only
   b. In the couple's own language or with the use of interpreters
   c. Exclusively by clinical geneticists
   d. Through written materials only, without face-to-face sessions

4. **Which category of PGD/PGS involves patients with repeated IVF failure?**
   a. High-risk PGD
   b. Preimplantation genetic screening (PGS)
   c. Preimplantation genetic diagnosis
   d. None of the above

5. **What is an essential aspect of patient counseling for preimplantation genetic diagnosis and preimplantation genetic screening?**
   a. The counseling should be directive
   b. Patients should be counseled by a nonprofessional
   c. The patient should be given only verbal information
   d. The counseling should be nondirective and conducted by suitably qualified professionals

6. **What is recommended regarding the testing for genetic disorders in PGD?**
   a. Testing should be done for all genetic disorders
   b. Testing should only be done for genetic disorders previously characterized for that couple
   c. Testing should only be done for genetic disorders previously identified in the population
   d. Testing is not necessary in PGD

7. **What should patients be counseled about regarding the decision-making process in PGD/PGS?**
   a. Decision making about the disposition of affected embryos or undiagnosed embryos
   b. Decision making about only the financial aspects of the procedure
   c. Decision making about only the ethical aspects of the procedure
   d. Decision making about the potential positive outcomes only

8. **Who is recommended for psychological evaluation?**
   a. Patients who refuse PGD/PGS procedures
   b. Patients with a history of reproductive failure or traumatic experiences
   c. All patients who are undergoing PGD/PGS procedures
   d. Patients who have successfully undergone PGD/PGS procedures

9. **What is the recommended status for the centers performing laboratory tests?**
   a. They should be approved by a local authority
   b. They should be approved by the State or a competent authority in the State

c. They should be approved by an international authority
d. They do not need to be approved

10. **What should be discussed with patients undergoing HLA testing?**
    a. The probability of all embryos being suitable for transfer
    b. The fate of unaffected, non-HLA-matched embryos
    c. The cost of HLA testing only
    d. The legal implications of HLA testing

11. **What documentation is recommended for IVF/PGD centers?**
    a. Genetic counseling report and original results of DNA testing
    b. Original results of DNA testing only
    c. Genetic counseling report only
    d. No documentation is necessary

12. **What is recommended regarding the culture and biopsy of embryos for PGD/PGS?**
    a. All cumulus cells should be left intact before biopsy
    b. Only cleavage-stage biopsy should be performed
    c. The embryo and blastomere identity should be checked throughout the procedure
    d. There is no need to check the embryo and blastomere identity

13. **What is the recommendation regarding the removal of cumulus cells during PGD/PGS?**
    a. They should not be removed
    b. They should be partially removed
    c. They should all be removed
    d. The decision to remove them should be made case by case

14. **What is the acceptable timing for the removal of the first polar body?**
    a. Between 18 and 22 h postinsemination
    b. Between 36 and 42 h post-hCG injection
    c. Immediately postinsemination
    d. Immediately post-hCG injection

15. **What is the recommended procedure for removing polar bodies?**
    a. Manual extraction   b. Aspiration
    c. Laser removal   d. Mechanical excision

16. **Which day postinsemination is recommended for a blastocyst biopsy?**
    a. Day 3   b. Day 4
    c. Day 5 or 6 d. Day 7

17. **How many cells are recommended to be removed safely during cleavage stage embryo biopsy?**
    a. One or two cells   b. Three or four cells
    c. Five or six cells   d. Seven or eight cells

18. **What is recommended for use in biopsy procedure for maintaining pH, osmolality, and temperature?**
    a. Standard IVF culture medium
    b. Commercial biopsy medium
    c. Acidified tyrode's solution
    d. "Home-brew" calcium, magnesium-free biopsy medium

19. **Which of the following probe sets is recommended for aneuploidy screening?**
    a. At least two chromosome pairs from 13, 14, 15, 16, 18, 21, 22, X and Y
    b. At least three chromosome pairs from 13, 14, 15, 16, 18, 21, 22, X and Y
    c. At least four chromosome pairs from 13, 14, 15, 16, 18, 21, 22, X and Y
    d. At least five chromosome pairs from 13, 14, 15, 16, 18, 21, 22, X and Y

20. **What is recommended to ensure transfer of the correct embryos?**
    a. Analyzing signals by two independent observers
    b. Analyzing signals by three independent observers
    c. Analyzing signals by a single observer
    d. Analyzing signals by the embryologist only

21. **Which of the following measures can be taken to reduce allelic dropout (ADO) during polymerase chain reaction or assay design?**
    a. Reducing denaturation temperatures
    b. Choosing suitable DNA polymerases
    c. Decreasing the use of lysis buffers
    d. Enlarging product size and primer sequence design

22. **What is recommended for identifying ADO when setting up any new test?**
    a. Incorporation of unlinked markers
    b. The use of a microsatellite or SNP as the marker
    c. Biopsy of a single cell
    d. Independent analysis of three cells

23. **In PCR protocols, what is recommended over conventional PCR due to its higher level of sensitivity?**
    a. Nested PCR   b. Multiplex PCR
    c. Fluorescent PCR d. Real-time PCR

24. **Which method is recommended for quality control and quality assurance in PGD and PGS?**
    a. Periodic external proficiency testing/assessment
    b. Random external proficiency testing/assessment
    c. Only internal quality control and quality assurance
    d. No specific quality control method is required

25. **What is the recommended maximum number of embryos to be transferred in favorable prognosis patients according to professional societies in Europe and the USA?**
    a. One
    b. Two
    c. Three
    d. Four

ANSWERS

1. **d.** Clinical genetics unit, IVF unit, and diagnostic testing laboratories
   The guidelines state that a PGD program requires the involvement of a clinical genetics unit, an IVF unit, and diagnostic testing laboratories.

2. **c.** Intracytoplasmic sperm injection
   ICSI is recommended as the method for insemination when performing a PCR-based diagnostic test on single embryonic cells.

3. **b.** In the couple's own language or with the use of interpreters
   The guidelines recommend that counseling should be conducted in the couple's own language or interpreters should be used.

4. **b.** Preimplantation genetic screening
   PGS is carried out for infertile patients undergoing IVF with the aim of increasing IVF pregnancy rates. This includes patients with repeated IVF failure.

5. **d.** The counseling should be nondirective and conducted by suitably qualified professionals.
   It is recommended that the patient has nondirective counseling with a suitably qualified professional(s) that includes the pertinent issues related to PGD/PGS.

6. **b.** Testing should only be done for genetic disorders previously characterized for that couple.
   Testing should be done only for genetic disorders previously characterized for that couple and for which testing is available.

7. **a.** Decision making about the disposition of affected embryos or undiagnosed embryos.
   Patients should be counseled about decision making concerning the disposition of affected embryos or undiagnosed embryos.

8. **b.** Patients with a history of reproductive failure or traumatic experiences.
   A psychological evaluation for patients is recommended with a history of reproductive failure, traumatic experiences, or couples for whom the team has concerns regarding the welfare of existing/future children or psychological well-being/mental capacity of future parents.

9. **b.** They should be approved by the State or a competent authority in the State.
   The centers in which laboratory tests are performed should be approved by the State or a competent authority in the State.

10. **b.** The fate of unaffected, non-HLA-matched embryos.
    The guidelines suggest that for HLA testing, the fate of unaffected, non-HLA-matched embryos should be discussed.

11. **a.** Genetic counseling report and original results of DNA testing.
    The guidelines recommend that the following documents, where applicable, should be made available to the IVF/PGD center: genetic counseling report, original results of DNA testing, and other relevant documentation.

12. **c.** The embryo and blastomere identity should be checked throughout the procedure.
    The guidelines strongly recommend that the embryo and blastomere identity is checked throughout the procedure so the diagnostic results can be unequivocally linked to specific embryos.

13. **c.** They should all be removed.
    Cumulus cells are removed before biopsy as these cells can contaminate both FISH and PCR diagnosis.

14. **b.** Between 36 and 42 h post-hCG injection
    The first polar body can be removed from the oocyte on the day of oocyte collection, which typically falls between 36 and 42 hours post-hCG injection.

15. **b.** Aspiration
    Polar bodies are typically removed via aspiration, which allows for a safe and effective procedure.

16. **c.** Day 5 or 6
    Blastocyst biopsy is recommended on the morning of day 5 or 6 postinsemination.

17. **a.** One or two cells
    The decision to remove one or two cells is based on many factors including the embryo cell number and the accuracy and reliability of the diagnostic test used.

18. **d.** "Home-brew" calcium, magnesium-free biopsy medium
    A calcium and magnesium-free biopsy medium is recommended to maintain pH, osmolality and temperature during the biopsy procedure.

19. **d.** At least five chromosome pairs from 13, 14, 15, 16, 18, 21, 22, X and Y
    For aneuploidy screening, a probe set of at least five chromosome pairs from 13, 14, 15, 16, 18, 21, 22, X and Y is recommended.

20. **a.** Analyzing signals by two independent observers
    Signals should be analyzed by two independent observers and discrepancies should be adjudicated by a third observer, when possible.

21. **b.** Choosing suitable DNA polymerases
    Rationale: The use of suitable DNA polymerases, increased denaturation temperatures, use of lysis buffers, and modification of primer sequence and product size can all contribute to minimizing ADO during PCR or assay design.

22. **b.** The use of a microsatellite or SNP as the marker.
    Rationale: The incorporation of linked markers is recommended when setting up any new test, especially to identify ADO. The marker ideally should be intragenic and could be a microsatellite or a single nucleotide polymorphism (SNP).

23. **c.** Fluorescent PCR
    Rationale: The guidelines recommend fluorescent PCR over conventional PCR, as it has a higher level of sensitivity and can reduce the likelihood of contamination and misdiagnosis due to errors in tube transfer.

24. **a.** Periodic external proficiency testing/assessment
    Rationale: The guidelines recommend the implementation of a voluntary system with proficiency testing/assessment performed at least annually for quality control and assurance in PGD and PGS.

25. **b.** Two
    Rationale: A maximum of two embryos should be transferred in favorable prognosis patients to avoid multiple gestations in routine IVF.

REFERENCES

1. Harton GL, Magli MC, Lundin K, Montag M, Lemmen J, Harper JC; European Society for Human Reproduction and Embryology (ESHRE) PGD Consortium/Embryology Special Interest Group. ESHRE PGD Consortium/Embryology Special Interest Group. best practice guidelines for polar body and embryo biopsy for preimplantation genetic diagnosis/screening (PGD/PGS). Hum Reprod. 2011;26(1):41-6.
2. Thornhill AR, deDie-Smulders CE, Geraedts JP, Harper JC, Harton GL, Lavery SA, et al.; ESHRE PGD Consortium. ESHRE PGD Consortium. Best practice guidelines for clinical preimplantation genetic diagnosis (PGD) and preimplantation genetic screening (PGS). Hum Reprod. 2005;20(1):35-48.

Chapter 78: Mullerian Anomalies

Shelly Agarwal

QUESTIONS

1. **A 17-year-old patient comes with complaints of primary amenorrhea. On examination, her height is in normal range and has well developed breast and pubic hair, with dimpling of vagina. Ultrasound reveals absent uterus.**
   Likely diagnosis is:
   a. Turner's syndrome
   b. Klinefelter's syndrome
   c. Gonadal agenesis
   d. Mullerian agenesis

2. **Following anomalies arise as a result of lateral fusion defect of the paired Mullerian ducts, *except*:**
   a. Bicornuate uterus
   b. Uterus didelphys
   c. Transverse vaginal septum
   d. Septate uterus

3. **A 19-year-old girl comes with complaints of primary amenorrhea with well-developed breast and grade II pubarche. The most likely diagnosis is:**
   a. Turner's syndrome
   b. Gonadal dysgenesis
   c. Mullerian agenesis
   d. Testicular feminization syndrome

4. **Ultrasound evaluation for Mullerian anomalies can be best timed during:**
   a. Menstrual phase
   b. Postmenstrual
   c. Preovulatory phase
   d. Secretory phase

5. **A 28-year-old woman, married for 4 years, comes with complaints of primary infertility. On workup, baseline investigations of both the partners are normal. Hysterosalpingogram (HSG) is performed. The report is attached as follows (refer to the figure next).**

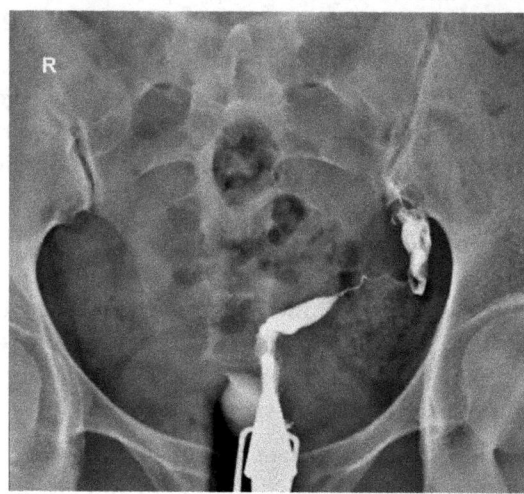

Source: Radiopaedia.org

   Your possible inference is all, *except*:
   a. Patient has good obstetrical outcomes when compared to uterus didelphys
   b. Malpresentations are common
   c. Pregnancy carries a risk of preterm labor
   d. Cervical incompetence is common and cerclage is indicated

6. **Which imaging technique is the preferred investigation for diagnosing any type of Mullerian anomalies?**
   a. Hysterosalpingography
   b. 3D ultrasound
   c. Magnetic resonance imaging (MRI)
   d. Saline infusion sonography

7. **Disorders of vertical fusion include all, *except*:**
   a. Transverse vaginal septum
   b. Uterus didelphys
   c. Cervical agenesis
   d. Imperforate hymen

8. **Which of the statement is incorrect regarding Mullerian Anomalies Classification (MAC), 2021?**
   a. T-shaped uterus is included as a uterine morphology in MAC 2021
   b. Septate uterus is defined as having an internal indentation depth >10 mm combined with an internal indentation angle <90°
   c. Normal/arcuate uterus has an internal indentation depth ≤10 mm and an internal indentation angle >90°
   d. Bicornuate uterus is defined as having an external fundal indentation depth >10 mm combined with an internal indentation angle >90°

9. **A 16-year-old girl presents with severe dysmenorrhea. An ultrasound scan showed a left unicornuate uterus with a right noncommunicating rudimentary horn distended with blood and right hematosalpinx. The most appropriate management for the same will be:**
   a. Excision of the rudimentary horn
   b. Hysterectomy
   c. Medical management with Dienogest
   d. Medical management with continuous oral contraceptive pills (OCPs)

10. **Diethylstilbestrol rarely causes:**
    a. Perifimbrial cyst
    b. Renal anomalies
    c. Clear cell cancer of vagina
    d. Vaginal adenosis

11. **A 35-year-old female presented to gyne outpatient department (OPD) with secondary infertility. As a part of infertility workup, hysterosalpingogram was performed.**

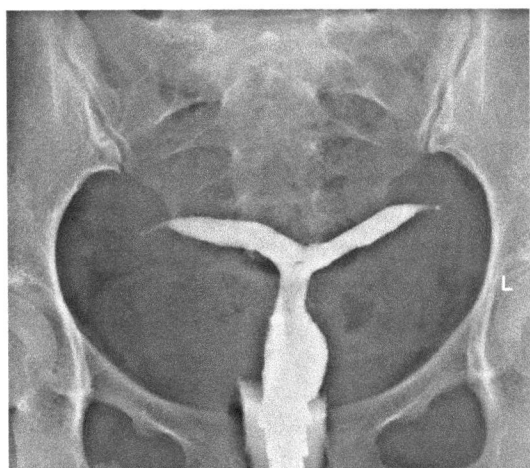

Source: Radiopedia

The angle between two uterine horns was estimated as 112°. The likely diagnosis is:
   a. Uterus didelphys
   b. Subseptate uterus
   c. Septate uterus
   d. Bicornuate uterus

12. **Identify the uterine anomaly.**
    a. Unicornuate uterus with a rudimentary horn
    b. Bicornuate uterus
    c. Septate uterus
    d. Uterus didelphys

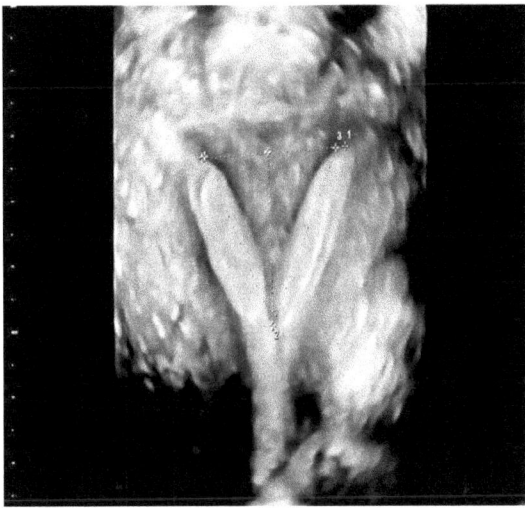

Source: Ultrasound in obstetrics and gynecology

13. **A 15-year-old girl presents in gyne OPD with complaints of primary amenorrhea and cyclic lower abdominal pain. The patient has well developed secondary sexual characters. On examination, there is partial agenesis of vagina with the presence of uterus. The likely diagnosis is:**
    a. MRKH (Mayer-Rokitansky-Küster-Hauser)
    b. Testicular feminization syndrome
    c. Vertical fusion defect
    d. Herlyn-Werner-Wunderlich syndrome

14. **A 29-year-old women, married for 1 year is anxious to conceive. She visits your gyne OPD with an ultrasound report of uterus didelphys. The most important indication for surgical repair (metroplasty) for this congenital anomaly will be:**
    a. Infertility
    b. Dysmenorrhea
    c. Heavy menstrual bleeding
    d. Recurrent pregnancy loss

15. **A patient with recurrent pregnancy loss undergoes a transcervical lysis of uterine septum. When should you allow her to conceive?**
    a. Immediately following operative hysteroscopy
    b. At least 2 months after the procedure
    c. At least 6 months after the procedure
    d. At least 1 year after the procedure

16. **A 19-year-old patient comes with complaints of primary amenorrhea. On examination, she has well-developed breast and pubic hair with dimpling of vagina. Ultrasound reveals absent uterus. Ideal time to repair for vaginal agenesis will be:**
    a. At birth
    b. At puberty
    c. Before marriage
    d. As soon as diagnosis is made

17. **Uterine septum is surgically excised from fundus in:**
    a. Strassman utriculoplasty
    b. Tompkin's operation
    c. Modified Jones metroplasty
    d. Hysteroscopic septal resection

18. **OHVIRA (obstructed hemivagina and ipsilateral renal anomaly) syndrome is unilateral obstructed hemivagina and ipsilateral renal agenesis associated with:**
    a. Unicornuate uterus
    b. Bicornuate uterus
    c. Septate uterus
    d. Uterus didelphys

19. **A 36-year-old female with complaints of secondary infertility and history of repeated pregnancy losses comes for evaluation. Workup shows a septate uterus on hysteroscopy. An abdominal unification operation is performed.**
    Which of the following is not correct regarding metroplasty?
    a. Scar after unification is not as strong as the scar formed after cesarean
    b. Endomyometritis is a common complication after cesarean section but is not common after uterine unification
    c. Elective cesarean is recommended to patients having abdominal metroplasty
    d. Patients can deliver vaginally after a metroplasty by hysteroscope or resectoscope

20. **See next a hysteroscopic image of patient with recurrent spontaneous abortions. The likely pathology is:**

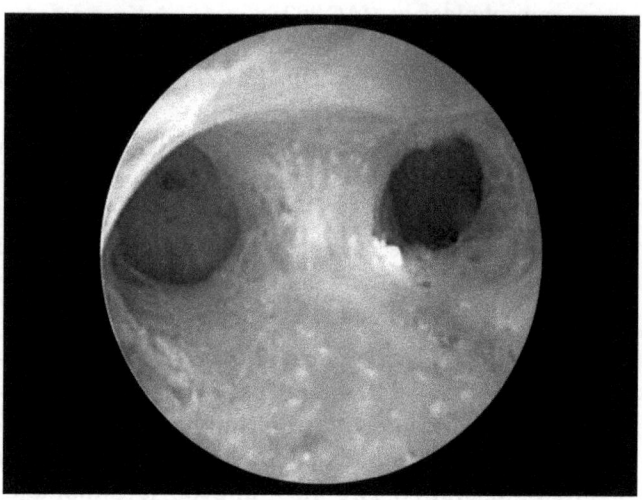

Source: ScienceDirect.com

    a. Normal uterine cavity   b. Arcuate uterus
    c. Asherman's syndrome   d. Septate uterus

21. **All of the following statements regarding classification of uterine anomalies are correct, *except*:**
    a. According to AFS-1988, diagnosis of septate uterus is based on subjective interpretation of anatomical type, using the coronal aspect of the uterus and without any measurable criteria
    b. According to ESHRE/ESGE (European Society of Human Reproduction and Embryology/European Society for Gynaecological Endoscopy) 2016, septate uterus diagnosed by external indentation depth is less, and internal indentation depth is greater, than 50% of uterine wall thickness, when uterine wall thickness is measured above interostial/intercornual line suggest that uterine wall thickness is the best objective benchmark for strict definition of uterine morphology
    c. According to ASRM (American Society for Reproductive Medicine), 2016, septate uterus is diagnosed by external fundal indentation depth is <1 cm, while internal fundal indentation depth is ≥1 cm
    d. According to Mullerian Anomalies Classification 2021, a septate uterus is defined as having an internal indentation depth >10 mm combined with an internal indentation angle <90°

CHAPTER 78: Mullerian Anomalies

22. **Which is the most common uterine anomaly?**
    a. Bicornuate uterus
    b. Septate uterus
    c. Unicornuate uterus
    d. Arcuate uterus

23. **Most common uterine malformation associated with renal anomalies is:**
    a. Bicornuate uterus
    b. Uterus didelphys
    c. Unicornuate uterus
    d. Septate uterus

24. **The most common congenital uterine anomaly which causes recurrent pregnancy loss is:**
    a. Septate uterus
    b. Uterine agenesis
    c. Bicornuate uterus
    d. Unicornuate uterus

25. **Ovary develops from:**
    a. Mullerian duct
    b. Genital tubercle
    c. Genital ridge
    d. Sinovaginal bulbs

26. **Vaginal epithelium is derived from:**
    a. Endoderm of urogenital sinus
    b. Endoderm of genital ridge
    c. Mesoderm of urogenital sinus
    d. Mesoderm of genital ridge

27. **Gartner duct is the remanent of the following embryological structure:**
    a. Mullerian duct
    b. Wolffian duct
    c. Genital tubercle
    d. Epoophoron

28. **A patient with primary infertility, anxious to conceive, comes to gynae OPD. Hysterosalpingography is performed which is suggestive of right unicornuate uterus. Considering its association with renal anomalies, an ultrasound upper abdomen is performed. The likelihood of finding a renal anomaly would be:**
    a. On right side
    b. On left side
    c. On both right or left side
    d. Could be either right or left side

29. **A 17-year-old female with primary amenorrhea visits gyne OPD. She has well-developed breast, but absent uterus and blind vagina. The next investigation to aid in diagnosis will be:**
    a. Serum follicle-stimulating hormone (FSH) and luteinizing hormone (LH) levels
    b. Karyotyping
    c. Gonadal biopsy
    d. Diagnostic laparoscopy

30. **SRY gene is located on:**
    a. Short arm of X chromosome
    b. Long arm of X chromosome
    c. Short arm of Y chromosome
    d. Long arm of Y chromosome

ANSWERS

1. **d.** In this patient, secondary sexual characteristics are well developed. Hence ovaries are not affected. Absence of uterus and dimpling of vagina suggest failure of paramesonephric duct to develop or in other words "Mullerian agenesis". This condition is also known as Mayer-Rokitansky-Küster-Hauser syndrome.
   [Reference: Rock JA, Breech LL. Surgery for anomalies of the Mullerian ducts. In: Rock JA, Jones HW III (Eds). Te Linde's Operative Gynecology, 10th edition. Philadelphia: Lippincott Williams & Wilkins; 2008. pp. 545-6]

2. **c.** Bicornuate uterus, uterus didelphys. and septate uterus are result of lateral fusion defect, whereas transverse vaginal septum, imperforate hymen, cervical agenesis, cervical dysgenesis, and partial vaginal agenesis are result of vertical fusion defect.
   [Reference: Rock JA, Breech LL. Surgery for anomalies of the Mullerian ducts. In: Rock JA, Jones HW III (Eds). Te Linde's Operative Gynecology, 10th edition. Philadelphia: Lippincott Williams & Wilkins; 2008. p. 539]

3. **d.** In case of a female presenting with primary amenorrhea with well-developed breast, but absent uterus and blind vagina, we primarily have to differentiate between MRKH (Mayer-Rokitansky-Küster-Hauser) (which is due to Mullerian agenesis) and testicular feminization syndrome, also known as androgen insensitivity syndrome or AIS (X-linked recessive gene defect where there is insensitivity to androgen receptor gene). In both these conditions, patient is phenotypically a female, but is genotypically different. Patients with MRKH are 46,XX while those with AIS are 46,XY. Grade II pubarche means scanty pubic hair which occurs in testicular feminization syndrome due to tissue receptor defect for normal androgens.
   (Reference: Konar H, Dutta DC. Disorders of sexual development. DC Dutta's Textbook of Gynecology,

8th edition. New Delhi: Jaypee Brothers Medical Publishers; 2020. p. 371)

4. **d.** At this time, endometrium is bright and echogenic and easy to visualize; therefore, more appropriate for evaluating congenital anomalies of the uterus.
(Reference: Hoffman B, Schorge J, Bradshaw K, Halvorson L, Schaffer J, Corton M. Anatomic disorders. William's Gynecology, 3rd edition. New York: McGraw-Hill Education; 2016. p. 418)

5. **a.** Unicornuate uterus has poor pregnancy outcomes. Abnormal shape, insufficient muscle mass of the uterus, reduced uterine volume, and inability to expand may explain poor reproductive performance.
[Reference: Rock JA, Breech LL. Surgery for anomalies of the Mullerian ducts. In: Rock JA, Jones HW III (Eds). Te Linde's Operative Gynecology, 10th edition. Philadelphia: Lippincott Williams & Wilkins; 2008. p. 574]

6. **c.** Magnetic resonance imaging is currently the preferred investigation for imaging Mullerian anomalies. It provides a clear delineation of both external and internal uterine anatomy and has reported an accuracy of up to 100%.

    Three-dimensional sonography can provide uterine image from virtually any angle. The coronal view can be constructed and help in evaluating internal and external uterine contours. Research suggest good concordance between 3D transvaginal ultrasonography (TVS) and magnetic resonance imaging, but MRI is still preferred for imaging complex defects.

    Hysterosalpingography and saline infusion sonography poorly define the external contour of the uterus and is used in women undergoing fertility evaluation.
(Reference: Hoffman B, Schorge J, Bradshaw K, Halvorson L, Schaffer J, Corton M. Anatomic disorders. William's Gynecology, 3rd edition. New York: McGraw-Hill Education; 2016. p. 418)

7. **b.** Uterus didelphys; it is a result of lateral fusion defect.
[Reference: Rock JA, Breech LL. Surgery for anomalies of the Mullerian ducts. In: Rock JA, Jones HW III (Eds). Te Linde's Operative Gynecology, 10th edition. Philadelphia: Lippincott Williams & Wilkins; 2008. p. 539]

8. **a.** T-shaped uterus is not included as a uterine morphology in MAC 2021.
[Reference: American Society for Reproductive Medicine. ASRM Mullerian Anomalies Classification (MAC 2021). (online) Available from: https://connect.asrm.org/education/asrm-mac-2021 (Last accessed December, 2023)]

9. **a.** In this case, there is a right noncommunicating rudimentary horn which is distended with blood along with right hematosalpinx. The management should aim at preserving fertility as retrograde menstruation would result in pelvic endometriosis and subsequent infertility. Hence excision of the rudimentary horn and ipsilateral tube is indicated.
[Reference: Rock JA, Breech LL. Surgery for anomalies of the Mullerian ducts. In: Rock JA, Jones HW III (Eds). Te Linde's Operative Gynecology, 10th edition. Philadelphia: Lippincott Williams & Wilkins; 2008. p. 577]

10. **b.** Diethylstilbestrol rarely causes renal anomalies.
(Reference: Hoffman B, Schorge J, Bradshaw K, Halvorson L, Schaffer J, Corton M. Anatomic disorders. William's Gynecology, 3rd edition. New York: McGraw-Hill Education; 2016. p. 423)

11. **d.** Widely diverging horns seen on ultrasonography (USG) may suggest bicornuate uterus. An intercornual angle >105° suggests bicornuate uterus, whereas angle <75° indicates a septate uterus. However, magnetic resonance imaging or 3D sonography is necessary to define fundal contour and for internal and external uterine assessment.
(Reference: Hoffman B, Schorge J, Bradshaw K, Halvorson L, Schaffer J, Corton M. Anatomic disorders. William's Gynecology, 3rd edition. New York: McGraw-Hill Education; 2016. p. 422)

12. **c.** Widely diverging horns seen on ultrasonography (USG) may suggest bicornuate uterus. An intercornual angle >90° suggests bicornuate uterus, whereas angle <90° indicates a septate uterus. In this case intercornual angle is 55° and a septal length of 3 cm, hence likely to be a septate uterus.
[Reference: American Society for Reproductive Medicine. ASRM Mullerian Anomalies Classification (MAC 2021). (online) Available from: https://connect.asrm.org/education/asrm-mac-2021 (Last accessed December, 2023)]

13. **c.** Vertical fusion defect like partial vaginal agenesis transverse vaginal septum and imperforate hymen present with primary amenorrhea. The primary symptom is monthly lower abdominal pain suggestive of cryptomenorrhea.

    In MRKH (Mayer-Rokitansky-Küster-Hauser), patients present with well-developed secondary characters with absent vagina and absent or small or bipartite uterus. In testicular feminization, patients are genotypically 46,XY. They will have well-developed breast, but scanty pubic hair. Ovaries and uterus will be absent on ultrasound.

    Herlyn-Werner-Wunderlich syndrome, also known as OHVIRA or obstructed hemivagina and ipsilateral renal anomaly, usually presents with double uterus with unilateral obstructed hemivagina and ipsilateral renal agenesis. Patient has menstruation, but complaints of progressively increasing pelvic pain during menstruation and hematocolpos on obstructed side.
    (Reference: Hoffman B, Schorge J, Bradshaw K, Halvorson L, Schaffer J, Corton M. Anatomic disorders. William's Gynecology, 3rd edition. New York: McGraw-Hill Education; 2016. pp. 417-9)

14. **d.** Of all the uterine anomalies (except arcuate uterus), uterus didelphys is associated with the best possibility of successful pregnancy. Therefore, indication of surgical treatment is limited to patients with recurrent pregnancy loss or adverse pregnancy outcomes occurring due to the anomaly.
    [Reference: Rock JA, Breech LL. Surgery for anomalies of the Mullerian ducts. In: Rock JA, Jones HW III (Eds). Te Linde's Operative Gynecology, 10th edition. Philadelphia: Lippincott Williams & Wilkins; 2008. p. 567]

15. **b.** After transcervical lysis of uterine septum, a 2-month delay before attempting to conceive is suggested to allow complete resorption of the septum.
    (Reference: Rock JA, Breech LL. Surgery for anomalies of the Mullerian ducts. In: Rock JA, Jones HW III (Eds). Te Linde's Operative Gynecology, 10th edition. Philadelphia: Lippincott Williams & Wilkins; 2008. p. 569)

16. **c.** *[Reference: Rock JA, Breech LL. Surgery for anomalies of the Mullerian ducts. In: Rock JA, Jones HW III (Eds). Te Linde's Operative Gynecology, 10th edition Philadelphia: Lippincott Williams & Wilkins; 2008. p. 547]*

17. **c.** Septal excision is done in Modified Jone's operation; whereas in Tompkin's operation uterine fundus is incised in midline and then septum is removed. Strassman operation is a procedure of choice for unification of two endometrial cavities of an externally divided uterus, both bicornuate and uterus didelphys.
    [Reference: Rock JA, Breech LL. Surgery for anomalies of the Mullerian ducts. In: Rock JA, Jones HW III (Eds). Te Linde's Operative Gynecology, 10th edition. Philadelphia: Lippincott Williams & Wilkins; 2008. pp. 570-2]

18. **d.** The triad of uterine didelphys, obstructed hemivagina, and ipsilateral renal anomaly is known as OHVIRA syndrome, and also Herlyn-Werner-Wunderlich syndrome.
    (Reference: Hoffman B, Schorge J, Bradshaw K, Halvorson L, Schaffer J, Corton M. Anatomic disorders. William's Gynecology, 3rd edition. New York: McGraw-Hill Education; 2016. p. 417)

19. **a.** Scar after unification is as strong as, if not stronger than, the scar formed after cesarean. The biological conditions in which healing occurs are entirely different.
    [Reference: Rock JA, Breech LL. Surgery for anomalies of the Mullerian ducts. In: Rock JA, Jones HW III (Eds). Te Linde's Operative Gynecology, 10th edition. Philadelphia: Lippincott Williams & Wilkins; 2008. p. 574]

20. **d.** We can appreciate that uterine cavity is divided into two parts by a thick septa in between. Also the visual appreciation suggests the angle of indentation to be <90°. Hence the pathology is septate uterus.
    [Reference: American Society for Reproductive Medicine. ASRM Mullerian Anomalies Classification (MAC 2021). (online) Available from: https://connect.asrm.org/education/asrm-mac-2021 (Last accessed December, 2023)]

21. **c.** Uterus is septate if: according to ESHRE/ESGE (European Society of Human Reproduction and Embryology/European Society for Gynaecological Endoscopy) 2016, external indentation depth is less, and internal indentation depth is >50% of uterine wall thickness, when uterine wall thickness is measured above interostial/intercornual line.

    According to CUME (Congenital Uterine Malformation by Experts) 2018, external fundal indentation depth is <1 cm, while internal fundal indentation depth is ≥1 cm.

According to ASRM (American Society for Reproductive Medicine) 2016, internal fundal indentation depth is ≥1.5 cm, with acute angle of internal indentation, and external fundal indentation depth is <1 cm.

According to MAC 2021, a septate uterus is defined as having an internal indentation depth >10 mm combined with an internal indentation angle <90°.
[Reference: Ludwin A, Tudorache S, Martins WP. ASRM Mullerian Anomalies Classification 2021: a critical review. Ultrasound Obstet Gynecol. 2022;60(1):7-21]

22. **b.** Septate uterus is the most common type of congenital uterine anomaly in about 35% of cases, followed by bicornuate uterus in 26% cases.

Mullerian anomalies	Incidence
Septate uterus	35%
Bicornuate uterus	26%
Arcuate uterus	18%
Unicornuate uterus	10%
Uterus didelphys	8%

(Reference: Konar H, Dutta DC. Congenital malformation of female genital organs. DC Dutta's Textbook of Gynecology, 8th edition. New Delhi: Jaypee Brothers Medical Publishers; 2020. p. 36)

23. **c.** Urinary tract anomalies are often associated with unicornuate uterus. On the side opposite to the unicornuate uterus, there may be a horseshoe kidney or pelvic kidney or hypoplastic kidney or an absent kidney.
[Reference: Rock JA, Breech LL. Surgery for anomalies of the Mullerian ducts. In: Rock JA, Jones HW III (Eds). Te Linde's Operative Gynecology, 10th edition. Philadelphia: Lippincott Williams & Wilkins; 2008. p. 574]

24. **a.** Septate uterus is associated with a markedly increased incidence of spontaneous abortion rates. This is likely due to partial or complete implantation on a largely avascular septum, from distortion of uterine cavity, and from associated cervical and endometrial abnormalities. Based on operative experience of septal defects, the blood supply to the fibromuscular septum appears to be markedly reduced when compared with normal myometrium.

(Reference: Hoffman B, Schorge J, Bradshaw K, Halvorson L, Schaffer J, Corton M. Anatomic disorders. William's Gynecology, 3rd edition. New York: McGraw-Hill Education; 2016. p. 422)
[Rock JA, Breech LL. Surgery for anomalies of the Mullerian ducts. In: Rock JA, Jones HW III (Eds). Te Linde's Operative Gynecology, 10th edition. Philadelphia: Lippincott Williams & Wilkins; 2008. p. 567]

25. **c.** At 5th week intrauterine, the gonadal ridges can be recognized as thickenings of the coelomic cavity just medial to mesonephric tubules. Gonadal differentiation into testis or ovary does not occur until 6th week of development.
(Reference: Hoffman B, Schorge J, Bradshaw K, Halvorson L, Schaffer J, Corton M. Anatomic disorders. William's Gynecology, 3rd edition. New York: McGraw-Hill Education; 2016. p. 404)
(Rock JA, Breech LL. Surgery for anomalies of the Mullerian ducts. In: Rock JA, Jones HW III (Eds). Te Linde's Operative Gynecology, 10th edition. Philadelphia: Lippincott Williams & Wilkins; 2008. p. 541)

26. **a.** Vaginal epithelium is derived from endoderm of urogenital sinus.
[Reference: Rock JA, Breech LL. Surgery for anomalies of the Mullerian ducts. In: Rock JA, Jones HW III (Eds). Te Linde's Operative Gynecology, 10th edition. Philadelphia: Lippincott Williams & Wilkins; 2008. p. 541]

27. **b.** The cranial part of Wolffian ducts can persist as epoophoron of the ovarian hilum; the caudal parts can persist as Gartner's duct.
[Reference: Rock JA, Breech LL. Surgery for anomalies of the Mullerian ducts. In: Rock JA, Jones HW III (Eds). Te Linde's Operative Gynecology, 10th edition. Philadelphia: Lippincott Williams & Wilkins; 2008. p. 541]

28. **b.** Urinary tract anomalies are often associated with unicornuate uterus. On the side opposite to the unicornuate uterus, there may be a horseshoe kidney or pelvic kidney or hypoplastic kidney or an absent kidney.
[Reference: Rock JA, Breech LL. Surgery for anomalies of the Mullerian ducts. In: Rock JA, Jones HW III (Eds). Te Linde's Operative Gynecology, 10th edition.

Philadelphia: Lippincott Williams & Wilkins; 2008. p. 574]

29. b. In case of a female presenting with primary amenorrhea with well-developed breast, but absent uterus and blind vagina, we primarily have to differentiate between MRKH (Mayer-Rokitansky-Küster-Hauser) (which is due to Mullerian agenesis) and androgen insensitivity syndrome (AIS) (X-linked recessive gene defect where there is insensitivity to androgen receptor gene). In both of these conditions, patient is phenotypically a female, but is genotypically different. Patients with MRKH are 46,XX while those with AIS are 46,XY. Hence, karyotype is the next investigation of choice.

(Reference: Konar H, Dutta DC. Amenorrhea. DC Dutta's Textbook of Gynecology, 8th edition. New Delhi: Jaypee Brothers Medical Publishers; 2020. p. 379)

30. c. Short arm of Y chromosome

(Reference: Konar H, Dutta DC. Disorders of sexual development. DC Dutta's Textbook of Gynecology, 8th edition. New Delhi: Jaypee Brothers Medical Publishers; 2020. p. 367)

Chapter 79

Fibroid

Deepa Chaudhary

QUESTIONS

1. **Which of the following risk factors is associated with increase in prevalence of fibroid?**
   a. Hyperestogenism
   b. Vitamin D Deficiency
   c. Obesity
   d. All of the above

2. **The United States Food and Drug Administration (USFDA) notes that occult uterine cancers such as sarcomas are found in approximately 1 in 225 to 1 in 580 women who undergo myomectomy or hysterectomy. Which of the following statements are false regarding perioperative assessment of fibroid for ruling out malignancy or leiomyosarcoma?**
   a. Leiomyosarcoma is found in approximately 1 in 495 to 1 in 1,100 women undergoing surgery for myomas
   b. Endometrial adenocarcinoma is the most common malignancy observed in women with fibroids and abnormal uterine bleeding
   c. Fibroid size and rate of growth are not predictive: a rapidly growing leiomyoma in a premenopausal woman is not predictive of malignancy
   d. Masses greater than 20 gestational weeks' size are not associated with increased risk of uterine sarcoma in premenopausal women
   e. None of the above

3. **A 36-year-old G2P2 presents for her well-woman examination. She has had two spontaneous vaginal deliveries without complications. Her largest child weighed 3,500 g at birth. Her menstrual cycle is regular and has never had an abnormal Pap smear. She does not smoke, but drinks about four times per week. Her weight is 70 kg. Her vital signs are normal. On pelvic examination uterus is enlarged to 20 weeks' size, is nontender, and does not cause the patient any dyspareunia or discomfort. Which of the following statements is true regarding management of asymptomatic fibroid?**
   a. There is no specific leiomyoma size that requires intervention in women who are asymptomatic
   b. Surgery is indicated for prophylactic symptom prevention as there are no reliable predictors of symptom development
   c. Surgical intervention is indicated solely to exclude the possibility of sarcoma
   d. All of the above

4. **Which of the following measures helps in minimum blood loss during laparoscopic myomectomy?**
   a. The use of intravenous vasopressin
   b. The use of unidirectional and bidirectional barbed suture
   c. The use of intravenous tranexamic acid
   d. The use of intravenous ascorbic acid

5. **An important determinant of the safety and feasibility of hysteroscopic myomectomy is the "myometrial-free margin". True about it is:**
   a. This cannot be evaluated via saline infusion sonography
   b. It is important to have at least a 1-cm thick margin from the lesion to the endometrial surface if hysteroscopic resection is planned
   c. Knowing this, the surgeon can gauge the complexity of hysteroscopic myomectomy, the degree of myometrial involvement, and the likelihood of completing the procedure in one setting
   d. None of these

6. A 35-year-old woman presents to you for routine well-woman examination. She has had two normal vaginal deliveries and is healthy. She smokes one pack of cigarettes per day. She is having heavy menstrual bleeding. Her last menstrual period was 3 weeks ago. During the pelvic examination, you notice that uterus is enlarged to 10–12 weeks' size. Transvaginal ultrasound shows type-2 intracavitary fibroid of size 4 cm size. Which of the following is the false regarding hysteroscopic myomectomy recommendation to this patient?
   a. To be removed hysteroscopically by experienced surgeons
   b. Informed consent for a two-staged hysteroscopic surgery in patients
   c. There is increased recovery, complications, and complete resection in women with fibroids > 3 cm
   d. Surgeons should consider pharmacologically decreasing the size of the myoma with a GnRH agonist or selective progesterone receptor modulators (SPRMs)

7. What is the STEP-W submucosal fibroid classification system?
   a. It was given by Lasmar et al. in 2011
   b. It is used for laparoscopic myomectomy
   c. Low score is good for laparoscopic myomectomy
   d. The STEP-W classification considers shape, topography, extension of the fibroid base, depth of fibroid penetration, and the lateral wall involvement

8. True about NICE (National Institute for Health and Care Excellence) recommendation for power morcellation are all, *except*:
   a. For people who are postmenopausal or over 50, this procedure should not be used
   b. For people who are premenopausal or 50 or under, this procedure should only be used with special arrangements for clinical governance, consent, and audit or research
   c. This procedure should only be done by a surgeon with specific training in laparoscopic surgery
   d. The committee noted that laparoscopic power morcellation for the treatment of fibroids is the subject of a safety communication from the United States Food and Drug Administration (FDA). In this communication, the FDA encourages the use of additional labeling on laparoscopic power morcellator devices to warn of the risks of disseminating malignant and benign uterine tissue. It also advises using containment systems
   e. None of the above

Questions 9 to 16
Match each figure with the correct description. Each option may be used once, more than once, or not at all.
   a. Highly cellular leiomyoma
   b. Leiomyoma with bizarre nuclei
   c. Leiomyosarcoma
   d. Suprapubic containment system with trocar inserted
   e. Robotic port placement with suprapubic Gelport device
   f. Bipolar loop resection of fibroid
   g. Tissue retrieval system with aperture adjacent to leiomyoma
   h. A catheter is placed around the lower uterine segment in order to occlude the uterine vessels
   i. A vascular clamp is placed across the ovarian vessels

9.

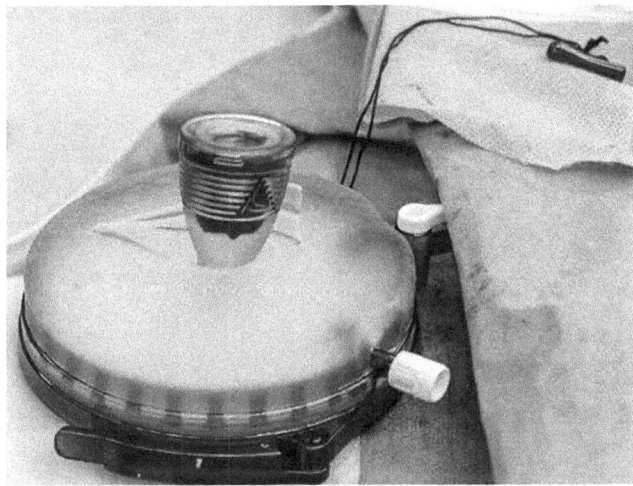

10.

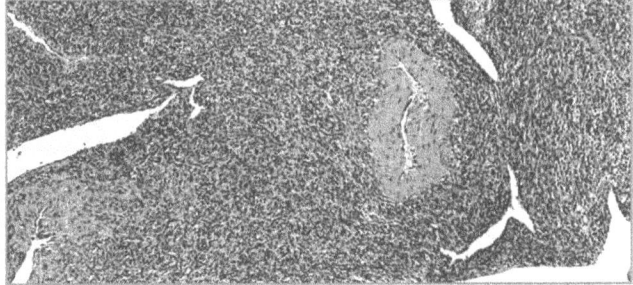

448 SECTION 2: Gynecology

11.

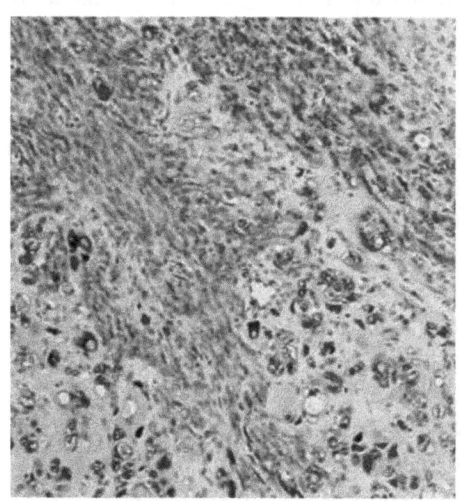

14.

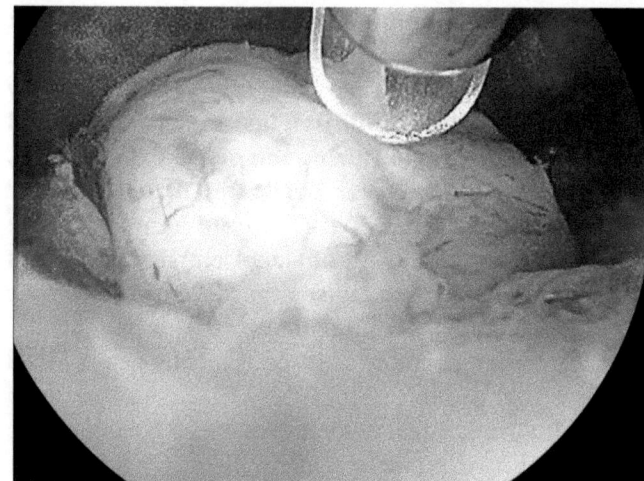

12.

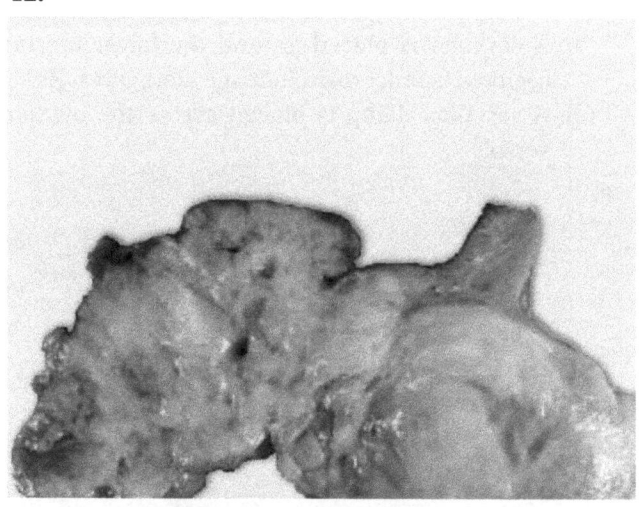

15.

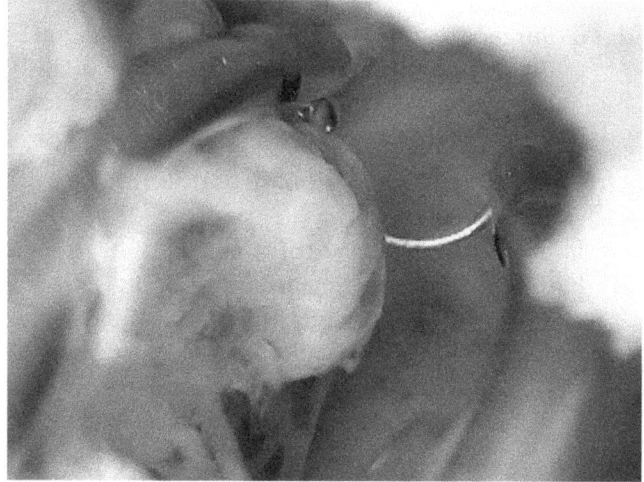

13.

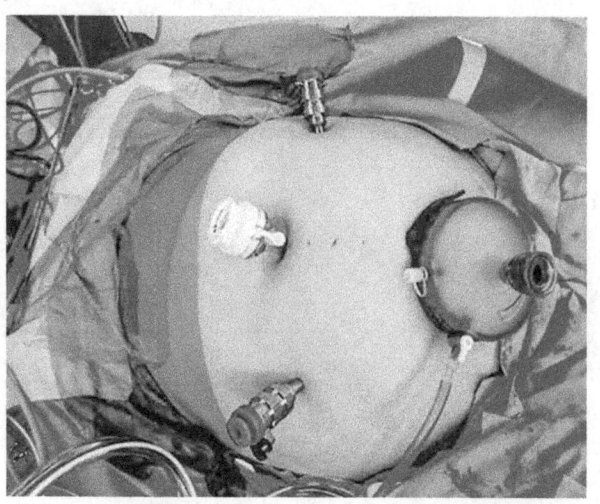

16.

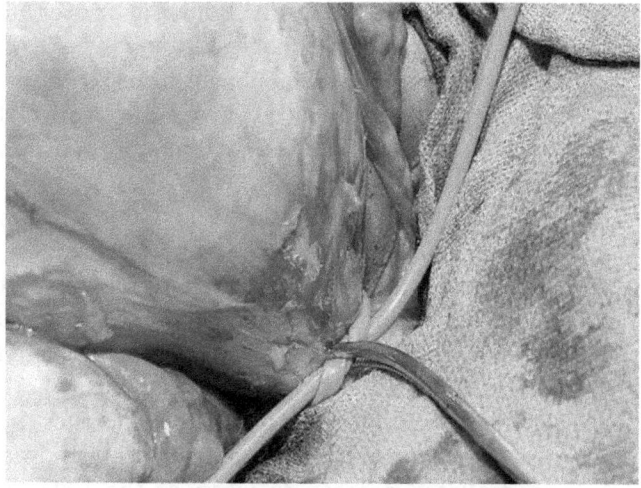

17. A 28-year-old G3P0 has a history of severe menstrual cramps, prolonged, heavy periods, chronic pelvic pain, and painful intercourse. All of her pregnancies were spontaneous abortions in the first trimester. A 3D transvaginal ultrasound, which she just had as part of the evaluation for recurrent abortion, showed a submucosal fibroid polyp of 2 × 2 cm. You have recommended hysteroscopic removal of fibroid. Which of the following statements is correct regarding role of fibroids in pregnancy outcome?
    a. The risk ratio of spontaneous abortion due to fibroid is 1.6:7.8
    b. The impact of a fibroid on reproductive outcome not does depend on the location of the fibroid
    c. Studies have demonstrated that intramural fibroids were associated with decreased implantation, clinical pregnancy, and ongoing pregnancy
    d. Only (a)
    e. Both (a) and (c)

Questions 18 to 24
Match the drugs with the most appropriate effect and/or side effects. Each option may be used once, more than once, or not at all.
    a. Decreases blood loss but no effect on fibroid size or volume
    b. Decreases fibroid size, volume, and blood loss during menstrual cycle
    c. No effect on blood loss or fibroid size
    d. Causes hot flushes
    e. Causes amenorrhea and osteomalacia
    f. Causes endometrial hyperplasia
    g. Decreases fibroid size and volume

18. Levonorgestrel-releasing intrauterine system (LNG-IUS)
19. Ulipristal acetate (UPA) is a selective progesterone receptor modulator.
20. Gonadotropin-releasing hormone antagonist
21. Gonadotropin-releasing hormone agonists
22. Mifepristone
23. Tranexamic acid
24. Nonsteroidal anti-inflammatory drugs (NSAIDs)
25. Regarding diagnostic accuracy of various imaging modality for fibroid, which of the following statement is true:
    a. Submucous fibroids were best identified with magnetic resonance imaging (MRI) (sensitivity 100%, specificity 91%)
    b. The preoperative diagnosis of uterine sarcoma may be possible with serum lactate dehydrogenase (LDH) and LDH isoenzyme 3 measurements along with gadolinium-enhanced diethylenetriamine pentaacetic acid (Gd-DTPA) dynamic MRI was reported to be highly accurate
    c. Both of the above
    d. None of the above

26. True statement regarding etiopathogenesis of fibroid is:
    a. Genetic differences between fibroids and leiomyosarcomas (LMSs) indicate that LMSs do not result from the malignant degeneration of fibroids
    b. Only estrogen hormone appear to promote the development of fibroids
    c. First-degree relatives of women with fibroids have a 1.5 times increased risk of developing fibroids
    d. A prospective study found that the risk of fibroids increased 1% with each 10 kg increase in body weight, and with increasing body mass index (BMI)

27. Prognostic factors related to new appearance of fibroids all are true, *except:*
    a. New appearance of fibroids is not more common following laparoscopic myomectomy when compared with abdominal myomectomy
    b. New fibroids would be expected to form as age increases, even following myomectomy
    c. The 10-year clinical new appearance rate for women who subsequently gave birth was 16%, but for those women who did not the rate was 28%
    d. None of the above

28. Uterine artery embolization (UAE) is an effective treatment for selected women with uterine fibroids. While counseling the patient regarding this modality you will explain:
    a. The effects of UAE on early ovarian failure, fertility, and pregnancy are unclear
    b. Persistent fever should be managed with antibiotics
    c. Failure to respond to antibiotics may indicate sepsis, which needs to be aggressively managed with hysterectomy
    d. All of the above

29. A fixed-dose combination of relugolix/estradiol/norethisterone (also known as norethindrone) acetate (Ryeqo®; Myfembree®) is:
    a. USFDA approved for the management of heavy menstrual bleeding associated with uterine fibroids

b. Given in intramuscular depot form
c. Can be given for lifelong treatment
d. Not well tolerated due to severe vasomotor symptoms

30. **The clinical evidence for relugolix–estradiol–norethisterone acetate came from two identical phase 3 randomized controlled trials, LIBERTY 1 and LIBERTY 2. The key inclusion criteria in the trials were all,** *except:*
    a. Being premenopausal
    b. Age 18–50 years
    c. Irregular menstrual periods
    d. A cycle of 21–38 days
    e. Diagnosis of fibroids confirmed with ultrasonography

ANSWERS

1. **d.** All of the above

2. **e.** None of the above.
   Unfortunately, even the most diligent preoperative assessments cannot completely exclude the possibility of leiomyosarcoma or other malignancy. It is important to recognize that endometrial adenocarcinoma is the most common malignancy observed in women with fibroids and abnormal uterine bleeding. Therefore, endometrial sampling is recommended prior to surgery in the setting of abnormal bleeding.
   (Reference: Handa VL, Le LV. Te Linde's Operative Gynecology, 12th edition. New York: Wolters Kluwer; 2019. p. 525)

3. **a.** There is no specific leiomyoma size that requires intervention in women who are asymptomatic. Surgery is not indicated for prophylactic symptom prevention as there are no reliable predictors of symptom development. Intervention can be considered in asymptomatic women who desire future fertility and have a submucosal leiomyoma amenable to hysteroscopic surgery.
   Another potential indication for surgery in asymptomatic women is the presence of moderate or severe hydronephrosis from ureteral compression.
   Surgical intervention is not indicated solely to exclude the possibility of sarcoma.
   (Reference: Handa VL, Le LV. Te Linde's Operative Gynecology, 12th edition. New York: Wolters Kluwer; 2019. p. 527)

4. **b.** The use of unidirectional and bidirectional barbed suture
   Table 18.3 lists the possible medical interventions that can reduce blood loss at myomectomy. Combinations of these interventions, such as intramyometrial vasopressin plus vaginal or rectal misoprostol, may have an additive effect. Low quality evidence for intravenous tranexamic acid and ascorbic acid.

TABLE 18.3: Perioperative Medical Measures to Reduce Intraoperative Blood Loss

Agent	Mean difference in blood loss versus placebo	Need for blood transfusion
Intramyometrial vasopressin[b]	245 mL	Decrease need
Intramyometrial bupivacaine and epinephrine[a]	68 mL	No effect
Vaginal misoprostol[b]	97 mL	No effect
Vaginal dinoprostone[a]	131 mL	Decrease need
Gelatin thrombin matrix[a]	545 mL	Decrease need
Fibrin sealant patch[a]	26 mL	No effect
Intravenous ascorbic acid[a]	411 mL	No effect
Intravenous tranexamic acid[a]	243 mL	No effect

Not all drugs are available in all countries. Also, some medications are not FDA approved for these indications.
[a]Low-quality evidence. [b]Moderate-quality evidence.
Source: Data from Kongnyuy E, Wiysonge CS. Interventions to reduce haemorrhage during myomectomy for fibroids. Cochrane Database Syst Rev 2014;(8):CD005355.

(Reference: Handa VL, Le LV. Te Linde's Operative Gynecology, 12th edition. New York: Wolters Kluwer; 2019. pp. 527-8)

5. **c.** Knowing this, the surgeon can gauge the complexity of hysteroscopic myomectomy, the degree of myometrial involvement, and the likelihood of completing the procedure in one setting.
   An important determinant of the safety and feasibility of hysteroscopic myomectomy is the "myometrial-free margin". This can be evaluated via saline infusion sonography or MRI. Although uterine remodeling occurs during operative hysteroscopy, it is important to have at least 1-cm thick margin from the lesion to the serosal surface if hysteroscopic resection is planned. Knowing this, the surgeon can gauge the

complexity of hysteroscopic myomectomy, the degree of myometrial involvement, and the likelihood of completing the procedure in one setting.
(Reference: Handa VL, Le LV. Te Linde's Operative Gynecology, 12th edition. New York: Wolters Kluwer; 2019. p. 28)

6. **c.** Chances of incomplete resection are high with FIGO (International Federation of Gynecology and Obstetrics) type 1 and 2 with size ≥3 cm.
(Reference: Handa VL, Le LV. Te Linde's Operative Gynecology, 12th edition. New York: Wolters Kluwer; 2019. p. 529)

7. **a.** Given by Lasmar RB et al. in 2011
The STEP-W classification considers size, topography, extension of the fibroid base, depth of fibroid penetration, and the lateral wall involvement. Each factor is assigned a point value. A low score of 0 to 4 (low complexity) is associated with safety and successful removal of the fibroid in one hysteroscopic setting. A score of 5 or 6 is considered high complexity, and may require a two-stage hysteroscopic procedure. A score of 7 to 9 is considered not amenable to treatment hysteroscopically

Step-w submucosal broid classi cation system

Size (cm)	Topo-graphy	Extension of the Base	Penetr-ation	Lateral wall	Total
0	<2	Low	<1/3	0	+1
1	>2 to 5	Middle	>1/3 to 2/3	<50%	
2	>5	Upper	>2/3	>50%	
Score	+	+	+	+	+
Score	Group	Complexity and therapeutic options			
0 to 4	I	Low-complexity hysteroscopic myomectomy			
5 to 6	II	High-complexity hysteroscopic myomectomy, concider two-step hysteroscopic myomectomy			
7 to 9	III	Consider alternatives to the hysteroscopic technique			

Step-w: size, topography, extension, penetration, wall: GnRH: gonodotropin-relesing hormine
(Reference: Lasmar RB, Xinmei Z, Indman PD, Celeste RK, Di Spiezio Sardo A. Feasibility of a new system of classification of submucous myomas: a multicenter study. Fertil Steril. 2011;95:2073-7)
Lasmar RB, Xinmei Z, Indman PD, et al. Feasibility of a new system of classification of submucous myomas: a multicenter study. Fertil Steril 2011; 95:2073

8. **e.** None of the above
[Reference: National Institute for Health and Care Excellence. (2021). Laparoscopic removal of uterine fibroids with power morcellation. Interventional procedures guidance (IPG703). (online) Available from: https://www.nice.org.uk/guidance/ipg703 (Last accessed December, 2023)]

9. **d.** Suprapubic containment system with trocar inserted

10. **a.** Highly cellular leiomyoma; the tumor is highly cellular resembling an endometrial stromal tumor, however, it shows fascicular growth as well as large and thick-walled blood vessels characteristic of smooth-muscle tumors.
Reference: Kurman R J, Carcangiu M L, Herrington C S, Young R H. WHO Classification of Tumours of Female Reproductive Organs WHO Classification of Tumours, 4th edition, volume 6. Lyon: International Agency for Research on Cancer; 2014.

11. **b.** Leiomyoma with bizarre nuclei. The bizarre nuclei alternate with areas of conventional leiomyoma; mitotic activity is typically low but karyorrhectic nuclci, which may mimic atypical mitotic figures, are common.
Reference: Kurman R J, Carcangiu M L, Herrington C S, Young R H. WHO Classification of Tumours of Female Reproductive Organs WHO Classification of Tumours, 4th edition, volume 6. Lyon: International Agency for Research on Cancer; 2014.

12. **c.** Leiomyosarcoma is the most common uterine sarcoma accounting for 1–2% of all uterine malignancies with an incidence of 0.3–0.4/100,000 women per year.
(Reference: Kurman RJ, Carcangiu ML, Herrington CS, Young RH. WHO Classification of Tumours of Female Reproductive Organs WHO Classification of Tumours, 4th edition, volume 6. Lyon: International Agency for Research on Cancer; 2014)

13. **e.** Robotic port placement with suprapubic Gelport device

14. **g.** Tissue retrieval system with aperture adjacent to leiomyoma
15. **f.** Bipolar Loop resection of fibroid
16. **h.** A catheter is placed around the lower uterine segment in order to occlude the uterine vessels
    (Reference: Handa VL, Le LV. Te Linde's Operative Gynecology, 12th edition. New York: Wolters Kluwer; 2019)
17. **e.** Both (a) and (c)
    Various systematic reviews have demonstrated that the location and size of fibroid plays important role in fertility outcomes.
    [References: Tolani AD, Kadambari, Desai H, Donthi S, Deendayal M. Fibroid and infertility: when to suggest myomectomy? In: Rooma S, Advincula A, Joseph K (Eds). Fibroid Uterus: Surgical Challenges in Minimal Access Surgery, 1st edition. Boca Raton: CRC Press; 2021]
    [Pritts EA, Parker WH, Olive DL. Fibroids and infertility: an updated systematic review of the evidence. Fertil Steril. 2009;91(4):1215-23]
    [Sunkara SK, Khairy M, El-Toukhy T, Khalaf Y, Coomarasamy A. The effect of intramural fibroids without uterine cavity involvement on the outcome of IVF treatment: a systematic review and meta-analysis. Hum Reprod. 2010;25(2):418-29]
    [Yan L, Yu Q, Zhang YN, Guo Z, Li Z, Niu J, et al. Effect of type 3 intramural fibroids on in vitro fertilization-intracytoplasmic sperm injection outcomes: a retrospective cohort study. Fertil Steril. 2018;109(5):817-22.e2]
18. **a.**
19. **b, d.**
20. **b, d.**
21. **b, d, f.**
22. **g, f.**
23. **a.**
24. **c.** *(Reference: Berek JS. Berek & Novak's Gynecology, 16th edition. Philadelphia: Wolters Kluwer; 2019)*
25. **c.** *(Reference: Berek JS. Berek & Novak's Gynecology, 16th edition. Philadelphia: Wolters Kluwer; 2019)*
26. **a.** *(Reference: Berek JS. Berek & Novak's Gynecology, 16th edition. Philadelphia: Wolters Kluwer; 2019)*
27. **d.** None of the above
    The Prognostic Factors Related to New Appearance of Fibroids (Page-577- Reference-Berek and Novek's Gynaecology 16th edition)are as follows:
    Age: Given that the incidence of fibroids increases with increasing age, 4 per 1,000 woman-years for 25 to 29 year olds and 22 per 1,000 for 40 to 44 year olds, new fibroids would be expected to form as age increases, even following myomectomy.
    [Reference: (Peddada SD, Laughlin SK, Miner K, et al. Growth of uterine leiomyomata among premenopausal black and white women. Proc Natl Acad Sci USA. 2008;105(50):19887-92)]
    Subsequent Childbearing -The 10-year clinical new appearance rate for women who subsequently gave birth was 16%, but for those women who did not the rate was 28%.
    [Reference: Candiani GB, Fedele L, Parazzini F, et al. Risk of recurrence after myomectomy. Br J Obstet Gynecol 1991;98(4):385-9)]
    Laparoscopic myomectomy: New appearance of fibroids is not more common following laparoscopic myomectomy when compared with abdominal myomectomy. Eighty-one women randomized to either laparoscopic or abdominal myomectomy were followed with TVS every 6 months for at least 40 months.
    [(Reference: Spies JB, Sacks D. Credentials for uterine artery embolization. J Vasc Interv Radiol. 2004;15(2): P-111-3)]
    Number of fibroids initially removed: After at least 5 years of follow-up, 27% of women who initially had a single fibroid removed had clinically detected new fibroids and 59% of women with multiple fibroids initially removed had new fibroids (151).
    Gonadotropin-releasing hormone agonists: Preoperative treatment with GnRH-a decreases fibroid volume and may make smaller fibroids harder to identify during surgery. A randomized study found that 3 months following abdominal myomectomy, 5 (63%) of 8 women in the GnRH group had fibroids less than 1.5 cm detected sonographically, while only 2 of 16 (13%) untreated women had small fibroids detected (157).
28. **d.** All of the above
    Uterine artery embolization (UAE) is an effective treatment for selected women with uterine fibroids. The effects of UAE on early ovarian failure, fertility, and pregnancy are unclear. Interventional radiologists advise against the procedure for women considering future fertility. Appropriate candidates for UAE include women who have bothersome symptoms to warrant hysterectomy or myomectomy. American College of Obstetricians and Gynecologists (ACOG) recommends that women considering UAE have a thorough evaluation with a gynecologist to

help facilitate collaboration with the interventional radiologist and that responsibility of caring for the patient be clear. Tissue hypoxia secondary to UAE causes postprocedural pain that usually requires pain management in the hospital for 1 day. NSAID medications are usually taken for 1 to 2 weeks, and many women return to normal activity within 1 to 3 weeks. Approximately 5% to 10% of women have pain for longer than 2 weeks. Ten percent of women require readmission to the hospital for postembolization syndrome, characterized by diffuse abdominal pain, nausea, vomiting, low-grade fever, malaise, anorexia, and leukocytosis. Treatment with intravenous fluids, NSAID medications, and pain management usually leads to resolution of symptoms within 2 to 3 days (170). Persistent fever should be managed with antibiotics. Failure to respond to antibiotics may indicate sepsis, which needs to be aggressively managed with hysterectomy. (Page-577- Reference- Berek and Novek's gynaecology 16th edition)
(Reference: Berek and Novek's Gynaecology. 16th edition, Page 577)

29. **a.** USFDA approved for the management of heavy menstrual bleeding associated with uterine fibroids. Relugolix is a gonadotropin-releasing hormone (GnRH) receptor antagonist that decreases serum estradiol and progesterone concentrations to postmenopausal levels. The addition of estradiol/ norethisterone acetate to relugolix ameliorates relugolix-induced bone loss and hot flush. In the two phase 3 LIBERTY trials, relugolix + estradiol/ norethisterone substantially decreased menstrual bleeding and improved a range of other uterine fibroid symptoms in women with uterine fibroids-associated heavy menstrual bleeding. The combination was generally well tolerated, with vasomotor symptoms being the most common adverse reaction. Treatment with this combination for over up to 2 years did not induce a clinically meaningful bone loss in the majority of women. Relugolix/estradiol/ norethisterone acetate, with its convenient once-daily administration, is a useful addition to current pharmacological treatment options for premenopausal women with symptomatic uterine fibroids.
[Reference: Syed YY. Relugolix/Estradiol/Norethisterone (Norethindrone) Acetate: A Review in Symptomatic Uterine Fibroids. Drugs. 2022;82(15):1549-56]

30. **c.** Irregular menstrual periods
[Reference: National Institute for Health and Care Excellence. (2022). Relugolix–estradiol–norethisterone acetate for treating moderate to severe symptoms of uterine fibroids. Technology appraisal guidance (TA832). (online) Available from: https://www.nice.org.uk/guidance/ta832 (Last accessed December, 2023)].

Chapter 80: Endocrinology of Reproduction

Nidhi Sharma Chauhan, Rajshree Dayanand Katke

QUESTIONS

1. Which of the following is false regarding prolactin?
   a. Thyrotropin-releasing hormone (TRH) has a stimulatory effect on prolactin
   b. Gene expression of prolactin is stimulated by estrogen
   c. Prolactin levels are highest in the midmorning hours
   d. Prolactin is not under positive hypothalamic control unlike follicle-stimulating hormone (FSH)

2. Which of the following statements is correct?
   a. FSH pulses can be measured as an indication of gonadotropin-releasing hormone (GnRH) pulsatile secretion
   b. Luteinizing hormone (LH) and FSH pulse can both be measured as an indication of GnRH pulsatile secretion
   c. LH pulses only can measured as an indication of GnRH pulsatile secretion
   d. All the above

3. Which of the following hormones has a higher production during the luteal phase?
   a. Estradiol
   b. LH
   c. Progesterone
   d. Estrone

4. All of the following options are true, *except:*
   a. Endorphins inhibit the release of gonadotropin-releasing hormone
   b. Ovarian sex steroids increase secretion of endorphins
   c. Endorphins increase the release of GnRH
   d. Dysphoria may be caused by a premenstrual withdrawal in endogenous opiates

5. What percentage of testosterone and estradiol are in the free from in women?
   a. 1, 2
   b. 1, 1
   c. 2, 1
   d. 2, 2

6. The blood levels of the hormone progesterone in the preovulatory phase in the adult female is:
   a. 1–1.5 ng/mL
   b. <1 ng/mL
   c. 2–3 ng/mL
   d. 3–3.5 ng/mL

7. Majority of the dihydrotestosterone (DHT) in females is derived from:
   a. Testosterone
   b. Dehydroepiandrosterone
   c. Androstenedione
   d. Dehydroepiandrosterone sulfate (DHEAS)

8. The most potent androgen is:
   a. Testosterone
   b. Dehydroepiandrosterone sulfate
   c. Dihydrotestosterone
   d. Androstenedione

9. Oocyte is arrested in which phase of prophase?
   a. Zygotene
   b. Leptotene
   c. Diplotene
   d. Pachytene

10. The most common cause of thyrotoxicosis in pregnancy is:
    a. Goiter
    b. Grave's disease
    c. TSH hypersecretion
    d. Gestational trophoblastic disease

11. Which of the following statement is false?
    a. Maternal thyroid-stimulating hormone (TSH) and human chorionic gonadotropin (hCG) reach a nadir at 10 weeks
    b. Euthyroid infertile women do not benefit from thyroid hormone treatment
    c. Free triiodothyronine (T3) and thyroxine (T4) increase in pregnancy
    d. Antithyroid antibodies are measured in women with elevated TSH but normal free T4

12. Which is the most important inhibitor of primordial follicle growth?
    a. Inhibin
    b. Anti-Mullerian hormone (AMH)
    c. Activin
    d. FSH

13. Aromatization in the granulosa cells is by the action of:
    a. LH
    b. FSH
    c. AMH
    d. Estrogen

14. Antral follicles which yield healthy oocytes do not have the following:
    a. High FSH receptors
    b. High estrogen levels
    c. Androgenic milieu
    d. Low androgen/estrogen ratio

15. Which of the following statements is false?
    a. Low levels of estrogen have a positive feedback on FSH
    b. Low levels of estrogen have a negative feedback on FSH
    c. Low levels of estrogen have a positive feedback on LH
    d. Both (a) and (c)

16. Which of the following is a derivative of the genital ridge?
    a. Fallopian tubes
    b. Ovary
    c. Uterus
    d. Vagina

17. At what gestation does AMH lead to regression of the Mullerian ducts?
    a. 8 weeks
    b. 20 weeks
    c. 18 weeks
    d. 28 weeks

18. Most severe and the rarest form of congenital adrenal hyperplasia is:
    a. P450 oxidoreductase deficiency
    b. 21 hydroxylase deficiency
    c. Congenital lipoid adrenal hyperplasia
    d. 17-hydroxylase deficiency

19. Which of the following has an X-linked pattern of inheritance?
    a. Complete androgen insensitivity syndrome
    b. Congenital adrenal hyperplasia
    c. Klinefelter syndrome
    d. Kallmann syndrome

20. Which of the following is the most probable karyotype in a 17-year-old girl with primary amenorrhea with Tanner stage 4 breast development. Axillary and pubic hair also age appropriately. Vagina is a blind ending pouch. Sonography of pelvis shows an absent uterus with normal ovaries?
    a. 46,XY
    b. 46,XX
    c. 45,X
    d. 46,XXY

21. The most probable diagnosis of a 14-year-old girl with primary amenorrhea with prepubertal breast development, Tanner 2 pubic hair, blind vaginal pouch, and karyotype 46,XY; she has hypertension with hyponatremia and hypokalemia. Hormonal assay: Hypergonadotropic hypogonadism.
    a. Swyer syndrome
    b. Androgen insensitivity syndrome
    c. 17 alpha hydroxylase deficiency
    d. Steroid 5 alpha reductase deficiency

22. Which of the following statements is false for Androgen insensitivity syndrome?
    a. 40% of patients can have de novo mutations
    b. It always follows Mendelian inheritance pattern
    c. X-linked recessive
    d. Can result from variety of inactivating mutations in the androgen receptor (AR) gene

23. Which of the following statements is false in regard with puberty?
    a. Juvenile pause is the interval between infancy and puberty when hypothalamic–pituitary–gonadal (HPG) axis lies dormant
    b. The pulsatile secretion of GnRH is completely abolished during the juvenile phase
    c. Low amplitude gonadotropin secretion can be detected in prepubertal children as young as 5 years old
    d. Early stage of puberty has a nocturnal rise of LH

456 SECTION 2: Gynecology

24. Regarding adrenarche, which of the following statements is untrue?
    a. Starts around 6 years of age
    b. It is dependent on the maturation of the hypothalamic–pituitary–gonadal axis
    c. Biochemical indicator of adrenarche in girls is dehydroepiandrosterone sulfate
    d. Clinically recognized as pubic hair development

25. Treatment of idiopathic central precocious puberty is:
    a. Long-acting GnRH agonists
    b. Short-acting GnRH agonists
    c. GnRH antagonists
    d. None of the above

26. Majority of the estrogen in maternal urine is from:
    a. Maternal ovary
    b. Peripheral conversion
    c. Fetal androgens
    d. Maternal androgens

27. Long half-life of hCG is due to:
    a. Galactosamine
    b. Fructose
    c. Mannose
    d. Sialic acid

28. Hyperprolactinemia does not present as:
    a. Secondary amenorrhea
    b. Primary amenorrhea
    c. Precocious puberty
    d. Delayed puberty

29. Which of the following is a false statement?
    a. Serial dilution samples should be taken when there is a suspicion of a large pituitary tumor and mildly elevated prolactin levels
    b. Assay specific values are higher in women than men
    c. Dynamic testing of prolactin is required due to its pulsatile secretion
    d. Metoclopramide may cause significant elevation in prolactin levels

30. Lifespan of the sperm and its ability to fertilize is:
    a. 3–5 days
    b. 3–5 weeks
    c. 3–5 hours
    d. 7–9 hours

ANSWERS

1. **c.** Prolactin levels are highest during sleep. Thyrotropin-releasing hormone stimulates prolactin secretion. Neuroendocrine agents originating in the hypothalamus have a positive stimulatory effect on growth hormone, follicle-stimulating hormone, luteinizing hormone, adrenocorticotropic hormone (ACTH), thyroid-stimulating hormone, and not prolactin.
   (Reference: Fritz MA, Speroff L. Clinical Gynecologic Endocrinology and Infertility, 8th edition. Philadelphia: Lippincott Williams & Wilkins; 2011. p. 162)

2. **c.** Measurement of luteinizing hormone pulses is used an indication of gonadotropin-releasing hormone pulsatile secretion as the long half-life of follicle-stimulating hormone.
   (Reference: Strauss JF III, Barbieri RL, Gargiulo AR. Yen & Jaffe's Reproductive Endocrinology. Physiology, Pathophysiology, and Clinical Management, 8th edition. Philadelphia: Elsevier; 2019. p. 9)

3. **c.** During the luteal phase production of progesterone increase to 20–30 mg/day.
   In the preovulatory phase progesterone production is <1 mg/day.
   (Reference: Fritz MA, Speroff L. Clinical Gynecologic Endocrinology and Infertility, 8th edition. Philadelphia: Lippincott Williams & Wilkins; 2011. p. 46)

4. **c.** Endorphins inhibit gonadotropin-releasing hormone release within the hypothalamus resulting in inhibition of gonadotropin secretion.
   B endorphins are five to ten times more potent than morphine.
   Endorphin levels peak during the luteal phase and are at lowest level during menses.
   Dysphoria experienced by some women in the premenstrual phase of cycle may be related to a withdrawal of endogenous opiates.
   (Reference: Infertility manual Kamini A Rao Second Edition Page 23)

5. **b.** While circulating in the blood, majority of the principal sex steroids, estradiol and testosterone, is bound to a protein carrier, known as SHBG produced mainly by the liver. Another 30% is loosely bound to

albumin, leaving only about 1% unbound and free. A very small percentage also binds to corticosteroid-binding globulin.
(Reference: Fritz MA, Speroff L. Clinical Gynecologic Endocrinology and Infertility, 8th edition. Philadelphia: Lippincott Williams & Wilkins; 2011. p. 43)

6. **b.** In the preovulatory phase in adult females, in all prepubertal females and in the normal male, the blood levels of progesterone are at the lower limits of immunoassay sensitivity: <1 ng/mL

    After ovulation, during the luteal phase progesterone ranges from 3 to 15 ng/mL.
    (Reference: Fritz MA, Speroff L. Clinical Gynecologic Endocrinology and Infertility, 8th edition. Philadelphia: Lippincott Williams & Wilkins; 2011. p. 46)

7. **c.** In women, because the production rate of androstenedione is greater than testosterone, blood dihydrotestosterone is primarily derived from androstenedione and partly from dehydroepiandrosterone. Thus, in women, the skin production of DHT is predominantly influenced by androstenedione.
    (Reference: Fritz MA, Speroff L. Clinical Gynecologic Endocrinology and Infertility, 8th edition. Philadelphia: Lippincott Williams & Wilkins; 2011. p. 48)

8. **c.** Dihydrotestosterone is the most potent androgen that cannot be aromatized to estradiol. It is non-aromatizable androgen.
    (Reference: Strauss JF III, Barbieri RL, Gargiulo AR. Yen & Jaffe's Reproductive Endocrinology. Physiology, Pathophysiology, and Clinical Management, 8th edition. Philadelphia: Elsevier; 2019. p. 291)

9. **c.** Oocytes are arrested in the diplotene stage of prophase of first meiotic division.
    (Reference: Strauss JF III, Barbieri RL, Gargiulo AR. Yen & Jaffe's Reproductive Endocrinology. Physiology, Pathophysiology, and Clinical Management, 8th edition. Philadelphia: Elsevier; 2019. p. 134)

10. **b.** The most common cause of thyrotoxicosis in pregnancy is Graves' disease.
    (Reference: Strauss JF III, Barbieri RL, Gargiulo AR. Yen & Jaffe's Reproductive Endocrinology. Physiology, Pathophysiology, and Clinical Management, 8th edition. Philadelphia: Elsevier; 2019. p. 605)

11. **b.** For patients with elevated thyroid-stimulating hormone but normal free T4, it is worth measuring antithyroid antibodies. A positive test identifies those who are likely to become clinically hypothyroid.
    (Reference: Guidelines for the treatment of hypothyroidism: Prepared by the American Thyroid Association Task Force on Thyroid Hormone Replacement. Thyroid. 2014;24:1670-751)

    In pregnancy: Increase in thyroid-binding globulin (TBG) leads to decrease in free triiodothyronine (T3) and thyroxine (T4). TSH reaches a nadir at 10 weeks.
    (Reference: Fritz MA, Speroff L. Clinical Gynecologic Endocrinology and Infertility, 8th edition. Philadelphia: Lippincott Williams & Wilkins; 2011. p. 898)

12. **b.** Anti-Müllerian hormone negatively regulates primordial follicle activation.
    (Reference: Strauss JF III, Barbieri RL, Gargiulo AR. Yen & Jaffe's Reproductive Endocrinology. Physiology, Pathophysiology, and Clinical Management, 8th edition. Philadelphia: Elsevier; 2019. p. 136)

13. **b.** An aromatase enzyme system acts to convert androgens to estrogens and is a factor limiting ovarian estrogen production.

    Aromatization is induced or activated through the action of FSH.

    FSH acts on granulosa cells to stimulate aromatization of androgens to estrogens.
    (Reference: Strauss JF III, Barbieri RL, Gargiulo AR. Yen & Jaffe's Reproductive Endocrinology. Physiology, Pathophysiology, and Clinical Management, 8th edition. Philadelphia: Elsevier; 2019. p. 76)

14. **c.** Antral follicles most likely to house a healthy oocyte have:
    - Highest estrogen concentrations
    - Highest FSH receptors
    - Lowest androgen/estrogen ratios

    (References: Fritz MA, Speroff L. Clinical Gynecologic Endocrinology and Infertility, 8th edition. Philadelphia: Lippincott Williams & Wilkins; 2011. p. 206
    Infertility manual Kamini A Rao Second Edition Page 23)

15. **d.** The secretion of FSH is very sensitive to negative inhibitory effects of estrogen even at low levels.

    At higher levels, estrogen combines with inhibin for a suppression of FSH that is profound and sustained.

At low levels, estrogen imposes a negative feedback relationship with LH.

At higher levels, however, estrogen exerts a positive stimulatory feedback effect on LH release.
(References: Fritz MA, Speroff L. Clinical Gynecologic Endocrinology and Infertility, 8th edition. Philadelphia: Lippincott Williams & Wilkins; 2011. p. 210.

Infertility manual Kamini A Rao Second Edition Page 23)

16. **b.** Ovaries are derived from the genital ridge.

    Rest fallopian tubes, uterus, and upper portion of vagina are derivatives of the Mullerian duct.
    (Reference: Fritz MA, Speroff L. Clinical Gynecologic Endocrinology and Infertility, 8th edition. Philadelphia: Lippincott Williams & Wilkins; 2011. p. 341)

17. **a.**

18. **c.** Congenital lipoid adrenal hyperplasia is the rarest and most severe form of congenital adrenal hyperplasia (CAH).
    (Reference: Fritz MA, Speroff L. Clinical Gynecologic Endocrinology and Infertility, 8th edition. Philadelphia: Lippincott Williams & Wilkins; 2011. p. 371)

19. **a.** *[Reference: The androgen receptor (AR) gene is located on the X chromosome (Xq12)].*

    Complete AIS follows an X-linked recessive pattern of inheritance.

20. **b.** *(Reference: Strauss JF III, Barbieri RL, Gargiulo AR. Yen & Jaffe's Reproductive Endocrinology. Physiology, Pathophysiology, and Clinical Management, 8th edition. Philadelphia: Elsevier; 2019. p. 207)*

21. **c.** *(Reference: Fritz MA, Speroff L. Clinical Gynecologic Endocrinology and Infertility, 8th edition. Philadelphia: Lippincott Williams & Wilkins; 2011. p. 369)*

22. **b.** *(Reference: Fritz MA, Speroff L. Clinical Gynecologic Endocrinology and Infertility, 8th edition. Philadelphia: Lippincott Williams & Wilkins; 2011. p. 373)*

23. **b.** *(Reference: Fritz MA, Speroff L. Clinical Gynecologic Endocrinology and Infertility, 8th edition. Philadelphia: Lippincott Williams & Wilkins; 2011. p. 393)*

24. **b.** *(Reference: Fritz MA, Speroff L. Clinical Gynecologic Endocrinology and Infertility, 8th edition. Philadelphia: Lippincott Williams & Wilkins; 2011. pp. 397-8)*

25. **a.** *(Reference: Appelbaum HL. Abnormal Female Puberty: A Clinical Casebook. New York: Springer International Publishing; 2016)*

26. **c.** *(Reference: Strauss JF III, Barbieri RL, Gargiulo AR. Yen & Jaffe's Reproductive Endocrinology. Physiology, Pathophysiology, and Clinical Management, 8th edition. Philadelphia: Elsevier; 2019. p. 256)*

27. **d.** *(Reference: Fritz MA, Speroff L. Clinical Gynecologic Endocrinology and Infertility, 8th edition. Philadelphia: Lippincott Williams & Wilkins; 2011. p. 287)*

28. **c.** *(Reference: Fritz MA, Speroff L. Clinical Gynecologic Endocrinology and Infertility, 8th edition. Philadelphia: Lippincott Williams & Wilkins; 2011. p. 447)*

29. **c.** *[Reference: Melmed S, Casanueva FF, Hoffman AR, Kleinberg DL, Montori VM, Schlechte JA, et al. Diagnosis and treatment of hyperprolactinemia: An Endocrine Society Clinical Practice Guideline. J Clin Endocrinol Metab. 2011;96(2):273-88]*

30. **a.** *(Reference: Fritz MA, Speroff L. Clinical Gynecologic Endocrinology and Infertility, 8th edition. Philadelphia: Lippincott Williams & Wilkins; 2011. p. 1156)*

Chapter 81

Menstruation

Urvashi Verma, Rekha Rani

QUESTIONS

1. Which of the following regarding Anti-Müllerian hormone (AMH) is incorrect?
   a. AMH is a marker of ovarian reserve
   b. AMH declines at menopause
   c. AMH is increased in polycystic ovarian reserve
   d. AMH is produced by theca cells

2. Which of the following is correct?
   a. Luteinizing hormone (LH) receptors are present on theca cells
   b. Follicle-stimulating hormone (FSH) receptors are present on granulosa cells
   c. For follicular recruitment growth selection and dominance both FSH and LH is required
   d. All the above

3. Which hormone is produced by corpus luteum?
   a. Estrogen
   b. Progesterone
   c. FSH
   d. LH

4. Primary source of progesterone is:
   a. Fetus
   b. Endometrium
   c. Corpus luteum
   d. Placenta

5. What will be most probable diagnosis in a 17-year-old girl with normal stature, no thelarche, raised FSH and LH, 46,XX with primary amenorrhea?
   a. Testicular feminizing syndrome
   b. Gonadal dysgenesis
   c. Kallmann syndrome
   d. Turner syndrome

6. When does the ovary contain maximum number of oogonia?
   a. At birth
   b. Third month of intrauterine life
   c. Fifth month of intrauterine life
   d. Seventh month of intrauterine life

7. On which day of menstruation cycle one should test for follicle-stimulating hormone (FSH) for appropriate diagnosis before commencing treatment?
   a. Second to fifth day of menstruation
   b. 14th day of menstruation
   c. 21st day of menstruation
   d. Any day of menstruation

8. What is the sequence of puberty changes in a normal girl?
   a. Thelarche, pubarche, menarche
   b. Pubarche, thelarche, menarche
   c. Pubarche, menarche, thelarche
   d. Menarche, thelarche, pubarche

9. Which of the following is suggestive of ovulation?
   a. Basal body temperature drop at least 0.5°C in the second half of the cycle
   b. Day 21 estrogen level is elevated
   c. Progesterone level on day 10 of the cycle is elevated
   d. Regular cycle with dysmenorrhea

10. The luteal phase of the menstrual cycle is associated with:
    a. High luteinizing hormone level
    b. High progesterone levels
    c. High prolactin level
    d. Low basal body temperature

11. The follicular phase of menstrual cycle is characterized by:
    a. Endometrial gland proliferation
    b. Decreased ovarian estradiol production
    c. Progesterone dominance
    d. A fixed length of 8 days

12. A sample of cervical mucus is taken on day 12 of the menstrual cycle. The mucus is thin, clear, and stretchy. It is placed on a slide and allow to air dry. When placed under microscopic, what would you, *expect*?
    a. Calcium citrate
    b. Clear fields, devoid of bacteria cell
    c. Thick mucus with background bacteria
    d. A fixed pattern characteristic of estrogen

13. Estrogen hormone is produced from all of the following organs, *except*:
    a. Corpus luteum
    b. B Anterior pituitary (anterior lobe of hypophysis)
    c. Placenta
    d. Testes

14. The midcycle luteinizing hormone (LH) surge:
    a. Enhances thecal cell androgen production
    b. Luteinizes granulose cells
    c. Initiates resumption of meiosis
    d. Facilitates oocyte expulsion
    e. All of the above

15. An involuted corpus luteum becomes a hyalinized mass known as a:
    a. Corpus albicans
    b. Corpus granulosa
    c. Graafian follicle
    d. Corpus atretica

16. Which of the following is the best method to predict the occurrence of ovulation?
    a. Thermogenic shift in basal body temperature
    b. Luteinizing hormone (LH) surge
    c. Endometrial decidualization
    d. Profuse, thin, acellular cervical mucous

17. Luteal phase deficiency:
    a. Has inadequate luteal progesterone production
    b. Has inadequate follicular estrogen production
    c. Can be corrected by estrogen
    d. Associated with delayed menstruation

18. On examination of endometrial tissue obtained from a biopsy reveals simple columnar epithelium with no subnuclear vacuoles. The stroma is edematous and tortuous gland contains secretions. These findings are consistent with which stage of menstrual cycle?
    a. Mid-proliferative
    b. Late proliferative
    c. Early secretory
    d. Mid-secretory

19. Ovulation occurs:
    a. 36 hours after luteinizing hormone (LH) surge
    b. 6–8 hours after LH surge
    c. After prolactin surge
    d. After follicles ripened in the ovary

20. Regarding estrogen hormone:
    a. It is produced in corpus luteum
    b. It is responsible for secretory changes in endometrium
    c. It is mainly secreted as Estriol by the ovary
    d. It cannot be detected in the blood of post-menopausal woman

21. Regarding human chorionic gonadotropin, all of the following are true, *except*:
    a. It is produced by the placenta
    b. Reversible for the maintenance of corpus luteum
    c. Its level doubles every 48 hours in ectopic pregnancy
    d. Reaches a peak concentration in maternal serum by 10 weeks' gestation

22. Endometrial changes during the menstrual cycle:
    a. The basal layer of the endometrium is responsive to hormonal stimulation
    b. The functional layer of the endometrium remains intact throughout menstrual cycle
    c. The increased thickness of the endometrium during the proliferative phase is due to estrogen action
    d. Estrogen induces secretory changes in the endometrium and reduces mitotic activity
    e. The zona compacta and spongiosum layer the basal layer of the endometrium

23. Inadequate luteal phase is associated with all of the following, *except*:
    a. Insufficient secretion on follicle-stimulating hormone (FSH) in the antecedent follicular phase
    b. Induction of ovulation with clomiphene citrate
    c. Induction of ovulation with human menopausal gonadotropins
    d. Administration of progesterone in the luteal phase

24. In the days after ovulation, all of the following occurs, *except*:
    a. The basal temperature rises
    b. The endometrium undergoes secretory changes
    c. The plasma progesterone concentration falls
    d. Cervical mucous becomes more viscous and scanty

25. The following hormones are secreted from the anterior pituitary gland, *except*:
    a. Follicle-stimulating hormone (FSH)
    b. Human chorionic gonadotropin (hCG)
    c. Luteinizing hormone (LH)
    d. Thyroid-stimulating hormone (TSH)

26. Ovulation may be indicated by all the following, *except*:
    a. Endometrial biopsy revealing secretary changes
    b. Elevation in prolactin
    c. Changing of cervical mucous to thick and scanty
    d. Progesterone level > 6.5 ng/mL

27. Which of the following is the primary source of estrogen?
    a. Theca interna cells
    b. Theca externa cells
    c. Granulosa cells
    d. Interstitial cells

28. Gonadotropin-releasing hormone (GnRH) stimulates the release of:
    a. Opiate peptides
    b. Adrenocorticotropic hormone (ACTH)
    c. Luteinizing hormone (LH)
    d. Growth hormone

29. Effect of estrogen on the cervical mucous:
    a. Increase the glycoprotein level and thus allow the penetration of the sperms
    b. Decrease the watery content
    c. Mucus plug formation
    d. Reduces mobility of sperm

30. Raised follicle-stimulating hormone (FSH) levels are found in all of the following conditions, *except*:
    a. Postmenopausal women
    b. Turner's syndrome
    c. Women on combined oral contraceptive pills
    d. Gonadal dysgenesis

31. Estrogen have all of the following actions, *except*:
    a. Produce proliferation of the endometrium
    b. Development of secondary sexual characteristics
    c. Fusion of the epiphysis
    d. Perimenopausal women who had hysterectomy with bilateral salpingo-oophorectomy

32. Which of the following pubertal events in is not mediated by gonadal estrogen production?
    a. Menstruation
    b. Pubic hair growth
    c. Breast development
    d. Skeletal growth

33. Which of the following statement regarding prolactin is true?
    a. Prolactin levels decrease shortly after sleep
    b. Prolactin levels increase levels increase after ingesting high glucose meals
    c. Prolactin levels decrease during surgery
    d. Prolactin levels increase during stress

34. Besides infertility, the most common symptoms of a luteal phase defect:
    a. Vaginal dryness
    b. Early abortion
    c. Tubal occlusion
    d. Breast tenderness

35. At which point in the menstrual cycle is a women most fertile?
    a. Day 1–5
    b. Day 9–16
    c. Day 17–21
    d. Day 22–28

ANSWERS

1. d.
2. d. *[Reference: Raju GA, Chavan R, Deenadayal M, Gunasheela D, Gutgutia R, Haripriya G, et al. Luteinizing hormone and follicle stimulating hormone synergy: A review of role in controlled ovarian hyperstimulation. J Hum Reprod Sci. 2013;6(4):227-34]*

3. c.	4. c.	5. b.	6. c.
7. a.	8. a.	9. d.	10. b.
11. a.	12. d.	13. b.	14. e.
15. a.	16. b.	17. a.	18. d.
19. a.	20. a.	21. c.	22. c.
23. a.	24. c.	25. b.	26. b.
27. c.	28. c.	29. a.	30. c.
31. d.	32. b.	33. d.	34. b.
35. b.			

Chapter 82: Abnormal Uterine Bleeding

Renu Gupta, Pavika Lal

QUESTIONS

1. **All are second-generation endometrial ablation techniques, *except*:**
   a. Microwave endometrial ablation
   b. Thermal balloon ablation
   c. Hydrothermal ablation
   d. Roller ball ablation

2. **All of the following statements are true regarding the physiology of menstruation, *except*:**
   a. Classical concept of ischemic necrosis of the endometrium as the initiation of menses has been shifted to enzymatic autodigestion of endometrium
   b. Histologically early menstruating endometrium exhibit coagulative necrosis instead of focal necrosis
   c. Hypoxia inducible factor 1 (HIF-1) is rarely detected in shedding menstrual endometrium
   d. End of menses is due to constriction of spiral arterioles along with coagulation and re-epithelization

3. **All are true for post-pill amenorrhea, *except*:**
   a. Failure to resume menstruation within 6 months after discontinuation of oral contraceptive pill (OCP)
   b. Associated with low levels of gonadotropins with mild-to-moderate elevation of prolactin
   c. Treatment is only required when pregnancy is desired
   d. FSH and LH levels should always be done for establishing the diagnosis

4. **All are true about Pictorial Blood Assessment Chart (PBAC), *except*:**
   a. Most widely used semiquantitative method to assess menstrual blood and record number of tampons/towels used
   b. More than 100 points signify heavy menstrual bleeding
   c. For each completely saturated pad and tampon, a score of 10 and 5 points is assigned respectively
   d. Sensitivity and specificity of PBA score is approximately, 90% and 100% respectively

5. **Which of the following is a feature of endometrial polyp on color Doppler transvaginal sonography (TVS)?**
   a. Pedicle artery sign
   b. Ring of fire sign
   c. Swiss cheese appearance sign
   d. Increased endometrial thickness

6. **All are true during the normal menstrual cycle, *except*:**
   a. The cyclical changes of the endometrium proceed in an orderly fashion in response to hormonal production
   b. Stratum functionalis is the source of endometrial regeneration after each menses
   c. During the proliferative phase, the endometrial glands changes from low columnar pattern to pseudostratified pattern just prior to ovulation
   d. Progressive decrease in estrogen receptor concentration in endometrial cells in latter half of cycle leading to decrease in estrogen induced DNA synthesis

7. **All are true about abnormal uterine bleeding (AUB) in adolescent age group, *except*:**
   a. Initial anovulation is due to immature hypothalamic pituitary ovarian axis
   b. The elder the age at menarche, the sooner the regulated cycles are established
   c. Possibility of pregnancy must be considered when an adolescent is seeking treatment for AUB

d. Screening with chlamydial infection is recommended in adolescent presenting with heavy menstrual bleeding (HMB)

8. **Following tests should be done in adolescent presenting with heavy menstrual bleeding, *except*:**
   a. Urine pregnancy test
   b. Prothrombin time/activated partial thromboplastin time (PT/aPTT)
   c. Screening of sexually transmitted disease (STD) from cervical or urine specimens
   d. Cervical cytology

9. **Which of the following is the most common cause of primary amenorrhea?**
   a. Pure gonadal dysgenesis
   b. MRKH (Mayer-Rokitansky-Küster-Hauser) syndrome
   c. Robert's uterus
   d. Transverse vaginal septum

10. **Miss Y, P0^{+0} 17-year-old female, came with complaint of primary amenorrhea. On examination, although her breast were well developed but she had absence of both pubic and axillary hair. On local examination, external genitalia was apparently normal and vagina was blind and short. On per rectal examination, uterus was not palpable. What will be the most probable karyotype?**
    a. 46,XX
    b. 46,XXY
    c. 46,XO
    d. 46,XY

11. **Irreversible side effect of danazol is:**
    a. Acne
    b. Deepening of voice
    c. Formation of ovarian cysts
    d. Increased facial hair

12. **Anovulatory bleeding in polycystic ovary syndrome (PCOS) is due to:**
    a. Increase in serum luteinizing hormone (LH) levels in early follicular phase due to increase in both LH pulse frequency and amplitude
    b. Increase in serum LH Level in early follicular phase due to increase in only LH pulse frequency
    c. Increase in serum LH level in early luteal phase due to increase in LH pulse frequency and amplitude
    d. Increase in serum LH level and follicle-stimulating hormone (FSH) level in early luteal phase

13. **In estrogen breakthrough bleeding, all are true, *except*:**
    a. Low level of chronic estrogen exposure results in intermittent spotting which is usually light in volume
    b. Low level of chronic estrogen exposure results in heavy bleeding
    c. High level of estrogen exposure results in amenorrhea followed by acute episodes of profuse bleeding
    d. Usually observed in patients with chronic anovulation

14. **All are characteristics of progesterone breakthrough bleeding, *except*:**
    a. Occurs when ratio of progesterone to estrogen is high
    b. Bleeding usually is irregular and light in volume with variable duration
    c. Seen in association with progesterone-only contraceptive (POP), implants, and depot medroxyprogesterone acetate (DMPA)
    d. May follow after bilateral oophorectomy during follicular phase of cycle

15. **All of the following are incorrect about PALM COEIN [Polyp, Adenomyosis, Leiomyoma (fibroid), or Malignancy or hyperplasia] or nonstructural (Coagulopathy, Ovulatory dysfunction, Endometrial, Iatrogenic, Not classified) classification, *except*:**
    a. A method of categorizing the results of investigation of women with abnormal uterine bleeding in the reproductive years
    b. An algorithm designed to lead to a diagnosis of the cause of abnormal uterine bleeding
    c. Appropriate for diagnosing women with postmenopausal bleeding
    d. An acronym for a set of symptoms that may or may not contribute to the cause of abnormal uterine bleeding in the reproductive years

16. **All are absolute contraindications of uterine artery embolization, *except*:**
    a. Cervical fibroid
    b. Concurrent use of GnRH agonist
    c. Severe renal insufficiency
    d. Adenomyosis

17. **Mechanism of action of high-dose estrogen when given to arrest acute episodes of bleeding:**
    a. Leads to vasoconstriction of the small capillaries in the endometrium
    b. Promotes rapid endometrial growth to cover the denuded endometrial surface
    c. Promotes the production of prostaglandins
    d. Helps in expulsion of retained clots

18. **All are causes of anovulatory bleeding, *except*:**
    a. Hyperprolactinemia
    b. Anorexia nervosa
    c. Obesity
    d. Chronic kidney/liver disease
    e. Pelvic tuberculosis

19. **Mrs. X P0^{+4} with history of recurrent abortions and curettages came with complaint of scanty menses and oligomenorrhea. Her last menstrual period (LMP) was 2 months back but her urine pregnancy test was negative. On sequential treatment with estrogen and progesterone no bleeding occurred. What is the most probable diagnosis?**
    a. Polycystic ovary syndrome (PCOS)
    b. Septate uterus
    c. Asherman syndrome
    d. Secondary cervical stenosis

20. **Regarding ulipristal acetate usage the following are incorrect, *except*:**
    a. Endometrial changes are reversible following cessation of therapy
    b. Epithelial proliferation has been shown
    c. Stromal proliferation has been shown
    d. The significance of progesterone receptor-associated endometrial changes (PAEC) is well known

21. **A 26-year-old woman presented with complaint of secondary amenorrhea. She did not complaint of any significant physical, emotional, or nutritional stress. Progestin challenge test was negative. USG showed thin endometrium and small ovaries. Hormonal profile: thyroid-stimulating hormone (TSH)—2.3 mIU/L, prolactin—20 mg/dL, follicle-stimulating hormone (FSH)—25 IU/L, and estradiol (E2)—20 pg/dL. All the following investigations are justified, *except*:**
    a. Karyotyping
    b. Anti-CYP21 antibodies
    c. FMR1 permutation testing
    d. Magnetic resonance imaging (MRI) head

22. **Perimenopausal transition is associated with?**
    a. High follicle-stimulating hormone (FSH), high luteinizing hormone (LH)
    b. Low FSH, high LH
    c. High FSH, normal LH
    d. Normal FSH, normal LH

23. **With regard to irregular menstrual cycles, which of the following is incorrect?**
    a. Normal in first year postmenarche
    b. >1 to <3 year postmenarche, cycles are considered irregular if they come >35 days' interval
    c. >3 years postmenarche to perimenopausal cycles coming at intervals <21 days' cycles are considered irregular
    d. <8 cycles per year are considered abnormal

24. **Which of the following is not true with respect to fibroids?**
    a. Women interested in pregnancy should not be offered uterine artery embolization as a treatment option
    b. Posterior uterine incision is preferred to remove fibroids during myomectomy to minimize formation of postoperative adhesions
    c. In unexplained infertility, submucosal fibroids should be removed in order to improve conception and pregnancy rates
    d. A hysterosalpingography (HSG) is not an appropriate test to evaluate and classify fibroids

25. **The critical level of body fat required for the onset and regularity of menstrual function corresponds to:**
    a. 17% for menarche and 22% for regular menstruation
    b. 27% for menarche and 22% for regular menstruation
    c. 17% for menarche and 27% for regular menstruation
    d. 22% for menarche and 17% for regular menstruation

26. **All are true about irregular bleeding that occurs in female who are using hormonal contraception, *except*?**
    a. Breakthrough bleeding occurs in first 1–3 months of oral contraceptive pill (OCP) use
    b. It should always be first managed by counseling and reassurance
    c. Screening for sexually transmitted disease (STD) should be considered in such patients
    d. Change to implants and progesterone-releasing intrauterine contraceptive device (IUCD) do not offer any relief over combined oral contraceptive (COC) in such cases

27. **The most common bleeding disorder in female presenting with heavy menstrual bleeding:**
    a. Factor VIII deficiency
    b. Bernard–Soulier syndrome
    c. Von Willebrand factor deficiency
    d. Glanzmann syndrome

28. **All are true about endometrial polyp associated with postmenopausal bleeding, *except*:**
    a. Asymptomatic endometrial polyp <2 cm in diameter should be removed
    b. Hysteroscopy offers the highest diagnostic accuracy for endometrial polyps
    c. Transvaginal ultrasound (TVUS) should be the imaging modality of choice
    d. Removal of asymptomatic polyp in premenopausal female should be considered in patients with risk factors for endometrial carcinoma

29. **Suspicion of coagulation dysfunction in case of a female presenting with heavy menstrual bleeding includes all, *except*:**
    a. History of postpartum hemorrhage (PPH) especially >24 hours
    b. History of hemorrhage from ovarian cyst
    c. History of prolonged bleeding after dental extraction or epistaxis
    d. Oral or gastrointestinal bleeding in presence of anatomic lesions

30. **Diagnosis of adenomyosis and leiomyoma require careful evaluation. Which of the following is true?**
    a. Multiple small uterine lesions with uniform echo structure are common in leiomyosarcomas
    b. The presence of fan-shaped shading is sufficient to diagnose adenomyosis
    c. Magnetic resonance imaging (MRI) is the first choice for diagnosis and mapping of myomas
    d. Small polyps and myomas can be removed by use of small dimensional hysteroscopes

ANSWERS

1. **d.** First-generation, commonly referred to as hysteroscopic techniques, require hysteroscopic visualization of the uterine cavity during the procedure. Examples in this group include endometrial laser ablation (ELA), transcervical resection of the endometrium (TCRE), and rollerball endometrial ablation. Second- and third-generation approaches, frequently referred to as non-hysteroscopic techniques, – do not require direct visualization of the uterine cavity during the procedure. Examples of second-generation techniques include thermal balloon endometrial ablation (Cavaterm®, Thermachoice®), microwave endometrial ablation (MEA®, Microsulis®), hydrothermal ablation (Hydro ThermAblator®), bipolar radiofrequency endometrial ablation (Novasure®, Minerva®), and endometrial cryotherapy (Cerene®, Her Option®). An example of a third-generation technique is Thermachoice III®. First-generation techniques (ELA, TCRE, rollerball endometrial ablation) and second-generation approaches (thermal balloon endometrial ablation, microwave endometrial ablation, hydrothermal ablation, bipolar radiofrequency endometrial ablation, endometrial cryotherapy) are of equivalent efficacy for heavy menstrual bleeding. Second-generation techniques are associated with shorter operating times and are performed more often under local rather than general anesthesia.
(Reference: Bofill Rodriguez M, Lethaby A, Grigore M, Brown J, Hickey M, Farquhar C. Endometrial resection and ablation techniques for heavy menstrual bleeding. Cochrane Database Syst Rev. 2019;1: CD001501)

2. **b.** *[Reference: Malik R, Radhika A G. Regulation of menstrual cycle. In: Malik R, Radhika A G (Eds). Berek & Novak's Gynecology South Asian Edition. Gurugram: Wolters Kluwer (India) Pvt. Ltd.; 2021. p. 523]*

3. **d.** Post-pill amenorrhea is a relatively uncomplicated medical problem to diagnose and treat, but it is imperative to exclude pituitary tumors or serious endocrinological abnormalities before treatment is begun. It is the failure to resume menstruation within 6 months after discontinuation of oral contraceptives. Objectively, a pattern of hypothalamic deficiency may be found, which usually consists of low values for the gonadotropic and ovarian hormones and mild-to-moderate elevations of prolactin. Treatment is required only if pregnancy is desired. Two very effective drugs are available that can be safely administered are bromocriptine and clomiphene. Women not desiring pregnancy at the time can be managed with reassurance in the expectation of a spontaneous return of menstruation and with periodic follow-ups.

[Reference: Rojas-Walsson R, Cardoso R. Diagnosis and management of post-pill amenorrhea. J Fam Pract. 1981;13(2):165-9]

4. **c.** The Pictorial Blood Assessment Chart (PBAC) score has a sensitivity of 91%, a specificity of 100%, positive predictive value (PPV) of 100%, and negative predictive value (NPV) of 85.5%. The chart consists of images representing lightly, moderately, and heavily stained sanitary towels (scored as 1, 5, and 20 respectively) and tampons (scored as 1, 5, or 10 respectively); passage of clots (assigned ascending scores from 1 to 5) and episodes of flooding are also recorded. Heavy menstrual bleeding is defined as PBAC score >100.
   [Reference: Halimeh S, Rott H, Kappert G. PBAC score: an easy-to-use tool to predict coagulation disorders in women with idiopathic heavy menstrual bleeding. Haemophilia. 2016;22(3):e217-20]

5. **a.** Endometrial polyps are a common cause of abnormal uterine bleeding. Ultrasound is the most accepted investigation to evaluate them. Color Doppler can depict vascularity of the endometrial polyp which is usually a single feeding vessel. This "pedicle artery sign" was described by Timmerman et al. as visualization of the feeding blood vessel of the endometrial polyp. Multiple feeding vessels are nonspecific and can be seen in endometrial hyperplasia, endometrial cancer, submucous fibroids, and even in some endometrial polyps. However, a rim-like vessel pattern in an endometrial lesion suggests the diagnosis of a submucosal fibroid. The pedicle artery sign on transvaginal color Doppler sonography was found to have sensitivity of 86.67%, accuracy of 86.67%, and positive predictive value of 100%.
   [Reference: Amreen S, Singh M, Choh NA, Saldanha C, Gojwari TA. Doppler evaluation of endometrial polyps. EJRNM. 2018;49(3):850-3]

6. **b.** Stratum spongiosum is the source of endometrial regeneration after each menses.
   [Reference: Malik R, Radhika AG. Regulation of menstrual cycle. In: Malik R, Radhika A G (Eds). Berek & Novak's Gynecology South Asian Edition. Gurugram: Wolters Kluwer (India) Pvt. Ltd.; 2021. p. 523]

7. **b.** The younger the age at menarche, the sooner the regulated cycles are established.
   [Reference: Malik R, Radhika A G. Adolescent abnormal uterine bleeding. In: Malik R, Radhika A G (Eds). Berek & Novak's Gynecology South Asian Edition. Gurugram: Wolters Kluwer (India) Pvt. Ltd.; 2021. p. 179]

8. **d.** Cervical cytology testing is generally not appropriate for adolescents, particularly at an emergency or urgent visit for excessive bleeding.
   [Reference: Malik R, Radhika AG. Diagnosis of adolescent abnormal uterine bleeding. In: Malik R, Radhika A G (Eds). Berek & Novak's Gynecology South Asian Edition. Gurugram: Wolters Kluwer (India) Pvt. Ltd.; 2021. p. 181]

9. **a.** Pure gonadal dysgenesis

10. **d.** Androgen insensitivity syndrome (AIS) is typically characterized by evidence of feminization (i.e., under masculinization) of the external genitalia at birth, abnormal secondary sexual development in puberty, and infertility in individuals with a 46,XY karyotype.

11. **b.** Weight gain, acne, flushing, sweating, voice changes (hoarseness, change in pitch), abnormal growth of body hair (in women), vaginal dryness/irritation, or decreased breast size may occur.

12. **a.** [Reference: Malik R, Radhika A G. Polycystic ovary syndrome. In: Malik R, Radhika A G (Eds). Berek & Novak's Gynecology South Asian Edition. Gurugram: Wolters Kluwer (India) Pvt. Ltd.; 2021. p. 153, 180]

13. **b.** (Reference: Natarajan P, Pandiyan R, Thanikachalam P. Abnormal uterine bleeding. Speroff's Clinical Gynecologic Endocrinology and Infertility, 1st South Asia edition. Gurugram: Wolters Kluwer India Pvt. Ltd.; 2023. p. 525)

14. **d.** (Reference: Natarajan P, Pandiyan R, Thanikachalam P. Abnormal uterine bleeding. Speroff's Clinical Gynecologic Endocrinology and Infertility, 1st South Asia edition. Gurugram: Wolters Kluwer India Pvt. Ltd.; 2023. p. 525)

15. **a.** It is not appropriate for diagnosing women with postmenopausal bleeding.

16. **d.**

Contraindications of uterine fibroid embolization (UFE):
- Viable active pregnancy
- Active endometritis
- Malignancy of the uterus/cervix without concurrent surgical treatment planned

- Postmenopausal patient with bleeding of undiagnosed etiology
- Fibroid that is already infarcted [based on (MRI) magnetic resonance imaging]
- Fibroid that is smaller than 1 cm
- Fibroid with pedunculated morphology (such as stalk width <50% of the maximum width)
- Fibroid located in the cervix
- Concurrent use of a gonadotropin-releasing hormone agonist
- Prior pelvic radiation therapy
- Immunocompromised state
- Fibroid growth resulting in overall uterus size equivalent or greater than the expected size at 24 weeks gestation (uterus cranial aspect reaching the umbilicus)
- Severe contrast allergy
- Severe renal insufficiency not receiving dialysis therapy
- Uncorrectable coagulopathy

Of some controversy:
- Patient desire for future pregnancy
- Adenomyosis

[*Reference: Young M, Coffey W, Mikhail LN. Uterine fibroid embolization. In: StatPearls (Internet). Treasure Island (FL): StatPearls Publishing; 2023*]

17. **b.** (*Reference: Natarajan P, Pandiyan R, Thanikachalam P. Abnormal uterine bleeding. Speroff's Clinical Gynecologic Endocrinology and Infertility, 1st South Asia edition. Gurugram: Wolters Kluwer India Pvt. Ltd.; 2023. p. 537*)

18. **e.** Pelvic tuberculosis

19. **c.** Asherman syndrome occurs primarily after a dilation and curettage performed for elective termination of pregnancy, a missed or incomplete miscarriage, or to treat a retained placenta after delivery. It may occur with or without hemorrhage after delivery or elective termination of pregnancy. Less often, it results after a dilation and curettage for a non-obstetrical procedure for excessive bleeding, sampling for endometrial cancer, or removal of endometrial polyps. It can also occur after surgery to remove uterine fibroids.

20. **a.** Endometrial changes are reversible following cessation of therapy and were associated with no signs of epithelial and stromal proliferation. The significance of progesterone receptor-associated endometrial changes (PAEC) is unknown. PAEC can be observed in a significant number of untreated patients.

21. **d.** The diagnosis is premature ovarian insufficiency. Numerical and structural abnormalities like translocations, deletions, and mosaicism run high risk of premature ovarian failure.
(*Reference: Natarajan P, Pandiyan R, Thanikachalam P. Abnormal uterine bleeding. Speroff's Clinical Gynecologic Endocrinology and Infertility, 1st South Asia edition. Gurugram: Wolters Kluwer India Pvt. Ltd.; 2023. p. 464*)

22. **c.** (*Reference: Marshburn P, Hurst B. Menstrual disorders during the reproductive years. Disorders of Menstruation, 1st edition. Hoboken: Wiley-Blackwell; 2011. p. 47*)

23. **b.**
- >1 to <3 year postmenarche, cycles are considered irregular if they come <21 days' or >45 days' interval
- >3 year postmenarche to perimenopausal cycles coming at intervals <21 days or >35 days cycles are considered irregular.

[*Reference: Teede HJ, Misso ML, Costello MF, Dokras A, Laven J, Moran L, et al.; International PCOS Network. Recommendations from the international evidence-based guideline for the assessment and management of polycystic ovary syndrome. Hum Reprod. 2018;33(9):1602-18. in: Hum Reprod. 2019;34(2):388*]

24. **b.** [*Reference: Vilos GA, Allaire C, Laberge PY, Leyland N; Special Contributors. SOGC Clinical Practice Guideline. The management of uterine leiomyomas. J Obstet Gynaecol Can. 2015;37(2):157-78*]

25. **a.** (*Reference: Natarajan P, Pandiyan R, Thanikachalam P. Speroff's Clinical Gynecologic Endocrinology and Infertility, 1st South Asia edition. New Delhi: Wolters Kluwer India Pvt. Ltd.; 2023. p. 490*)
[*Balen A. Amenorrhoea. In: Balen A (Ed). Reproductive Endocrinology for the MRCOG and Beyond, 2nd edition. Cambridge: Cambridge University Press; 2007. p. 83*]

26. **d.** [*Reference: Solone M, Adams Hillard PJ. Adult gynecology: reproductive years. In: Malik R, Radhika AG (Eds). Berek & Novak's Gynecology South Asian Edition. Gurugram: Wolters Kluwer (India) Pvt. Ltd.; 2021. p. 193*]

27. **c.** Von Willebrand disease (VWD) is a common bleeding disorder that typically manifests with mucosal bleeding. Women with VWD are more likely to have bleeding symptoms related to the high prevalence of heavy menstrual bleeding.

28. **a.** *[Reference: Amreen S, Singh M, Choh N A, Saldanha C, Gojwari TA. Doppler evaluation of endometrial polyps. EJRNM. 2018;49(3):850-3]*

29. **d.** *[Reference: Solone M, Adams Hillard PJ. Adult gynecology: reproductive years. In: Malik R, Radhika AG (Eds). Berek & Novak's Gynecology South Asian Edition. Gurugram: Wolters Kluwer (India) Pvt. Ltd.; 2021. p. 193]*

30. **d.** Typical ultrasound features of myomas in the myometrium are a well-defined, round lesion. Shadowing is often present at the edge of myomas (edge shadows) or internal (fan-shaped shadowing). Features of leiomyosarcomas include a single large lesion with a heterogenic mixed echo structure. At least two of the characteristics of adenomyosis needs to be present to give a diagnosis of adenomyosis. Characteristics include asymmetry of uterine walls, a globally enlarged uterus, ill-defined myometrial mass, anechogenic cysts, small anechoic lacunae, linear striations and buds, irregular endometrial outline. Transvaginal ultrasound is first choice. Sonohysterography may be needed to determine the impact of myomas on the endometrial cavity. The numbers of myomas with diameter >1-1.5 cm should be counted, measured and mapped according to location and site (0-8). Three-dimensional ultrasonography may be advantageous in evaluation of a few myomas. In the presence of multiple myomas and when minimally invasive treatment options are planned, magnetic resonance imaging (MRI) may enable mapping of more myomas. The accuracy of measurements of 1-4 myomas are no more accurate on MRI than transvaginal sonography (TVS). Small-dimensional hysteroscopes are not optimal in the presence of bleeding and larger pathology, but can be used to remove small polyps and myomas.

Chapter 83

Premenstrual Syndrome

Vandana Solanki, Deepa Singh

QUESTIONS

1. Which one is true for premenstrual syndrome?
   i. Physical and behavioral symptoms
   ii. Cyclic
   iii. No symptom-free period
   iv. Prominent symptoms of irritability, dysphoria, and internal tension
   a. i, iii
   b. i, ii, iii
   c. I, Iv
   d. i, ii

2. Who first described premenstrual syndrome?
   a. Greene
   b. Dalton
   c. RT Frank
   d. Diego

3. Symptoms of premenstrual syndrome (PMS) typically arise during:
   a. Last 7–10 days of cycle
   b. First 7 days of cycle
   c. Last 4 and first 3 days of cycle
   d. Last 2 days of cycle

4. The diagnosis of premenstrual syndrome (PMS) and premenstrual dysphoric disorder (PMDD) depends on:
   i. Presence of physical symptoms
   ii. Timing
   iii. Severity
   iv. Exclusion of other diagnosis
   a. i, ii, iii
   b. i, ii, iv
   c. i, iii, iv
   d. i, ii, iii, iv

5. COPE, i.e., Calendar of Premenstrual Experience, has:
   a. 10 physical and 12 behavioral symptoms
   b. 12 physical and 10 behavioral symptoms
   c. 4 physical and 12 behavioral symptoms
   d. 10 physical and 12 behavioral symptoms

6. Which is the most popular survey for analysis of premenstrual syndrome (PMS)?
   a. MDQ (Menstrual Distress Questionnaire)
   b. PAF (Premenstrual Assessment Form)
   c. COPE (Calendar of Premenstrual Experience)
   d. PRISM (Prospective Record of the Impact and Severity of Menstruation)

7. The diagnosis of PMS require how much increase in symptoms 5 days before menses as compared to 5 days after onset of menses?
   a. 28%
   b. 30%
   c. 40%
   d. 50%

8. Premenstrual dysphoric disorder include:
   i. Somatic symptoms
   ii. Affective symptoms
   iii. Timing
   iv. Symptom-free period
   a. i, ii, iii, iv
   b. i, iv
   c. ii, iii, iv
   d. i, ii

9. Premenstrual syndrome is caused by disturbance in:
   a. Dopaminergic system
   b. GABAergic system
   c. Both
   d. None of the above

10. Premenstrual syndrome and premenstrual dysphoric disorder has most important role in pathophysiology of:
    a. Estrogen
    b. Progesterone
    c. Dopamine
    d. Serotonin

11. Effective treatment of premenstrual syndrome and premenstrual dysphoric disorder include:
    i. Selective serotonin reuptake inhibitor (SSRI) + Alprazolam
    ii. SSRI + GnRH (gonadotropin-releasing hormone) antagonist

iii. SSRI + GnRH agonist
iv. Alprazolam + OCP (oral contraceptive pill)
a. i, iii
b. i, ii, iv
c. i, ii
d. ii, iv

12. First-line treatment for premenstrual syndrome and premenstrual dysphoric disorder is:
a. Fluoxetine
b. Alprazolam
c. Venlafaxine
d. Oral contraceptive pill (OCP)

13. Gonadotropin-releasing hormone (GnRH) agonist mainly relieve symptoms like:
a. Depression
b. Anxiety
c. Physical symptoms
d. Dysphoria

14. Which one is true about oral contraceptive pill (OCP) action on PMS?
a. Relieve bloating and breast pain
b. Relieve mood symptoms
c. Relieve both somatic and mood symptoms
d. Just relieve behavioral symptoms

15. Women with PMS and PMDD who fails to respond to the treatment should be considered for:
i. Anxiety disorder
ii. Malingering
iii. Noncompliance
iv. Substance abuse
a. i, iv
b. ii, iii
c. i, iii
d. ii, iv

16. Causes of premenstrual syndrome is:
a. Endocrine event during menstrual phase
b. Abnormal response to normal cycle changes in ovarian steroid hormone level
c. Both
d. None

17. Who firstly used the term "premenstrual syndrome"?
i. Greene
i. Dalton
ii. Rupert
iii. Frank
a. i, ii
b. ii, iii
c. iii, iv
d. iv, i

18. Women who have no demonstrable symptom-free interval during _____ phase of cycle merit careful evaluation for a mood or anxiety disorder.
a. Luteal
b. Follicular
c. Menstrual
d. (b) and (c)

19. Calendar of Premenstrual Experience (COPE) uses _____ scale.
a. Nominal
b. Ordinal
c. Likert
d. Interval

20. Which is the most common menstrual problem?
a. Dysmenorrhea
b. Premenstrual dysphoric disorder
c. Premenstrual syndrome
d. Irregular menses

21. Which of the following is effective treatment of PMS and PMDD?
a. Alprazolam
b. Progesterone
c. Dietary restriction
d. Vitamins

22. True about fluoxetine treatment is:
i. Not well tolerated
ii. Daily dose of 20 mg OD
iii. Relieve somatic symptoms and mood symptoms
iv. Well tolerated
a. ii, iii, iv
b. i, ii, iii
c. iii, iv
d. ii, iv

23. Alprazolam relieves:
a. Depressive symptoms
b. Somatic symptoms
c. Both
d. None

24. Spironolactone act as a treatment of premenstrual syndrome because:
a. It has potassium-sparing effect
b. Being a diuretic
c. Structural similarity to steroid hormone
d. None

25. Which one is the oldest and simplest method of treatment of PMS and PMDD?
a. Oral contraceptive pill
b. Gonadotropin-releasing hormone agonist
c. Diet and exercise
d. Spironolactone

26. Treatment of choice with mild symptoms and significant socioeconomic dysfunction is:
a. Placebo
b. Selective serotonin reuptake inhibitor (SSRI)
c. Oral contraceptive pill
d. Aerobic exercise

27. What is second line of treatment if selective serotonin reuptake inhibitor fails?
a. Oral contraceptive pill
b. High-dose alprazolam
c. Low-dose alprazolam
d. Gonadotropin-releasing hormone antagonist

28. What is the key to effective management of premenstrual syndrome?
    a. Accurate diagnosis
    b. Level of steroid hormones
    c. Presence or absence of depression
    d. None

29. What are the most common side effects of selective serotonin reuptake inhibitor?
    a. Diminished sexual interest
    b. Sedation
    c. Fluid retention
    d. Addiction

30. Which are the symptoms of premenstrual syndrome?
    i. Hypersomnia
    ii. Anxiety
    iii. Depression
    iv. Insomnia

    a. i, ii, iii   b. i, ii, iv
    c. i, ii, iii, iv   d. ii, iii, iv

ANSWERS

1. **d.** i, ii
   The simplest definition of the premenstrual syndrome is that cyclic physical and behavioral symptoms which appear in the days preceding menses and interfere with work or lifestyle, followed by a symptom-free interval.
   (Reference: Fritz MA, Speroff L. Clinical Gynecologic Endocrinology and Infertility, 8th edition. Philadelphia: Lippincott Williams & Wilkins; 2011. p. 568)

2. **c.** RT Frank
   (Reference: Fritz MA, Speroff L. Clinical Gynecologic Endocrinology and Infertility, 8th edition. Philadelphia: Lippincott Williams & Wilkins; 2011. p. 569)

3. **a.** Last 7-10 days of cycle
   (Reference: Fritz MA, Speroff L. Clinical Gynecologic Endocrinology and Infertility, 8th edition. Philadelphia: Lippincott Williams & Wilkins; 2011. p. 569)

4. **d.** i, ii, iii, iv
   The diagnosis of both premenstrual syndrome and premenstrual dysphoric disorder depends on the presence of typical symptoms, their timings, severity, and the exclusion of other diagnosis.
   (Reference: Fritz MA, Speroff L. Clinical Gynecologic Endocrinology and Infertility, 8th edition. Philadelphia: Lippincott Williams & Wilkins; 2011. p. 570)

5. **d.** 10 physical and 12 behavioral.
   (Reference: Fritz MA, Speroff L. Clinical Gynecologic Endocrinology and Infertility, 8th edition. Philadelphia: Lippincott Williams & Wilkins; 2011. p. 570)

6. **b.** COPE (Calendar of Premenstrual Experience)
   (Reference: Fritz MA, Speroff L. Clinical Gynecologic Endocrinology and Infertility, 8th edition. Philadelphia: Lippincott Williams & Wilkins; 2011. p. 572)

7. **b.** 30%
   (Reference: Fritz MA, Speroff L. Clinical Gynecologic Endocrinology and Infertility, 8th edition. Philadelphia: Lippincott Williams & Wilkins; 2011. p. 572)

8. **c.** ii, iii, iv
   The diagnosis of premenstrual syndrome require both affective and somatic symptoms, the diagnosis of premenstrual dysphoric disorder can include but does not require somatic symptoms.
   (Reference: Fritz MA, Speroff L. Clinical Gynecologic Endocrinology and Infertility, 8th edition. Philadelphia: Lippincott Williams & Wilkins; 2011. p. 572)

9. **b.** GABAergic system
   The anxiolytic action of certain progesterone metabolites that act as a ligand for gamma-aminobutyric acid A (GABA$_A$) receptor and the effectiveness of alprazolam in relieving symptoms of premenstrual syndrome suggest that disorder might involve a disturbance in GABAergic system.
   (Reference: Fritz MA, Speroff L. Clinical Gynecologic Endocrinology and Infertility, 8th edition. Philadelphia: Lippincott Williams & Wilkins; 2011. p. 574)

10. **d.** Serotonin
    The weight of current evidence suggests strongly that premenstrual syndrome and premenstrual dysphoric disorder result from an abnormal or exaggerated effect of cyclic change in ovarian steroid hormone

on central neurotransmitter mechanism and that on serotonin in particular, plays an important role in pathophysiology.
(Reference: Fritz MA, Speroff L. Clinical Gynecologic Endocrinology and Infertility, 8th edition. Philadelphia: Lippincott Williams & Wilkins; 2011. p. 575)

11. **a.** i, iii
(Reference: Fritz MA, Speroff L. Clinical Gynecologic Endocrinology and Infertility, 8th edition. Philadelphia: Lippincott Williams & Wilkins; 2011. p. 576)

12. **a.** Fluoxetine
Fluoxetine in a daily dose of 20 mg has demonstrated sustained efficacy for relieving both somatic and mood symptoms and is generally well tolerated.
(Reference: Fritz MA, Speroff L. Clinical Gynecologic Endocrinology and Infertility, 8th edition. Philadelphia: Lippincott Williams & Wilkins; 2011. p. 576)

13. **b.** Physical symptoms
Gonadotropin-releasing hormone (GnRH) agonists generally are more effective in relieving irritability and physical symptoms than for treatment of prominent symptoms of depression and dysphoria.
(Reference: Fritz MA, Speroff L. Clinical Gynecologic Endocrinology and Infertility, 8th edition. Philadelphia: Lippincott Williams & Wilkins; 2011. p. 577)

14. **a.** Relieve bloating and breast pain
Oral contraceptive pill (OCP) helped to relieve breast pain and symptoms of bloating but had no detectable benefits for relieving mood symptoms.
(Reference: Fritz MA, Speroff L. Clinical Gynecologic Endocrinology and Infertility, 8th edition. Philadelphia: Lippincott Williams & Wilkins; 2011. p. 577)

15. **a.** i, iv
In women diagnosed with premenstrual syndrome or premenstrual dysphoric disorder who fail to respond to the treatment usually effective, it is important to consider underlying conditions such as major depression, generalized anxiety disorder, or substance abuse.
(Reference: Fritz MA, Speroff L. Clinical Gynecologic Endocrinology and Infertility, 8th edition. Philadelphia: Lippincott Williams & Wilkins; 2011. p. 572)

16. **b.** Abnormal response to normal cycle changes in ovarian steroid hormone level
(Reference: Fritz MA, Speroff L. Clinical Gynecologic Endocrinology and Infertility, 8th edition. Philadelphia: Lippincott Williams & Wilkins; 2011. p. 574)

17. **a.** i, ii
(Reference: Fritz MA, Speroff L. Clinical Gynecologic Endocrinology and Infertility, 8th edition. Philadelphia: Lippincott Williams & Wilkins; 2011. p. 569)

18. **b.** Follicular
Women who have no demonstrable symptom-free interval during the follicular phase merit careful evaluation for a mood or anxiety disorder.
(Reference: Fritz MA, Speroff L. Clinical Gynecologic Endocrinology and Infertility, 8th edition. Philadelphia: Lippincott Williams & Wilkins; 2011. p. 573)

19. **c.** Likert
(Reference: Fritz MA, Speroff L. Clinical Gynecologic Endocrinology and Infertility, 8th edition. Philadelphia: Lippincott Williams & Wilkins; 2011. p. 570)

20. **c.** PMS

21. **a.** Alprazolam
(Reference: Fritz MA, Speroff L. Clinical Gynecologic Endocrinology and Infertility, 8th edition. Philadelphia: Lippincott Williams & Wilkins; 2011. p. 576)

22. **a.** ii, iii, iv
Fluoxetine in a daily dose of 20 mg has demonstrated sustained efficacy for relieving both somatic and mood symptoms and is generally well tolerated.
(Reference: Fritz MA, Speroff L. Clinical Gynecologic Endocrinology and Infertility, 8th edition. Philadelphia: Lippincott Williams & Wilkins; 2011. p. 576)

23. **a.** Depressive symptoms
Alprazolam is another medication that may be useful in the treatment of premenstrual syndrome and premenstrual dysphoric disorder, although its effectiveness may be limited to the relief of depressive symptoms.
(Reference: Fritz MA, Speroff L. Clinical Gynecologic Endocrinology and Infertility, 8th edition. Philadelphia: Lippincott Williams & Wilkins; 2011. p. 577)

24. **c.** Structural similarity to steroid hormones
Spironolactone is a potassium-sparing diuretic having structural similarity to steroid hormones and is widely used in the treatment of premenstrual syndrome.
(Reference: Fritz MA, Speroff L. Clinical Gynecologic Endocrinology and Infertility, 8th edition. Philadelphia: Lippincott Williams & Wilkins; 2011. p. 576)

25. **a.** Oral contraceptive pill
These are one of the oldest and simplest method for treatment of premenstrual syndrome and premenstrual dysphoric disorder based on the idea of substituting a constant hormonal environment for the dynamic cyclic pattern of the normal menstrual cycle.
(Reference: Fritz MA, Speroff L. Clinical Gynecologic Endocrinology and Infertility, 8th edition. Philadelphia: Lippincott Williams & Wilkins; 2011. p. 577)

26. **d.** Aerobic exercises
When symptoms are mild and evidence of significant socioeconomic dysfunction is lacking patients can be advised to consider aerobic exercise as treatment.
(Reference: Fritz MA, Speroff L. Clinical Gynecologic Endocrinology and Infertility, 8th edition. Philadelphia: Lippincott Williams & Wilkins; 2011. p. 578)

27. **c.** Low-dose alprazolam
When selective serotonin reuptake inhibitor treatment proved unsuccessful low-dose alprazolam is a logical choice to try, although sedating effect may limit the usefulness.
(Reference: Fritz MA, Speroff L. Clinical Gynecologic Endocrinology and Infertility, 8th edition. Philadelphia: Lippincott Williams & Wilkins; 2011. p. 576)

28. **a.** Accurate diagnosis
The key to effective treatment of premenstrual syndrome and premenstrual dysphoric disorder is accurate diagnosis which rests primarily on the collection of objective evidence that patient's symptoms are clearly cyclic, as documented by use of calendar of premenstrual experience survey or other similar calendar-based screening tool over the interval spanning three menstrual cycles.
(Reference: Fritz MA, Speroff L. Clinical Gynecologic Endocrinology and Infertility, 8th edition. Philadelphia: Lippincott Williams & Wilkins; 2011. p. 575)

29. **a.** Diminished sexual interest
Sexual dysfunction including anorgasmia and diminished sexual interest is perhaps the most significant potential adverse effects of selective serotonin reuptake inhibitor treatment and women should be advised of specific possibility before treatment begins.
(Reference: Fritz MA, Speroff L. Clinical Gynecologic Endocrinology and Infertility, 8th edition. Philadelphia: Lippincott Williams & Wilkins; 2011. p. 578)

30. **c.** i, ii, iii, iv
(Reference: Fritz MA, Speroff L. Clinical Gynecologic Endocrinology and Infertility, 8th edition. Philadelphia: Lippincott Williams & Wilkins; 2011. p. 573)

Chapter 84: Postmenopausal Bleeding

Pushpa Lata Sankhwar

QUESTIONS

1. A 45-year-old woman complains of spotting following her menses for 5 months. Prior to starting treatment, you want to check if she is menopausal. On which day of the menstrual cycle, will you estimate her serum follicle-stimulating hormone (FSH) levels?
   a. On day 2–5 after last menstrual period
   b. On the day of her visit to doctor irrespective of her menses
   c. On day of menstruation
   d. Just before menstruation

2. What is the diagnostic value of serum follicle-stimulating hormone (FSH) in menopause?
   a. >50 µ/mL
   b. >40 µ/mL
   c. >30 µ/mL
   d. >20 µ/mL

3. A menopausal woman presents with complaints of hot flashes. Which of the following neurotransmitters are responsible for these symptoms?
   a. Serotonin and epinephrine
   b. Serotonin and norepinephrine
   c. Adrenaline and epinephrine
   d. Noradrenaline and epinephrine

4. A 53-year-old perimenopausal woman presents with episodes of sensation of intense heat which lasts for about 2–4 minutes associated with profuse sweating. What is the most effective treatment for her?
   a. Combined oral contraceptive pills
   b. Clonidine with cetirizine
   c. Estrogen therapy
   d. Danazol

5. A 54-year-old postmenopausal woman presented with complaints of dyspareunia and vaginal spotting. On examination, the vagina appeared pale with small petechiae. Transvaginal ultrasound reveals a 3-mm thick endometrium with no abnormality. Which among the following would be the next step in the management?
   a. Pipelle biopsy
   b. Estradiol-releasing vaginal ring
   c. Mirena intrauterine device
   d. Hysteroscopy

6. A 50-year-old woman presents with complaint of vaginal bleeding and mentions that her last menstrual period was 10 months ago. What is the minimum duration of amenorrhea for her to be considered as postmenopausal bleeding?
   a. 3 months   b. 6 months
   c. 9 months   d. 12 months

7. What is the investigation of choice in a 55-year-old woman who presents with postmenopausal bleeding?
   a. Pap smear
   b. Endometrial biopsy
   c. Ultrasonography
   d. CA-125 estimation

8. A 54-year primiparous obese woman presents to your OPD with a complaint of bleeding per vagina. She gives a history of cessation of menses 1 year back with irregularity at the fundus on sonography. What could be the next step?
   a. Pap smear
   b. Colposcopy
   c. Endometrial biopsy
   d. Hysteroscopy-guided biopsy

9. A 58-year-old postmenopausal woman presented with bleeding per vagina (PV). Hysteroscopic biopsy reveals complex endometrial hyperplasia with atypia. What is the risk of progression of this condition to cancer?
   a. 3%
   b. 8%
   c. 29%
   d. 54%

10. A 52-year-old postmenopausal woman has come to you with an USG report showing normal uterus with endometrial thickness of 7 mm and bilateral atrophic ovaries. What is the next step in her management?
    a. Follow up ultrasound after 3 months
    b. Hysterectomy
    c. Endometrial biopsy
    d. Progesterone therapy

11. A 62-year-old woman presents with vaginal bleeding 11 years after she attained menopause. An endometrial biopsy revealed adenocarcinoma. What is the gold standard method for staging her condition?
    a. MRI
    b. Surgery
    c. Endometrial biopsy
    d. Positron emission tomography (PET)-CT

12. Which of the following predisposes a patient to develop type 2 carcinoma endometrium?
    a. K-Ras mutation
    b. Premenopause age group
    c. *PTEN* mutation
    d. Atrophic endometrium

13. A 62-year-old woman with postmenopausal bleeding was diagnosed as a case of CA endometrium. Which lymph nodes are the most commonly involved in patients with endometrial carcinoma?
    a. Femoral
    b. Inguinal
    c. Para-aortic
    d. Paracolic

14. Which among the following is the mainstay of treatment in a patient diagnosed with stage III endometrial cancer?
    a. Surgery
    b. Surgery + Chemotherapy
    c. External beam radiotherapy
    d. Brachytherapy

15. Human papilloma virus (HPV) could be one of the causes of the cervical cancer. What is *not* true regarding human papilloma virus?
    a. E1 and E2 are viral proteins needed for replication
    b. E6 and E7 are viral proteins needed for malignant transformation
    c. E6 acts via the retinoblastoma gene
    d. HPV-16 is the most common serotype causing carcinoma cervix

16. Which of the following methods will you prefer for treatment of high-grade squamous intraepithelial lesion (HSIL) in a young lady?
    a. Cold knife conization
    b. Large loop excision of transformation zone
    c. Electrocoagulation
    d. Hysterectomy

17. You would suspect and evaluate for carcinoma cervix in patients presenting with which of the following condition?
    a. Menorrhagia
    b. Metrorrhagia
    c. Polymenorrhea
    d. Amenorrhea

18. A 58-year-old woman with postmenopausal bleeding presented to her gynecologist. She was diagnosed with CA cervix stage IB after evaluation. What is the treatment of choice for this patient?
    a. Type I hysterectomy
    b. Type II hysterectomy
    c. Type III hysterectomy
    d. Type IV hysterectomy

19. You are planning to administer radiotherapy to a 58-year-old woman with carcinoma cervix. What is the dose to be administered at point B?
    a. 5,000 cGY
    b. 6,000 cGY
    c. 7,000 cGY
    d. 8,000 cGY

20. A 65-year-old woman with postmenopausal bleeding was found to have a normal endometrium and a 2-cm endometrial polyp on hysteroscopic assessment. Which of the following is most appropriate next step?
    a. Expectant management
    b. Blind avulsion should be offered
    c. Hysteroscopic resection of polyp and endometrial biopsy
    d. Dilatation and curettage

21. The investigation of choice in a 55-year-old postmenopausal woman who has presented with postmenopausal bleeding is:
    a. Pap smear
    b. Fractional curettage
    c. Transvaginal bleeding
    d. CA-125 estimation

22. A menopausal woman presents with complaints of hot flushes. Which of the following neurotransmitters are responsible for symptoms?
   a. Serotonin and epinephrine
   b. Serotonin and norepinephrine
   c. Adrenaline and epinephrine
   d. Noradrenaline and epinephrine

23. A 58-year-old postmenopausal lady presented with complaints of dyspareunia and vaginal spotting. On examination, the vagina appeared pale with small petechiae. Transvaginal sonography (TVS) revealed a 3-mm thick endometrium with no abnormality. Which among the following would be next best step in management?
   a. Pipelle biopsy of vagina and antibiotics
   b. Colposcopy with vaginoscopic evaluation followed by local estradiol
   c. Mirena intrauterine device
   d. Hysteroscopy and oral progesterone

24. A 67-year-old woman is being screened for osteoporosis with a dual X-ray absorptiometry (DEXA) scan. Which of the following places are useful for detection of early rapid bone loss?
   a. Lumbar vertebrae
   b. Cervical vertebrae
   c. Shaft of femur
   d. Wrist

25. You are prescribing estrogen therapy for a perimenopausal woman with hot flushes. What is the minimum number of days in a month during which you should combine it with progesterone?
   a. 5–8 days   b. 10–12 days
   c. 14–16 days   d. 21–22 days

26. A 50-year-old woman presents with complaints of vaginal bleeding and mentions that her last menstrual period was 10 months ago. What is the minimum duration of amenorrhea for this to be considered postmenopausal bleeding?
   a. 3 months   b. 6 months
   c. 9 months   d. 12 months

27. A patient is planned to undergo hysteroscopic polypectomy using bipolar electrocautery. What is the ideal agent for distention?
   a. Glycine   b. Normal saline
   c. CO_2 d. 70% dextrose

28. A 48-year-old young lady [p2 + 0 (L2) – P2 + 0 (L2)], a known of case PCOS, presents with abnormal uterine bleeding. Her endometrial thickness was 18 mm on transvaginal sonography (TVS). Her endometrial sampling report came as atypical endometrial hyperplasia. The most appropriate treatment for this patient is:
   a. Observation
   b. Medroxy-progesterone depot
   c. Total abdominal hysterectomy (TAH) + Bilateral salpingectomy
   d. Levonorgestrel-releasing intrauterine system (LNG-IUS) insertion

29. A 58-year-old multipara woman was diagnosed to have grade 1 endometroid endometrial cancer without lymphovascular invasion based on histopathological examination (HPE) of specimen, who underwent surgery for abnormal uterine bleeding (AUB) without prior endometrial sampling. The total abdominal hysterectomy and bilateral salpingo-oophrectomy was done. What is next best management for her?
   a. Observation
   b. Completion of staging with pelvic and para-aortic lymph-node dissection
   c. Adjuvant chemoradiation
   d. Adjuvant radiation therapy

30. According to WHO global initiative to eliminate cancer cervix 90:70:90 triple pillar intervention:
   i. 90% of women screened using a high-performance screening test at the age of 35 and 45 years.
   ii. 70% of girls fully vaccinated with two doses of HPV vaccine by the age of 15 years
   iii. 90% of women detected with a cervical lesion should receive treatment and care.
   a. All three statements are true
   b. Only statement (i) is true
   c. Both statements (i) and (iii) are true
   d. Only statement (iii) is true

ANSWERS

1. **a.** *Correct explanation:* On day 2–5 after last menstrual period which is lowest in this phase.
   [Reference: Kumar S, Padubidri VG, Daftary SN (Eds). Shaw's Textbook of Gynecology, 17th edition. Gurugram (Haryana): Elsevier India; 2018. p. 86]

CHAPTER 84: Postmenopausal Bleeding 477

2. **b.** *Correct explanation:* >40 μ/mL
   [Reference: Hoffman B, Schorge J, Bradshaw K, Halvorson L, Schaffer J, Corton M (Eds). William's Gynecology, 3rd edition. New York: McGraw-Hill Education/Medical; 2016. p. 489]

3. **b.** *Correct explanation:* Serotonin and norepinephrine
   [Reference: Hoffman B, Schorge J, Bradshaw K, Halvorson L, Schaffer J, Corton M (Eds). William's Gynecology, 3rd edition. New York: McGraw-Hill Education/Medical; 2016. p. 476]

4. **c.** *Correct explanation:* Estrogen therapy as she is suffering from menopausal syndrome with vasomotor symptoms due to lack of estrogen.
   [Reference: Hoffman B, Schorge J, Bradshaw K, Halvorson L, Schaffer J, Corton M (Eds). William's Gynecology, 3rd edition. New York: McGraw-Hill Education/Medical; 2016. p. 495]

5. **b.** *Correct explanation:* Estradiol-releasing vaginal ring as she is suffering from genitourinary syndrome of menopause (GSM).
   [Reference: Berek JS (Ed). Berek and Novak's Gynecology, 16th edition. Philadelphia: Lippincott Williams and Wilkins; 2019. p. 891]

6. **d.** *Correct explanation:* 12 months
   (Reference: Williams Gynecology, 3rd Edition, Page 484)

7. **b.** *Correct explanation:* Endometrial biopsy will give the most accurate cause of her PMB.
   [Reference: Berek JS (Ed). Berek and Novak's Gynecology, 16th edition. Philadelphia: Lippincott Williams and Wilkins; 2019. p. 2372]

8. **d.** *Correct explanation:* Usually, fundal lesion is missed in endometrial biopsy so it is recommended to do the hysteroscopic-guided biopsy, if feasible.
   (Reference: Williams Gynecology, 3rd Edition, Page 312)

9. **c.** *Correct explanation:* 29%
   [Reference: Hoffman BL, Schorge JO, Halvorson LM, Hamid CA, Corton MM, Schaffer JI (Eds). William's Gynecology, 4th edition. New York: McGraw-Hill Education/Medical; 2020. p. 700]

10. **c.** *Correct explanation:* Go for endometrial biopsy as her endotracheal tube (ET) is 7 mm and needs evaluation, one can miss malignancy if left for observation.
    (Reference: Williams Gynecology, 4th Edition, Pages 704-5)

11. **b.** *Correct explanation:* Surgery
    (Reference: Williams Gynecology, 3rd Edition, Pages 656-7)

12. **d.** *Correct explanation:* Atrophic endometrium
    (Reference: Williams Gynecology, 3rd Edition, Pages 660-1)

13. **c.** *Correct explanation:* Para-aortic
    (Reference: Williams Gynecology, 3rd Edition, Pages 672-3)

14. **b.** *Correct explanation:* Surgery + Chemotherapy
    [Reference: FIGO (www.figo.org/cancer-corpus-uteri-0016166)]

15. **c.** *Correct explanation:* E6 acts via the retinoblastoma gene.
    [Reference: Berek JS (Ed). Berek and Novak's Gynecology, 16th edition. Philadelphia: Lippincott Williams and Wilkins; 2019. p. 2448]

16. **b.** *Correct explanation:* Large loop excision of transformation zone
    [Reference: Hoffman B, Schorge J, Bradshaw K, Halvorson L, Schaffer J, Corton M (Eds). William's Gynecology, 3rd edition. New York: McGraw-Hill Education/Medical; 2016. pp. 644, 988]

17. **b.** *Correct explanation:* Metrorrhagia
    [Reference: Hoffman B, Schorge J, Bradshaw K, Halvorson L, Schaffer J, Corton M (Eds). William's Gynecology, 3rd edition. New York: McGraw-Hill Education/Medical; 2016. p. 662]

18. **c.** *Correct explanation:* Type III hysterectomy
    [Reference: Hoffman B, Schorge J, Bradshaw K, Halvorson L, Schaffer J, Corton M (Eds). William's Gynecology, 3rd edition. New York: McGraw-Hill Education/Medical; 2016. pp. 669-72]

19. **b.** *Correct explanation:* 6,000 cGY
    [Reference: Berek JS (Ed). Berek and Novak's Gynecology, 16th edition. Philadelphia: Lippincott Williams and Wilkins; 2019. p. 2488]

20. **c.** *Correct explanation:* Hysteroscopic resection of polyp and endometrial biopsy
    (Reference: Williams Gynecology, 3rd Edition, Pages 702-3)

21. **b.** *Correct explanation:* Fractional curettage
    (Reference: Williams Gynecology, 3rd Edition, Pages 665-6)

22. **b.** *Correct explanation:* Serotonin and norepinephrine
    [Reference: Hoffman B, Schorge J, Bradshaw K, Halvorson L, Schaffer J, Corton M (Eds). William's Gynecology, 3rd edition. New York: McGraw-Hill Education/Medical; 2016. p. 476]

23. **b.** *Correct explanation:* Colposcopy with vaginoscopic evaluation followed by local estradiol
    [Reference: Berek JS (Ed). Berek and Novak's Gynecology, 16th edition. Philadelphia: Lippincott Williams and Wilkins; 2019. p. 891]

24. **a.** *Correct explanation:* Lumbar vertebrae
    [Reference: Hoffman B, Schorge J, Bradshaw K, Halvorson L, Schaffer J, Corton M (Eds). William's Gynecology, 3rd edition. New York: McGraw-Hill Education/Medical; 2016. p. 479]

25. **b.** *Correct explanation:* 10–12 days
    [Reference: Hoffman B, Schorge J, Bradshaw K, Halvorson L, Schaffer J, Corton M (Eds). William's Gynecology, 3rd edition. New York: McGraw-Hill Education/Medical; 2016. p. 482]

26. **d.** *Correct explanation:* 12 months
    (Reference: Williams Gynecology, 3rd Edition, Pages 496-7)

27. **b.** *Correct explanation:* Normal saline
    (Reference: Williams Gynecology, 3rd Edition, Pages 704-5)

28. **c.** *Correct explanation:* Total abdominal hysterectomy (TAH) + Bilateral salpingectomy
    [Reference: Berek JS (Ed). Berek and Novak's Gynecology, 16th edition. Philadelphia: Lippincott Williams and Wilkins; 2019]

29. **a.** *Correct explanation:* Observation
    (Reference: Williams Gyenecology, 3rd Edition, Pages 676-7)

30. **d.** *Correct explanation:* Only statement (iii) is true.
    [Reference: FIGO. (2021). FIGO Cancer Report, 2021. (online) Available from: https://www.figo.org/figo-cancer-report-2021 (Last accessed December, 2023)]

Chapter 85

Vaginal Infection and Pelvic Inflammatory Diseases

Suman Chaudhary, Ruchika Garg

QUESTIONS

A. BACTERIAL VAGINOSIS

1. **The normal vaginal pH is:**
   a. <4.5
   b. 4.5–5.5
   c. 5.5–6.5
   d. >6.5

2. **Which of the following is true?**
   a. The normal vaginal flora is anaerobic
   b. The most common bacteria in vagina is hydrogen peroxide producing lactobacilli
   c. Estrogen stimulated vaginal epithelial cells are rich in glucose
   d. The pH level of normal vagina is maintained by production of acetic acid

3. **Clue cells are:**
   a. Superficial vaginal epithelial cells with adherent bacteria usually *Gardnerella vaginalis*
   b. Superficial vaginal epithelial cells with adherent bacteria usually *Trichomonas vaginalis*
   c. Superficial cervical epithelial cells with adherent bacteria usually *Gardnerella vaginalis*
   d. Superficial cervical epithelial cells with adherent bacteria usually *Trichomonas vaginalis*

4. **Amsel's diagnostic criteria for bacterial vaginosis includes all, *except*:**
   a. Presence of fishy vaginal odor
   b. The pH of these secretions is <4.5
   c. The addition of KOH to vaginal secretions releases amine-like odor
   d. Vaginal secretions are gray and they thinly coat the vaginal wall

5. **Bacterial vaginosis is diagnosed by all, *except*:**
   a. Culture of *Gardnerella vaginalis*
   b. Amsel's diagnostic test
   c. Nugent's score
   d. Diagnostic test using pH and amines test cards

6. **Drug of choice for treatment of bacterial vaginosis is:**
   a. Tablet azithromycin 500 mg once a day for 5 days
   b. Tablet fluconazole 150 mg single dose
   c. Tablet metronidazole 500 mg twice times a day for 7 days
   d. Tablet secnidazole 2 g single dose

7. **All is true for treatment of bacterial vaginosis, *except*:**
   a. Tablet metronidazole 500 mg twice a day for 7 days is the treatment of choice
   b. Tablet clindamycin 300 mg twice daily for 7 days is also good alternative
   c. Metronidazole gel 0.75% one applicator (5 g) once daily for 5 days
   d. Treatment of male sexual partner is recommended

8. **Regarding the treatment of bacterial vaginosis all are true, *except*:**
   a. Oral treatment with metronidazole is the treatment of choice
   b. Many clinicians prefer intravaginal treatment to avoid systemic side effects such as mild-to-moderate gastrointestinal upset and unpleasant taste
   c. Treatment of the male sexual partner does not improve therapeutic response and therefore is not recommended
   d. The overall cure rate range from 50 to 65% with the metronidazole treatment regimens

B. TRICHOMONAS VAGINITIS

9. **All is true about trichomonas vaginitis, *except*:**
   a. It is the most prevalent nonviral sexually transmitted infection in united states

b. It is caused by an anaerobic bacteria, *Trichomonas vaginalis*
c. The transmission rate is high to the extent that 70% men acquire the disease after a single exposure
d. It often accompanies bacterial vaginosis (BV), which can be present in as many as 60% of patients with trichomonas vaginitis

10. **Colpitis macularis is associated with:**
    a. Trichomonas vaginitis
    b. Bacterial vaginosis
    c. Vaginal candidiasis
    d. Cancer cervix

11. **All are true about trichomonas vaginitis, *except*:**
    a. The whiff test may be positive
    b. The pH of vaginal secretions is could be variable or higher than 5.5
    c. Amsel's diagnostic criteria is used for its diagnosis
    d. Pregnant women with trichomonas vaginitis are at increased risk for premature rupture of the membranes and preterm delivery

12. **Trichomonas vaginitis is:**
    a. Associated with profuse purulent malodourous vaginal discharge that may be accompanied with pruritus
    b. Vaginal secretions are gray and they thinly coat the vaginal wall
    c. White curdy discharge is present
    d. The pH of the vagina is usually normal <4.5

13. **All is true about treatment of trichomonas vaginitis, *except*:**
    a. Metronidazole is the drug of choice
    b. Both a single dose 2 g orally or multidose 500 mg twice daily for 7 days are effective
    c. Metronidazole gel can be used for its treatment
    d. The treatment with metronidazole is highly effective with cure rates of 95%

14. **Women with trichomonas vaginitis who do not respond to initial therapy all can be done, *except*:**
    a. Should be treated with metronidazole 500 mg twice daily for 7 days again
    b. Sexual partner should be treated
    c. Retesting for *Trichomonas vaginalis* is recommended within 3 months
    d. Should be treated with clindamycin 300 mg twice daily for 7 days

15. **All can be used for treatment of trichomonas vaginitis, *except*:**
    a. Metronidazole 500 mg twice daily for 7 days
    b. Tinidazole 2 g orally in a single dose is another recommended regimen
    c. Sexual partner need not be treated
    d. Metronidazole 2 g single dose is also highly effective

C. VULVOVAGINAL CANDIDIASIS

16. **Factors that predisposes women to symptomatic vulvovaginal candidiasis (VVC) are all, *except*:**
    a. Pregnancy
    b. Diabetes
    c. Nonsteroidal anti-inflammatory drugs (NSAIDs) use
    d. Antibiotic use

17. **Which of the following statement is true about vulvovaginal candidiasis?**
    a. *Candida glabrata* is responsible for 85-90% of fungal vaginal infections
    b. *Candida* are dimorphic fungi which exist in two forms—blastospore and mycelium
    c. Blastopore causes the colonization and tissue invasion and mycelia are responsible for transmission and asymptomatic colonization
    d. Extensive areas of pruritus and inflammation are due to extensive invasion of the lower genital tract epithelial cells

18. **Complicated vulvovaginal candidiasis is true for all, *except*:**
    a. It is always caused by *Candida albicans*
    b. It is severe, recurrent infection
    c. Patients with immunocompromised state, e.g., diabetic and women with human immunodeficiency virus (HIV) are at increased risk
    d. Treatment with fluconazole 150 mg needs to be repeated after 72 hours

19. **Recurrent vulvovaginal candidiasis is defined as:**
    a. Four or more episodes in a year
    b. Five or more episodes in a year
    c. When it reoccurs within 3 months of treatment
    d. When it reoccurs within 6 months of treatment

20. **The treatment of choice of patients with recurrent vulvovaginal candidiasis consists of:**
    a. Inducing a remission of with fluconazole—150 mg every 3 days for three doses, patients should be maintained on a suppressive dose of fluconazole, 150 mg weekly for 6 months

b. Inducing a remission of with fluconazole—150 mg two doses at 3 days, patients should be maintained on a suppressive dose of fluconazole, 150 mg weekly for 3 months
c. Inducing a remission of with fluconazole—150 mg every 2 days for three doses, patients should be maintained on a suppressive dose of fluconazole, 150 mg weekly for 1 year
d. Inducing a remission of with fluconazole—150 mg every 3 days for three doses, patients should be maintained on a suppressive dose of fluconazole, 150 mg weekly for 1 year

D. PELVIC INFLAMMATORY DISEASE

21. All are true about cervicitis, *except:*
    a. *Neisseria gonorrhoeae* and *Chlamydia trachomatis* infect only the glandular epithelium
    b. *Trichomonas, Candida*, and herpes simplex virus (HSV) can cause inflammation of both ectocervix and endocervix
    c. The Gram stained slide of cervical mucopus will reveal the presence of an increased number of neutrophils (>30 per high-power field)
    d. Cervicitis is commonly associated with bacterial vaginosis, which, if not treated concurrently, leads to significant persistence of the symptoms and signs of cervicitis

22. True statement about treatment of cervicitis is:
    a. Treatment consists of an antibiotic regimen recommended for the treatment of uncomplicated lower genital tract infection with both chlamydia and gonorrhea
    b. Fluoroquinolone are recommended for the treatment of gonococcal cervicitis
    c. Treatment of sexual partner is usually not recommended
    d. Treatment of gonococcal cervicitis with single drug therapy is usually successful

23. Triad of the symptoms and signs used for pelvic inflammatory disease (PID) is:
    a. Abdominal pain, uterine tenderness, and fever
    b. Pelvic pain, cervical motion, and adnexal tenderness and presence of fever
    c. Abdominal pain, adnexal tenderness, and presence of malaise
    d. Backache, lower abdominal pain, and presence of fever

24. Additional criteria to increase the specificity of diagnosis of pelvic inflammatory disease are:
    a. Endometrial biopsy showing endometritis, leukocytosis, and positive Mantoux test
    b. Cervical biopsy showing cervicitis, leukocytosis, and raised C-reactive protein (CRP)
    c. Positive test for bacterial vaginosis, elevated CRP, and erythrocyte sedimentation rate (ESR) and presence of fever of >100.4°F
    d. Endometrial biopsy showing endometritis, elevated CRP and ESR and presence of fever of >100.4°F

25. Parenteral therapy for pelvic inflammatory disease is recommended in all, *except:*
    a. When diagnosis is uncertain
    b. There is pelvic abscess
    c. Presence of severe illness
    d. Presence of pelvic pain for chronically long duration

26. Regarding the treatment of pelvic inflammatory disease the true statement is:
    a. Inclusion of metronidazole in oral or parenteral regimen is recommended to provide antibiotics coverage against anaerobic organisms
    b. Treatment of PID should be started after confirmation of diagnosis only
    c. PID is usually associated with vaginitis which should also be treated simultaneously
    d. Partner treatment is not recommended in PID

CASE-BASED QUESTIONS

A. A 25-year-old, para 2 women usually has pain lower abdomen since 6 months, she got appendectomy done 3 months back for similar complaints but had no relief. She visited her gynecologist outpatient department (OPD) recently.

27. The true statement about her illness is:
    a. She is suffering from sexually transmitted infection, so partner treatment should be initiated first
    b. She should be admitted and given parenteral therapy
    c. She should undergo surgery again
    d. Bacterial vaginosis is usually present in these patients

28. The best next step in her management is:
    a. Perform a per speculum and per vaginal examination to detect the cervical motion tenderness

b. Start the oral antibiotic regime containing doxycycline and metronidazole
c. Perform a sonography to rule out any pelvic pathology and pelvic abscess
d. Admitting the patient for parenteral therapy and if needed surgery

B. A 32-year-old pregnant woman has complaints of discharge per vaginum with itching and burning sensations. She also complaints of white curd-like discharge per vaginum.

29. **The true statement about her illness:**
   a. She is suffering of a sexually transmitted infection
   b. It is a fungal infections caused by *Candida albicans*
   c. She is at increased risk of preterm labor and abortions
   d. She is having urinary tract infection too

30. **A per speculum examination of this woman will show:**
   a. White cottage cheese or curdy discharge
   b. Profuse purulent malodourous discharge
   c. Vaginal secretion has fishy odor
   d. Vaginal secretions are gray thinly coating vaginal wall

31. **On examination, all are true, *except*:**
   a. Testing of pH of vagina will show a pH of <5
   b. Whiff test is negative
   c. Colpitis macularis is typically present
   d. Saline preparation evaluation is normal

32. **The treatment of choice is:**
   a. Tablet fluconazole 150 mg single dose
   b. Tablet metronidazole 400 mg twice a day for 7 days
   c. Vaginal suppositories of clotrimazole 100 mg HS for 6 days
   d. Tablet clindamycin 300 mg twice a day for 7 days

C. A 30-year-old multiparous woman presents to gynecologist outpatient department with complaints of pelvic pain, fever, and pus-like discharge per vaginum. On examination there is mucopurulent discharge coming from cervical os and the cervical motion tenderness was present.

33. **What is the true statement regarding the etiology of this illness?**
   a. It is most commonly caused by sexually transmitted organism such as *Neisseria gonorrhoeae* and *Trichomonas vaginalis*
   b. When caused by *Chlamydia trachomatis* it is usually a severe illness
   c. It is associated with bacterial vaginosis causing organisms such as *Prevotella*, *Gardnerella vaginalis*, and *Peptostreptococcus*
   d. *Mycobacterium tuberculosis* never causes this illness

34. **All are true about it, *except*:**
   a. The diagnosis is traditionally based on the presence of triad of symptoms—pelvic pain, cervical motion, and adnexal tenderness and fever
   b. There is wide variation in symptoms and sign which makes the diagnosis of acute pelvic inflammatory disease difficult
   c. Cervical motion tenderness in these women suggests presence of peritoneal inflammation
   d. PID caused by chlamydia is very severe disease, usually treated with inpatient parenteral antibiotic treatment

35. **What is the best next step in management of this patient?**
   a. Ultrasonographic examination of whole abdomen and pelvis to diagnosis pelvic inflammatory disease
   b. High vaginal swab and endocervical swab culture and sensitivity
   c. Urethral swab culture and sensitivity of partner
   d. Laparoscopic examination to observe the pus exudate from fimbrial end to diagnose it

36. **The Centers for Disease Control and Prevention (CDC) recommended oral antibiotic regime for this patient is:**
   a. Tablet ofloxacin (200 mg) and ornidazole 500 mg twice a day for 7 days
   b. Tablet clindamycin 300 mg twice a day for 14 days
   c. Injection ceftriaxone 250 mg stat, tablet doxycycline 100 mg, and tablet metronidazole 400 mg twice a day for 14 days
   d. Tablet amoxicillin and clavulanic acid 625 mg thrice a day for 14 days

D. A 20-year-old newly married women complaints of profuse vaginal discharge with itching since 15 days. She also complaints of burning sensation at perineum, burning micturition, and dyspareunia. Her husband has complaints of soreness, redness, and swelling of penis after intercourse. On examination there is red vagina and red cervix (strawberry cervix) with profuse, purulent malodourous discharge.

CHAPTER 85: Vaginal Infection and Pelvic Inflammatory Diseases

37. What is the causative agent of this sexually transmitted infection?
    a. *Trichomonas vaginalis*
    b. *Candida albicans*
    c. *Neisseria gonorrhoeae*
    d. *Chlamydia trachomatis*

38. The causative agent is:
    a. Bacteria
    b. Fungus
    c. Protozoa
    d. Virus

39. Treatment of this infection is all, *except*:
    a. Metronidazole is the drug of choice—2 g single dose or 500 mg twice a day for 7 days
    b. Tinidazole 2 g orally in a single dose is another recommended regimen
    c. The sexual partner should be treated
    d. Metronidazole gel should be used for the treatment

ANSWERS

A. BACTERIAL VAGINOSIS

1. **a.** The pH level of the normal vagina is lower than 4.5, which is maintained by the production of lactic acid. Estrogen-stimulated vaginal epithelial cells are rich in glycogen. Vaginal epithelial cells break down glycogen to monosaccharides, which can be converted by the cells themselves, and lactobacilli to lactic acid.
(Reference: Berek JS. Berek & Novak's Gynecology, 16th edition. Philadelphia: Lippincott Williams and Wilkins; 2019)

2. **b.** The normal vaginal flora is mostly aerobic, with an average of six different species of bacteria, the most common of which is hydrogen peroxide producing estrogen-stimulated vaginal epithelial cells are rich in glycogen. Vaginal epithelial cells break down glycogen to monosaccharides, which can be converted by the cells themselves, and lactobacilli to lactic acid.
(Reference: Berek JS. Berek & Novak's Gynecology, 16th edition. Philadelphia: Lippincott Williams and Wilkins; 2019)

3. **a.** Normal vaginal secretions are floccular in consistency, white in color, and usually located in the dependent portion of the vagina (posterior fornix). Vaginal secretions can be analyzed by a wet-mount preparation. A sample of vaginal secretions is suspended in 0.5 mL of normal saline in a tube, transferred to a slide, covered with a slip, and assessed by microscopy. Some clinicians prefer to prepare slides by suspending secretions in saline placed directly on the slide. Secretions should not be placed on the slide without saline because this method causes drying of the vaginal secretions and does not result in a well-suspended preparation. Microscopy of normal vaginal secretions reveals many superficial 882 epithelial cells, few white blood cells (less than one per epithelial cell), and few, if any, clue cells. Clue cells are superficial vaginal epithelial cells with adherent bacteria, usually *Gardnerella vaginalis*, which obliterates the crisp cell border when visualized microscopically.
(Reference: Berek JS. Berek & Novak's Gynecology, 16th edition. Philadelphia: Lippincott Williams and Wilkins; 2019)

4. **b.** Bacterial vaginosis is diagnosed on the basis of the following findings: clinical criteria require three of the following signs or symptoms (Amsel's diagnostic criteria):
    - A fishy vaginal odor, which is particularly noticeable following coitus, and vaginal discharge are present
    - Vaginal secretions are gray and thinly coat the vaginal walls
    - The pH of these secretions is higher than 4.5 (usually 4.7–5.7)
    - Microscopy of the vaginal secretions reveals an increased number of clue cells, and leukocytes are conspicuously absent. In advanced cases of BV, >20% of the epithelial cells are clue cells.
    - The addition of KOH to the vaginal secretions (the "whiff" test) releases a fishy, amine-like odor.

(Reference: Berek JS. Berek & Novak's Gynecology, 16th edition. Philadelphia: Lippincott Williams and Wilkins; 2019)

5. **a.** Clinicians who are unable to perform microscopy should use alternative diagnostic tests such as a pH and amines test card, detection of *Gardnerella vaginalis* ribosomal ribonucleic acid (RNA), or Gram stain. Culture of *G. vaginalis* is not recommended as a diagnostic tool because of its lack of specificity.

The *Nugent score* is a Gram stain scoring system for vaginal swabs to diagnose bacterial vaginosis. The Nugent score is calculated by assessing for the presence of large gram-positive rods (*Lactobacillus* morphotypes; decrease in *Lactobacillus* scored as

0-4), small gram-variable rods (*Gardnerella vaginalis* morphotypes; scored as 0-4), and curved gram-variable rods (*Mobiluncus* spp. morphotypes; scored as 0-2). A score of 7-10 is consistent with bacterial vaginosis without culture. The Nugent score is now rarely used by physicians due to the time it takes to read the slides and requires the use of a trained microscopist.[1] Bacterial vaginosis diagnosis is done by evaluating the pH, the presences of *Lactobacillus* spp. versus a mixed flora consisting of *Gardnerella vaginalis*, *Bacteroides* spp., *Mobiluncus* spp., and *Mycoplasma hominis*.

[References: (1) Bennett JE, Dolin R, Blaser MJ. Mandell, Douglas, and Bennett's Principles and Practice of Infectious Diseases, 8th edition. Philadelphia, PA: Elsevier/Saunders; 2015. (2) Berek JS. Berek & Novak's Gynecology, 16th edition. Philadelphia: Lippincott Williams and Wilkins; 2019]

6. **c.** The following treatments are effective for bacterial vaginosis:
   - Metronidazole, an antibiotic with excellent activity against anaerobes but poor activity against lactobacilli, is the drug of choice for the treatment of BV. A dose of 500 mg administered orally twice a day for 7 days should be used.
   - Metronidazole gel, 0.75%, one applicator (5 g) intravaginally once daily for 5 days, may alternatively be prescribed.

   The overall cure rates range from 75 to 84% with the aforementioned regimens. Clindamycin in the following regimens is effective in treating BV:
   - Clindamycin ovules, 100 mg, intravaginally once at bedtime for 3 days
   - Clindamycin bioadhesive cream, 2%, 100 mg intravaginally in a single dose
   - Clindamycin cream, 2%, one applicator full (5 g) intravaginally at bedtime for 7 days
   - Clindamycin, 300 mg, orally twice daily for 7 days

   (Reference: Berek JS. Berek & Novak's Gynecology, 16th edition. Philadelphia: Lippincott Williams and Wilkins; 2019)

7. **d.** Treatment of the male sexual partner does not improve therapeutic response and therefore is not recommended. See explanation of question 6.

8. **d.** See explanation of question 6.

B. TRICHOMONAS VAGINITIS

9. **b.** Trichomonas vaginitis, the most prevalent nonviral sexually transmitted infection in the United States is caused by the sexually transmitted, flagellated parasite, *Trichomonas vaginalis*. The transmission rate is high; 70% of men contract the disease after a single exposure to an infected woman, which suggests that the rate of male-to-female transmission is even higher. The parasite, which exists only in trophozoite form, is an anaerobe that has the ability to generate hydrogen to combine with oxygen to create an anaerobic environment. It often accompanies bacterial vaginosis, which can be diagnosed in as many as 60% of patients with trichomonas vaginitis. *T. vaginalis* infection is associated with a two- to three-fold increased risk for human immunodeficiency virus acquisition.

(Reference: Berek JS. Berek & Novak's Gynecology, 16th edition. Philadelphia: Lippincott Williams and Wilkins; 2019)

10. **a.** Symptoms and signs may be much milder in patients with small inocula of trichomonads, and trichomonas vaginitis is often asymptomatic.
    - Trichomonas vaginitis is associated with a profuse, purulent, and malodorous vaginal discharge that may be accompanied by vulvar pruritus.
    - A purulent vaginal discharge may exude from the vagina.
    - In patients with high concentrations of organisms, a patchy vaginal erythema and colpitis macularis ("strawberry" cervix) may be observed.
    - The pH of the vaginal secretions could be variable or higher than 5.0.
    - Microscopy of the secretions reveals motile trichomonads and increased numbers of leukocytes.
    - Clue cells may be present because of the common association with bacterial vaginosis.
    - The whiff test may be positive.

    (Reference: Berek JS. Berek & Novak's Gynecology, 16th edition. Philadelphia: Lippincott Williams and Wilkins; 2019)

11. **c.** See explanation of question 10. Amsel's diagnostic criteria is used for diagnosis of bacterial vaginosis.

12. **a.** See explanation of question 10.
    Vaginal secretions are gray and they thinly coat the vaginal wall in bacterial vaginosis. White curdy discharge is present in vulvovaginal candidiasis. The pH of the vaginal secretion is variable or higher than 5.
    (Reference: Berek JS. Berek & Novak's Gynecology, 16th edition. Philadelphia: Lippincott Williams and Wilkins; 2019)

13. **c.** The treatment of trichomonas vaginitis can be summarized as follows:
    - Metronidazole is the drug of choice for treatment of vaginal trichomoniasis. Both a single dose (2 g orally) and a multidose (500 mg twice daily for 7 days) regimen are highly effective and have cure rates of about 95%.
    - Tinidazole 2 g orally in a single dose is another recommended regimen.
    - The sexual partner should be treated.
    - Women who do not respond to initial therapy should be treated again with metronidazole, 500 mg, twice daily for 7 days. If repeated treatment is not effective, the patient should be treated with a single 2 g dose of metronidazole once daily for 5 days or tinidazole, 2 g, in a single dose for 5 days.
    - Patients who do not respond to repeated treatment with metronidazole or tinidazole and for whom the possibility of reinfection is excluded should be referred for expert consultation. In these uncommon refractory cases, an important part of management is to obtain cultures of the parasite to determine its susceptibility to metronidazole and tinidazole.
    - Retesting for *T. vaginalis* is recommended within 3 months following initial treatment due to high rate of reinfection.
    - Metronidazole gel should not be used for the treatment of vaginal trichomoniasis.
    (Reference: Berek JS. Berek & Novak's Gynecology, 16th edition. Philadelphia: Lippincott Williams and Wilkins; 2019)

14. **d.** See the explanation of question 13.

15. **c.** See the explanation of question 13.

C. VULVOVAGINAL CANDIDIASIS

16. **c.** Factors that predispose women to the development of symptomatic VVC include antibiotic use, pregnancy, immunosuppressive states, and diabetes. Pregnancy and diabetes are associated with a qualitative decrease in cell-mediated immunity, leading to a higher incidence of candidiasis.
    (Reference: Berek JS. Berek & Novak's Gynecology, 16th edition. Philadelphia: Lippincott Williams and Wilkins; 2019)

17. **b.** An estimated 75% of women experience at least one episode of vulvovaginal candidiasis during their lifetimes. Nearly 45% of women will experience two or more episodes. Few are plagued with a chronic, recurrent infection.
    Candida albicans is responsible for 85–90% of vaginal yeast infections. Other species of *Candida*, such as *Candida glabrata* and *Candida tropicalis*, can cause vulvovaginal symptoms and tend to be resistant to therapy.
    Candida are dimorphic fungi existing as blastospores, which are responsible for transmission and asymptomatic colonization, and as mycelia, which result from blastospore germination and enhance colonization and facilitate tissue invasion. The extensive areas of pruritus and inflammation often associated with minimal invasion of the lower genital tract epithelial cells suggest that an extracellular toxin or enzyme may play a role in the pathogenesis of this disease. A hypersensitivity phenomenon may be responsible for the irritative symptoms associated with VVC, especially for patients with chronic, recurrent disease. Patients with symptomatic disease usually have an increased concentration of these microorganisms (>104 per mL) compared with asymptomatic patients.
    (Reference: Berek JS. Berek & Novak's Gynecology, 16th edition. Philadelphia: Lippincott Williams and Wilkins; 2019)

18. **a.** It is helpful to categorize women with vulvovaginal candidiasis as having either uncomplicated or complicated disease **(Table 1)**.

TABLE 1: Classification of vulvovaginal candidiasis.

Uncomplicated	Complicated
Sporadic or infrequent in occurrence	Recurrent symptoms
Mild to moderate symptoms	Severe symptoms
Likely to be *Candida albicans*	Non-albicans *Candida*
Immunocompetent women	Immunocompromised, e.g., diabetic women, HIV, immunosuppressive therapy

(*Source:* Sobel JD, Faro S, Force RW, Foxman B, Ledger WJ, Nyirjesy PR, et al. Vulvovaginal candidiasis: epidemiologic, diagnostic, and therapeutic considerations. Am J Obstet Gynecol. 1998;178:203-11.)

(*Reference: Berek JS. Berek & Novak's Gynecology, 16th edition. Philadelphia: Lippincott Williams and Wilkins; 2019*)

19. **a.** A small number of women develop recurrent vulvovaginal candidiasis (RVVC), defined as four or more episodes in a year. Non-albicans *Candida* species are observed in 10–20% of RVVC. These women experience persistent irritative symptoms of the vestibule and vulva. Burning replaces itching as the prominent symptom in patients with RVVC. The diagnosis should be confirmed by direct microscopy of the vaginal secretions and by fungal culture.

(*Reference: Berek JS. Berek & Novak's Gynecology, 16th edition. Philadelphia: Lippincott Williams and Wilkins; 2019*)

20. **a.** The treatment of patients with recurrent vulvovaginal candidiasis consists of inducing a remission of chronic symptoms with fluconazole (150 mg every 3 days for three doses). Patients should be maintained on a suppressive dose of this agent (fluconazole, 150 mg weekly) for 6 months. On this regimen, 90% of women with RVVC will remain in remission. After suppressive therapy, approximately half will remain asymptomatic. Recurrence will occur in the other half and should prompt reinstitution of suppressive therapy. Patients with RVVC should have a fungal culture performed to look for non-albicans *Candida*, and potential resistance to fluconazole. If recurrence persists or in patients with non-albicans *Candida*, boric acid 600 mg vaginal suppository is recommended for 2 weeks.

(*Reference: Berek JS. Berek & Novak's Gynecology, 16th edition. Philadelphia: Lippincott Williams and Wilkins; 2019*)

■ D. PELVIC INFLAMMATORY DISEASE

21. **b.** The ectocervical squamous epithelium is an extension of and is continuous with the vaginal epithelium. *Trichomonas*, *Candida*, and herpes simplex virus can cause inflammation of the ectocervix. Conversely, *Neisseria gonorrhoeae* and *Chlamydia trachomatis* infect only the glandular epithelium.

The diagnosis of cervicitis is based on the finding of a purulent endocervical discharge, generally yellow or green in color and referred to as "mucopus". Placement of the mucopus on a slide that can be Gram stained will reveal the presence of an increased number of neutrophils (>30 per high-power field). The presence of intracellular gram-negative diplococci, leading to the presumptive diagnosis of gonococcal endocervicitis, may be detected. If the Gram stain results are negative for gonococci, the presumptive diagnosis is chlamydial cervicitis.

22. **a.** Treatment of cervicitis consists of an antibiotic regimen recommended for the treatment of uncomplicated lower genital tract infection with both chlamydia and gonorrhea.

Dual therapy is recommended for the treatment of gonorrhea, and cefixime is no longer a first-line regimen.

Fluoroquinolone resistance is common in *Neisseria gonorrhoeae* isolates, and, therefore, these agents are no longer recommended for the treatment of women with gonococcal cervicitis. It is imperative that all sexual partners be treated with a similar antibiotic regimen. Cervicitis is commonly associated with BV, which, if not treated concurrently, leads to significant persistence of the symptoms and signs of cervicitis.

(*Reference: Berek JS. Berek & Novak's Gynecology, 16th edition. Philadelphia: Lippincott Williams and Wilkins; 2019*)

23. **b.** Traditionally, the diagnosis of PID is based on a triad of symptoms and signs, including pelvic pain, cervical motion and adnexal tenderness, and the presence of fever. It is recognized that there is wide variation in

many symptoms and signs among women with this condition, which makes the diagnosis of acute PID difficult. Many women with PID exhibit subtle or mild symptoms that are not readily recognized as PID. Consequently, delay in diagnosis and therapy probably contributes to the inflammatory sequelae in the upper reproductive tract. In the diagnosis of PID, the goal is to establish guidelines that are sufficiently sensitive to avoid missing mild cases but sufficiently specific to avoid giving antibiotic therapy to women who are not infected. Genitourinary tract symptoms may indicate PID; therefore, the diagnosis of PID should be considered in women with any genitourinary symptoms, including, but not limited to, lower abdominal pain, excessive vaginal discharge, menorrhagia, metrorrhagia, fever, chills, and urinary symptoms. Some women may develop PID without having overt symptoms. Pelvic organ tenderness, either uterine tenderness alone or uterine tenderness with adnexal tenderness, is present in patients with PID. Cervical motion tenderness suggests the presence of peritoneal inflammation, which causes pain when the peritoneum is stretched by moving the cervix and causing traction of the adnexa on the pelvic peritoneum. Direct or rebound abdominal tenderness may be present.
(Reference: Berek JS. Berek & Novak's Gynecology, 16th edition. Philadelphia: Lippincott Williams and Wilkins; 2019)

24. **d.** Clinical criteria for the diagnosis of pelvic inflammatory disease:
    - *Symptoms*: None necessary
    - *Signs*:
      - Pelvic organ tenderness
      - Leukorrhea and/or mucopurulent endocervicitis
    - *Additional criteria to increase the specificity of the diagnosis*:
      - Endometrial biopsy showing endometritis
      - Elevated C-reactive protein or erythrocyte sedimentation rate
      - Temperature higher than 38°C (100.4°F)
      - Leukocytosis
      - Positive test for gonorrhea or chlamydia
    - *Elaborate criteria*:
      - Ultrasound documenting tubo-ovarian abscess
      - Laparoscopy visually confirming salpingitis

Sexual partners of women with PID should be evaluated and treated for urethral infection with chlamydia or gonorrhea.
(Reference: Berek JS. Berek & Novak's Gynecology, 16th edition. Philadelphia: Lippincott Williams and Wilkins; 2019)

25. **d.** Therapy regimens for PID must provide empirical, broad-spectrum coverage of likely pathogens, including *N. gonorrhoeae*, *C. trachomatis*, *M. genitalium*, gram-negative facultative bacteria, anaerobes, and streptococci. An outpatient regimen of cefoxitin and doxycycline is as effective as an inpatient parenteral regimen of the same antimicrobials. Therefore, hospitalization is recommended only when the diagnosis is uncertain, pelvic abscess is suspected, clinical disease is severe, or compliance with an outpatient regimen is in question. Hospitalized patients can be considered for discharge when their fever has lysed.
(Reference: Berek JS. Berek & Novak's Gynecology, 16th edition. Philadelphia: Lippincott Williams and Wilkins; 2019)

26. **a.** All regimens used to treat PID should also be effective against *N. gonorrhoeae* and *C. trachomatis* because negative endocervical screening for these organisms does not rule out upper genital tract infection. Anaerobic bacteria have been isolated from the upper genital tract of women who have PID, and data from in vitro studies have revealed that some anaerobes (e.g., *Bacteroides fragilis*) can cause tubal and epithelial destruction. BV is often present among women who have PID. Addition of metronidazole to intramuscular or oral PID regimens more effectively eradicates anaerobic organisms from the upper genital tract. Until treatment regimens that do not cover anaerobic microbes have been demonstrated to prevent long-term sequelae (e.g., infertility and ectopic pregnancy) as successfully as the regimens that are effective against these microbes, using regimens with anaerobic activity should be considered. Treatment should be initiated as soon as the presumptive diagnosis has been made because prevention of long-term sequelae is dependent on early administration of recommended antimicrobials. For women with PID of mild or moderate clinical severity, parenteral and oral regimens appear to have similar efficacy. The decision of whether hospitalization is necessary

should be based on provider judgment and whether the woman meets any of the following criteria:
- Surgical emergencies (e.g., appendicitis) cannot be excluded
- Tubo-ovarian abscess
- Pregnancy
- Severe illness, nausea and vomiting, or oral temperature >38.5°C (101°F)
- Unable to follow or tolerate an outpatient oral regimen
- No clinical response to oral antimicrobial therapy

[Reference: Centers for Disease Control and Prevention. (2021). Sexually Transmitted Infections Treatment Guidelines, 2021. (online) Available from: https://www.cdc.gov/std/treatment-guidelines/default.htm. (Last accessed December, 2023)]

ANSWERS OF CASE-BASED QUESTIONS

27. d.	28. a.	29. b.	30. a.
31. c.	32. c.	33. c.	34. d.
35. a.	36. c.	37. a.	38. c.
39. d.			

Chapter 86: Hyperprolactinemia

Shubhra Agarwal

1. What are the forms of prolactin (PRL) in the basal state?
   a. Monomer
   b. Dimer
   c. Multimeric
   d. All of the above

2. Ahumada-Del Castillo syndrome comprise?
   a. Galactorrhea and headache
   b. Visual impairment and amenorrhea
   c. Galactorrhea and amenorrhea
   d. Amenorrhea and scotoma

3. Chiari-Frommel syndrome consists of:
   a. Galactorrhea and amenorrhea
   b. Scotoma and headache
   c. Hot flushes and decreased libido
   d. Extended postpartum galactorrhea and amenorrhea

4. Forbes-Albright syndrome consists of:
   a. Galactorrhea and amenorrhea associated with pituitary tumors
   b. Scotoma and headache
   c. Galactorrhea and amenorrhea with scotoma
   d. Burden and headache and visual impairment

5. Which of the following is a mechanism of action of PRL?
   a. Inhibits pulsatile gonadotropin hormone-releasing hormone (GnRH) reaction → inhibits luteinizing hormone (LH) and follicle-stimulating hormone (FSH) release → directly impairs gonadal steroidogenesis → primary and secondary amenorrhea
   b. Directly acts on gonadal → primary and secondary amenorrhea
   c. Decreases FSH which acts on gonads causing primary and secondary amenorrhea
   d. Inhibits inhibin B → acts on gonads causing primary and secondary amenorrhea

6. What is hook effect?
   i. Occurs when serum PRL levels are very high (5,000 ng/mL)
   ii. Increased amount causes antibody saturation in the immunoradiometric assay resulting in falsely low levels
   iii. Can be avoided using dilution
   iv. Occurs between 20 and 200 ng/mL with macroadenoma

   Which of the following is correct?
   a. i and iv
   b. ii and iii
   c. All of the above
   d. iii and iv

7. The sample for prolactin measurement should be withdrawn preferably:
   a. Midmorning
   b. At night
   c. Early morning
   d. Evening

8. How to avoid misdiagnosis with macroprolactin?
   a. Dilution of serum by repeating assay
   b. Pretreat serum with immunoglobulins
   c. Pretreat serum with polyethylene glycol
   d. Store the sample for 24 hours at −20°C

9. A patient presenting with galactorrhea, blurring of vision, and renal impairment suspected of pituitary adenoma is planned for magnetic resonance imaging (MRI). MRI should be done:
   a. With gadolinium
   b. Without gadolinium
   c. With maximum amount of gadolinium
   d. With minimal gadolinium

10. Which of the following statements is correct for a patient with idiopathic hyperprolactinemia?
    i. Serum PRL should be measured annually.
    ii. Raised serum PRL 20–100 ng/mL with no cause may have microadenomas not visible on imaging studies.
    iii. Dopamine agonists (DAs) are the mainstay of management.
    a. i and ii
    b. i, ii, and iii
    c. ii and iii
    d. All of the above

11. Which of the following DAs are ergot derivatives?
    a. Cabergoline and bromocriptine
    b. Quinagolide
    c. Pergolide
    d. All of the above

12. Which of the following drugs used in the treatment of hyperprolactinemia is withdrawn from the market due to association with valvular heart disease at high doses (3 mg/day) in patients with parkinsonism?
    a. Pergolide
    b. Quinagolide
    c. Both
    d. None

13. All the following drugs lead to hyperprolactinemia, *except*:
    a. Neuroleptics
    b. Antipsychotics
    c. Anti depressants
    d. PPI

14. Hyperprolactinemia may recur in … cases of macroprolactinoma within a year after treatment withdrawal.
    a. 26–65%
    b. 20–25%
    c. 20%
    d. 50%

15. Radiotherapy in hyperprolactinemia is reserved for:
    i. Patients not responding to DA therapy
    ii. Patients not cured by surgery
    iii. Malignant prolactinoma which is very rare
    iv. Patients with scotoma and bitemporal hemianopia

    Which is correct?
    a. i and ii
    b. i, ii, and iii
    c. ii and iv
    d. All of the above

16. A pregnant patient has microprolactinoma diagnosed prior to pregnancy on treatment with DA. Which of the following statements is correct?
    a. Continue DA therapy for at least 6 months
    b. Stop DA as soon as pregnancy is confirmed
    c. DA therapy should be continued till term
    d. Surgical treatment is advised

17. In a pregnant woman with macroadenomas, symptomatic tumor expansion occurs in:
    a. >75%
    b. 50%
    c. 20–30%
    d. <1%

18. Risk of progression of microadenoma to macroadenoma is:
    a. 50%
    b. 25%
    c. 7%
    d. 5%

19. Which of the following drugs is used for the treatment of hyperprolactinemia?
    a. Cabergoline
    b. Pergolide
    c. Quinagolide
    d. All of the above

20. Which of the following drugs causes psychotic reaction?
    a. Cabergoline
    b. Bromocriptine
    c. Quinagolide
    d. Pergolide

21. Macroadenomas are pituitary tumors larger than:
    a. 1 cm
    b. 5 cm
    c. 2.5 cm
    d. 3 cm

22. Isolated galactorrhea without raised PRL is seen in:
    a. 50%
    b. 20%
    c. 70%
    d. 80%

23. In patients with both galactorrhea and amenorrhea, how many patients have hyperprolactinemia?
    a. One-third
    b. Two-thirds
    c. Three-fourths
    d. All of the above

24. Osteopenia/osteoporosis in hyperprolactinemia is due to:
    a. Raised prolactin itself
    b. Hyperprolactinemia leading to estrogen deficiency
    c. Raised thyroid-stimulating hormone (TSH)
    d. None

25. A macroadenoma with hyperprolactinemia has reached normal levels following treatment with ergot alkaloid. A repeat MRI is indicated after:
    a. 1 month
    b. Annually
    c. 3 months
    d. 6 months

26. Which of the following statements is correct?
    a. Normal PRL level is an absolute proof of tumor response to treatment
    b. Resumption of menses is an absolute proof of tumor response to treatment
    c. Both a and b
    d. None of the above

27. Hyperprolactinemia in women with chronic renal failure occurs in:
    a. 20-75%
    b. 50%
    c. 5%
    d. 85%

28. After successful treatment of hyperprolactinemia, monitoring of PRL levels is necessary to ensure:
    a. Ongoing symptom relief
    b. Prevention of pituitary tumor recurrence
    c. Normalization of bone density
    d. Fertility restoration

29. Amenorrhea without galactorrhea is associated with hyperprolactinemia in:
    a. 15%   b. 40%
    c. 5%   d. 60%

30. Which of the following conditions is commonly associated with hyperprolactinemia?
    a. Polycystic ovary syndrome (PCOS)
    b. Diabetes mellitus
    c. Addison's disease
    d. Hypothyroidism

ANSWERS

1. **d.** In the basal state, three forms are released: (1) Monomer, (2) dimer, and (3) multimeric species. Larger species can be degraded into monomeric forms by reducing disulfide bonds.

2. **c.** Galactorrhea and amenorrhea are seen in 60% of patients.

3. **d.** Chiari-Frommel syndrome refers to extended postpartum galactorrhea and amenorrhea.

4. **a.** Forbes-Albright syndrome consists of galactorrhea and amenorrhea associated with a pituitary tumor.

5. **a.** The cessation of normal ovulatory processes resulting from elevated PRL levels is primarily caused by the suppressive effects of PRL, via hypothalamic mediation, on GnRH pulsatile release

6. **c.** *Hook effect:* Caution should be exercised in interpreting serum PRL concentrations between 20 and 200 ng/mL (20-200 μg/L SI units) in the presence of a macroadenoma because of falsely low values due to the "hook effect." It occurs when serum PRL levels are very high (5,000 ng/mL). Increased amount causes antibody saturation in the immunoradiometric assay, leading to falsely low levels. The artifact can be avoided by repeating the assay using a 1:100 dilution of serum.

7. **a.** Prolactin measurement should be withdrawn preferably midmorning. There is diurnal variation with the lowest levels occurring in midmorning.

8. **b.** Macroprolactin causes hyperprolactinemia through decreased prolactin clearance. Macroprolactin has decreased bioactivity. Misdiagnosis can be avoided by asking the laboratory to pretreat serum with polyethylene glycol to precipitate the macroprolactin before the immunoassay for prolactin in supernatant.

9. **b.** MRI for a patient with any degree of renal impairment should be done without gadolinium.

10. **d.** All of the above

11. **a.** Cabergoline and bromocriptine are ergot derivatives which act as DAs.

12. **a.** Recent studies reveal an increased risk of cardiac valve regurgitation in patients with Parkinson's disease who were treated with high doses of *cabergoline* or *pergolide* but not with *bromocriptine*. Higher doses and a longer duration of therapy were associated with a higher risk of valvulopathy.

13. **d.** The most common cause of elevated PRL levels is likely pharmacologic; most patients using antipsychotic medications and many other patients using agents with antidopaminergic properties will exhibit moderately elevated PRL levels. Neuroleptics, antipsychotics, anticonvulsants, antihistamines, opiates, antidepressants can all cause hyperprolactinemia.

14. **b.** Hyperprolactinemia may recur in 26-65% of cases of macroprolactinoma within a year after treatment withdrawal.

15. **b.** External radiation is associated with significant side effects including hypopituitarism, optic nerve damage, neurological dysfunction, and increased

risks of stroke and secondary brain tumors. Therefore, this option is reserved for patients not responding to DA therapy. Therefore this option is reserved for patients not responding to DA therapy, not cured by surgery or with malignant prolactinoma.

For patients not cured by surgery, malignant prolactinoma occurs, which is very rare.

16. **b.** Microprolactinomas—the risk of clinically relevant tumor expansion is <2% during pregnancy. Therefore, stop DA therapy as soon as pregnancy is confirmed. Advise the patient to report for urgent assessment in the event of a severe headache or visual disturbance. Serial PRL monitoring is not necessary.

17. **c.** Macroadenomas—symptomatic tumor expansion occurs in 20–30% of women. Both options can be offered, i.e., stopping DA therapy when pregnancy is confirmed, with close surveillance, or continuing DA in pregnancy.

18. **c.** Microadenomas rarely progress to macroadenomas. Six large series of patients with microadenomas reveal that, with no treatment, the risk for progression of microadenoma to a macroadenoma is only 7%.

19. **d.** Cabergoline in a dosage of 0.25–0.5 mg once or twice a week, bromocriptine, quinagolide, pergolide are the drugs that can be used to treat hyperprolactinemia. Cabergoline is the drug of choice, long acting with better compliance, superior in reducing prolactin secretion.

20. **b.** One rare adverse effect of *bromocriptine* is a psychotic reaction. Symptoms include auditory hallucinations, delusional ideas, and changes in mood that quickly resolve after discontinuation of the drug.

21. **a.** Macroadenomas are pituitary tumors that are larger than 1 cm in size.

22. **a.** Prolactin levels may be within the normal range in nearly 50% of patients. In these cases whether caused by a prior transient episode of hyperprolactinemia or other unknown factors the sensitivity of breast to lactotropic stimulus engendered by normal prolactin level is sufficient to cause galactorrhea.

23. **b.** In patients with both galactorrhea and amenorrhea, approximately two-thirds will have hyperprolactinemia; in that group, approximately one-third will have a pituitary adenoma.

24. **b.** Hyperprolactinemia-induced estrogen deficiency, rather than prolactin itself, is the major factor in the development of osteopenia.

25. **d.** If serum prolactin levels remain normal for 2–3 years and the MRI does not show any tumor mass, then the drug can be stopped. Follow-up then includes every 3 monthly serum prolactin levels for the first year and then annually. An MRI of the brain is done if prolactin levels increase above normal.

26. **d.**

27. **a.** Hyperprolactinemia in women with chronic renal failure occurs in 20–75%.

28. **b.** After 1 year of treatment, the dose of dopamine agonist can be reduced. If serum prolactin levels remain normal for 2–3 years and the MRI does not show any tumor mass, then the drug can be stopped.

29. **a.** Amenorrhea without galactorrhea is associated with hyperprolactinemia in 15% of patients.

30. **d.** When prolactin levels are found to be elevated, hypothyroidism and medications should first be ruled out as a cause.

REFERENCES

1. Peterson RK, Link MC. Peterson M. Endocrine disorders. In: Berek JS (Eds). Berek and Novak's Gynecology, 16th edition. Philadelphia: Wolters Kluwer; 2019. pp. 1957-74.
2. Rao KA, Rao VA, Devi R. Endocrine disorders affecting reproduction. In: A Rao (Ed). Principles and Practice of Assisted Reproductive Technology, 2nd edition. New Delhi: Jaypee Brothers Medical Publishers (P) Ltd; 2019. pp. 148-57.

Chapter 87: Prolapse Uterus: Part 1

Beena Kumari, Rajshree Dayanand Katke

QUESTIONS

1. **Middle part of posterior vaginal wall prolapse lead to:**
   a. Enterocoele
   b. Urethrocele
   c. Rectocele
   d. None of the above

2. **Uterovaginal (UV) prolapse is:**
   a. Descent of the uterus primarily followed by vaginal inversion
   b. First vaginal prolapse followed by dragging down of uterus
   c. Both vagina and uterus prolapsed simultaneously
   d. None of the above

3. **Vaginal rugae are lost in:**
   a. Distension cystocele
   b. Displacement cystocele
   c. Both a and b
   d. Only in third-degree cystocele

4. **Cystocele is restricted in the space between:**
   a. Submeatal sulcus and transverse sulcus
   b. Transverse sulcus and bladder sulcus
   c. Submeatal sulcus and bladder sulcus
   d. External urethral meatus and bladder sulcus

5. **Q-tip test is used to test:**
   a. Occult stress urinary incontinence
   b. Urethral hypermobility
   c. Tone of perineal body
   d. None of the above

6. **The site(s) of decubitus ulcer in UV prolapse is (are):**
   a. Vagina
   b. Cervix
   c. Both a and b
   d. Uterus

7. **Gellhorn pessary is a type of:**
   a. Support pessary
   b. Space-occupying pessary
   c. Both a and b
   d. None of the above

8. **Which of the following is a posterior sling surgery?**
   a. Purandare's sling surgery
   b. Khanna's sling surgery
   c. Joshi's sling surgery
   d. Both a and c

9. **Which of the following is not a step of Fothergill's repair?**
   a. Anterior colporrhaphy
   b. Amputation of cervix
   c. Shortening of cardinal ligament and reattachment to the posterior aspect of cervix
   d. Posterior colpoperineorrhaphy

10. **In which McCall's culdoplasty does the suture pass through the posterior vaginal wall?**
    a. Internal
    b. External
    c. Both a and b
    d. None of the above

11. **De Lancy's level III support defect will lead to:**
    a. Urethral hypermotility
    b. Cystocele
    c. Both a and b
    d. Enterocele

12. **Bonney test is positive in:**
    a. Stress urinary incontinence
    b. Urge incontinence
    c. Neurogenic urinary incontinence
    d. None of the above

13. **Plication of uterosacral ligament and fixation to vaginal vault is called:**
    a. McCall's culdoplasty
    b. Moschcowitz operation
    c. Halban method
    d. None of the above

14. **Which of the following organ prolapse is not an etiology of pelvic organ prolapse?**
    a. Marfan's syndrome
    b. Undernutrition
    c. Obesity
    d. Prolonged first stage of labor

15. **Which of the following is true regarding staging of pelvic organ prolapse quantification?**
    a. *Stage 3:* Most distal portion of prolapse <1 cm below hymen but total vaginal length (TVL) <2 cm
    b. *Stage 3:* Most distal portion of prolapse >1 cm below hymen but TVL >2 cm
    c. *Stage 3:* Most distal portion of prolapse >1 cm below hymen but TVL <2 cm
    d. None of the above

16. **As per the Baden–Walker halfway system, Grade I UV descent is:**
    a. Normal position for each respective site
    b. Descent is halfway to the hymen
    c. Descent is halfway after the hymen
    d. Descent is halfway to introitus

17. **Osteitis is a complication of which of the following operations of UV prolapse?**
    a. Purandare sling
    b. Khanna sling
    c. LeFort colpocleisis
    d. Fothergill repair

18. **Which of the following is not a support of uterus?**
    a. Endopelvic fascia
    b. Broad ligament
    c. Arcus tendinous fascia
    d. Perineal body

19. **Which of the following muscles are not attached to perineal body?**
    a. Deep transverse perineal
    b. Sphincter urethrae
    c. Ischiocavernosus
    d. All of the above

20. **Which of the following is not a sign of a well-fitted pessary?**
    a. No descent on cough/valsalva
    b. One finger can be inserted between pessary and vaginal side wall
    c. Fitted at the level of ischial tuberosity
    d. Not visible when labia are separated

21. **Which of the following regarding uterine descent is not correct?**
    a. First-degree descent—cervix descends below its normal level on straining—gut does not protrude from the vulva
    b. First-degree descent—cervix descends below its normal level on straining and protrudes from the vulva
    c. Second-degree descent—cervix reaches up to vulva on straining
    d. Procidentia—whole uterus on prolapsed outside vulva

22. **Which of the following is a cause of urge incontinence?**
    a. Detrusor instability
    b. Increased parasympathetic activity
    c. Urinary tract infection
    d. All of the above

23. **Which of the following is the cause of UV prolapse?**
    a. Aging
    b. Estrogen deprivation
    c. Collagen abnormalities
    d. Increase in abnormal pressure
    e. Trauma during vaginal delivery
    f. All of the above

24. **Which of the following is not a posterior vaginal wall defect?**
    a. Enterocele
    b. Rectocele
    c. Perineal body descent
    d. Perineal tear

25. **Which of the following is not an indication for the use of pessary?**
    a. When childbearing is intended in the near future
    b. Refusal of operation by patient
    c. Prolapse with pregnancy
    d. Nonhealing decubitus ulcer

26. **All the following are complications associated with pessary, *except*:**
    a. Bacterial vaginitis ulceration of vaginal wall
    b. Cervicitis
    c. Reduction of prolapse
    d. Strangulation of prolapsed tissue

27. **Management of third-degree prolapse in a 27 year P1T0 can be all, *except*:**
    a. Vaginal hysterectomy
    b. Fothergill surgery
    c. Sling surgery
    d. Ring pessary

28. **Which of the following is a common symptom in women with vaginal or uterine prolapse?**
    a. Upper deck pair
    b. Urinary incontinence
    c. Diarrhea
    d. Excessive moisture in the vaginal mucosa

29. Which of the following is not a prerequisite for continence?
    a. Internal urethral sphincter at levator ani
    b. Pressure >20 cm of H_2O
    c. Urethrovesical angle >100°
    d. Tone of pelvic floor muscles

30. Which of the following is the cause and management of decubitus ulcers?
    a. Friction, glycerine and acriflavine dressing, respectively
    b. Venous congestion, magnesium sulfate dressing, respectively
    c. Malignant changes of prolapsed part, vaginal hysterectomy followed by chemotherapy, respectively
    d. Venous congestion, glycerine and acriflavine dressing, respectively

ANSWERS

1. c.	2. a.	3. a.	4. b.
5. b.	6. c.	7. c.	8. b.
9. c.	10. b.	11. a.	12. a.
13. a.	14. d.	15. c.	16. b.
17. a.	18. b.	19. c.	20. c.
21. b.	22. d.	23. f.	24. a.
25. d.	26. c.	27. a.	28. b.
29. a.	30. b.		

Chapter 88: Prolapse Uterus: Part II

Ruchika Garg

ETIOLOGY, SUPPORTS OF UTERUS, CLASSIFICATION, RISK FACTORS, SYMPTOMS, EXAMINATION, AND DIFFERENTIAL DIAGNOSIS

Savita Somalwar, Kanchan Dwidmuthe

QUESTIONS

1. All the following are risk factors for genital prolapse, *except:*
   a. Multiparty
   b. Inadequate spacing
   c. Proper puerperal rehabilitation
   d. Chronic cough

2. Which of the following statements is not true for prolapse?
   a. Descent of the cervix up to the introitus is 2° descent
   b. Procidentia is when the whole of the uterus lies outside the introitus
   c. Descent of the upper third of the posterior vaginal wall is enterocele
   d. Descent of the lower two-thirds of the anterior vaginal wall is urethrocele

3. All the following statements are true in the pelvic organ prolapse (POP) quantification system, *except:*
   a. Hymen is the reference point
   b. Total vaginal length is measured with maximal straining
   c. Genital hiatus is measured from the midpoint of the external urinary meatus to the midpoint of the posterior fourchette
   d. Perineal body is measured from the midpoint of the posterior fourchette to the midpoint of the anus

4. Women with prolapse can present with all of the following symptoms, *except:*
   a. Mass coming out of vagina
   b. Fullness in vagina
   c. Backache
   d. Diarrhea

5. In women with prolapse, occult stress incontinence is examined with:
   a. Reducing prolapse
   b. Without reducing prolapse
   c. Both a and b
   d. None of the above

6. Decubitus ulcer is managed with:
   a. Packing of prolapse with glycerin, acriflavine, or ring pessary
   b. Packing of prolapse with glycerin and acriflavine along with pessary
   c. Douching with antiseptic solution
   d. Both b and c

7. Which of the following is not an aggravating factor for prolapse?
   a. Chronic cough
   b. Chronic constipation
   c. Obesity
   d. Diarrhea

8. All the following are sulci on the anterior vaginal wall, *except:*
   a. Submeatal sulcus
   b. Transverse vaginal sulcus
   c. Bladder sulcus
   d. Suprameatal sulcus

9. In women with POP and urethral hypermobility, the resting urethral angle is greater than:
   a. 15°
   b. 20°
   c. 25°
   d. 30°

10. **As per the modified Oxford scale, grade 5 tone of levator ani means:**
    a. A flicker under finger
    b. A weak contraction or increase in tension without any discernible lift or squeeze
    c. Good pelvic contraction causing elevation of the posterior vaginal wall against resistance and indrawing of the perineum
    d. Strong contraction of the pelvic floor against strong resistance

11. **Integrity of the pudendal nerve is tested by:**
    a. Anal reflex
    b. Bulbocavernosus reflex
    c. Both a and b
    d. None of the above

12. **All the following features differentiate Gartner duct cyst from cystocele, *except*:**
    a. Well defined
    b. Reducible
    c. Absence of cough impulse
    d. Absence of vaginal rugosities

13. **In congenital elongation of the cervix, the vaginal fornices are:**
    a. Deep and narrow   b. Shallow and narrow
    c. Deep and wide   d. Shallow and wide

14. **Which of the following is not an indication for the use of pessary?**
    a. Prolapse in the first trimester
    b. Healing of decubitus ulcer
    c. Women unfit for surgery
    d. Women willing for surgery

15. **Level 1 support of DeLancey support system of the pelvic organ includes:**
    a. Endopelvic fibromuscular tissue
    b. Uterosacral and cardinal ligament
    c. Levator ani muscle
    d. Levator fascia

16. **Level 2 defect of DeLancey support of pelvic organs causes:**
    a. Enterocele   b. Uterine descent
    c. Vault prolapse   d. Cystocele

17. **Origin of the uterosacral ligament is from:**
    a. S2 to S4 sacral vertebrae
    b. S5 sacral vertebrae
    c. Coccyx
    d. Cervix and posterior part of the cervix

18. **Point Aα in the Pelvic Organ Prolapse Quantification (POPQ) system of classification of prolapse corresponds to:**
    a. Point on posterior wall 3 cm from hymen
    b. Point on anterior wall 3 cm from hymen
    c. Nondependent portion of rest of anterior wall
    d. Nondependent portion of rest of posterior wall

19. **Which of the following points in the POPQ system of classification of prolapse is omitted if the cervix is absent?**
    a. Point C   b. Point D
    c. Point Ap   d. Point Bp

20. **Stage 3 of POP according to POPQ classification is:**
    a. Complete to nearly complete eversion of vagina
    b. The most distal portion of prolapse is >1 cm above the level of the hymen
    c. The most distal portion of prolapse is <1 cm proximal or distal to the plane of hymen
    d. The most distal position of prolapse is <1 cm below the plane of the hymen but no further than 2 cm less than the total vaginal length

21. **Urethral hypermobility is present when:**
    a. Resting urethral angle is >30°
    b. Resting urethral angle is >50°
    c. Resting urethral angle is <30°
    d. Urethral angle is <50°

22. **Normally, external os of the cervix lies:**
    a. At the level of ischial spine
    b. At the level of hymen
    c. Above ischial spine
    d. 2 cm below ischial spine

23. **Enterocele is a result of defect in which of the following DeLancey levels?**
    a. Level 1   b. Level 2
    c. Level 3   d. All of the above

24. **Which of the following is a type of anterior vaginal wall prolapse?**
    a. Cystocele   b. Urethrocele
    c. Cystourethrocele   d. All of the above

ANSWERS

1. **c.** Proper puerperal rehabilitation i.e taking adequate rest, avoiding lifting heavy weights as well as Kegel's exercises can help in preventing genital prolapse.

2. **d.** According to Shaw's classification of prolapse, descent of upper two thirds of anterior vaginal wall is cystocele and descent of lower one third anterior vaginal wall is urethrocele.

3. **b.**

4. **d.**

5. **a.**

6. **a.** Decubitus ulcer occurs due to descent of cervix from normal anatomical position and interference in circulation. Packing of prolapse with glycerin, acriflavine or insertion of pessary helps in keeping cervix in anatomical position and healing of decubitus ulcer. So either treatment is required and not both simultaneously.

7. **d.**

8. **d.**

9. **d.**

10. **d.**

11. **c.**

12. **b.**

13. **a.**

14. **d.**

15. **b.** The support system for the uterus and vagina has been described as consisting of three levels

    Level I refers to the uterosacral/cardinal ligament complex, which serve to maintain the vaginal length and axis.

    Level II support consists of the paravaginal attachments of the lateral vagina and endopelvic fibromuscular connective tissue to the arcus tendineus and levator fascia that maintain the midline position of the vagina.

    Level III support pertains to the distal vagina and is made up of the muscles and connective tissue surrounding the distal vagina and perineum.

    - Damage to Level I supports causes uterine descent, enterocele and vault descent.
    - Damage to Level II supports causes cystocele, rectocele.
    - Damage to Level III supports causes urethrocele, gaping introitus and deficient perineum

16. **d.**

17. **a.**

18. **b.** *The POP-Q examination* provides a standardized measurement system to allow for more accurate assessments of postoperative outcome and to ensure uniform, reliable, and site specific descriptions of POP. POPQ Classification uses nine points as mentioned below.

    - *Aa:* Anterior wall 3 cm from hymen –3 cm to +3 cm
    - *Ba:* Most dependent portion of rest of anterior wall –3 cm to +TVL
    - *C:* Cervix or vaginal cuff ±TVL
    - *D:* Posterior fornix (if no prior hysterectomy) ±TVL or omitted
    - *Ap:* Posterior wall 3 cm from hymen –3 cm to +3 cm
    - *Bp:* Most dependent portion of rest of posterior wall.
    - *Genital hiatus (GH):* Measured from the middle of the external urethral meatus to the posterior midline hymen.
    - *Perineal body:* Measured from the posterior margin of the genital hiatus to the mid-anal opening.
    - *Total vaginal length (TVL):* It is the greatest depth of the vagina in centimeters when the vaginal apex is reduced to its full normal position.

    All measurements except the total vaginal length are measured during maximal straining.

19. **b.**

20. **d.**

21. **a.**

22. **a.**

23. **a.**

24. **d.** Shaw's classification of uterovaginal prolapse
    A. *Anterior vaginal wall*
       Upper two-thirds: Cystocele
       Urethrocele
       Lower one third – Urethrocele
    B. *Posterior vaginal wall*
       Upper one-third - Enterocele (pouch of Douglas hernia)
       Lower two-thirds- Rectocele

MANAGEMENT

Anuja Bhalerao, Sheela Jain

QUESTIONS

1. All the following are restorative surgical procedures for the management of prolapse, *except*:
   a. Shirodkar's operation
   b. Ward Mayo's operation
   c. Manchester operation
   d. Purandare's operation

2. Which of the following is not a complication of Fothergill's operation?
   a. Injury to the bladder and rectum
   b. Urinary retention or cystitis
   c. Hemorrhage
   d. Enterocele formation

3. Mesh surgery is contraindicated in all, *except*:
   a. Hypertensive patient
   b. Uncontrolled diabetes
   c. Obese patient
   d. Active pelvic infection

4. Which of the following statements is incorrect regarding Purandare's cervicopexy operation?
   a. It is indicated in congenital or nulliparous patients.
   b. Facial strips of rectus sheath are stitched to the posterior surface of the cervix
   c. Cervix is amputated below the internal os
   d. It may be combined with the Moschcowitz procedure

5. Which of the following is not an advantage of Shirodkar's sling operation?
   a. It is anatomically the most correct operation
   b. It provides a dynamic support
   c. It provides a strong bony support
   d. There is no tendency to enterocoele formation

6. Virkud's classification of sling operation is based on all of the following, *except*:
   a. Position of support
   b. Type of support
   c. Type of loop formed
   d. Whether fascia or mesh is used

7. All the following are the complications of mesh surgery in prolapse, *except*:
   a. Fistula formation
   b. Urinary incontinence
   c. Hemorrhage
   d. Dyspareunia

8. In Khanna's sling operation, the lateral ends of the mersilene tape are anchored to:
   a. Sacrospinous ligament
   b. Anterior superior iliac spine
   c. Posterior superior iliac spine
   d. Sacral promontory

9. Which of the following statements is incorrect regarding hysteropexy?
   a. Sacrospinous ligament fixation may be done
   b. Cystoscopy must be done after uterosacral suspension
   c. Usually, unilateral sacrospinous fixation is done
   d. Uterosacral suspension cannot be done laparoscopically

10. Which of the following statements is not true about Fothergill's repair?
    a. It is the treatment of choice in young women desirous of pregnancy
    b. Anterior colporrhaphy is combined with amputation of the cervix
    c. Mackenrodt's ligaments are sutured in front of the cervix
    d. Shirodkar modified this surgery by suturing uterosacral ligament in front of the cervix

11. All the following statements are true about Purandare's sling operation, *except*:
    a. The uterus becomes retroverted and there is a tendency to enterocele formation
    b. It is easy to perform and provides a strong static support
    c. If very tight, there is a risk of bowel entrapment between the uterus and anterior abdominal wall
    d. Tape anchored anteriorly may be damaged at subsequent cesarean

12. Differential diagnoses of something coming out of vagina are all, *except*:
    a. Bartholin's cyst
    b. Gärtner duct cyst
    c. Fibroid and polyp
    d. Prolapse

13. Which of the following statements is false?
    a. Vault prolapse is when the top of the vagina descends into or out of the vagina posthysterectomy
    b. Uterine prolapse is graded as first degree (within the vagina) to third degree (at the introitus)
    c. Rectocele is rectum prolapsed with the posterior vaginal wall
    d. Enterocele contains the small bowel

14. **All the following are surgical management options that preserve the uterus, *except*:**
    a. Ward Mayo's operation
    b. Sling surgeries
    c. Sacrohysteropexy
    d. Le Fort's operation

15. **In a young prolapse, all the following are performed, *except*:**
    a. Sling surgeries
    b. Sacrocolpopexy
    c. Le Fort's operation
    d. Ward Mayo's operation

16. **Vaginal hysterectomy (VH) is:**
    a. Clean
    b. Clean-contaminated
    c. Infected
    d. Contaminated

17. **What are the ways to reduce ureteric injury during VH?**
    a. Downward traction on the cervix helps displace the ureters laterally and superiorly
    b. Downward traction on the cervix helps displace the ureters medially
    c. While securing the uterine arteries, double clamp is preferred over single clamp
    d. Both b and c

18. **Which of the following statements is false?**
    a. Sacrospinous ligament fixation has high rates of sciatic nerve injury
    b. During uterosacral ligament suspension, the most common complication is ureteral obstruction
    c. Pelvic pain is a unique complication of synthetic mesh used in POP surgeries
    d. None of the above

19. **Which of the following statements is false regarding Le Fort colpocleisis?**
    a. Reserved for elderly women or medically compromised
    b. Lateral drainage channels are not created
    c. Indicated when women are no longer sexually active
    d. Transvaginal ultrasonography (TVS), Pap smear, and endometrial biopsy should be done before surgery

20. **Which of the following statements is false regarding posthysterectomy vaginal vault prolapse (PHVP)?**
    a. Routine urodynamic assessment is recommended
    b. Clinician should work as part of pelvic floor multidisciplinary team
    c. MaCall culdoplasty at the time of VH is effective in preventing subsequent PHVP
    d. Sacrospinous fixation at the time of VH should be considered when the vault descends to introitus during closure

21. **The surgery of choice in a sexually active young lady with vault prolapse is:**
    a. Sacrocolpopexy
    b. Sacrospinous fixation
    c. Le Fort's repair
    d. Colpocleisis

22. **Identify the given instrument.**

    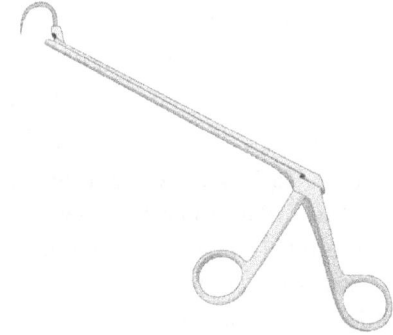

    a. Miya hook
    b. Grass hook
    c. Manson hook
    d. Mayo hook

23. **Identify the false statement.**
    a. Identification of loss of pelvic floor support, if any, and its management during hysterectomy where indication is not prolapse
    b. During abdominal hysterectomy, suturing of parametrium with angles of vaginal vault is not useful
    c. During VH, repair of enterocele and tightening of uterosacral and Mackenrodt's ligament with vaginal vault help prevent prolapse
    d. Fixing uterosacral ligament with vaginal vault in McCall culdoplasty during VH prevents prolapse

ANSWERS

1. **b.** Ward Mayo operation is vaginal hysterectomy for prolapse uterus.
   Shirodkar's and Purandare's operation are sling surgeries while in Manchester operation amputation

of cervix is done and Mackenrodt ligaments are attached in front of cervix. In these three surgeries, we try to restore the level of uterus which has descended down.

2. **d.** The cervix is amputated and the cut ends of Mackenrodt ligaments are sutured in front of the cervix. This does not predispose to enterocoele formation.

3. **a.**

4. **b.**

5. **b.** Shirodkar's sling operation provides a static support, because using the tape, the cervix is fixed to the lumbosacral fascia.

6. **d.** Virkud's classification of sling operation is based on position of support – whether from anterior or posterior, type of support – whether dynamic or static and type of loop formed – whether closed or open.

7. **c.**

8. **b.** In Khanna's sling operation, lateral ends of mersilene tape are anchored to the anterior superior iliac spine.

9. **d.**

10. **a.** Fothergill's operation is not the treatment of choice in women desirous of pregnancy because amputation of cervix may lead to secondary infertility, incompetent cervical os, recurrent abortions or preterm delivery. Excessive fibrosis may cause cervical stenosis and dystocia during labor.

11. **b.** It provides a dynamic support because the ends of the tape on either side are attached to external oblique aponeurosis and not to any bony structure.

12. **a.**

13. **b.**

14. **a.**

15. **c.** Le Forte's operation is partial colpoclesis and is done in older women who are sexually inactive.

16. **b.** In vaginal hysterectomy peritoneum is opened and hence it is clean-contaminated.

17. **a.**

18. **d.**

19. **b.**

20. **a.**

21. **a.**

22. **a.** Miya hook is a ligature carrier and makes sacrospinous ligament fixation easier and safer during prolapse surgery.

23. **b.**

Chapter 89: Urogynecology

Vineeta, Rashmi Bala, Priyanka Rai

QUESTIONS

1. **The principle of Burch colposuspension is:**
   a. To attach the paravaginal fascia to the pectineal ligament
   b. To attach the bladder neck to the pectineal line
   c. To attach the bladder neck to the pectineal ligament
   d. To attach the paravaginal fascia to the pectineal line

2. **All the following are included in the conservative management of overactive bladder (OAB), except:**
   a. Botulinum toxin A
   b. Bladder retraining
   c. Anticholinergic drugs
   d. None of the above

3. **Which of the following statements regarding physiology of urine storage is false?**
   a. Alpha-adrenergic contraction of urethral smooth muscle prevents leakage
   b. Activation of parasympathetic transmission leads to reduced detrusor pressure
   c. The urethral sphincter receives somatic innervation from the pudendal nerve
   d. Sympathetic fibers in the superior hypogastric plexus communicates with alpha- and beta-adrenergic receptors

4. **Regarding medications that can cause incontinence, which of the following pair is wrong?**
   a. Nifedipine—Inhibits bladder contraction—urinary retention
   b. Phenylephrine—Internal urethral sphincter contraction—urinary retention
   c. Tricyclic antidepressant—Inhibits bladder contraction—urinary retention
   d. Prazosin—Internal urethral sphincter contraction—urinary retention

5. **DeLancey level of support system includes all of the following, except:**
   a. Level III—lateral vaginal wall attachment to arcus tendinous fascia pelvis
   b. Level I— Mackenrodt and uterosacral ligament at the level of cervix and upper vagina
   c. Level II - lateral vaginal wall attachment to arcs tendinous rectovaginalis
   d. None of the above

6. **All of the following are the cystoscopic features of interstitial cystitis, except:**
   a. Glomerulations
   b. Mucosal leucoplakia
   c. Hydrodistension of bladder
   d. Terminal hematuria

7. **The Food and Drug Administration (FDA)-approved intravesical drug for interstitial cystitis is:**
   a. Elmiron
   b. Hydroxyzine
   c. Dimethyl sulfoxide (DMSO)
   d. Phenazopyridine

8. **The theory proposed by De Lancey about stress urinary incontinence is:**
   a. Integral theory of continence
   b. Epithelial hypersensitivity theory
   c. Hammock theory
   d. Myogenic theory

9. **The incorrect statement about stress urinary incontinence (SUI) is:**
   a. Pregnancy increases the risk of SUI
   b. White women have less prevalence than Hispanic Asian or black women
   c. Urodynamics is no longer necessary prior to treatment in pure SUI
   d. Prevalence peaks in the fifth decade

10. **What is false about OAB?**
    a. OAB is associated with urgency, frequency, and nocturia
    b. OAB is free from the micturition center
    c. OAB is associated with the absence of urinary tract infection (UTI)
    d. Multiple sclerosis, Parkinson's, and spinal cord injury are associated with OAB

11. **Management for voiding dysfunction included all, except:**
    a. Chondroitin sulfate
    b. Self-catheterization
    c. Neuromodulation
    d. Alfa- and beta-blockers

12. **Percutaneous tibial nerve stimulation (PTNS) is approved by FDA for the treatment of:**
    a. OAB
    b. SUI
    c. Voiding dysfunction
    d. Vesicovaginal fistula

13. **Complications of untreated urethral diverticulum (UD) are all, except:**
    a. Abscess
    b. Incontinence
    c. Stone formation
    d. Stricture

14. **Classical triad of UD includes:**
    a. Dysuria, postmicturition dribbling, and dyspareunia
    b. Dysuria, urgency, and frequency
    c. Dysuria, postmicturition dribbling, and urgency
    d. Dysuria, dyspareunia, and hematuria

15. **Treatment for UD includes all of the following, except:**
    a. Endoscopic deroofing
    b. Diverticulectomy
    c. Marsupialization
    d. Partial ablation of diverticulum sac

16. **Which of the following investigations is used to diagnose bladder pain syndrome (BPS)?**
    a. Urodynamic study
    b. Cystoscopy and hydrodistension
    c. Potassium sensitivity test
    d. None of the above

17. **Which of the following is the preferred sequence in the management of BPS?**
    a. Bladder/food diary, exercise > oral amitriptyline > oral cyclosporine A > intravesical DMSO > neuromodulation
    b. Bladder/food diary, exercise > oral amitriptyline > intravesical botulinum toxin A > neuromodulation > oral cyclosporine A
    c. Bladder/food diary, exercise > oral amitriptyline > neuromodulation > intravesical botulinum toxin A > oral cyclosporine A
    d. None of the above

18. **Which of the following statements is false about the Latzko procedure?**
    a. It can be performed for a small posthysterectomy fistula
    b. The vesical edge of the fistula is dissected
    c. The posterior vaginal wall becomes the posterior bladder wall
    d. Prolonged catheterization is not required following this procedure

19. **Which of the following structures is most likely to get damaged with the retropubic midurethral sling procedure?**
    a. Pudendal artery
    b. Pudendal nerve
    c. Inferior epigastric artery
    d. Inferior epigastric nerve

20. **Which of the following muscles is not used in muscle transposition during the repair of a complete perineal tear?**
    a. Gracilis muscle
    b. Sartorius muscle
    c. Gluteus muscle
    d. Bulbocavernosus muscle

21. **A 53-year-old G2P2 healthy woman attends clinic with the complaint of increased frequency of urine during nighttime with around 4–5 episodes. She also complains of a sudden urge to void for which she needs to rush to the toilet with few episodes of leakage of urine. Her urine dipstick does not show white blood cell (WBC), red blood cells (RBC), bacteria, or protein and the culture is negative. What is the most likely diagnosis of this patient?**
    a. Genuine stress incontinence
    b. Urge incontinence
    c. Overflow incontinence
    d. Neurogenic bladder

22. **In reference to question no. 21, what should be the next best treatment plan for her?**
    a. Vaginal estrogen cream
    b. Perform Kegel exercise
    c. Perform urodynamic study
    d. Maintain bladder diary and bladder training

23. What is the next plan of action after failed conservative management of urge incontinence?
    a. Oxybutynin
    b. Amitriptyline
    c. Voiding cystourethrogram
    d. Intravesical DMSO

24. How to diagnose occult SUI prior to surgery for prolapse?
    a. Ask the patient to wear a pessary and look for urinary incontinence symptoms.
    b. Urodynamic study prior to surgery
    c. Cough stress test after reduction of the prolapse
    d. All of the above

25. Which of the following statements is false in case of vaginal mesh exposure following transobturator tape (TOT) surgery for SUI?
    a. Likely to occur in the setting of vaginal injury at the time of mesh placement
    b. It can occur when the initial suburethral incision and paraurethral dissection are too close to the vaginal epithelium
    c. Watchful waiting is not an option for women who are asymptomatic with mesh exposure
    d. Topical estrogen is used in small mesh exposure

26. Which among the following is not a risk factor for incontinence?
    a. Smoking
    b. High body mass index (BMI)
    c. Functional impairment
    d. Hypertension

27. Postvoid residual (PVR) volume is increased in all, except:
    a. Neurogenic bladder   b. Recurrent UTI
    c. SUI   d. Prolapse

28. Chassar Moir technique is used for:
    a. SUI
    b. OAB
    c. Vesicovaginal fistula
    d. Urinary diversion procedures

29. Agents used as bulking agent in urethral bulking procedures include all, except:
    a. Polydimethylsiloxane silicone
    b. Calcium hydroxyapatite
    c. Pyrolytic carbon-coated beads
    d. Autologous fat

30. Urodynamic study is absolutely indicated for all of the following conditions, except:
    a. Before surgical treatment for pure SUI
    b. Before surgical treatment for urge incontinence
    c. Before surgical treatment of patients with neurological component for incontinence
    d. Before surgical treatment for frail elderly and children

ANSWERS

1. **a.** Abdominal anti-incontinence procedures attempt to correct SUI by stabilizing the anterior vaginal wall and ureterovesical junction in a retropubic location. Burch procedure, also known as retropubic urethropexy, uses the strength of the pectineal ligament (Cooper's ligament) to stabilize the anterior vaginal wall and anchor the wall to the skeletal framework of the pelvis. The Burch colposuspension uses suture to affix the paravaginal tissues to Cooper's ligament.
   [Reference: Hoffman BL, Schorge JO, Halvorson LM, Hamid CA, Corton MM, Schaffer JI (Eds). Surgeries for pelvic floor disorders. Williams Gynecology, 4th edition. New York: McGraw Hill; 2020. p. 1091]

2. **a.** For women with OAB thalassotherapy who have not responded to nonsurgical management or treatment with medication (anticholinergics), offer urodynamic investigation to determine whether detrusor overactivity (DO) is causing her symptoms. If DO is causing her symptoms, offer an invasive procedure in the form of bladder wall injection with botulinum toxin type A.
   [Reference: National Institute for Health and Care Excellence (NICE). (2018). Urinary incontinence in neurological disease: assessment and management. Clinical guideline CG148. London: NICE; 2018 [online]. Available from https://www.nice.org.uk/guidance/cg148 (Last accessed December, 2023)]

3. **b.** When the appropriate time for bladder emptying arises, sympathetic stimulation is reduced, and parasympathetic stimulation is triggered via the pontine micturition center. Specifically, neural impulses carried in the pelvic nerves stimulate acetylcholine release and lead to detrusor muscle contraction. Concurrent with detrusor stimulation, acetylcholine also stimulates muscarinic receptors in

the urethra and leads to outlet relaxation for voiding, while sympathetic outflow through the pudendal null to the urethral outlet is inhibited.
[Reference: Hoffman BL, Schorge JO, Halvorson LM, Hamid CA, Corton MM, Schaffer JI (Eds). Urinary incontinence. Williams Gynecology, 4th edition. New York: McGraw Hill; 2020. p. 545]

4. **d.** Prazosin is an alpha-adrenergic blocker which causes internal urethral sphincter relaxation, hence causing urinary leakage.
[Reference: Hoffman BL, Schorge JO, Halvorson LM, Hamid CA, Corton MM, Schaffer JI (Eds). Urinary incontinence, Williams Gynecology. 4th edition. New York: McGraw Hill; 2020. p. 523]

5. **d.** Level I support is the attachment of the cardinal and the uterosacral ligaments to the cervix and upper vagina. Level II support consists of paravaginal attachments that are contiguous with the cardinal/uterosacral complex at the ischial spine. These are the connective tissue attachments of the lateral vagina anteriorly to the arcus tendinous fascia pelvis and posteriorly to the arcus tendinous rectovaginalis. Level III support is composed of the perineal body, superficial and deep perineal muscles, and fibromuscular connective tissue. Collectively, these support the distal one-third of the vagina and introitus.
[Reference: Hoffman BL, Schorge JO, Halvorson LM, Hamid CA, Corton MM, Schaffer JI (Eds). Pelvic organ prolapse. Williams Gynecology, 4th edition. New York: McGraw Hill; 2020. p. 541]

6. **b.** The NIDDK (National Institute of Diabetes, Digestive and Kidney Disease) criteria include all, except mucosal leukoplakia.
(Reference: Berek JS. Urinary tract. Berek & Novak's Gynecology Essentials, 1st edition. Philadelphia: Wolters Kluwer; 2020)

7. **c.** All drugs are used for intravesical installation for interstitial cystitis but DMSO is the only drug which is FDA approved.
(Reference: Berek JS. Urinary tract. Berek & Novak's Gynecology Essentials, 1st edition. Philadelphia: Wolters Kluwer; 2020)

8. **c.** Hammock theory is proposed by DeLancey as support of the bladder neck and urethra to be an intact vaginal wall at the base of the bladder.

(Reference: Berek JS. Urinary tract. Berek & Novak's Gynecology Essentials, 1st edition. Philadelphia: Wolters Kluwer; 2020)

9. **b.** Race has been shown to have a variable effect on urinary incontinence by subtype. White women have a higher prevalence and incidence than Hispanic Asian and black women.
(Reference: Berek JS. Urinary tract. Berek & Novak's Gynecology Essentials, 1st edition. Philadelphia: Wolters Kluwer; 2020)

10. **b.** Any abnormality in the pathway between the micturition center and the bladder may lead to OAB.
(Reference: Berek JS. Urinary tract. Berek & Novak's Gynecology Essentials, 1st edition. Philadelphia: Wolters Kluwer; 2020)

11. **a.** Chondroitin sulfate is used for BPS and not for voiding dysfunction.
(Reference: Berek JS. Urinary tract. Berek & Novak's Gynecology Essentials, 1st edition. Philadelphia: Wolters Kluwer; 2020)

12. **a.** In 2000, FDA approved PTNS for the treatment of OAB.
(Reference: Berek JS. Urinary tract. Berek & Novak's Gynecology Essentials, 1st edition. Philadelphia: Wolters Kluwer; 2020)

13. **d.** Urinary tract infection, abscess, stone formation, incontinence, and neoplasm are the complications of untreated UD. Stricture usually follows surgery for UD.
(Reference: Archer R, Blackman J, Stott M, Barrington J. Urethral diverticulum. The Obstet Gynaecol. 2015;17:125-9)

14. **a.** The classical triad of UD includes dysuria, postmicturition dribbling, and dyspareunia.
(Reference: Archer R, Blackman J, Stott M, Barrington J. Urethral diverticulum. The Obstet Gynaecol. 2015;17:125-9)

15. **d.** *(Reference: Archer R, Blackman J, Stott M, Barrington J. Urethral diverticulum. The Obstet Gynaecolo. 2015;17:125-9)*

16. **d.** Bladder pain syndrome is a chronic pain syndrome and the principles of management of chronic pain should be used in the initial assessment of the condition. BPS is a diagnosis of exclusion, and other conditions should be excluded. Bladder biopsies

and hydrodistension are not recommended for the diagnosis of BPS. Cystoscopy does not confirm or exclude the diagnosis of BPS but is required to exclude other conditions that mimic BPS. Potassium sensitivity test, urodynamic assessment, and urinary biomarkers should not be used to diagnose BPS.
[Reference: Management of Bladder Pain Syndrome: Green-top Guideline No. 70. BJOG. 2017. 124(2):e46-e72]

17. **b.**
- *First-line treatment:* Conservative—analgesia, stress relief, dietary modification, exercise, physical therapy, and support groups
- *Second-line treatment:* Oral—cimetidine and amitriptyline. If it fails, refer to the pain team and/or clinical psychologist.
- *Third-line treatment:* Intravesical—DMSO, heparin, botulinum toxin A, chondroitin sulfate, lidocaine, and hyaluronic acid
- *Fourth-line treatment:* Neuromodulation and oral cyclosporine

Fifth-line treatment: Cystoscopy and hydrodistension
[Reference: Management of Bladder Pain Syndrome: Green-top Guideline No. 70. BJOG. 2017. 124(2):e46-e72]

18. **b.** Typically simple, small fistulas near the vaginal apex (e.g., posthysterectomy) can be repaired using the Latzko technique, while larger, more complex fistulas (e.g., fistula from obstructed labor) may require more extensive dissection. In the Latzko technique of partial colpocleisis, the bladder is mobilized circumferentially from the surrounding tissue, but the fistula tract is not excised as it is imbricated into the bladder cavity with closure of the fistula.
(Reference: Handa VL, Van Le L. Vesicovaginal and rectovaginal fistula. Te Linde's Operative Gynecology. Philadelphia: Wolters Kluwer; 2019. p. 947)

19. **c.**

20. **d.** *(Reference: Handa VL, Van Le L. Vesicovaginal and rectovaginal fistula. Te Linde's Operative Gynecology ebook, 12th edition. Philadelphia: Wolters Kluwer; 2019. p. 963)*

21. **b.** *[Reference: Nice Guidance-Urinary incontinence and pelvic organ prolapse in women: management: © NICE (2019) Urinary incontinence and pelvic organ prolapse in women: management. BJU Int. 2019;123(5):777-803]*

22. **d.** *[Reference: Nice Guidance-Urinary incontinence and pelvic organ prolapse in women: management: © NICE (2019) Urinary incontinence and pelvic organ prolapse in women: management. BJU Int. 2019;123(5):777-803]*

23. **a.** For women with overactive bladder that has not responded to non-surgical

   For women with overactive bladder that has not responded to non-surgical management or treatment with medicine and who wish to discuss further treatment options:
   1. Offer urodynamic investigation to determine whether detrusor overactivity is causing her overactive bladder symptoms and
   2. If detrusor overactivity is causing her overactive bladder symptoms, offer an invasive procedure in line with the recommendation on bladder wall injection in the section on botulinum toxin type A and the recommendation in the section on urinary diversion

[Reference: Nice Guidance-Urinary incontinence and pelvic organ prolapse in women: management: © NICE (2019) Urinary incontinence and pelvic organ prolapse in women: management. BJU Int. 2019;123(5):777-803]

24. **d.** Occult SUI is a phenomenon in which pelvic organ prolapse obstructs the urethra, thus making the presence of underlying SUI. This phenomenon is thought to unmask SUI after prolapse surgery. Surgery for SUI can be performed at the time of surgery for prolapse. There are three different approaches to considering and managing occult SUI, and the approach taken may vary according to the preferences and concerns of an individual patient. This can be done with prolapse reduction during a cough stress test or urodynamic evaluation or by having the patient wear a pessary.
(Reference: Handa VL, Van Le L. Mid urethral sling and surgery for stress urinary incontinence. Te Linde's Operative Gynecology ebook, 12th edition. Philadelphia: Wolters Kluwer; 2019. p. 913)

25. **c.** Treatment options include topical vaginal estrogen, trimming of mesh in office, surgical management, and watchful waiting. Some small exposures may

be asymptomatic. Watchful waiting is appropriate following full disclosure of the exposure to the patient and in the absence of infection, dyspareunia, or bothersome bleeding.
(Reference: Handa VL, Van Le L. Mid urethral sling and surgery for stress urinary incontinence. Te Linde's Operative Gynecology ebook, 12th edition. Philadelphia: Wolters Kluwer; 2019. p. 897)

26. **d.** *[Reference: Hoffman BL, Schorge JO, Halvorson LM, Hamid CA, Corton MM, Schaffer JI (Eds). Urinary incontinence, Williams Gynecology, 4th edition. New York: McGraw Hill; 2020. p. 513]*

27. **c.** PVR is normal or reduced in women with SUI.
[Reference: Hoffman BL, Schorge JO, Halvorson LM, Hamid CA, Corton MM, Schaffer JI (Eds). Urinary incontinence. Williams Gynecology, 4th edition. New York: McGraw Hill; 2020. p. 524]

28. **c.**

29. **d.** Autologous fat is not used as it is no better than saline placebo.
(Reference: Handa VL, Van Le L. Mid urethral sling and surgery for stress urinary incontinence. Te Linde's Operative Gynecology ebook, 12th edition. Philadelphia: Wolters Kluwer; 2019. p. 909)

30. **a.** According to NICE (National Institute for Health and Care Excellence) guidelines, urodynamic testing is not recommended if pure SUI has been diagnosed based on history and examination unless there is a suggestion of voiding dysfunction, anterior compartment prolapse, or previous failed surgical management.
[Reference: National Institute for Health and Care Excellence (NICE). Urinary incontinence in neurological disease: assessment and management. Clinical guideline CG148. London: NICE; 2018. [online] Available from https://www.nice.org.uk/guidance/cg148 (Last accessed December, 2023)]

Chapter 90

Contraception

Suchi Jain, Ruchika Garg

QUESTIONS

1. According to the National Family Health Survey 5 (NFHS-5), the total unmet need for contraception in India is almost (15–49 years):
   a. 4.3
   b. 9.4
   c. 15.3
   d. 50.2

2. According to NFHS-5, the most common method for family planning used in India is:
   a. Condom
   b. Oral pills
   c. Intrauterine contraceptive device (IUCD)
   d. Female sterilization

3. In India, the unmet need of family planning in the age group of 15–19 years (adolescents) is almost:
   a. 27%
   b. 40%
   c. 13%
   d. 9.3%

4. Currently, the replacement level fertility rate in India is:
   a. 2.17 births per woman
   b. 2.15 births per woman
   c. 2.13 births per woman
   d. 2.19 births per woman

5. Which of the following countries has the lowest total fertility rate (TFR)?
   a. Japan
   b. South Korea
   c. United Kingdom
   d. Australia

6. Which of the following states in India has the highest TFR?
   a. Goa
   b. Bihar
   c. Uttar Pradesh
   d. Arunachal Pradesh

7. Which of the following statements is false about levonorgestrel-releasing intrauterine system (LNG-IUS) Jaydess/Skyla?
   a. It can be used in nulliparous
   b. It has 13.5 mg LNG released @ 6–10 microgram/day
   c. It is licensed for a use of 5–7 years
   d. It has a silver ring

8. Which of the following statements is false about GyneFix intrauterine implant?
   a. It is nonhormonal
   b. Its main advantage is flexibility
   c. It acts by reducing sperm motility and inhibiting implantation
   d. None of the above

9. The lowest ectopic pregnancy rate is seen with:
   a. CuT 200
   b. Mirena
   c. Progestasert
   d. CuT 380A

10. Which of the following statements is false about Zoely combined oral contraceptive pill (COCP)?
    a. It has fourth-generation progesterone as nomegestrol acetate (NOMAC) and ethinyl estradiol as hemihydrate
    b. It is taken as a 24/4 regimen
    c. Withdrawal bleeding is lesser or absent
    d. It has lesser contraceptive efficacy than OCPs having drospirenone and ethinylestradiol

11. Which of the following is an ultralow dose oral contraceptive pill (OCP)?
    a. Femilon
    b. Minesse
    c. Yasmin
    d. Ovral L

12. Which of the following OCPs contains estradiol valerate?
    a. Minesse
    b. Qlaira
    c. Zoely
    d. Loette

13. Which of the following statements is not true about combination injectable contraceptive (CIC)?
    a. Injection Cyclofem has DMPA (depot medroxyprogesterone acetate) 25 mg with estradiol cypionate 5 mg
    b. It is taken at 3 months interval
    c. It is given within 5 days of menses
    d. Mesigyna is also a CIC

14. Which of the following statements is not true about Evra patch?
    a. It contains segesterone acetate + ethinyl estradiol
    b. It is applied weekly for 3 weeks and then 1 week off
    c. Extended regimen can be used for fewer episodes of withdrawal bleeding
    d. None of the above

15. Which of the following is false about postpartum intrauterine contraceptive device (PPIUCD) insertion?
    a. PPIUCD should not be inserted between 48 hours and 6 weeks after birth
    b. Postplacental insertion means within 30 minutes of placental delivery
    c. Manual correction of the angle between the uterus and vagina is an important step
    d. It can be done within 48 hours of delivery

16. Which of the following is a type of "Twelve-hour progestogen-only pill (POP)?"
    a. Norgeston   b. Cerazette
    c. Femulen   d. Noriday

17. Which of the following is not a progesterone-only contraceptive?
    a. Injection DMPA
    b. Injection NET-EN (norethisterone enanthate)
    c. Injection Mesigyna
    d. Norplant

18. Which of the following is an example of extended-use OCP?
    a. Seasonale
    b. Lybrel
    c. Both a and b
    d. None of the above

19. The extended-use OCP Seasonale contains:
    a. 84 days active pills + 7 days inactive pills
    b. 84 days active pills + 7 days low-dose estrogen pills
    c. Full-year active pills with no inactive pills
    d. None of the above

20. Which of the following does not belong to the World Health Organization (WHO) category 4 for OCP?
    a. Valvular heart disease with pulmonary hypertension
    b. Breastfeeding at 4 weeks postpartum
    c. Epilepsy
    d. Liver tumors

21. An example of biodegradable implant contraception is:
    a. Capronor
    b. Jadelle
    c. Norethindrone Annuelle
    d. Both a and c

22. Which of the following statements is true about Mirena?
    a. The chance of ectopic pregnancy is very low
    b. Nulliparity is not a contraindication
    c. It is comparable to endometrial ablation in heavy menstrual bleeding (HMB)
    d. All of the above

23. Which of the following statements is not true about centchroman?
    a. It is a selective estrogen receptor modulator (SERM)
    b. It mainly acts by inhibiting embryonic implantation
    c. It inhibits ovulation
    d. It can be given to lactating women

24. Which of the following statements is false about OCP?
    a. Failure rate is low: 0.1 per hundred woman-years (HWY) use
    b. Zoely and Qlaira have enzyme-inducing effects and so cannot be used with antibiotics
    c. It protects against ovarian, endometrial, and colorectal cancer
    d. It should be avoided if there is history of breast cancer

25. Which of the following is a method of transcervical sterilization?
    a. Adiana   b. Quinacrine pellet
    c. Essure   d. All of the above

26. Which of the following statements is true about Essure?
    a. It is a method of transcervical sterilization done hysteroscopically
    b. Its success rate is similar to surgical sterilization
    c. Tubes are blocked permanently
    d. All of the above

27. Which of the following statements is false about Fibroplant?
    a. It is LNG-IUS
    b. It should not be used as hormone replacement therapy (HRT) for postmenopausal women
    c. It is smaller than Mirena
    d. It can be used in perimenopausal women

28. The failure rate of OCPs in the first year of correct and consistent use is:
    a. 0.5%   b. 1.5%
    c. 0.3%   d. 1.0%

29. What is the age range for intrauterine device (IUD) insertion?
    a. 16–30 years
    b. 21–35 years
    c. 25–45 years
    d. No age limit

30. Which is the most commonly used method of contraception in India?
    a. Oral pills
    b. CuT
    c. Female sterilization
    d. Condom

31. According to available evidence, the effectiveness of female sterilization in first year use is:
    a. 1.5 pregnancy per 100 women
    b. 0.5 pregnancy per 100 women
    c. 1.1 pregnancy per 100 women
    d. None of the above

32. Which of the following statements is not true about Today sponge?
    a. It is a form of barrier contraception
    b. Before insertion, it should be soaked in water
    c. It should be inserted up to 24 hours before coitus
    d. It should be removed soon after coitus is over

33. Which of the following is a female barrier contraceptive?
    a. Vaginal contraceptive film (VCF)
    b. Dutch cap
    c. Today sponge
    d. All of the above

34. Which of the following is unmedicated IUCD?
    a. Nova T   b. Mahua ring
    c. Lippes loop   d. CuT 380A
    e. Both b and c

35. In which of the following methods of sterilization is the segment of tubal loop not excised?
    a. Pomeroy's technique
    b. Modified Pomeroy's technique
    c. Madlener's technique
    d. Kroener's technique

36. Which of the following methods of sterilization has the lowest failure rate?
    a. Laparoscopic sterilization
    b. Pomeroy's technique
    c. Irving technique
    d. Madlener's technique

37. Which of the following is not a method of emergency contraceptive?
    a. LNG 1.5 mg single dose within 72 hours of coitus
    b. Two tablets Ovral L taken within 72 hours
    c. Ulipristal 30 mg within 5 days
    d. None of the above

38. Which of the following is an ideal method of injectable contraceptive?
    a. Injection Antara 150 mg 3 monthly
    b. Injection NET-EN 200 mg 2 monthly
    c. Depo-subQ provera-104 mg given subcutaneously
    d. All of the above

39. Which of the following IUCD can be used as HRT in postmenopausal women?
    a. Mirena   b. Uniplant
    c. Fibroplant   d. None of the above

40. Which of the following can be used to assess the efficacy of contraception?
    a. Life table analysis
    b. Pearl index
    c. Fertility awareness method
    d. Both a and b

ANSWERS

1. b.
2. d.
3. a.
4. c.
5. b.
6. b.
7. c. [Reference: Malhotra N, Malhotra J. Jeffcoate's Principles of Gynaecology, 9th edition. New Delhi:

8. d. [Reference: Malhotra N, Malhotra J. Jeffcoate's Principles of Gynaecology, 9th edition. New Delhi: Jaypee Brothers Medical Publishers (P) Ltd; 2018. p. 982]

8. d. [Reference: Malhotra N, Malhotra J. Jeffcoate's Principles of Gynaecology, 9th edition. New Delhi: Jaypee Brothers Medical Publishers (P) Ltd; 2018. p. 985]

9. b. [Reference: Malhotra N, Malhotra J. Jeffcoate's Principles of Gynaecology, 9th edition. New Delhi: Jaypee Brothers Medical Publishers (P) Ltd; 2018. p. 993]

10. d. [Reference: Malhotra N, Malhotra J. Jeffcoate's Principles of Gynaecology, 9th edition. New Delhi: Jaypee Brothers Medical Publishers (P) Ltd; 2018. p. 996]

11. b. [Reference: Malhotra N, Malhotra J. Jeffcoate's Principles of Gynaecology, 9th edition. New Delhi: Jaypee Brothers Medical Publishers (P) Ltd; 2018. p. 996]

12. b. [Reference: Malhotra N, Malhotra J. Jeffcoate's Principles of Gynaecology, 9th edition. New Delhi: Jaypee Brothers Medical Publishers (P) Ltd; 2018. p. 996]

13. b. [Reference: Konar H. DC Dutta's Textbook of Gynecology, 7th edition. New Delhi: Jaypee Brothers Medical Publishers (P) Ltd; 2016. p. 415]

14. a. [Reference: Malhotra N, Malhotra J. Jeffcoate's Principles of Gynaecology, 9th edition. New Delhi: Jaypee Brothers Medical Publishers (P) Ltd; 2018. p. 997]

15. b. [Reference: Malhotra N, Malhotra J. Jeffcoate's Principles of Gynaecology, 9th edition. New Delhi: Jaypee Brothers Medical Publishers (P) Ltd; 2018. p. 1020]

16. b. [Reference: Malhotra N, Malhotra J. Jeffcoate's Principles of Gynaecology, 9th edition. New Delhi: Jaypee Brothers Medical Publishers (P) Ltd; 2018. p. 1006]

17. c. [Reference: Konar H. DC Dutta's Textbook of Gynecology, 7th edition. New Delhi: Jaypee Brothers Medical Publishers (P) Ltd; 2016. p. 415]

18. c. [Reference: Malhotra N, Malhotra J. Jeffcoate's Principles of Gynaecology, 9th edition. New Delhi: Jaypee Brothers Medical Publishers (P) Ltd; 2018. p. 1001]

19. a. [Reference: Malhotra N, Malhotra J. Jeffcoate's Principles of Gynaecology, 9th edition. New Delhi: Jaypee Brothers Medical Publishers (P) Ltd; 2018. p. 1001]

20. c. [Reference: Malhotra N, Malhotra J. Jeffcoate's Principles of Gynaecology, 9th edition. New Delhi: Jaypee Brothers Medical Publishers (P) Ltd; 2018. p. 1000]

21. d. [Reference: Malhotra N, Malhotra J. Jeffcoate's Principles of Gynaecology, 9th edition. New Delhi: Jaypee Brothers Medical Publishers (P) Ltd; 2018. p. 1010]

22. d. [Reference: Malhotra N, Malhotra J. Jeffcoate's Principles of Gynaecology, 9th edition. New Delhi: Jaypee Brothers Medical Publishers (P) Ltd; 2018. p. 1013]

23. c. [Reference: Malhotra N, Malhotra J. Jeffcoate's Principles of Gynaecology, 9th edition. New Delhi: Jaypee Brothers Medical Publishers (P) Ltd; 2018. p. 1017]

24. b. (Reference: Page 1006, Jeffcoat, 9th edition page 401, DCD, Gynae, 7th edition)

25. d. [Reference: Konar H (Ed). DC Dutta's Textbook of Gynecology, 7th edition. New Delhi: Jaypee Brothers Medical Publishers (P) Ltd; 2016. p. 416]

26. d. [Reference: Konar H. DC Dutta's Textbook of Gynecology, 7th edition. New Delhi: Jaypee Brothers Medical Publishers (P) Ltd; 2016. p. 416.

27. b. [Reference: Konar H. DC Dutta's Textbook of Gynecology, 7th edition. New Delhi: Jaypee Brothers Medical Publishers (P) Ltd; 2016. p. 416]

28. c. [Reference: UNFPA. (2013) Certificate Course on Contraception in Clinical Practice. P. 18. (online) Available from: https://india.unfpa.org/en/publications/certificate-course-contraception-clinical-practice?page=18 (Last accessed December, 2023).

Certificate Course on Contraception in Clinical Practice, UNFPA (United Nations Population Fund)]

29. d. [Reference: Certificate Course on Contraception in Clinical Practice, UNFPA (United Nations Population Fund)]

30. c. [Reference: Certificate Course on Contraception in Clinical Practice, UNFPA (United Nations Population Fund)]

31. **b.** (UNFPA, 22)

32. **d.** *[Reference: Malhotra N, Malhotra J. Jeffcoate's Principles of Gynaecology, 9th edition. New Delhi: Jaypee Brothers Medical Publishers (P) Ltd; 2018. p. 977]*

33. **d.** *[Reference: Malhotra N, Malhotra J. Jeffcoate's Principles of Gynaecology, 9th edition. New Delhi: Jaypee Brothers Medical Publishers (P) Ltd; 2018. p. 977]*

34. **e.** *[Reference: Malhotra N, Malhotra J. Jeffcoate's Principles of Gynaecology, 9th edition. New Delhi: Jaypee Brothers Medical Publishers (P) Ltd; 2018. p. 981]*

35. **c.** *[Reference: Konar H. DC Dutta's Textbook of Gynecology, 7th edition. New Delhi: Jaypee Brothers Medical Publishers (P) Ltd; 2016. p. 408]*

36. **b.** *[Reference: Konar H. DC Dutta's Textbook of Gynecology, 7th edition. New Delhi: Jaypee Brothers Medical Publishers (P) Ltd; 2016. p. 411]*

37. **b.** *[Reference: Konar H. DC Dutta's Textbook of Gynecology, 7th edition. New Delhi: Jaypee Brothers Medical Publishers (P) Ltd; 2016. p. 404]*

38. **d.** *[Reference: Konar H. DC Dutta's Textbook of Gynecology, 7th edition. New Delhi: Jaypee Brothers Medical Publishers (P) Ltd; 2016. p. 403]*

39. **c.** *[Reference: Konar H. DC Dutta's Textbook of Gynecology, 7th edition. New Delhi: Jaypee Brothers Medical Publishers (P) Ltd; 2016. p. 416]*

40. **d.** *[Reference: Malhotra N, Malhotra J. Jeffcoate's Principles of Gynaecology, 9th edition. New Delhi: Jaypee Brothers Medical Publishers (P) Ltd; 2018. p. 966]*

Chapter 91: Vulvodynia

Richa Singh, Shaifali Singh

QUESTIONS

1. Which of the following subtypes of vulvodynia primarily affects the vestibular glands and is characterized by severe pain upon touch or pressure?
   a. Provoked vestibulodynia (PVD)
   b. Generalized vulvodynia
   c. Vulvar atrophy
   d. Neurological vulvodynia

2. Which part of the female genitalia is primarily affected by vulvodynia?
   a. Vagina
   b. Clitoris
   c. Labia
   d. Cervix

3. What is the most common symptom of vulvodynia?
   a. Vaginal discharge
   b. Itching
   c. Burning or stinging pain
   d. Swelling

4. Vulvodynia is typically diagnosed through:
   a. Blood tests
   b. Pap smear
   c. Physical examination
   d. X-rays

5. Which of the following is NOT a subtype of vulvodynia?
   a. PVD
   b. Generalized vulvodynia
   c. Vaginismus
   d. Clitorodynia

6. Which of the following is a known risk factor for vulvodynia?
   a. Frequent sexual intercourse
   b. Using scented hygiene products
   c. Smoking
   d. Regular exercise

7. How is PVD characterized?
   a. Pain during sexual intercourse
   b. Constant pain in the vulva
   c. Pain during urination
   d. Itching and redness

8. Which type of healthcare provider is typically involved in the diagnosis and treatment of vulvodynia?
   a. Cardiologist
   b. Gynecologist
   c. Dentist
   d. Dermatologist

9. Treatment for vulvodynia may include:
   a. Antibiotics
   b. Hormone therapy
   c. Physical therapy
   d. All of the above

10. Which of the following may exacerbate symptoms of vulvodynia?
    a. Wearing loose-fitting clothing
    b. Using water-based lubricants
    c. Stress and anxiety
    d. Avoiding spicy foods

11. Vulvodynia can lead to difficulties in:
    a. Digestion
    b. Walking
    c. Sexual activity
    d. Vision

12. What percentage of women are estimated to be affected by vulvodynia?
    a. <1%
    b. Approximately 5%
    c. Around 20%
    d. >50%

13. Which of the following is a potential complication of untreated vulvodynia?
    a. Skin cancer
    b. Chronic pelvic pain
    c. Migraines
    d. Hearing loss

14. Which age group is most commonly affected by vulvodynia?
    a. Adolescents
    b. Young adults
    c. Middle-aged women
    d. Elderly women

15. What is the main goal of treatment for vulvodynia?
    a. Immediate pain relief
    b. Permanent cure
    c. Symptom management and improved quality of life
    d. Prevention of other gynecological conditions

16. Which of the following is NOT a recommended self-care measure for vulvodynia?
    a. Using mild, fragrance-free soap
    b. Avoiding tight-fitting clothing
    c. Frequent use of scented bath products
    d. Applying cool compresses

17. Vulvodynia is a psychological disorder.
    a. True
    b. False

18. What is the typical duration of pain required for the diagnosis of vulvodynia?
    a. Less than 1 week
    b. At least 1 month
    c. At least 1 year
    d. There is no specific duration requirement

19. What percentage of women with vulvodynia experience pain during sexual intercourse?
    a. None
    b. Approximately 10%
    c. About 50%
    d. All of them

20. Which of the following can be used to help manage pain in vulvodynia?
    a. Hot baths
    b. Ice packs
    c. Electrical stimulation
    d. All of the above

21. Which neurotransmitter is thought to play a role in the pain associated with vulvodynia?
    a. Dopamine
    b. Serotonin
    c. Acetylcholine
    d. Norepinephrine

22. What is the primary purpose of the Q-tip test in diagnosing vulvodynia?
    a. To measure vaginal pH
    b. To detect signs of infection
    c. To identify painful areas in the vulvar vestibule
    d. To assess cervical position

23. Which of the following is a common trigger for vulvodynia symptoms?
    a. Fresh air
    b. Sunlight
    c. Emotional stress
    d. Drinking water

24. How is generalized vulvodynia different from PVD?
    a. It affects only the inner labia
    b. It causes pain throughout the entire vulvar area
    c. It is not associated with sexual activity
    d. It is caused by a bacterial infection

25. Vulvodynia can be completely cured in all cases.
    a. True
    b. False

26. Which type of vulvodynia primarily affects postmenopausal women?
    a. Essential vulvodynia
    b. Secondary vulvodynia
    c. Neurological vulvodynia
    d. Menopausal vestibulodynia

27. The primary symptom of vulvodynia is:
    a. Vaginal dryness
    b. Muscle weakness
    c. Chronic vulvar pain
    d. Frequent urination

28. What is the primary purpose of topical medications in treating vulvodynia?
    a. To cure the condition
    b. To provide temporary pain relief
    c. To prevent bacterial infections
    d. To promote fertility

29. Vulvodynia can impact a woman's ability to become pregnant.
    a. True
    b. False

30. What is the first-line treatment for vulvodynia?
    a. Surgery
    b. Psychotherapy
    c. Topical anesthetics
    d. Conservative measures and physical therapy

ANSWERS

1. a.	2. c.	3. c.	4. c.
5. c.	6. b.	7. a.	8. b.
9. d.	10. c.	11. c.	12. b.
13. b.	14. c.	15. c.	16. c.
17. b.	18. d.	19. d.	20. d.
21. d.	22. c.	23. c.	24. b.
25. b.	26. d.	27. c.	28. b.
29. a.	30. d.		

REFERENCES

1. Jones HA, Rock JM (Eds). Vulvovaginal disease: diagnosis and management. Te Linde's Operative Gynecology, 11th edition. Philadelphia: Lippincott Williams and Wilkins; 2015.
2. Hoffman BL, Schorge JO, Halvorson LM, Hamid CA, Corton MM, Joseph I. Schaffer JI. Williams Gynecology, 4th edition. New York: McGraw-Hill; 2021.
3. Fritz MA, Speroff L. Clinical Gynecologic Endocrinology and Infertility, 8th edition. Philadelphia: Lippincott Williams and Wilkins; 2010.
4. Konar H, Dutta DC. Dutta's Textbook of Obstetrics, 7th edition. New Delhi: Jaypee Brothers Medical Publishers (P) Ltd; 2013.
5. Malhotra N, Malhotra J, Saxena R, Bora NM. Jeffcoate's Principles of Gynaecology, 9th edition. New Delhi: Jaypee Brothers Medical Publishers (P) Ltd; 2019.
6. Padubidri VG, Daftary SN, Kumar S. Shaw's Textbook of Gynaecology, 18th edition. Amsterdam: Elsevier; 2023.

Chapter 92: Contraception Miscellaneous

Vidya Thobbi

QUESTIONS

1. Which of the following statements accurately describes population dynamics?
   a. It refers to the study of population interactions with their environment
   b. It focuses solely on the study of animal populations
   c. It refers to the study of population genetics
   d. It focuses solely on the study of human populations

2. Which of the following methods is considered a form of hormonal contraception?
   a. Condoms
   b. Intrauterine devices (IUDs)
   c. Birth control pills
   d. Tubal ligation

3. A 23-year-old woman comes to clinic with history of unprotected intercourse 2 days ago. Which of the following will you prescribe as a single-dose contraception?
   a. Levonorgestrel 0.75 mg
   b. Ethinyl estradiol 50 µg
   c. Levonorgestrel 1.5 mg
   d. Norgestrel 0.25 mg

4. Which of the following contraceptive methods has the highest effectiveness rate in preventing pregnancy?
   a. Condoms
   b. Birth control pills
   c. Intrauterine devices (IUDs)
   d. Diaphragms

5. A 40-year-old male patient underwent a vasectomy. What is the failure rate of this procedure?
   a. 0.5%
   b. 0.15%
   c. 3%
   d. 1%

6. What is the dose of ulipristal for emergency contraception?
   a. 60 µg
   b. 3 mg
   c. 30 mg
   d. 30 µg

7. A nulliparous woman has been using "TODAY SPONGE" as a contraceptive. What does it contain?
   a. Nonoxynol-9
   b. Octoxynol-8
   c. Menfegol
   d. Tergitol

8. Identify the contraceptive shown in the given image.
   a. Male condoms
   b. Female condom
   c. Diaphragm
   d. Cervical cap

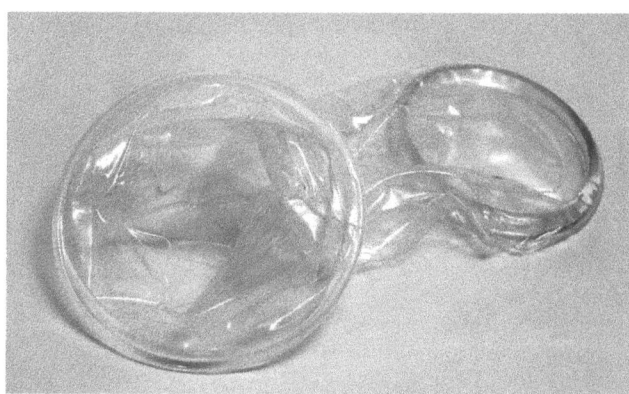

9. Which of the following is the most effective reversible method of contraception?
   a. Combined pill
   b. Norplant
   c. Mini pill
   d. Mirena

10. Which of the following methods of contraception is reversible for men?
    a. Vasectomy
    b. SUPPRELIN® LA implant
    c. Intrauterine device (IUD)
    d. Birth control pills

11. Which of the following is *not* the mechanism of action of the device given in the image below?
    a. Chronic endometrial infection
    b. Increase the motility of tubes
    c. Enzymatic changes to prevent implantation
    d. Formation of cervical mucous plug

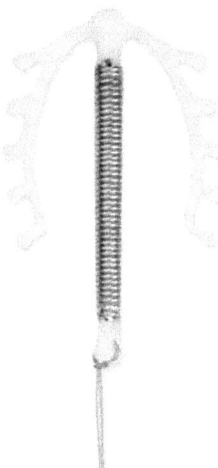

12. You are inserting Nova-T in a patient for spacing of births. This device contains:
    a. Copper and silver
    b. Copper and aluminum
    c. Only copper
    d. Copper and selenium

13. A young woman who is using a cervical diaphragm asks for an alternative contraception. You suggest a recently launched contraceptive Phexxi®. What is its composition?
    a. Lactic acid, citric acid, and potassium bitartrate
    b. Ascorbic acid, citric acid, and calcium bitartrate
    c. Lactic acid, ascorbic acid, and potassium bitartrate
    d. Ascorbic acid, lactic acid, and calcium bitartrate

14. Which of the following is *not* an advantage of norgestimate oral contraceptive pills (OCPs)?
    a. Reduces venous thrombosis
    b. Less metabolic side effects
    c. Reduces acne and hirsutism
    d. Lesser cardiovascular risk

15. A patient has come to your clinic for contraceptive advice, as she has a family history of breast cancer. You suggest oral contraceptive to her. What is the initial dose of this drug?
    a. 30 mg on day 1 of cycle
    b. 60 mg on day 1 of cycle
    c. 60 mg on day 14 of cycle
    d. 30 mg on day 14 of cycle

16. You are prescribing nonoxynol-9 jelly to a woman using a cervical diaphragm for contraception. What is the mechanism of action?
    a. Acrosomal enzyme inhibition
    b. Cervical enzyme alteration
    c. Glucose uptake inhibition by sperms
    d. Disruption of cell membrane

17. Fimbriectomy is also known as:
    a. Pomeroy's technique
    b. Uchida's procedure
    c. Kroener's procedure
    d. Irving's procedure

18. Intrauterine contraceptive device (IUCD) insertion is being considered in a multiparous woman who wants long-term contraception. This method of contraception is absolutely contraindication in all of the following, *except:*
    a. Uterine leiomyomas
    b. Suspected pregnancy
    c. HIV infection
    d. Pelvic inflammatory disease

ANSWERS

1. **a.** It refers to the study of population interactions with their environment.
2. **c.** Birth control
3. **c.** Levonorgestrel 1.5 mg
4. **c.** Intrauterine devices (IUDs)
5. **b.** 0.15%
6. **c.** 30 mg
7. **a.** Nonoxynol-9
8. **b.** Female condom
9. **b.** Norplant
10. **b.** SUPPRELIN® LA implant
11. **d.** Formation of cervical mucous plug
12. **a.** Copper and silver
13. **a.** Lactic acid, citric acid, and potassium bitartrate
14. **a.** Reduces venous thrombosis
15. **a.** 30 mg on day 1 of cycle
16. **d.** Disruption of cell membrane
17. **c.** Kroener's procedure
18. **c.** HIV infection

Chapter 93: Premature Ovarian Insufficiency

Ritu Sharma, Pinky Mishra

QUESTIONS

1. **Amenorrhea with loss of ovarian activity before the age of 40 years is termed as:**
   a. Low ovarian reserve
   b. Ovarian failure
   c. Premature ovarian insufficiency (POI)
   d. Early menopause

2. **The most common symptom of premature ovarian insufficiency in adolescents is:**
   a. Vaginal dryness
   b. Hot flushes
   c. Amenorrhea/oligomenorrhea
   d. Urogenital symptoms

3. **Incidence of premature ovarian insufficiency in amenorrheic women is:**
   a. 2–10%
   b. 15–20%
   c. 0.05–1%
   d. 20–30%

4. **The most common cause of premature ovarian insufficiency is:**
   a. Genetic abnormalities
   b. Autoimmune disorders
   c. Chemoradiation
   d. Idiopathic

5. **Baseline investigation to diagnose premature ovarian insufficiency are:**
   a. Follicle-stimulating hormone (FSH), estradiol, thyroid-stimulating hormone (TSH), and prolactin
   b. FSH, antral follicle count, anti-müllerian hormone (AMH), and estradiol
   c. AMH, inhibin B, FSH, and TSH
   d. Serial estradiol levels, AMH, inhibin B, and FSH

6. **Diagnosis of premature ovarian insufficiency is made when:**
   a. Two reports of serum follicle-stimulating hormone levels >25 IU/L at 4 weeks interval
   b. Single report of serum FSH levels >40 mIU/mL
   c. Two reports of serum FSH levels >25 mIU/mL at 6 weeks interval
   d. Two reports of serum FSH levels >40 mIU/L at 4 weeks interval

7. **Upon diagnosis of premature ovarian insufficiency, following investigations are recommended:**
   a. Fragile X premutations
   b. Screening for anti-thyroid peroxidase (TPO) antibodies and adrenocortical antibodies
   c. Karyotyping
   d. All of the above

8. **Diagnostic marker for autoimmune premature ovarian insufficiency is:**
   a. 21-OH antibodies/adrenal cortex autoantibody (ACA)
   b. Anti-thyroid peroxidase antibodies
   c. Antinuclear antibody (ANA)
   d. Rheumatoid arthritis (RA) factor

9. **Life expectancy in untreated premature ovarian insufficiency is reduced due to:**
   a. Osteoporosis
   b. Cardiovascular disease
   c. Endocrinopathies
   d. None of the above

10. **Incorrect statement about premature ovarian insufficiency in adolescent population is:**
    a. POI is associated with increased risk of cardiovascular mortality
    b. Risk of cardiovascular adverse effects are further potentiated by hormone therapy
    c. No standard screening regimen is available for cardiovascular risk assessment
    d. Annual blood pressure (BP) and weight monitoring; and 5 yearly lipid profile is warranted

11. The primary goal of management in premature ovarian insufficiency is to:
    a. Restore normal ovarian function
    b. Prevent complications associated with estrogen deficiency
    c. Achieve pregnancy through assisted reproductive technologies
    d. Eliminate symptoms of menopause

12. Ms X was diagnosed with premature ovarian insufficiency at the age of 16 years. Her breast development is in Tanner stage II. Hormone therapy in the girl would include:
    a. Sequential estrogen-progesterone therapy
    b. Slow incremental dose of estrogen followed by progesterone
    c. Slow incremental dose of progesterone followed by estrogen
    d. Continuous estrogen-progesterone therapy

13. Find the incorrect statement:
    a. Bisphosphonates should not be used for a prolonged period in adolescent premature ovarian insufficiency with low bone mineral density (BMD)
    b. BMD in adolescent POI should be done at diagnosis; if low initially and estrogen therapy initiated, repeated 5 yearly
    c. BMD in adolescent POI should be done at diagnosis, if normal initially and estrogen therapy initiated, it should be repeated 5 yearly
    d. Hormone therapy is the preferred choice for low bone mass in POI

14. What is the first-line therapy for the low bone mass in women with premature ovarian insufficiency?
    a. Bisphosphonates
    b. Calcium
    c. Vitamin D_3
    d. Hormone therapy (HT)

15. Chance of spontaneous conception despite diagnosis of premature ovarian insufficiency is:
    a. 1–2%
    b. 5–10%
    c. 10–15%
    d. 15–20%

16. Spontaneous pregnancies in idiopathic premature ovarian insufficiency are at:
    a. Increased risk of obstetric complications
    b. Increased risk of neonatal complications
    c. Fetomaternal risk is comparable with general population
    d. Increased risk of congenital anomalies in fetus

17. A woman with premature ovarian insufficiency is keen on conception; which of the following option is preferred for enhancing her fertility:
    a. Ovulation induction
    b. Intrauterine insemination (IUI)
    c. In vitro fertilization (IVF)
    d. Oocyte donation

18. Women who undergo cancer treatment and are at risk of premature ovarian insufficiency may consider:
    a. Oocyte/ovarian cryopreservation (egg freezing) before treatment
    b. Hormone replacement therapy after treatment
    c. In vitro fertilization using donor eggs
    d. All of the above

19. Pregnancies in following women with premature ovarian insufficiency who survived cancer are at high risk, *except*:
    a. Cancer survivors who have received anthracycline-based chemotherapy
    b. Cancer survivors who have received nonanthracycline-based chemotherapy
    c. Cancer survivors who have received alkylating agent-based chemotherapy
    d. Cancer survivors who have received radiation to uterus

20. The risk of developing premature ovarian insufficiency due to cancer treatment is influenced by:
    a. The type of chemotherapy drugs used
    b. The radiation dose received during radiotherapy
    c. The age at which treatment was received
    d. All of the above

21. Which type of cancer treatment is more likely to cause ovarian damage?
    a. Chemotherapy
    b. Radiotherapy
    c. Both chemotherapy and radiotherapy have an equal risk
    d. Neither chemotherapy nor radiotherapy pose a risk

22. In Turner syndrome (TS), estrogen replacement therapy is recommended for:
    a. Enhancing fertility
    b. Correcting growth hormone deficiency
    c. Preventing osteoporosis and cardiovascular complications
    d. Managing autoimmune disorders

23. **Cognitive impairment associated with iatrogenic premature ovarian insufficiency primarily affects:**
    a. Memory and executive functions
    b. Language and communication skills
    c. Motor coordination and balance
    d. Vision and spatial awareness

24. **The management of cognitive impairment in women with premature ovarian insufficiency may include:**
    a. Hormone replacement therapy (HRT)
    b. Cognitive training and exercises
    c. Regular physical exercise
    d. All of the above

25. **Incorrect statement about use of hormone therapy in premature ovarian insufficiency is:**
    a. It is cardioprotective
    b. It improves bone health
    c. It prevents cognitive impairment
    d. It increases the risk of breast cancer

26. **To reduce the risk of thromboembolism associated with hormone therapy:**
    a. HT is preferred over combined oral contraceptives
    b. Transdermal route is preferred over oral route
    c. None of the above
    d. Both of the above

27. **All doses of progesterone can be used in hormone replacement therapy, *except*:**
    a. 2.5 mg of medroxyprogesterone acetate (MPA) is used daily for 12 days each month
    b. 10 mg of MPA is used daily for 12 days each month
    c. 200 mg of micronized progesterone daily for 12 days each month
    d. 100 mg of oral micronized progesterone continuously for at least 12 weeks

28. **Micronized progesterone used in hormone replacement therapy in comparison to synthetic progesterone:**
    a. Have a better thromboembolic safety profile
    b. Have a better cardiovascular safety profile
    c. Pose a higher risk of breast cancer
    d. Does not protect endometrium from mitogenic effect of estrogens

29. **All of the following progesterones can be used in hormone replacement therapy, *except*:**
    a. Intrauterine levonorgestrel-releasing intrauterine system (LNG-IUS)
    b. Intramuscular depot medroxyprogesterone acetate
    c. Oral medroxyprogesterone acetate
    d. Oral micronized progesterone

30. **In carriers of women with BRCA1 and BRCA2 mutations after risk reducing salpingo-oophorectomy, use of short-term combined hormone therapy is associated with:**
    a. Increased risk of breast cancer
    b. Increased risk of endometrial cancer
    c. Both of the above
    d. None of the above

ANSWERS

1. **c.** Premature ovarian insufficiency is defined by loss of ovarian activity before the age of 40 years, represented by menstrual disturbances for ≥4 months associated with raised gonadotropin levels and low estradiol levels. Ovarian insufficiency is termed premature at or below 40 years of age as it is 2 SD from mean menopausal age (50 ± 4 years). Ovarian reserve encompasses both the quantity and quality of primordial follicles. Low ovarian reserve is a condition in which the ovary loses its normal reproductive potential. Early menopause is natural menopause in the 40–44 age group. "Premature ovarian insufficiency", "primary ovarian insufficiency", and "primary ovarian failure" terms were previously used synonymously. Due to the unpredictable ovarian function resulting in spontaneous conception in 5–10% of these cases; and negative connation attached to term "failure", term "insufficiency" is preferred by the National Institutes of Health (NIH). Further since "primary" and "secondary" terms being used in amenorrhea relation to menarche, to avoid the confusion "premature" term is preferred. Hence the European Society of Human Reproduction and Embryology (ESHRE) guideline development group (GDG) recommends the use of terminology "premature ovarian insufficiency" for this condition.[1]

2. **c.** Though the mentioned symptoms are commonly experienced by women with POI; but young women with primary amenorrhea, who have never been exposed to estrogen, rarely experience symptoms of hypoestrogenism at presentation, implying that estrogen withdrawal and not the estrogen deficiency

is responsible for these symptoms. The diagnosis in young women is therefore often delayed. These women should also be counseled regarding the genetic predisposition; risk and prevention of future fertility issues, associated comorbidities; and long-term sequelae-cardiovascular diseases, and osteoporosis. Psychological counseling required in adolescents with POI due to associated loss of self-esteem and emotional disturbances.[2]

3. **a.** Overall prevalence of POI increases gradually from 0.01% in <20 years, 0.1% in <30 years to 1% in <40 years; the incidence of POI in amenorrheic women is 2-10%.[2]

4. **d.** The most common cause of premature ovarian insufficiency is idiopathic which accounts for 90% of cases. In the remaining, the etiology includes:
   - Genetic abnormalities 10-12%, with majority involving X-chromosome—Turner syndrome 45XO/mosaic 45X/46XX (lost X-chromosome with/without gonadal dysgenesis), fragile-X syndrome 13-26% due to premutation in *FMR1* gene for fragile X (alteration in X-chromosome), and monosomy X
   - Autoimmune POI (adrenal autoimmunity 50-80%; thyroid autoimmunity 14-27%)
   - Infections (mumps oophoritis 3-7%)
   - Iatrogenic causes (surgery, radiotherapy, chemotherapy, and pelvic vein embolization)
   - Environmental factors

   A detailed menstrual, medical, and family history along with thorough physical examination help in clinching the diagnosis.[1]

5. **a.** Premature ovarian insufficiency is characterized by hypergonadotropic hypogonadism. Those women with irregular menstruation for ≥4 months, thorough evaluation is important so as not to miss POI cases as they adversely affect the bone health in young women. The initial laboratory evaluation for suspected premature ovarian insufficiency includes measurements of basal FSH and basal estradiol; and tests to rule out most common causes such as pregnancy, hypothyroidism, and hyperprolactinemia. If POI is confirmed then we go for further workup. Anti-müllerian hormone is not sufficiently discriminative for a diagnosis of POI as it may be low in women with regular cycles as well as in premenopausal women (may become undetectable approximately 5 years before the menopause). Inhibin B due to significant intermenstrual variability and poor predictive value is also not recommended for diagnosis. There is no evidence to include antral follicle count (AFC) (AFC < 5) as ovarian function may fluctuate resulting in intermittent follicular activity. There is no evidence to include laparoscopy, with or without ovarian biopsies. Consensus after diagnosis suggests going for karyotyping, *FMR1* premutations, 21-hydroxylase (CYP21), pelvic ultrasound, and other investigations as suggested to establish the underlying cause.[1]

6. **a.** The cutoff values of FSH used to diagnose POI differs in the literature varying from 25 to 40 mIU/L. Since autoimmune POI, an important etiology of POI, has been reported to express FSH levels lower than the proposed cutoff values, ESHRE GDG (2015) decided to use a cut off level of FSH >25 IU/L which is more than the normal physiological range even at the preovulatory peak. Hence the women <40 years of age with menstrual irregularities for ≥4 months, with two reports of serum FSH levels >25 IU/L at 4 weeks interval will be diagnosed to have POI. The estradiol levels are below 50 pg/mL in POI.[1]

7. **d.** After diagnosis of POI, etiology of POI needs to be ascertained in young women by a geneticist. Chromosomal abnormalities are detected in 10-12% of women diagnosed with POI. Fragile-X syndrome is an X-linked inherited condition caused by a mutation of the fragile-X mental-retardation 1 *(FMR1)* gene for fragile X. Women among whom karyotyping is normal, 6% will have premutation (55-200 repeats) of *FMR1* gene. Women who carry the premutation (55-200 repeats) of *FMR1* gene have an increased risk of 13-26% to develop POI. Fragile-X premutation have a prevalence of 0.8-7.5% in women with sporadic POI and up to 13% in women with a positive family history. Due to associated mental retardation, ataxia, developmental delay in children, Fragile-X testing is indicated for the family members to identify the carriers, and hence the risk of developing POI in the carriers as well in their subsequent progeny. In women with detectable Y chromosomal material, gonadectomy is recommended. With regards to autoimmune POI, autoimmune Addison's disease (60-80% of patients) and thyroid autoimmunity (14-27%) contribute to the major cases; and endocrinologist opinion for the same should be sought.[2]

8. **a.** Premature ovarian insufficiency shows important association with certain autoimmune disorders constituting autoimmune polyendocrine syndrome (APS). Autoimmune Addison's disease (50-80%) is the most common cause responsible for autoimmune POI followed by autoimmune Hashimoto thyroiditis (14-27%). Hence ACA, more specifically 21-hydroxylase autoantibodies (21-OH Ab) appear to be the marker with the highest diagnostic sensitivity for autoimmune POI; and if positive, refer to endocrinologist for further workup (ACTH stimulation test). Thyroid peroxidase autoantibodies (TPO-Ab) should also be assayed for autoimmune thyroiditis; if positive, annual thyroid-stimulating hormone is recommended. If both are absent, no need for retesting unless one becomes symptomatic.

    Undetected diabetes is prevalent in 2.5% cases. Rarely associated autoimmune disorders include systemic lupus erythematosus (SLE), rheumatoid arthritis, multiple sclerosis, and myasthenia gravis; immune thrombocytopenic purpura, autoimmune hemolytic anemia, pernicious anemia; coeliac disease, inflammatory bowel diseases, primary biliary cirrhosis, glomerulonephritis; Sjögren's syndrome, vitiligo, and alopecia areata.[1]

9. **b.** The women with POI are at increased risk of cardiovascular morbidity and mortality. This is due to the metabolic and endothelial changes that occur due to estrogen deprivation. In a prospective US cohort study there was 50% increase in the ischemic heart disease related deaths in women who developed menopause at the age from 35 to 40 years compared to women who attained menopause at 49-51 years. In another study, it was found that after 39 years of age, delay of menopause for every year reduces cardiovascular mortality by 2%.

    Cardiovascular morbidity and mortality is further increased in women with POI with Turner syndrome due to associated aortic aneurysm, aortic stenosis and coarctation of aorta. If initial imaging for cardiovascular pathology is negative in Turner syndrome, focused imaging at transition to adulthood, before conception, or if hypertension develops is recommended or routine screening 5-10 yearly may be advised. The maternal mortality rate is estimated to be approximately 3.5%, attributed to aortic arch or aortic valve abnormalities. The risk of aortic dissection is increased by two to five times during pregnancy in women with Turner syndrome. Annual blood pressure, weight, lipid profile, and hemoglobin A1c (HbA1c) status assessment is advised.[1]

10. **b.** There has been an increased risk of cardiovascular disease and mortality in women with POI. No screening regimes are yet approved to reduce this risk; however, annual BP monitoring and 5 yearly lipid profile monitoring is recommended. Hormone therapy is not associated with an additional risk of cardiovascular adverse effects in adolescent population with POI; instead it has been reported to have beneficial effects on blood pressure, insulin resistance, plasma lipids (reducing atherosclerotic plaque), catecholamine (preventing coronary constriction), and endothelial function. Available observational and nonrandomized intervention studies have shown a decrease in myocardial infarction risk, improved endothelial function, and no increased risk of ischemic heart disease or cardiovascular disease-associated mortality in those using estrogen replacement. Hence, early initiation of hormone therapy and continuation until the natural age of menopause is strongly recommended in women with POI to control future risk of cardiovascular disease. The cardiovascular risk can be further reduced by stopping smoking, regular exercise, and attaining a healthy weight.[2]

11. **b.** The POI is hypogonadotropic estrogen-deficient state which is associated with short- and long-term complications. Hormone therapy in POI women aims to maintain endogenous serum levels of estradiol of about 100 pg/mL, the normal premenopausal levels achieved by functional ovaries. Estrogen supplementation will take care of secondary complications. It is recommended to continue HT until the age of natural menopause (average age of 51 years). HT in POI replaces the normal premenopausal hormonal levels required to support cardiovascular health, bone health, and sexual health; while in menopausal HT, the goal is to relieve menopausal symptoms only. So, HT in POI includes higher doses of estrogen than that in menopausal women. Oral contraceptive pills (OCPs) containing even higher doses of estrogen (required for ovulation suppression) than the replacement dose in HT, have more risk of thromboembolism, hence not included in first line

management. Compared to OCPs this risk can be further reduced by giving HT via transdermal route eliminating first pass effect on liver. Also OCPs reduce the meagre chance of spontaneous conception in those wanting to conceive.[3]

12. **b.** In girls with absent or incomplete breast development, estrogen should be initiated first by 12 years of age and increased slowly followed by administration of graduated progesterone to prevent tubular breast formation associated with combined formulations. One may start with 6.25 µg/day of 17-beta estradiol transdermal or 0.25 mg/day of micronized oral estradiol; increasing the dose gradually every 3–6 months over the course of 2 years with end point to attain an adult dose or when spontaneous menses ensues. This is followed by addition of cyclic progesterone-oral micronized progesterone 100–200 mg/day for 12–14 days each month, to ensure endometrial protection. More physiological estrogen levels are achieved with transdermal estradiol, hence preferred.[3]

13. **c.** Bone mass evaluation at diagnosis of POI should be considered in all patients; and hormone therapy is recommended first-line therapy for managing BMD. The value of repeat dual X-ray absorptiometry (DEXA) scan in those with normal BMD and estrogen therapy initiated is limited; however, BMD should be repeated 5 yearly if osteoporosis is detected initially. With persistently low BMD, estrogen therapy should be reevaluated for the dose and route as well as secondary causes of BMD loss may be considered. In adolescents, there is no clear evidence to support more frequent BMD assessments owing to unclear implications of low BMD with low risk of fracture in this population and option for long-term management.

Owing to the long half-life of bisphosphonates, safety and fertility concerns; and fetal toxicity risk (following spontaneous conception/following donor eggs in vitro fertilization) arise in young women with POI; and hence their long-term use in young women is not recommended.[3]

14. **d.** Women with POI have reduced bone mineral density, and this has been associated with the degree and duration of estrogen deficiency; as well as the age of onset of POI (as maximum bone mass is attained by 30 years of age). Low bone mass in women with POI is best managed by hormone therapy, unlike in postmenopausal women where bisphosphonates is the accepted first-line therapy. Owing to lack of sufficient data on safety and fertility in young women with long term use of bisphosphonates, it is not preferred in POI. Risk of fracture can be further reduced by balanced diet with adequate calcium and vitamin D intake; cessation of smoking and limited alcohol intake; and weight-bearing exercise to maintain healthy weight.[3]

15. **b.** In POI though the fertility is markedly compromised, it may not be absolute as spontaneous ovulation is observed in 25% of women with POI, spontaneous conception in 5–10%. So, those who do not want to conceive should be counseled to use contraceptives to avoid unwanted pregnancies. Barrier contraceptives and intrauterine contraceptive devices (IUCDs) are preferred over oral contraceptive pills; as OCPs in POI show reduced efficacy in inhibiting ovulation due to the persistent elevated serum gonadotropin levels. Also instead of oral progesterone only contraceptives, levonorgestrel-releasing intrauterine system is preferred in these patients. Those who would like to conceive, should be thoroughly investigated for blood pressure, kidney function tests, and thyroid function tests.[2]

16. **c.** Compared to the general population, spontaneous pregnancies in women with idiopathic POI do not show any higher obstetric morbidity or neonatal risk—abortions, prematurity, low birth weight, stillbirth, etc., though the data is limited. The risk is not increased in case of spontaneous pregnancies after most of chemotherapy agents as well. A pilot study of 20 cases and 20 age-matched controls, examining the aneuploidy rates in embryos from women with prematurely declining ovarian function (not POI) showed this to be the same as that for women with age-appropriate ovarian function.[1]

17. **d.** In women with POI, interventions that can reliably increase ovarian activity are lacking; hence natural conception/conception via assisted reproductive technology (ART) using one's own oocytes is not suggested. Oocyte donation is the recommended treatment in women with POI wishing to conceive. Risk of aneuploidy in the fetus will depend on age of donor. Those considering oocyte donation from siblings should undergo preconception counseling explaining the potential risk of genetic mutations in

families; hence oocyte donor suspected of POI should be fully investigated prior to donation. IVF with preconception genetic diagnosis is recommended to prevent transgenerational transmission of genetic mutations in families. The male fetuses are at more risk depending on CGG repeats length. Referral to reproductive endocrinologist for fertility preservation is the best option before POI gets established. Further pregnancies resulting from oocyte donation should be kept under supervision of a high-risk obstetrics unit because of associated obstetrical complications. In women undergoing surgery, or chemoradiation, cryopreservation of oocytes, embryos, or ovarian tissue can be attempted; surgical transposition of ovaries may also be offered. Option of adoption may also be kept open. The management options need to be individualized. The recent research focus is on stem cell technology, and on in vitro activation (IVA) followed by autotransplantation of ovarian tissue.[1]

18. **d.** Regular monitoring of ovarian function is important in women who have undergone cancer treatment to detect early signs of premature ovarian insufficiency, to guide decisions regarding fertility preservation options and managing hormonal imbalances. Cardiologist consultation in preconceptional period is recommended in women with POI surviving cancer and in women with POI with Turner syndrome due to associated cardiovascular mortality and morbidity.[1]

19. **b.** Anthracyclines (doxorubicin) and alkylating agents (cyclophosphamide, chlorambucil, busulfan) are cardiotoxic drugs, hence cardiologist opinion should be sought prior to conception in women with POI who have received anthracycline or alkylating-based chemotherapy. Anthracyclines shows cardiotoxicity at all doses, with significant effect at a cumulative dose between 250 and 300 mg/m^2. Combined chemoradiotherapy further increases the risk leading to exacerbation of preexisting cardiac dysfunction resulting in peripartum cardiomyopathy and heart failure. Abdominopelvic radiotherapy is reported to adversely affect the uterine function and obstetrical outcome. The effect being directly proportional to the dose as well as the age at treatment. It has shown to increase the risk of abortions, preterm labor, uterine rupture, placenta accreta syndrome, postpartum hemorrhage; fetal growth restriction (FGR), stillbirth, and neonatal complications.[4]

20. **d.** Both chemotherapy and radiotherapy causes "acute ovarian failure" which may or may not be transient. Age and type of adjuvant chemotherapy appear to be the primary determinants of premature ovarian insufficiency with age being the independent determinant. In older women, the median time to onset of ovarian failure is shorter (2-4 months versus 6-16 months, respectively), and is less likely to be reversible than that in younger women (50% versus 10%, respectively). With combination adjuvant chemotherapy, risk of menopause is again higher in women age older than 40 years than younger ones (49-100% versus 21-71% in younger women). The ovarian response to irradiation depends on the radiation area, age as well as dose. An ovarian dose of 4 Gy in women over 40 years of age is associated with higher incidence of POI as compared to young women (100% versus 30%, respectively); in young women dose of ≥10 Gy is significantly associated with ovarian failure. Pelvic irradiation in the prepubertal girl may result in arrested uterine growth, and increased incidence of abortions and preterm labor in future pregnancy.[4]

21. **b.** With radiotherapy damage is extensive and irreversible; whereas with chemotherapy there are chances of reversal. Damage increases further if woman receives both radiotherapy and chemotherapy.[1]

22. **c.** Hormone replacement therapy in girls with Turner syndrome address the specific challenges with additional aspects that need to be taken into account, like the need for puberty induction, and potentially severe implications on bone, cardiovascular, and neurological health. There is associated increased incidence of thyroid disorders and hypertension as well; so preconception consultation with cardiologist and endocrinologist is recommended.[1]

23. **a.** Surgical menopause in young women subsequent to bilateral oophorectomy results in neuritic plaque formation, which is associated with an increased risk of cognitive decline and Alzheimer's disease. The younger the age of surgery, the rapid is the cognitive decline. Hormone therapy has shown protective effect on neurocognition by reducing cognitive decline; however, HT does not reverse Alzheimer's disease neuropathology. It is recommended to initiate HT within 5 years of surgical menopause, and continued for 10 years; however, in older age (>60 years), HT should be used with caution as it has been found to

increase the risk for dementia and vascular disease. Since in women with premature ovarian insufficiency with intact ovaries, the evidence on cognitive function is conflicting and scarce; the management in such cases follows the above recommendation.[4]

24. **d.** Hormone treatment in association with lifestyle management should be the ideal management for cognitive impairment in women with premature ovarian insufficiency and to reduce the age-related risk for vascular diseases. Lifestyle management options—cessation of smoking, exercise, and eating a healthy diet; will help in lowering abdominal fat, hypertension, hyperlipidemia, and insulin resistance risk. Since smoking is associated with early menopause, it should be stopped in women prone to POI.[1]

25. **d.** Hormone therapy in POI protects the cardiovascular health, bone health, and prevent cognitive impairment. Though the dose of estrogen in HT in POI is more than that in HT for menopausal women, it is not found to increase the risk of breast cancer in women with POI. It has been reported that breast cancer risk increases with increasing age at menopause, and is lowest in women experiencing menopause before the age of 40 years. The accepted rationale is that in young women with POI, HT aims to maintain physiological levels similar to that in age-matched women with normal ovarian estrogen production; hence should not have a higher risk of breast cancer than the latter. Studies evaluating the incidence of breast cancer among menopausal women exposed and unexposed to hormone replacement therapy, have reported nonsignificantly lower incidence among women exposed to HRT in the age groups 40-44 [relative risk (RR) 0.56, 95% confidence interval (CI) 0.07-2.01] and 45-49 (RR 0.62, 95% CI 0.62-1.22); and reported significantly higher incidence among women over 50 years exposed to HRT [RR 1.19 (95% CI 0.96-1.46) for ages 50-54 years; RR 3.71 (95% CI 2.16-5.94) for ages 65-67 years] as compared to unexposed women. Further increased breast density, as assessed by mammography, in postmenopausal women is associated with increased breast cancer risk. Hence, implying that the risk of breast cancer is directly related to age and breast density.[3]

26. **d.** Since the estrogen dose in combined oral contraceptives is higher and provides supraphysiological levels, the risk of thromboembolism is more with oral contraceptive pill than that with HT. As the transdermal route of estrogen eliminates the first pass effect of liver, it is associated with reduced risk of thromboembolism compared with oral route. Estradiol preparations include 17-beta estradiol 1-2 mg/day orally, or 100 µg/day transdermal; or conjugated equine estrogen 0.625-1.25 mg/day. 17-beta estradiol is preferred estrogen preparation. Transdermal route is also preferred in women with premature ovarian insufficiency with obesity, migraine, hypertension, and prior deep vein thrombosis (DVT). The genitourinary symptoms need local estrogen therapy apart from systemic therapy.[3]

27. **a.** Women with premature ovarian insufficiency and an intact uterus taking estrogen replacement require progestogen therapy to protect against estrogen derived risk of endometrial carcinoma. Dose of progestogen required depends on the dose of estrogen and the regimen (i.e., continuous combined or sequential). Continuous regimens require a minimum dose of 1 mg of oral norethisterone daily or 2.5 mg medroxyprogesterone acetate or 100 mg micronized oral progesterone at moderate to high doses of estrogen. Sequential regimens require 10 mg MPA or 200 mg micronized oral progesterone for a minimum of 10-12 days per month.[3]

28. **b.** The available evidence from postmenopausal women is in support of natural micronized progesterone with better cardiovascular safety profile and lower breast cancer risk when compared to synthetic progestogens. Unopposed estrogen therapy is associated with 10-50% incidence endometrial hyperplasia per year. Regarding protecting the endometrium from hyperplasia caused by 0.625 mg/day conjugated equine estradiol (CEE), a randomized controlled trial demonstrated that in oral dose of 200 mg/day for 12 days per month, micronized natural progesterone was as good as 10 mg/day medroxyprogesterone acetate for 12 days per month, or 2.5 mg MPA every day; however some studies favor oral MPA.[3]

29. b. Progestogens can be administered via the oral, transdermal (as a patch), or intrauterine routes. Subdermal implants and intramuscular depot preparations are also available, although these are licensed as contraceptive devices and no data exists for their use in HRT for endometrial protection.[3]

30. d. Risk of epithelial ovarian cancer in patients who are positive for BRCA1 and BRCA2 is increased to the extent of 39–58% and 13–29%, respectively. Risk-reducing salpingo-oophorectomy RRSO is recommended typically between 35 and 40 years in patients with BRCA1; and between 40 and 45 years in patients with BRCA2, since onset of ovarian cancer is delayed by 8–10 years in the latter. Being young, women with BRCA1 and 2 carriers after RRSO requires combined HT. It has been reported that short term HT use in these women neither increase the risk of breast cancer nor the risk of endometrial cancer. HT is contraindicated in breast cancer survivors.[3]

REFERENCES

1. Webber L, Davies M, Anderson R, Bartlett J, Braat D, Cartwright B, Cifkova R, et al. European Society for Human Reproduction and Embryology (ESHRE). Guideline Group on POI. ESHRE Guideline: management of women with premature ovarian insufficiency. Hum Reprod. 2016;31(5):926-37.
2. Committee Opinion No.605. Primary Ovarian insufficiency in adolescent and young women. Obstet Gynecol. 2014;123:193-7.
3. Committee Opinion No. 698: Hormone Therapy in Primary Ovarian Insufficiency. Obstet Gynecol. 2017;129:e134-41.
4. Torrealday S, Kodaman P, Pal L. Premature Ovarian Insufficiency—an update on recent advances in understanding and management. F1000Res. 2017;6:2069.

Chapter 94

Myomectomy

Kanchan Rani, Divya Suman

QUESTIONS

1. **What are the indications of open abdominal myomectomy?**
   a. Symptomatic intramural, transmural or subserosal leiomyomas in whom future childbearing is desired and a hysteroscopic or laparoscopic myomectomy is not feasible
   b. Symptomatic intramural, transmural or subserosal leiomyomas with coexisting cervical or uterine carcinoma
   c. Symptomatic intramural, transmural or subserosal leiomyomas with sever medical comorbidities
   d. All of them

2. **What are the risk factors for increased blood loss?**
   a. Fibroids large in size
   b. Fibroids multiple in number
   c. Fibroids low in the pelvis
   d. All of them

3. **Which is true for the role of gonadotropin-releasing hormone (GnRH) agonists in the management of fibroid?**
   a. For patients who strongly prefer a transverse rather than a vertical incision and in whom uterine size reduction is anticipated to enable adequate surgical exposure through such an incision
   b. It may obscure the tissue plane between the fibroid and normal myometrium and make enucleation more challenging
   c. GnRH effects on smaller fibroids may also obscure identification during surgery, and these persistent myomas may cause symptoms in the future
   d. All of them

4. **Which is not true for incisions for open myomectomy?**
   a. A vertical abdominal incision is used whenever possible
   b. The uterine incisions may be either vertical or transverse
   c. Anterior uterine incisions are associated with fewer adnexal adhesions than posterior incisions
   d. All of them

5. **Which is true for preventing bleeding in open abdominal myomectomy?**
   a. A tourniquet is placed around the lower uterine segment to limit blood loss
   b. Vascular clamps on the infundibulopelvic ligaments may also be used
   c. Injection of vasopressin just below the pseudocapsule of myoma
   d. All of them

6. **Which is true for the closure?**
   a. Closure of a myometrial defect that is >2 cm deep often requires two layers to achieve adequate tissue apposition and hemostasis
   b. The serosa is closed as a baseball stitch with monocryl to decrease exposure of suture and adhesion formation
   c. Both of them
   d. None of them

7. **Which is not true regarding different kind of myomas?**
   a. Hysteroscopic myomectomy is the procedure of choice for patients with primarily intracavitary leiomyomas
   b. Removal of submucosal myomas during open abdominal myomectomy requires transmural myometrial dissection

c. Removal of a cervical fibroid through a vaginal colpotomy incision is better to perform
d. For those with submucosal myomas and myomas in multiple other locations, both hysteroscopic and abdominal/laparoscopic myomectomy may be required

8. What are the complications of myomectomy?
   a. Hemorrhage
   b. Adhesive disease
   c. Visceral injury
   d. All of them

9. Which is not true for follow-up and postoperative advice?
   a. Patients require 4-6 weeks for recuperation after abdominal myomectomy is done
   b. Resumption of vaginal intercourse should be prohibited for 4-6 weeks
   c. Patients are encouraged to resume their normal daily activities as quickly as is comfortable
   d. None of them

10. Which is not true for counseling about future fertility after myomectomy?
    a. Should wait from 3-6 months before attempting to conceive
    b. If a patient is having difficulty conceiving following a myomectomy, early assessment of the uterine cavity and fallopian tubes with a hysterosalpingogram is advisable
    c. Myomectomy appears to be associated with an increased risk of uterine rupture during subsequent pregnancy
    d. None of them

11. What does preoperative counseling for myomectomy includes?
    a. Preparing for potential blood loss
    b. Role of GnRH agonist (if indicated)
    c. Thromboprophylaxis
    d. All of them

12. What are the indications of cesarean section myomectomy?
    a. Prevention of necrobiosis
    b. Fibroids of lower uterine segment causing difficulty to access the baby
    c. Forbids causing difficulty in uterine wound closure
    d. All of them

13. What are the possible complications of cesarean myomectomy?
    a. Hemorrhage
    b. Cesarean hysterectomy
    c. Postoperative fever
    d. All of them

14. What are the possible techniques to prevent hemorrhage during cesarean myomectomy?
    a. Uterine thorniest
    b. Bilateral uterine artery ligation
    c. Electrocautery
    d. All of them

15. Cesarean myomectomy should be avoided in intramural myomas within fundus or cornua of uterus.
    a. True
    b. False

ANSWERS

1. **a.** In general, open abdominal myomectomy is performed for patients with symptomatic intramural, transmural, or subserosal leiomyomas in whom future childbearing is desired and a hysteroscopic or laparoscopic myomectomy is not feasible. The abdominal approach is also reasonable for some type 2 fibroids. Open abdominal myomectomy is contraindicated in patients in whom laparotomy is contraindicated (e.g., medical comorbidities). Myomectomy is also contraindicated in patients with coexisting cervical or uterine carcinoma.
[Reference: Management of Symptomatic Uterine Leiomyomas: ACOG Practice Bulletin, Number 228. Obstet Gynecol. 2021;137(6):e100-e115]

2. **d.** Risk factors for increased blood loss include fibroids that are large, multiple in number, or those located low in the pelvis (e.g., cervical fibroid). It is seen that major complications (e.g., hemorrhage, visceral injury, and failure to complete the planned procedure) were associated with fibroid size ≥5 or removal of >3 fibroids.
(Reference: Sizzi O, Rossetti A, Malzoni M, Minelli L, La Grotta F, Soranna L, et al. Italian multicenter study on complications of laparoscopic myomectomy. J Minim Invasive Gynecol. 2007;14:453-62)

3. **d.** Routine administration of GnRH agonist prior to open myomectomy is not recommended. But for patients who strongly prefer a transverse rather than a vertical incision and in whom uterine size reduction is anticipated to enable adequate surgical exposure through such an incision.
[References: (1) Lethaby A, Puscasiu L, Vollenhoven B. Preoperative medical therapy before surgery for uterine fibroids. Cochrane Database Syst Rev. 2017;11:CD000547. (2) Bustos López HH, Miranda

Rodríguez JA, Kably Ambe A, Serviere Zaragoza C, Espinoza de los Monteros A, Alvarado Durán A. Preoperative management of uterine leiomyomatosis using pituitary gonadotropin-releasing hormone analogues. Ginecol Obstet Mex. 1995;63:356-64]

4. **a.** A low transverse abdominal incision (e.g., Pfannenstiel and Maylard) is used whenever possible. Compared with a large vertical incision (e.g., to the umbilicus or above), transverse incisions decrease postoperative pain and improve scar cosmesis.
[Reference: Parker WH. (2023). Uterine Fibroids (Leiomyomas): Laparoscopic Myomectomy and Other Laparoscopic Treatments. (online) Available from: https://www.uptodate.com/contents/uterine-fibroids-leiomyomas-laparoscopic-myomectomy-and-other-laparoscopic-treatments. (Last accessed December, 2023)]

5. **d.** All these techniques should be individualized and used according to the expertise of surgeons.
[Reference: Parker WH. (2023). Uterine Fibroids (Leiomyomas): Laparoscopic Myomectomy and Other Laparoscopic Treatments. (online) Available from: https://www.uptodate.com/contents/uterine-fibroids-leiomyomas-laparoscopic-myomectomy-and-other-laparoscopic-treatments. (Last accessed December, 2023)]

6. **c.** Closure of the myometrial defects with running unlocked layers of 0-Vicryl (polyglactin 910) suture on a circle taper needle is done.
[Reference: Parker WH. (2023). Uterine Fibroids (Leiomyomas): Laparoscopic Myomectomy and Other Laparoscopic Treatments. (online) Available from: https://www.uptodate.com/contents/uterine-fibroids-leiomyomas-laparoscopic-myomectomy-and-other-laparoscopic-treatments. (Last accessed December, 2023)]

7. **c.** Hysteroscopic myomectomy is the procedure of choice for patients with primarily intracavitary leiomyomas [the International Federation of Gynecology and Obstetrics (FIGO) type 0, type 1, or some type 2]. However, for those with submucosal myomas and myomas in multiple other locations, both hysteroscopic and abdominal/laparoscopic myomectomy may be required.

    Cervical or broad ligament myomas are a common finding and are often proximal to the ureter or major pelvic vessels. Removal of a cervical fibroid through a vaginal colpotomy incision is rarely performed.
(Reference: Bhandari S, Ganguly I, Agarwal P, Singh A, Gupta N. Effect of myomectomy on endometrial cavity: a prospective study of 51 cases. J Hum Reprod Sci. 2016;9:107-11)

8. **d.** The average volume of blood loss for open abdominal myomectomy varies across studies from approximately 200–800 mL. Adhesion formation after myomectomy has been well documented. Factors associated with adhesive disease are posterior location of a removed myoma and the presence of sutures.
[References: (1) Sawin SW, Pilevsky ND, Berlin JA, Barnhart KT. Comparability of perioperative morbidity between abdominal myomectomy and hysterectomy for women with uterine leiomyomas. Am J Obstet Gynecol. 2000;183:1448. (2) Schüring AN, Garcia-Rocha GJ, Schlösser HW, Greb RR, Kiesel L, Schippert C. Perioperative complications in conventional and microsurgical abdominal myomectomy. Arch Gynecol Obstet. 2011;284:137-44. (3) Dubuisson JB, Fauconnier A, Chapron C, Kreiker G, Nörgaard C. Second look after laparoscopic myomectomy. Hum Reprod. 1998;13:2102-6]

9. **b.** Decisions regarding resumption of vaginal intercourse are made by the patient; there are no medical restrictions on sexual activity. The follow-up visit includes an evaluation for potential complications and an examination of the abdomen and incision.
[References: (1) Minig L, Trimble EL, Sarsotti C, Sebastiani MM, Spong CY. Building the evidence base for postoperative and postpartum advice. Obstet Gynecol. 2009;114:892-900. (2) Nygaard IE, Hamad NM, Shaw JM. Activity restrictions after gynecologic surgery: is there evidence? Int Urogynecol J. 2013;24:719-24]

10. **d.** Myomectomy appears to be associated with an increased risk of uterine rupture during subsequent pregnancy, but it is difficult to ascertain the degree of risk and whether entering the uterine cavity adds to this risk. Thus, timing and route of delivery must be individualized based on the degree and location of the prior myomectomy. In general, cesarean birth is recommended for patients in which the myomectomy

was extensive or complicated; a trial of labor may be an option for patients in whom the myomectomy was unlikely to have significantly compromised the myometrium.

[References: (1) Tsuji S, Takahashi K, Imaoka I, Sugimura K, Miyazaki K, Noda Y. MRI evaluation of the uterine structure after myomectomy. Gynecol Obstet Invest. 2006;61:106-10. (2) Wallach EE, Vlahos NF. Uterine myomas: an overview of development, clinical features, and management. Obstet Gynecol. 2004;104:393-406]

11. **d.** The patient should receive all the information regarding risks and complications and she should be given the choices.
[Reference: Parker WH. (2023). Uterine Fibroids (Leiomyomas): Laparoscopic Myomectomy and Other Laparoscopic Treatments. (online) Available from: https://www.uptodate.com/contents/uterine-fibroids-leiomyomas-laparoscopic-myomectomy-and-other-laparoscopic-treatments. (Last accessed December, 2023)]

12. **d.** *(Reference: Awoleke JO. Myomectomy during caesarean birth in fibroid-endemic, low resource settings. Obstet Gynecol Int. 2013;2013:520834)*

13. **d.** *[Reference: Kaymak O, Ustunyurt E, Okyay RE, Kalyonc S, Mollamahmutoglu L. Myomectomy during cesarean section. Int J Gynecol Obstet. 2005;89(2):90-3]*

14. **d.** Any of these techniques can be used according to the demand and the expertise of operating surgeon.
[Reference: Sapmaz E, Celik H, Altungül A. Bilateral ascending uterine artery ligation vs. tourniquet use for hemostasis in cesarean myomectomy. A comparison J Reprod Med. 2003;48(12):950-4]

15. **a.** Fibroids situated at fundus or cornua are not intended to produce any difficulty in delivering the baby and if tried to remove may cause severe complications so, they are better to leave during cesarean section.
[Reference: Hassiakos D, Christopoulos P, Vitoratos N, Xarchoulakou E, Vaggos G, Papadias K. Myomectomy during cesarean section: a safe procedure? Ann New York A Cad Sci. 2006;1092(1):408-13]

Chapter 95

Ovarian Hyperstimulation Syndrome: Part 1

Kanchan Rani, Divya Suman

QUESTIONS

1. Which among the following is not responsible for clinical features of ovarian hyperstimulation syndrome (OHSS)?
   a. Exposure of hyperstimulated ovaries to human chorionic gonadotropin (hCG) leads to the production of proinflammatory mediators
   b. Vascular endothelial growth factor (VEGF) and a variety of cytokines are likely to be involved in the development of this condition
   c. These proinflammatory mediators cause a decrease in vascular permeability and a prothrombotic effect
   d. In response to hCG, VEGF appears to mediate the vascular permeability of OHSS

2. Which of the following is not true for the clinical features of OHSS?
   a. There is loss of fluid in the third space
   b. There is hypovolemia
   c. There is increased serum osmolality
   d. There is hyponatremia

3. Which of the following is true for the incidence of OHSS?
   a. Mild OHSS has been estimated in one-third of cycles
   b. Combined incidence of moderate or severe OHSS varies from 3.1 to 8%
   c. Both a and b
   d. None of the above

4. There is an increased risk of OHSS in women with:
   a. History of OHSS
   b. Polycystic ovary syndrome (PCOS)
   c. Increased anti-Müllerian hormone (AMH) levels
   d. All of the above

5. Which of the following is not true for the diagnosis of OHSS?
   a. There may be a preceding history of an excessive ovarian response to stimulation, but the absence of such a history does not rule out a diagnosis of OHSS
   b. The typical presentation is abdominal distension and discomfort following the trigger injection used to promote final follicular maturation prior to oocyte retrieval
   c. Early OHSS usually presents within 7 days of the hCG injection, used to promote final follicular maturation prior to oocyte retrieval
   d. Late OHSS typically presents 15 or more days after the hCG injection and is usually associated with an excessive ovarian response

6. Which of the following statements is true for the management of OHSS?
   a. The combination of elevated hematocrit and reduced serum osmolality and sodium is indicative of OHSS
   b. Ovarian hyperstimulation syndrome by itself is not commonly associated with severe pain, pyrexia, or signs of peritonism. It requires clinical review and investigation to rule out underlying complications.
   c. Both a and b
   d. None of the above

7. What management is appropriate in the outpatient setting for patients with OHSS?
   a. Nonsteroidal anti-inflammatory agents for pain relief
   b. Paracentesis of ascitic fluid should not be strictly carried out on an outpatient basis
   c. Thromboprophylaxis should be provided
   d. Oral opiates should be avoided

8. If conception occurs with OHSS, endogenous hCG can lead to a worsening of OHSS, whereas, in the absence of pregnancy, recovery is usually complete by the time of the withdrawal bleed.
   a. True
   b. False

9. When should women with OHSS be admitted?
   a. Unable to achieve satisfactory pain control
   b. Unable to attend for regular outpatient follow-up
   c. Unable to maintain adequate fluid intake due to nausea
   d. Any of the above

10. How should women with OHSS be monitored?
    a. Body weight, abdominal girth, and fluid intake and output should be measured on a daily basis with C-reactive protein levels
    b. Depending on the clinical features, arterial blood gases, ECG, chest X-ray, and other imaging may be required
    c. Both a and b
    d. None of the above

11. What is not true for the appropriate management of fluid balance in OHSS?
    a. Fluid replacement by the oral route should be used for hydration wherever practicable to correct intravascular dehydration
    b. Vigorous intravenous fluid therapy with crystalloids is the mainstay for fluid management in OHSS
    c. Women with persistent hemoconcentration despite volume replacement with intravenous colloids may need invasive monitoring, and this should be managed with anesthetic input
    d. Diuretics should be avoided, but they may have a role in a multidisciplinary setting if oliguria persists despite all other efforts

12. How should ascites and effusions should be managed in OHSS?
    a. Paracentesis should be carried out only abdominally under ultrasound guidance
    b. Intravenous crystalloid therapy should be considered for women who have large volumes of fluid removed by paracentesis
    c. Both a and b
    d. None of the above

13. Which among these is not an indication of paracentesis in OHSS?
    a. Severe abdominal distension and abdominal pain secondary to ascites
    b. Shortness of breath and respiratory compromise secondary to ascites and increased intra-abdominal pressure
    c. Oliguria despite adequate volume replacement, secondary to increased abdominal pressure causing reduced renal perfusion
    d. Mild abdominal pain with abdominal bloating and ovarian size less than 8 cms

14. Which among these is not true for the management of thrombosis in OHSS?
    a. Women with severe or critical and moderate OHSS should be evaluated for predisposing risk factors for thrombosis and prescribed either antiembolism stockings or low-molecular-weight heparin (LMWH) if indicated
    b. The duration of LMWH prophylaxis should be individualized according to patient-risk factors and outcome of treatment
    c. In addition to the usual symptoms and signs of venous thromboembolism (VTE), thromboembolism should be suspected in women with OHSS who present with unusual neurological symptoms, even if they present several weeks after apparent improvement in OHSS
    d. For women with severe OHSS who conceive, thromboprophylaxis should be considered at least until the end of the first trimester

15. Surgery is only indicated in patients with OHSS if there is a coincident problem such as adnexal torsion, ovarian rupture, or ectopic pregnancy.
    a. True
    b. False

ANSWERS

1. **c.** Exposure of ovaries to hCG or luteinizing hormone (LH) following controlled ovarian stimulation (COS) by follicle-stimulating hormone (FSH) underlies most cases of OHSS. Exposure of hyperstimulated ovaries to hCG leads to the production of proinflammatory mediators. Chief among these is vascular endothelial growth factor (VEGF), but a variety of cytokines are likely to be involved in the pathogenesis and clinical features of OHSS. The occurrence of ovarian enlargement with the local and systemic effects of proinflammatory mediators, including increased vascular permeability and a prothrombotic effect, is responsible for the clinical features of OHSS.

[Reference: Braat DD, Schutte JM, Bernardus RE, Mooij TM, van Leeuwen FE. Maternal death related to IVF in the Netherlands 1984-2008. Hum Reprod. 2010;25(7):1782-6]

2. **c.** Increased vascular permeability leads to loss of fluid into the third space, manifesting as ascites or, less commonly, pleural and pericardial effusions. Women with severe OHSS demonstrate hypovolemia, with a typical loss of 20% of their calculated blood volume in the acute phase of OHSS. Accompanying this hypovolemia is reduced serum osmolality and sodium.
[Reference: Evbuomwan IO, Davison JM, Murdoch AP. Coexistent hemoconcentration and hypo-osmolality during superovulation and in severe ovarian hyperstimulation syndrome: a volume homeostasis paradox. Fertil Steril. 2000;74(1):67-72]

3. **c.** It is known that the incidence of OHSS varies between different types of fertility treatment, with treatments involving greater degrees of ovarian stimulation being associated with a higher incidence. In cycles of conventional in vitro fertilization (IVF), mild OHSS has been estimated to affect around one-third of cycles, while the combined incidence of moderate or severe OHSS varies from 3.1 to 8%.
[References: Kupka MS, Ferraretti AP, de Mouzon J, Erb K, D'Hooghe T, Castilla JA, et al.; European IVF-Monitoring Consortium, for the European Society of Human Reproduction and Embryology (ESHRE). Assisted reproductive technology in Europe, 2010: results generated from European registers by ESHRE. Hum Reprod. 2014;29(10):2099-113]

4. **d.** Certain patient and cycle characteristics increase the risk of OHSS; women with a previous history of OHSS, PCOS, increased antral follicle count (AFC), or high levels of AMH are at an increased risk of OHSS.
[Reference: Al-Inany HG, Youssef MA, Aboulghar M, Broekmans F, Sterrenburg M, Smit J, et al. GnRH antagonists are safer than agonists: an update of a Cochrane review. Hum Reprod Update 2011;17(4):435]

5. **d.** The time of presentation following trigger injection divides patients into two groups: Early and late OHSS. 'Early' OHSS usually presents within 7 days of the hCG injection and is usually associated with an excessive ovarian response. 'Late' OHSS typically presents 10 or more days after the hCG injection and is usually the result of endogenous hCG derived from an early pregnancy. The preceding ovarian response in these women may be unremarkable. Late OHSS tends to be more prolonged and severe than early OHSS.
[Reference: Mathur RS, Akande AV, Keay SD, Hunt LP, Jenkins JM. Distinction between early and late ovarian hyperstimulation syndrome. Fertil Steril. 2000;73(5):901-7]

6. **c.** The symptoms of OHSS are not specific, and there are no diagnostic tests for the condition. Hence, care must be taken to exclude other serious conditions that may present in a similar manner but require very different management. The presence of severe pain, pyrexia, or signs of peritonism should lead to a thorough clinical review and investigation to rule out other diagnoses. Important differential diagnoses include pelvic infection, pelvic abscess, appendicitis, ovarian torsion or cyst rupture, bowel perforation, and ectopic pregnancy.
[Reference: Evbuomwan I. The role of osmoregulation in the pathophysiology and management of severe ovarian hyperstimulation syndrome. Hum Fertil (Camb). 2013;16(3):162-7]

7. **c.** Women undergoing outpatient management of OHSS should be appropriately counseled and provided with information regarding fluid intake and output monitoring. In addition, they should be provided with contact details to access advice.

Nonsteroidal anti-inflammatory agents should be avoided, as they may compromise renal function.

Women with severe OHSS being managed on an outpatient basis should receive thromboprophylaxis with LMWH. The duration of treatment should be individualized, taking into account risk factors and whether or not conception occurs.

Paracentesis of ascitic fluid may be carried out on an outpatient basis by the abdominal or transvaginal route under ultrasound guidance.

There is insufficient evidence to support the use of GnRH antagonists or dopamine agonists in treating established OHSS.
[References: Shrivastav P, Nadkarni P, Craft I. Day care management of severe ovarian hyperstimulation syndrome avoids hospitalization and morbidity. Hum Reprod 1994;9(5):812-4.

Lincoln SR, Opsahl MS, Blauer KL, Black SH, Schulman JD. Aggressive outpatient treatment of ovarian hyperstimulation syndrome with ascites using transvaginal culdocentesis and intravenous albumin minimizes hospitalization. J Assist Reprod Genet. 2002;19(4):159-63.

Shukla U, Deval B, Hamoda H, Savvas M, Narvekar N. A programme of outpatient surveillance for women at risk of severe OHSS following IVF: a prospective follow-up review of 99 cases. Hum Fertil (Camb). 2011;14(Suppl 1):7]

8. **a.** In the majority of women with OHSS, the condition is self-limiting. The object of monitoring is to identify women who suffer an increasing severity of OHSS and may require further measures. In most women, the condition resolves over a period of 7–10 days.
   (Reference: Nouri K, Tempfer CB, Lenart C, Windischbauer L, Walch K, Promberger R, et al. Predictive factors for recovery time in patients suffering from severe OHSS. Reprod Biol Endocrinol. 2014;12:59)

9. **d.** There is variability in the threshold for hospital admission between practitioners and it is not possible to be categorical about criteria for admission. The value of admission lies in the possibility of closer monitoring, ease of intervention, and availability of a multidisciplinary input. This is crucial in the care of women with critical OHSS, who may be at an imminent risk of complications or who have already developed complications that may require intensive care.
   [Reference: Practice Committee of the American Society for Reproductive Medicine. Ovarian hyperstimulation syndrome. Fertil Steril. 2008;90(Suppl 5):S188-93]

10. **c.** Recovery is signaled by a diuresis, normalization of hematocrit, and a reduction in abdominal girth and body weight. C-reactive protein levels have been shown to correlate with other markers of OHSS such as abdominal girth and weight and may have a role in monitoring.
    [Reference: Nowicka MA, Fritz-Rdzanek A, Grzybowski W, Walecka I, Niemiec KT, Jakimiuk AJ. C-reactive protein as the indicator of severity in ovarian hyperstimulation syndrome. Gynecol Endocrinol. 2010;26(6):399-403]

11. **b.** Vigorous intravenous fluid therapy with crystalloids has the potential of worsening ascites in the presence of increased capillary permeability. Hence, the oral route should be used for hydration wherever practicable. Some patients may need effective analgesia and antiemetics in order to be able to maintain adequate fluid balance. However, acutely dehydrated women may need intravenous fluid therapy to correct fluid balance, followed by oral fluids to maintain hydration. Crystalloids are useful for the initial correction of dehydration in women who are unable to maintain adequate oral intake. There are theoretical advantages to using colloids rather than crystalloids for initial rehydration.
    [Reference: Royal College of Obstetricians and Gynaecologists. The management of ovarian hyperstimulation syndrome, Green-Top Guideline No. 5. London: RCOG; 2016. (online) Available from https://www.rcog.org.uk/media/or1jqxbf/gtg_5_ohss.pdf (Last accessed December, 2023)]

12. **d.** Paracentesis should be carried out under ultrasound guidance to avoid trauma to the enlarged, vascular ovaries. Both abdominal and transvaginal routes are well described. Abdominal paracentesis allows the insertion of an indwelling catheter and this may minimize the need for repeating the procedure. Intravenous colloid therapy should be considered for women who have large volumes of fluid removed by paracentesis.
    [Reference: Royal College of Obstetricians and Gynaecologists. The management of ovarian hyperstimulation syndrome, Green-Top Guideline No. 5. London: RCOG; 2016. (online) Available from https://www.rcog.org.uk/media/or1jqxbf/gtg_5_ohss.pdf (Last accessed December, 2023)]

13. **d.** Mild abdominal pain with abdominal bloating and ovarian size less than 8 cms
    These are symptoms of mild OHSS and ascites is not seen in this stage so paracentesis is neither required nor indicated.
    [Reference: Royal College of Obstetricians and Gynaecologists. The management of ovarian hyperstimulation syndrome, Green-Top Guideline No. 5. London: RCOG; 2016. (online) Available from https://www.rcog.org.uk/media/or1jqxbf/gtg_5_ohss.pdf (Last accessed December, 2023)]

14. **a.** Women with severe or critical OHSS and those admitted with OHSS must receive LMWH prophylaxis. However, women with moderate OHSS should be evaluated for predisposing risk factors.

[References: Royal College of Obstetricians and Gynaecologists. Reducing the Risk of Venous Thromboembolism during Pregnancy and the Puerperium. Green-Top Guideline No. 37a. London: RCOG; 2015. (online) Available from https://www.rcog.org.uk/media/m4mbpjwi/gtg-no37a-2015_amended-2023.pdf (Last accessed December, 2023).
ESHRE Capri Workshop Group. Venous thromboembolism in women: a specific reproductive health risk. Hum Reprod Update 2013;19(5):471-82]

15. **a.** Hyperstimulated ovaries are likely to be highly vascular and liable to damage on handling. The risk of ovarian torsion or rupture appears to be increased in women with OHSS, particularly in the presence of pregnancy. In rare cases of critical OHSS, termination of pregnancy has been reported in the situation of progressive thrombosis despite anticoagulation.

[Reference: Royal College of Obstetricians and Gynaecologists. The Management of Ovarian Hyperstimulation Syndrome. Green-Top Guideline No. 5. London: RCOG; 2016. (online) Available from https://www.rcog.org.uk/media/or1jqxbf/gtg_5_ohss.pdf (Last accessed December, 2023)]

Chapter 96: Ovarian Hyperstimulation Syndrome: Part 2

Athulya Shajan

QUESTIONS

1. What is the typical presentation of a patient with ovarian hyperstimulation syndrome (OHSS)?
   a. Abdominal distention and discomfort following a high-protein diet
   b. Abdominal distention and discomfort following intense physical activity
   c. Abdominal distention and discomfort following the trigger injection used to promote final follicular maturation prior to oocyte retrieval
   d. Abdominal distention and discomfort following an unrelated surgical procedure

2. What is "late" ovarian hyperstimulation syndrome typically associated with?
   a. High hCG levels from an early pregnancy
   b. A severe infection
   c. A history of endometriosis
   d. Advanced age

3. Which of the following features would be indicative of severe ovarian hyperstimulation syndrome?
   a. Ovarian size of <8 cm
   b. Clinical ascites and hematocrit >0.45
   c. Nausea and mild abdominal pain
   d. No ultrasound evidence of ascites

4. Where should women at risk of ovarian hyperstimulation syndrome be informed to report their symptoms?
   a. The nearest accident and emergency department
   b. Their local general practitioner
   c. The licensed center providing their fertility treatment
   d. A specialized OHSS hotline

5. Which of the following tests may be indicated in the examination and investigation of women with suspected ovarian hyperstimulation syndrome?
   a. Full blood count
   b. Hematocrit
   c. Liver function tests
   d. All of the above

6. What are the typical symptoms of ovarian hyperstimulation syndrome?
   a. Shortness of breath, persistent cough, and chest pain
   b. Abdominal bloating, abdominal discomfort/pain, and reduced urine output
   c. Weight loss, frequent urination, and increased thirst
   d. Severe headache, blurred vision, and dizziness

7. What are the two groups of ovarian hyperstimulation syndrome based on the time of presentation following the trigger injection?
   a. Early and late OHSS
   b. Mild and severe OHSS
   c. Stage 1 and stage 2 OHSS
   d. Acute and chronic OHSS

8. Which women are considered suitable for outpatient care in the context of ovarian hyperstimulation syndrome?
   a. Only women with mild OHSS
   b. Only women with moderate OHSS
   c. Women with mild or moderate OHSS, and selected cases with severe OHSS
   d. All women diagnosed with OHSS, regardless of severity

9. Which medication should be avoided in women diagnosed with ovarian hyperstimulation syndrome, as it may compromise renal function?
   a. Aspirin
   b. Nonsteroidal anti-inflammatory agents (NSAIDs)
   c. Paracetamol
   d. Opioids

10. Which patient factor does not increase the risk of developing ovarian hyperstimulation syndrome?
    a. A previous history of OHSS
    b. Polycystic ovary syndrome
    c. Low levels of anti-Müllerian hormone (AMH)
    d. High number of antral follicles on ultrasound

11. Which of the following complications may occur in severe ovarian hyperstimulation syndrome?
    a. Renal failure
    b. Gastrointestinal bleeding
    c. Liver damage
    d. Memory loss

12. Which symptom should prompt an urgent review in women with ovarian hyperstimulation syndrome being managed on an outpatient basis?
    a. Mild abdominal discomfort
    b. Increased thirst
    c. Worsening OHSS symptoms
    d. Slight weight gain

13. When is surgery indicated in patients with ovarian hyperstimulation syndrome?
    a. In all cases of OHSS
    b. If there is a coincident problem such as adnexal torsion, ovarian rupture, or ectopic pregnancy
    c. If thrombosis is suspected
    d. If there is respiratory compromise

14. What is the reported incidence of ovarian hyperstimulation syndrome in conventional IVF cycles?
    a. 1.1%
    b. 3.1%
    c. 8%
    d. 33%

15. Ovarian hyperstimulation syndrome is more likely to occur in women with:
    a. Previous history of OHSS
    b. Polycystic ovary syndrome
    c. Increased antral follicle count (AFC)
    d. All of the above

16. Which treatment approach has shown a reduced risk of ovarian hyperstimulation syndrome in IVF cycles?
    a. Gonadotropin-releasing hormone (GnRH) agonists
    b. Clomifene
    c. Gonadotropin-releasing hormone antagonists
    d. Monofollicular ovulation induction with gonadotropins

17. What is the most common complication of IVF treatment?
    a. Ectopic pregnancy
    b. Preeclampsia
    c. Ovarian hyperstimulation syndrome
    d. Thrombosis

18. What is the recommended management for women with mild or moderate ovarian hyperstimulation syndrome?
    a. Inpatient care
    b. Outpatient care
    c. Intravenous colloid therapy
    d. Gonadotrophin-releasing hormone antagonists

19. What is the recommended treatment for women with severe ovarian hyperstimulation syndrome being managed on an outpatient basis?
    a. Gonadotropin-releasing hormone antagonists
    b. Thromboprophylaxis with low-molecular-weight heparin
    c. Paracentesis of ascitic fluid
    d. Diuretics

20. How should women with ovarian hyperstimulation syndrome being managed on an outpatient basis be monitored?
    a. Daily review
    b. Review every 2–3 days
    c. Review every 7 days
    d. Weekly review

21. What is the typical loss of blood volume in the acute phase of ovarian hyperstimulation syndrome?
    a. 5% of calculated blood volume
    b. 10% of calculated blood volume
    c. 15% of calculated blood volume
    d. 20% of calculated blood volume

22. What is the primary treatment approach for ovarian hyperstimulation syndrome?
    a. Intravenous fluids and paracentesis
    b. Administration of nonsteroidal anti-inflammatory drugs

c. Surgical intervention
d. Outpatient management with appropriate counseling, monitoring, and potential thromboprophylaxis

23. **Which of the following signs may indicate a worsening of ovarian hyperstimulation syndrome?**
    a. Decreased abdominal distention
    b. Increased urine output
    c. Weight loss
    d. Shortness of breath and tachycardia

24. **When should hospital admission be considered for a patient with ovarian hyperstimulation syndrome?**
    a. When the patient is unable to maintain adequate fluid intake due to nausea
    b. When the patient shows signs of improving OHSS
    c. When the patient is able to achieve satisfactory pain control
    d. When the patient prefers to be managed at home

25. **Which analgesics are suitable for relieving the symptoms of ovarian hyperstimulation syndrome?**
    a. Nonsteroidal anti-inflammatory drugs
    b. Aspirin
    c. Paracetamol and oral opiates
    d. Morphine injections

26. **How should the risk of thrombosis be managed in patients with severe ovarian hyperstimulation syndrome?**
    a. Administering LMWH prophylaxis
    b. Regular physical exercise
    c. High-dose aspirin therapy
    d. Withdrawing all medications to prevent drug interactions

27. **How should women with ovarian hyperstimulation syndrome be monitored in an inpatient setting?**
    a. Daily assessment, tracking changes in the severity of the disease
    b. Bi-weekly assessments with blood tests
    c. No special monitoring is needed
    d. Weekly ultrasound to check the ovaries

28. **What is the potential risk associated with pregnancies complicated by ovarian hyperstimulation syndrome?**
    a. Reduced risk of preeclampsia
    b. Increased risk of preeclampsia and preterm delivery
    c. No known risks associated with pregnancies
    d. High risk of multiple pregnancies

29. **When is paracentesis indicated in the management of ovarian hyperstimulation syndrome?**
    a. As a routine procedure for all women with OHSS
    b. Only if the woman has severe abdominal pain
    c. When there is shortness of breath and respiratory compromise
    d. When there is oliguria despite adequate volume replacement

30. **What should women with severe or critical ovarian hyperstimulation syndrome receive as prophylaxis?**
    a. Antibiotics
    b. Diuretics
    c. Thromboprophylaxis with LMWH
    d. Hormone therapy

ANSWERS

1. **c.** Ovarian hyperstimulation syndrome typically presents with abdominal distention and discomfort following the trigger injection used to promote final follicular maturation prior to oocyte retrieval.

2. **a.** "Late" OHSS typically presents 10 or more days after the hCG injection and is usually the result of endogenous hCG derived from an early pregnancy.

3. **b.** Clinical ascites and hematocrit >0.45 are indicative of severe OHSS. The other options are indicative of mild or moderate OHSS.

4. **c.** Women should be informed to report their symptoms to the licensed center providing their fertility treatment.

5. **d.** Full blood count, hematocrit and liver function tests are all part of the investigation of women with suspected OHSS, along with several other tests.

6. **b.** Abdominal bloating, abdominal discomfort/pain, reduced urine output.
    OHSS typically presents with abdominal distention and discomfort. Other symptoms may include reduced urine output, nausea and vomiting, breathlessness, and swelling in the legs or vulva.

7. **a.** Early and late OHSS
    OHSS can be categorized into "Early" OHSS, which usually presents within 7 days of the hCG injection, and "Late" OHSS that typically presents 10 or more days after the hCG injection.

8. **c.** Women with mild or moderate OHSS, and selected cases with severe OHSS

Outpatient management is considered appropriate for women with mild or moderate OHSS, and in selected cases of severe OHSS where close monitoring and immediate access to inpatient care are ensured.

9. **b.** Nonsteroidal anti-inflammatory drugs/agents (NSAIDs)
   NSAIDs are to be avoided in women diagnosed with OHSS because they may potentially impair renal function, which is already a concern in severe cases of the syndrome.

10. **c.** Low levels of anti-Müllerian hormone
    Elevated levels of AMH, not low levels, are associated with an increased risk of OHSS. AMH is a marker of ovarian reserve, and higher levels are often found in women with polycystic ovary syndrome, who are at an increased risk of OHSS.

11. **a.** Renal failure
    In severe cases of OHSS, life-threatening complications such as renal failure, acute respiratory distress syndrome, hemorrhage from ovarian rupture, and thromboembolism can occur.

12. **c.** Worsening OHSS symptoms
    Women with OHSS being managed on an outpatient basis should be reviewed urgently if they develop symptoms or signs of worsening OHSS, as the condition can quickly escalate and may require inpatient management.

13. **b.** If there is a coincident problem such as adnexal torsion, ovarian rupture, or ectopic pregnancy
    Rationale: Surgery is only indicated in patients with OHSS if there is a coincident problem such as adnexal torsion, ovarian rupture, or ectopic pregnancy and should be performed by an experienced surgeon.

14. **c.** 8%
    Rationale: The combined incidence of moderate or severe OHSS in conventional IVF cycles varies from 3.1 to 8%.

15. **d.** All of the above
    Rationale: Women with a previous history of OHSS, polycystic ovary syndrome, increased antral follicle count, or high levels of anti-Müllerian hormone are at an increased risk of OHSS.

16. **c.** Gonadotropin-releasing hormone antagonists
    Rationale: Evidence from meta-analysis shows a reduced risk of OHSS in IVF cycles employing GnRH antagonists compared with cycles where GnRH agonists are used as part of the regimen for controlled ovarian hyperstimulation.

17. **c.** Ovarian hyperstimulation syndrome
    Rationale: OHSS is the most common complication of IVF treatment.

18. **b.** Outpatient care
    Rationale: Outpatient management is appropriate for women with mild or moderate OHSS.

19. **b.** Thromboprophylaxis with low-molecular-weight heparin
    Rationale: Women with severe OHSS being managed on an outpatient basis should receive thromboprophylaxis with low-molecular-weight heparin.

20. **b.** Review every 2–3 days
    Rationale: Women with OHSS being managed on an outpatient basis should be reviewed urgently if they develop symptoms or signs of worsening OHSS. In the absence of these, review every 2–3 days is likely to be adequate.

21. **d.** 20% of calculated blood volume
    Rationale: Women with severe OHSS demonstrate hypovolemia, with a typical loss of 20% of their calculated blood volume in the acute phase of OHSS.

22. **d.** Outpatient management with appropriate counseling, monitoring, and potential thromboprophylaxis.
    Management of OHSS in outpatient settings involves educating the patient, monitoring fluid intake and output, providing contact details for advice, and possibly administering thromboprophylaxis. NSAIDs should be avoided due to potential renal function compromise.

23. **d.** Shortness of breath and tachycardia.
    Shortness of breath, tachycardia, hypotension, reduced urine output, increased abdominal distention and pain, and elevated hematocrit are among the signs indicating worsening OHSS.

24. **a.** When the patient is unable to maintain adequate fluid intake due to nausea.
    Hospital admission should be considered for patients with OHSS if they are unable to maintain adequate fluid intake due to nausea, cannot achieve satisfactory pain control, show signs of worsening

OHSS despite outpatient intervention, or cannot attend regular outpatient follow-up.

25. **c.** Paracetamol and oral opiates.
Paracetamol and oral opiates are suitable for pain relief in OHSS. NSAIDs should be avoided as they might compromise renal function.

26. **a.** Administering LMWH prophylaxis.
Women with severe or critical OHSS should receive LMWH prophylaxis due to the increased risk of thromboembolism.

27. **a.** Daily assessment, tracking changes in the severity of the disease.
Women admitted with OHSS should be assessed at least once daily to track changes in the severity of the disease process by watching the vitals, urine output, abdominal girth, etc. and to identify any complications at an early stage.

28. **b.** Increased risk of preeclampsia and preterm delivery.
Pregnancies complicated by OHSS may have an increased risk of preeclampsia and preterm delivery.

29. **d.** When there is oliguria despite adequate volume replacement
Rationale: Paracentesis is indicated in the management of OHSS when there is oliguria despite adequate volume replacement, secondary to increased abdominal pressure causing reduced renal perfusion. Severe abdominal distention and pain and shortness of breath due to ascites and increased intra-abdominal pressure are other indications for paracentesis. It should be carried out under ultrasound guidance and can be performed abdominally or vaginally. (Evidence level 4)

30. **c.** Thromboprophylaxis with LMWH
Rationale: Women with severe or critical OHSS should receive thromboprophylaxis with low-molecular-weight heparin. The use of LMWH is important in reducing the risk of thromboembolism associated with severe OHSS. The duration of LMWH prophylaxis should be individualized according to patient risk factors and outcome of treatment. (Evidence level 3)

REFERENCES

1. The Royal College of Obstetricians and Gynaecologists Green top guideline number 5: the management of ovarian hyperstimulation syndrome. 2016.
2. The American Society of Reproductive Medicine. Ovarian hyperstimulation syndrome. Fertil Steril. 2008;90:S188-93.

Chapter 97

Thyroid in Pregnancy

Savita Somalwar, Anuja Bhalerao, Sheela Jain, Prabhat Agrawal

QUESTIONS

1. According to World Health Organization (WHO), daily recommended allowance of iodine during pregnancy and lactation is:
   a. 200 mg
   b. 250 mg
   c. 300 mg
   d. 350 mg

2. As per American Thyroid Association (ATA) 2017 guidelines, the lower limit of thyroid-stimulating hormone (TSH) in first trimester of pregnancy is:
   a. 0.1 mIU/L
   b. 0.2 mIU/L
   c. 0.3 mIU/L
   d. 0.4 mIU/L

3. As per American College of Obstetrics and Gynecology (ACOG), serum TSH in hypothyroid women desirous of conception should be:
   a. <0.5 mIU/L
   b. <1 mIU/L
   c. <1.5 mIU/L
   d. <2.5 mIU/L

4. As per American Thyroid Association 2017 guidelines the upper reference value of serum TSH in pregnancy, if population and trimester specific values are not available, is:
   a. 2.5 mIU/L
   b. 3 mIU/L
   c. 3.5 mIU/L
   d. 4 mIU/L

5. Pregnant euthyroid women with positive thyroid autoantibodies should be screened with serum TSH in:
   a. First trimester
   b. Second trimester
   c. Third trimester
   d. Each trimester

6. As per FOGSI (Federation of Obstetric and Gynaecological Societies of India) 2021 guidelines, dose of levothyroxine in pregnant women on treatment should be increased by:
   a. 30%
   b. 50%
   c. 70%
   d. 90%

7. In women with overt hypothyroidism dose of levothyroxine after delivery should be:
   a. Increased
   b. Same
   c. Decreased
   d. Same as prepregnant dose

8. In women with postpartum thyroiditis who have recovered fully, serum TSH should be done:
   a. Monthly
   b. 3 monthly
   c. 6 monthly
   d. Annually

9. Methimazole exposure in first trimester can lead to following fetal anomalies, *except*:
   a. Choanal atresia
   b. Esophageal atresia
   c. Aplasia cutis
   d. Ebstein anomaly

10. This is not a risk factor for postpartum thyroiditis:
    a. Type 1 diabetes mellitus (DM)
    b. Pulmonary tuberculosis
    c. History of postpartum thyroiditis in previous pregnancy
    d. Positive thyroid peroxidase antibody

11. Fetus starts producing thyroxine after:
    a. 12 weeks
    b. 14 weeks
    c. 16 weeks
    d. 18 weeks

12. In pregnancy hyperthyroidism can be treated with all these drugs, *except*:
    a. Propylthiouracil in first trimester
    b. Methimazole in second and third trimester
    c. Propylthiouracil in all trimesters
    d. Radioactive iodine 131

13. American Thyroid Association 2017 guidelines recommend levothyroxine therapy during pregnancy in all of the following, *except*:
    a. Thyroid-stimulating hormone ≥ 10 mIU/L
    b. Serum TSH upper level reference range (ULRR) 10 mIU/L and thyroid peroxidase (TPO) positive

c. Serum TSH ULRR 2.5 mIU/L and TPO negative
d. Both (a) and (b)

14. All these complications in pregnancy can lead to hyperthyroidism, *except*:
    a. Hyperemesis gravidarum
    b. Hydatidiform mole
    c. Multiple gestation
    d. Hashimoto's thyroiditis

15. Thyrotoxic phase of postpartum thyroiditis is usually managed with:
    a. Beta blockers   b. Antithionides
    c. Thyroidectomy   d. Thyroid ablation

16. All newborns should be screened with serum TSH:
    a. Immediately after birth   b. 2–5 days after birth
    c. 6–9 days after birth   d. 10–13 days after birth

17. Optimal time to do thyroidectomy in pregnant women if required is:
    a. First trimester   b. Second trimester
    c. Third trimester   d. Any trimester

18. This antithyroid drug cannot be given in lactating women:
    a. Methimazole   b. Propylthiouracil
    c. Radioactive iodine 131   d. Both (a) and (b)

19. All of these thyroid disorders require treatment during pregnancy, *except*:
    a. Subclinical hypothyroidism
    b. Overt hypothyroidism
    c. Overt hyperthyroidism
    d. Subclinical hyperthyroidism

20. Recommended dose of levothyroxine in pregnant women with overt hypothyroidism as per FOGSI 2021 guidelines is:
    a. 1.6–2 µg/kg/day   b. 2.6–3 µg/kg/day
    c. 3.6–4 µg/kg/day   d. 4.6–5 µg/kg/day

21. According to World Health Organization, iodine requirement in women of reproductive age group per day is:
    a. 50 mg   b. 100 mg
    c. 150 mg   d. 200 mg

22. Thyroid-releasing hormone (TRH) is produced by:
    a. Anterior pituitary   b. Posterior pituitary
    c. Hypothalamus   d. Adipose tissue

23. Thyroid stimulating hormone is produced by:
    a. Thyroid gland   b. Hypothalamus
    c. Anterior pituitary   d. Adipose tissue

24. Thyroid-binding globulin is produced in:
    a. Adipose tissue   b. Bone marrow
    c. Liver   d. Spleen

25. In subclinical hypothyroidism:
    a. Thyroid-stimulating hormone and free thyroxine (T4) both are reduced
    b. TSH is reduced and free T4 is normal
    c. TSH is reduced and free T4 is elevated
    d. TSH is elevated and free T4 is normal

26. In overt hypothyroidism:
    a. Thyroid-stimulating hormone is elevated and free thyroxine (T4) is reduced
    b. TSH is elevated and free T4 is normal
    c. TSH and free T4 both are elevated
    d. TSH and free T4 both are reduced

27. In overt hyperthyroidism:
    a. Thyroid-stimulating hormone is reduced and free thyroxine (T4) is elevated
    b. Both TSH and free T4 are elevated
    c. TSH is elevated and free T4 is reduced
    d. TSH and free T4 are reduced

28. Half-life of levothyroxine is:
    a. 3 days   b. 5 days
    c. 7 days   d. 9 days

29. All of the following drugs interfere with levothyroxine absorption, *except*:
    a. Aluminum hydroxide   b. Cholestyramine
    c. Sucralfate   d. Nifedipine

30. In women with hypothyroidism sex hormone-binding globulin (SHBG) is:
    a. Increased
    b. Decreased
    c. Same
    d. Increased and then decreased

31. Severe hyperthyroidism can lead to all, *except*:
    a. Weight gain   b. Amenorrhea
    c. Weight loss   d. Tremors

32. Women on propylthiouracil should be monitored with:
    a. Complete blood count   b. Renal function test
    c. Liver function test   d. Serum uric acid

33. Hyperthyroid women on treatment are monitored with:
    a. Serum TSH   b. Free T4
    c. Total T4   d. Serum TSH and free T4

CHAPTER 97: Thyroid in Pregnancy

34. **European 2021 guidelines recommend following thyroid tests in women with subfertility:**
    a. Serum TSH
    b. Free T3 and free T4
    c. TPO antibody
    d. Serum TSH and TPO antibody

35. **Screening TSH of male partner in subfertility is not required with:**
    a. Ejaculatory dysfunction
    b. Erectile dysfunction
    c. Normal semen parameters
    d. Altered semen parameters

ANSWERS

1. **b.**
2. **a.** As per American Thyroid Association (ATA) 2017 guidelines, the lower limit of serum TSH in first, second and third trimesters is 0.1 mIU/L, 0.2 mIU/L and 0.3 mIU/L respectively.
3. **d.**
4. **d.**
5. **d.**
6. **a.**
7. **d.**
8. **d.**
9. **d.**
10. **b.**
11. **a.**
12. **d.** Radioactive iodine 131 is contraindicated in pregnancy.
13. **c.**
14. **d.**
15. **a.**
16. **b.**
17. **b.**
18. **c.**
19. **d.** Subclinical hyperthyroidism does not require treatment in pregnancy, while subclinical hypothyroidism, overt hypothyroidism and overt hyperthyroidism requires treatment in pregnancy.
20. **a.**
21. **c.**
22. **c.**
23. **c.**
24. **c.**
25. **d.** In subclinical hypothyroidism serum TSH is increased but Free T4 is normal whereas in overt or clinical hypothyroidism serum TSH is elevated and free T4 is reduced.
26. **a.**
27. **a.** In subclinical hyperthyroidism serum TSH is reduced and Free T4 is normal whereas in overt hyperthyroidism serum TSH is reduced and free T4 is elevated.
28. **c.**
29. **d.**
30. **b.**
31. **a.**
32. **c.** Propylthiouracil can cause liver failure.
33. **b.**
34. **d.**
35. **c.**

Chapter 98: Cervical Cancer

Monica Agrawal

QUESTIONS

1. Invasive cervical carcinoma <4 cm in greatest dimension and involving upper two-thirds of vagina without parametrial invasion is stage:
   a. IB3
   b. IIA1
   c. IIA2
   d. IIIA

2. Patients with pelvic and/or para-aortic lymph node metastases irrespective of primary tumor size or local pelvic spread are designated as having stage:
   a. IIIA disease
   b. IIIB disease
   c. IIIC disease
   d. IVA disease

3. The incidence of invasive cervical cancer associated with pregnancy is:
   a. 1.2 in 10,000
   b. 2.2 in 10,000
   c. 3.2 in 10,000
   d. 4.2 in 10,000

4. The most sensitive imaging examination for depicting metastases to the retroperitoneal lymph nodes in invasive cervical carcinoma is:
   a. PET
   b. MRI
   c. Integrated PET/CT
   d. CT scan

5. According to the Global Cancer Observatory (GLOBOCAN) 2020, estimated global burden of cervical cancer in India is:
   a. 11%
   b. 21%
   c. 24%
   d. 30%

6. Cryotherapy for cervical intraepithelial neoplasia is acceptable when:
   a. Endocervical sampling is positive
   b. CIN 1 has persisted for 24 months
   c. Colposcopy is inadequate
   d. Recurrent CIN 2/3

7. Preferred treatment for CIN 3 is:
   a. Cryotherapy
   b. Laser ablation
   c. Loop electrosurgical excision procedure (LEEP)
   d. Thermal coagulation

8. Atypical vessels characteristic of invasive cervical cancer include all, *except:*
   a. Looped
   b. Branching
   c. Mosaic
   d. Reticular

9. The American College of Obstetricians and Gynecologists (ACOG) recommends that women not initiate cervical cancer screening regardless of the onset of sexual activity unless they are:
   a. 19 years
   b. 20 years
   c. 21 years
   d. 22 years

10. The nonavalent HPV vaccine protects up to 96.7% for HPV disease related to following genotypes, *except:*
    a. 31
    b. 33
    c. 45
    d. 53

11. Most common symptom occurring in patients with cancer cervix is:
    a. Asymptomatic
    b. Malodorous vaginal discharge
    c. Weight loss
    d. Vaginal bleeding

12. Percentage of women with squamous cervical carcinoma detected to have HPV infection is:
    a. 85%
    b. 90%
    c. 95%
    d. 99%

13. Ideal candidates for radical trachelectomy, a surgical management option for women with invasive cervical cancer who desire uterine preservation and fertility have tumor size:
    a. <1 cm
    b. <2 cm
    c. <3 cm
    d. <4 cm

14. **Risk factors for development of cervical cancer are all of the following, *except*:**
    a. Age <16 years at first intercourse
    b. Nulliparous women
    c. Cigarette smoking
    d. Chronic immune suppression

15. **The 5-year survival rate for stage I cancer of the cervix with either radiation therapy or radical hysterectomy is approximately:**
    a. 95%   b. 90%
    c. 85%   d. 80%

16. **Appropriate treatment for 52-year-old female, parity 5, living 5, depth of stromal invasion <3 mm with no lymphovascular space invasion is:**
    a. Simple extrafascial hysterectomy
    b. Modified radical trachelectomy
    c. Modified radical hysterectomy
    d. Chemoradiation

17. **HPV vaccines need to be kept at:**
    a. −18°C (Freezer)   b. −4°C
    c. 2–8°C   d. 20–25°C

18. **Most common type of HPV found in women with normal cytology, CIN 2, and CIN 3 is:**
    a. Type 16   b. Type 18
    c. Type 31   d. Type 35

19. **Which type of HPV is more specific for invasive tumors?**
    a. Type 16   b. Type 18
    c. Type 35   d. Type 51

20. **Advantages to the use of surgery instead of radiotherapy are all, *except*:**
    a. Urologic fistula 1–2%
    b. Vaginal stenosis
    c. Ovaries can be conserved
    d. Bladder atony in 3%

21. **Modified radical hysterectomy (type II) differs from the radical hysterectomy (type III) in all of the following ways, *except*:**
    a. The uterine artery is transected at the level of the ureter, thus preserving the ureteral branch to the ureter
    b. The anterior vesicouterine ligament is divided, but the posterior vesicouterine ligament is conserved
    c. Removal of most of the uterosacral and cardinal ligaments
    d. A smaller margin of vagina is removed

22. **The hysterectomy described by Wertheim's is often referred to as:**
    a. Extrafascial hysterectomy
    b. Type III radical hysterectomy
    c. Modified radical hysterectomy
    d. Extended radical hysterectomy

23. **In type IV radical hysterectomy, all of the following are removed, *except*:**
    a. Periureteral tissue
    b. Portions of distal ureter and bladder
    c. Superior vesicle artery
    d. Three-fourths of the vagina

24. **In classical 2D cervix brachytherapy in cervical cancer, usual doses delivered to point A are:**
    a. 4,000–5,000 cGy   b. 5,000–6,000 cGy
    c. 6,000–7,000 cGy   d. 7,000–8,000 cGy

25. **The tolerance dose of irradiation for the urinary bladder and rectum is:**
    a. <5,000 cGy   b. <6,000 cGy
    c. <7,000 cGy   d. <8,000 cGy

26. **In cervix brachytherapy, point A is defined as:**
    a. 2 cm superior to the external cervical os and 2 cm lateral to the internal uterine canal
    b. 3 cm superior to the external cervical os and 2 cm lateral to the internal uterine canal
    c. 2 cm superior to the external cervical os and 3 cm lateral to the internal uterine canal
    d. 3 cm superior to the external cervical os and 3 cm lateral to the internal uterine canal

27. **In cervix brachytherapy, point B is defined as:**
    a. 2 cm lateral to point A
    b. 3 cm lateral to point A
    c. 4 cm lateral to point A
    d. 5 cm lateral to point A

28. **High dose rate (HDR) isotope most often used for modern 3 D brachytherapy is:**
    a. Cesium-137   b. Platinum-195
    c. Technetium-99   d. Iridium-192

29. **Chemotherapeutic agent of choice for Stage IIB to Stage IIIB invasive cervical cancer is:**
    a. Cisplatin   b. 5-Fluorouracil
    c. Hydroxyurea   d. Carboplatin

30. **Treatment of choice if para-aortic lymph nodes are involved in invasive cervical cancer is:**
    a. Radical hysterectomy with pelvic lymphadenectomy

b. Chemoradiation, pelvic field radiation
c. Chemoradiation, pelvic + extended field radiation + systemic chemotherapy
d. Chemoradiation, pelvic + extended field radiation + pelvic exenteration

31. **In Stage I A1 of cervical cancer with <3 mm invasion incidence of pelvic lymph node metastasis is:**
    a. <1 %
    b. <2 %
    c. <3 %
    d. <5 %

32. **All of the following is true about cervical cancer, *except*:**
    a. Patients with the large cell type of carcinoma, with or without keratinization, have a better prognosis than those with the small cell variant
    b. Cervical cancer is a clinically staged disease
    c. There are an increasing number of cervical adenocarcinomas reported in women in their 20s and 30s
    d. In the 2018 staging system, horizontal spread is no longer considered in Stage IA

ANSWERS

1. **b.** Stage IIA1
2. **c.** IIIC disease
   (Reference: 2018 FIGO Staging System for Uterine Cervical Cancer)
   FIGO = International Federation of Gynecology and Obstetrics

Stage	Description
I	Carcinoma is strictly confined to the cervix (extension to the uterine corpus should be disregarded)
IA	Invasive carcinoma that can be diagnosed only with microscopy, with maximum depth of invasion <5 mm
IA1	Stromal invasion <3 mm in depth
IA2	Stromal invasion ≥3 mm and <5 mm in depth
IB	Invasive carcinoma confined to the uterine cervix, with measured deepest invasion ≥5 mm
IB1*	Tumor measures <2 cm in greatest dimension
IB2*	Tumor measures ≥2 cm and <4 cm in greatest dimension
IB3*	Tumor measures ≥4 cm in greatest dimension
II	Carcinoma invades beyond the uterus, but has not extended onto the lower third of the vagina or to the pelvic wall

Contd...

Contd...

Stage	Description
IIA	Limited to the upper two-thirds of the vagina without parametrial involvement
IIA1	Tumor measures <4 cm in greatest dimension
IIA2	Tumor measures ≥4 cm in greatest dimension
IIB	With parametrial involvement but not up to the pelvic wall
III	Carcinoma involves the lower third of the vagina and/or extends to the pelvic wall and/or causes hydronephrosis or nonfunctioning kidney and/or involves pelvic and/or para-aortic lymph nodes
IIIA	Involves the lower third of the vagina, with no extension to the pelvic wall
IIIB	Extension to the pelvic wall and/or hydronephrosis or nonfunctioning kidney from tumor
IIIC*	Involvement of pelvic and/or para-aortic lymph nodes, irrespective of tumor size and extent†
IIIC1*	Pelvic lymph node metastasis only
IIIC2*	Para-aortic lymph node metastasis
IV	Carcinoma has extended beyond the true pelvis or has involved (biopsy-proven) the mucosa of the bladder or rectum
IVA	Spread to adjacent pelvic organs
IVB	Spread to distant organs

Note: Imaging and pathologic analysis, where available, can be used to supplement clinical findings for all stages.
*Indicates stages that are new from the 2009 FIGO system.
†Stage IIIC should be annotated with r (radiology) or p (pathologic analysis) to indicate the method used to allocate this stage. Imaging modality or pathologic technique should also be documented.

3. **a.** 1.2 in 10,000
   (Reference: Radhika AG, Malik R. Berek and Novak's Gynecology, South Asia Edition, 16th edition. Gurugram: Wolter Kluwer; 2022. p. 1082)

4. **c.** Integrated PET/CT
   (Reference: Lee SI, Atri M. 2018 FIGO Staging System for Uterine Cervical Cancer: Enter Cross-sectional Imaging. Radiology. 2019;292:15-24)

   Retroperitoneal lymph node metastases: The 2018 FIGO staging system explicitly states that the status of the pelvic and para-aortic lymph nodes (stage IIIC) can be determined with imaging. PET/CT, MRI, and CT are the imaging options. Other option for nodal evaluation is surgical and includes lymphadenectomy or sentinel node biopsy, the latter limited to sites where the necessary surgical and pathologic expertise are available. Although surgery is more sensitive, imaging is less morbid in avoiding the short- and long-term complications of lymphadenectomy.

Positron emission tomography (PET)/CT is the most sensitive imaging examination for detection of lymphadenopathy. A meta-analysis of 72 studies involving 5,042 women found that PET demonstrates a higher sensitivity (75%) and comparable specificity (98%) to MRI (sensitivity of 56% and specificity of 93%) and CT (sensitivity of 58% and specificity of 92%).
[Reference: Choi HJ, Ju W, Myung SK, Kim Y. Diagnostic performance of computer tomography, magnetic resonance imaging, and positron emission tomography or positron emission tomography/computer tomography for detection of metastatic lymph nodes in patients with cervical cancer: meta-analysis. Cancer Sci. 2010;101(6):1471-9]

In a paired comparison, a multicenter prospective trial of 153 women showed that PET/CT is more sensitive than is CT alone, especially in depicting lymph nodes in the para-aortic stations. Detection of lymphadenopathy that extends beyond the pelvis into the para-aortic region is clinically significant, not only because it upstages the patient, but it also expands the fields for radiation therapy.
[Reference: Atri M, Zhang Z, Dehdashti F, Lee SI, Ali S, Marques H, et al. Utility of PET-CT to evaluate retroperitoneal lymph node metastasis in advanced cervical cancer: results of ACRIN6671/GOG0233 trial. Gynecol Oncol. 2016;142(3):413-9]

CT versus PET/CT in detecting abdominal retroperitoneal metastases in uterine cervical cancer

Parameter	FDG PET/CT	CT	p value
Sensitivity (%)	50 (44, 56)	42 (36, 48)	0.05
Specificity (%)	85 (80, 89)	89 (84, 92)	0.21

If PET/CT is unavailable, then CT or MRI is a second-line alternative with both modalities demonstrating similar diagnostic performance.

5. **c.** 21%
(Reference: GLOBOCAN India 2020 database, collated by the International Agency for Research on Cancer and hosted by the Global Cancer Observatory)

More than 58% of all cases of cervical cancer globally were estimated in Asia followed by Africa (20%), Europe (10%) and Latin America (10%) and more than half of deaths were estimated in Asia (58%) followed by Africa (22%), and Latin America (9%). 39% of all cases occurred in China (18%) and India (21%) and 40% of total deaths from cervical cancer (17% in China; 23% in India).

6. **b.** CIN 1 has persisted for 24 months
(Reference: Radhika AG, Malik R. Berek and Novak's Gynecology, South Asia Edition, 16th edition. Gurugram: Wolter Kluwer; 2022. p. 407)

Cryotherapy should be considered acceptable therapy when the following criteria are met:
- CIN 1 that has persisted for 24 months
- Small lesion
- Ectocervical location only
- Negative endocervical sample
- No endocervical gland involvement on biopsy

7. **c.** LEEP
(Reference: Radhika AG, Malik R. Berek and Novak's Gynecology, South Asia Edition, 16th edition. Gurugram: Wolter Kluwer; 2022. p. 408)

Treatment of CIN 2 and 3: All CIN 2 and 3 lesions require treatment in women 21 years of age and older. This recommendation is based on a meta-analysis showing that CIN 2 progresses to CIS in 20% of cases and to invasion in 5%. Progression of CIS to invasion is 5%.

In recognition of the small but real risk for preterm birth, young women <20 years may be offered a program of surveillance with cytology and colposcopy at 6-month intervals with treatment only for persistence at 24 months. The heterogeneity of CIN 2 lesions is significant and regression rates are higher than for CIN 3. The histological distinction between CIN 2 and CIN 3 remains subjective and these diagnoses are combined in the 2006 Consensus Guidelines.

Although CIN can be treated with a variety of techniques, the preferred treatment for CIN 2 and 3 is LEEP. This allows a specimen to be sent for evaluation and enables the pathologist to identify occult microinvasive cancer or adenomatous lesions to ensure these lesions were treated adequately. The persistent and recurrent disease rate post-treatment is estimated at 4–10%.

Most of the excisional and ablative techniques used to treat CIN can be performed in an outpatient setting, which is one of the main objectives in the management of this disease.

8. **c.** Mosaic
(Reference: Radhika AG, Malik R. Berek and Novak's Gynecology, South Asia Edition, 16th edition. Gurugram: Wolter Kluwer; 2022. p. 1059)
Colposcopic examination is mandatory for patients with suspected early invasive cancer based on cervical cytology and a grossly normal-appearing cervix. Colposcopic findings that suggest invasion are—(1) abnormal blood vessels, (2) irregular surface contour with loss of surface epithelium, and (3) color tone change. Colposcopically directed biopsies may permit the diagnosis of frank invasion and thus avoid the need for diagnostic cone biopsy, allowing treatment to be administered without delay.

Abnormal blood vessels: Abnormal vessels may be looped, branched, or reticular. Abnormal looped vessels are the most common colposcopic finding and arise from the punctated and mosaic vessels present in cervical intraepithelial neoplasia (CIN). As the neoplastic growth process proceeds and the need for oxygen and nutrition increases, angiogenesis occurs as a result of tumor and local tissue production of vascular endothelial growth factor (VEGF), platelet-derived growth factor (PDGF), epidermal growth factor (EGF), and other cytokines, resulting in the proliferation of blood vessels and neovascularization. Punctate vessels push out over the surface of the epithelium in an erratic fashion, producing the looped, corkscrew, or J-shaped pattern of abnormal vessels characteristic of invasive disease. Abnormal blood vessels arise from the cervical stroma and are pushed to the surface as the underlying cancer invades. The normally branching cervical stromal vessels are best observed over nabothian cysts. In this area, the branches are generally at acute angles, with the caliber of vessels becoming smaller after branching, much like the arborization of a tree. The abnormal branching blood vessels seen with cancer tend to form obtuse or right angles, with the caliber sometimes enlarging after branching. Sharp turns, dilations, and luminal narrowing also characterize these vessels. The surface epithelium may be lost in these areas, leading to irregular surface contour and friability.

Abnormal reticular vessels represent the terminal capillaries of the cervical epithelium. Normal capillaries are best seen in postmenopausal women with atrophic epithelium. When cancer involves this epithelium, the surface is eroded, and the capillary network is exposed. These vessels are very fine and short and appear as small comma-shaped vessels without an organized pattern. They are not specific to invasive cancer; atrophic cervicitis may also have this appearance.

9. **c.** 21 years
[Reference: American College of Obstetricians and Gynecologists. Updated guidelines for management of cervical cancer screening abnormalities. Practice Advisory. Washington, DC: American College of Obstetricians and Gynecologists; 2020. (online) Available from: https://www.acog.org/clinical/clinical-guidance/practice-advisory/articles/2020/10/updated-guidelines-for-management-of-cervical-cancer-screening-abnormalities. (Last accessed December, 2023)]
The American College of Obstetricians and Gynecologists (ACOG) joins ASCCP and the Society of Gynecologic Oncology (SGO) in endorsing the US Preventive Services Task Force (USPSTF) cervical cancer screening recommendations.

USPSTF recommendations for routine cervical cancer screening:

Population*	Recommendation	USPSTF recommendation grade†
Aged less than 21 years	No screening	D
Aged 21–29 years	Cytology alone every 3 years*	A
Aged 30–65 years	Any one of the following: • Cytology alone every 3 years • FDA-approved primary hrHPV testing alone every 5 years • Cotesting (hrHPV testing and cytology) every 5 years	A

Contd...

Contd...

USPSTF recommendations for routine cervical cancer screening:

Population*	Recommendation	USPSTF recommendation grade†
Aged greater than 65 years	No screening after adequate negative prior screening results§	D
Hysterectomy with removal of the cervix	No screening in individuals who do not have a history of high-grade cervical precancerous lesions or cervical cancer	D

(FDA: Food and Drug Administration; hrHPV: high-risk human papillomavirus testing)

Note:
*These recommendations apply to individuals with a cervix who do not have any signs or symptoms of cervical cancer, regardless of their sexual history or HPV vaccination status. These recommendations *do not apply* to individuals who are at high risk of the disease, such as those who have previously received a diagnosis of a high-grade precancerous cervical lesion. These recommendations also do not apply to individuals with in utero exposure to diethylstilbestrol or those who have a compromised immune system (e.g., individuals with human immunodeficiency virus).

†Grade A denotes that "The USPSTF recommends the service. There is high certainty that the net benefit is substantial." A Grade D definition means that, "The USPSTF recommends against the service. There is moderate or high certainty that the service has no net benefit or that the harms outweigh the benefits." For more information on the USPSTF grades, see *https://www.uspreventiveservicestaskforce.org/Page/Name/grade-definitions*

‡Primary hrHPV testing is FDA approved for use starting at age 25 years, and ACOG, ASCCP, and SGO advise that primary hrHPV testing every 5 years can be considered as an alternative to cytology-only screening in average-risk patients aged 25–29 years.

§Adequate *negative prior screening test results* are defined as three consecutive negative cytology results, two consecutive negative co-testing results, or two consecutive negative hrHPV test results within 10 years before stopping screening, with the most recent test occurring within the recommended screening interval for the test used.

Source: Data from Curry SJ, Krist AH, Owens DK, Barry MJ, Caughey AB, Davidson KW, et al. Screening for cervical cancer: U.S. Preventive Services Task Force recommendation statement. U.S. Preventive Services Task Force. JAMA. 2018;320:674-86.

Age to initiate screening: The introduction of vaccines targeting the most common cancer-causing HPV genotypes has advanced the primary prevention of cervical cancer. As vaccination coverage increases and more vaccinated individuals reach the age to initiate cervical cancer screening, HPV prevalence is expected to continue to decline. This could prompt future changes to screening guidelines, such as raising the screening initiation age to 25 years, as is recommended in the recently updated ACS guidelines. Although HPV vaccination rates continue to improve, nationwide HPV vaccination coverage remains below target levels, and there are racial, ethnic, socioeconomic, and geographic disparities in vaccination rates. Cervical cancer screening rates also are below expectations, with the lowest levels reported among individuals younger than 30 years. Raising the screening start age to 25 years could increase the already high rate of underscreening among individuals aged 25–29 years and exacerbate existing health inequities in cervical cancer screening, incidence, morbidity, and mortality. Given these significant health equity concerns and the current suboptimal rates of cervical cancer screening and HPV vaccination, ACOG, ASCCP, and SGO continue to recommend initiation of cervical cancer screening at age 21 years.

10. **d.** 53

[Reference: American College of Obstetricians and Gynecologist. Human Papillomavirus Vaccination: ACOG Committee Opinion, Number 809. Obstet Gynecol. 2020;136(2):e15-e21]

Vaccine efficacy human papillomavirus vaccines are among the most effective vaccines available worldwide, with unequivocal data demonstrating >99% efficacy when administered to women who have not been exposed to that particular type of HPV. The HPV vaccine significantly reduces the incidence of anogenital cancer and genital warts in women and in men. Additionally, HPV vaccination may decrease the incidence of oropharyngeal cancer. In the United States, the prevalence of vaccine-type HPV infection decreased 71% among women aged 14–19 years between 2006 (when the quadrivalent HPV vaccine was introduced) and 2014. Additionally, a marked reduction in genital warts has occurred in countries with high HPV vaccine coverage.

The 9-valent HPV vaccine protects against >99% of HPV disease related to genotypes 6, 11, 16, and 18 and up to 96.7% for HPV disease related to genotypes 31, 33, 45, 52, and 58. This includes prevention of cervical, vaginal, vulvar, and anal disease caused by these HPV types. The HPV vaccine is a prophylactic vaccine used to prevent disease. Studies are ongoing currently as to whether it may be helpful to prevent recurrent disease, but current data does not support its use as a therapeutic vaccine.

11. **d.** Vaginal bleeding
(Reference: Radhika AG, Malik R. Berek and Novak's Gynecology, South Asia Edition, 16th edition. Gurugram: Wolters Kluwer; 2022. p. 1059)
Vaginal bleeding is the most common symptom occurring in patients with cancer cervix. Most often this is postcoital bleeding, but it may occur as irregular or postmenopausal bleeding. Patients with advanced disease may present with malodorous vaginal discharge, weight loss, or obstructive uropathy. In asymptomatic patients, cervical cancer is most commonly identified through evaluation of abnormal cytologic screening tests.

12. **d.** 99%
(Reference: Radhika AG, Malik R. Berek and Novak's Gynecology, South Asia Edition, 16th edition. Gurugram: Wolters Kluwer; 2022. p. 407)
The initiating event in cervical dysplasia and carcinogenesis is infection with HPV. HPV infection was detected in up to 99% of women with squamous cervical carcinoma. There are more than 100 different types of HPV, more than 30 of which can affect the lower genital tract. There are 15 high-risk HPV subtypes: two of the high-risk subtypes, 16 and 18 are found in up to 70% of cervical carcinomas.

13. **b.** <2 cm
(Reference: Radhika AG, Malik R. Berek and Novak's Gynecology, South Asia Edition, 16th edition. Gurugram: Wolters Kluwer; 2022. p. 1081)
Treatment of stages IB1, IB2, and IIA1 invasive cancer: Stage IB lesions are subdivided into stage IB1, which denotes lesions that have 5 mm or more of stromal invasion and are smaller than 2 cm in maximum diameter and Stage IB2 for lesions that are 2 cm or larger and less than 4 cm and IB3 that denotes lesions that are 4 cm or larger. Stage IIA1 disease involves the upper two-thirds of the vagina, but total lesion size is 4 cm or less. Patients with lesions 2 cm or less may be managed with either radical trachelectomy or a type III radical hysterectomy, with pelvic lymphadenectomy.
Radical trachelectomy should be restricted to candidates who desire future fertility with low-risk disease and a tumor size <2 cm. The para-aortic lymph node chain must be evaluated, especially if pelvic nodal disease is encountered. Adjuvant radiation therapy is recommended if intermediate risk factors are identified postoperatively. Adjuvant chemoradiation is indicated if high-risk features are found.

14. **b.** Nulliparous women
(Reference: Radhika AG, Malik R. Berek and Novak's Gynecology, South Asia Edition, 16th edition. Gurugram: Wolters Kluwer; 2022. p. 1058)
There are numerous risk factors for cervical cancer: young age at first intercourse (younger than 16 years), multiple sexual partners, cigarette smoking, race, high parity, low socioeconomic status, and chronic immune suppression. The relationship to oral contraceptive use was debated. Some investigators proposed that use of oral contraceptives might increase the incidence of cervical glandular abnormalities; however, this hypothesis was not consistently supported. Many of these risk factors are linked to sexual activity and exposure to sexually transmitted diseases. Infection with the herpes virus was thought to be the initiating event in cervical cancer; however, infection with human papillomavirus (HPV) was determined to be the causal agent in the development of cervical cancer, with herpes virus and *Chlamydia trachomatis* likely acting as cofactors. The role of human immunodeficiency virus (HIV) in cervical cancer is mediated through immune suppression. The Centers for Disease Control and Prevention described cervical cancer as an acquired immune deficiency syndrome (AIDS)-defining illness in patients infected with HIV.

15. **c.** 85%
(Reference: Radhika AG, Malik R. Berek and Novak's Gynecology, South Asia Edition, 16th edition. Gurugram: Wolters Kluwer; 2022. p. 1067)

Treatment options: The treatment of cervical cancer is similar to the treatment of any other type of malignancy in that both the primary lesion and potential sites of spread should be evaluated and treated. The therapeutic modalities for achieving this goal include primary treatment with surgery, radiotherapy, chemotherapy, or chemoradiation. Whereas radiation therapy can be used in all stages of disease, surgery is limited to patients with stage I to IIa disease. The 5-year survival rate for stage I cancer of the cervix is approximately 85% with either radiation therapy or radical hysterectomy.

A study using the National Cancer Institute's Surveillance Epidemiology and End Results data by an intent-to-treat analysis showed that patients in the surgery arm had an improved survival when compared with patients in the radiation arm. Optimal therapy consists of radiation, or surgery alone, to limit the increased morbidity that occurs when the two treatment modalities are combined. Recent improvements in the treatment of cervical carcinoma include adjuvant chemoradiation in patients discovered to have high-risk cervical carcinoma after radical hysterectomy and in patients with locally advanced cervical carcinoma.

16. **a.** Simple extrafascial hysterectomy
(Reference: Radhika AG, Malik R. Berek and Novak's Gynecology, South Asia Edition, 16th edition. Gurugram: Wolters Kluwer; 2022. p. 1081)

Simple (extrafascial) hysterectomy: Type I hysterectomy is an appropriate therapy for patients with stage IA1 tumors without lymph–vascular space invasion who are not desirous of future fertility. In such cases, lymphadenectomy is not recommended. If lymph–vascular space invasion is found, a modified radical hysterectomy with pelvic lymphadenectomy is appropriate and effective therapy.

17. **c.** 2–8°C
(Reference: World Health Organization. Comprehensive Cervical Cancer Control: A Guide to Essential Practice, 2nd edition. Geneva: World Health Organization; 2014)

HPV vaccine storage and the cold chain: HPV vaccines are sensitive to freezing; if frozen, they need to be discarded because they will no longer provide protection. Therefore, the following should be noted:
- They need to be kept at 2–8°C.
- HPV vaccines cannot be placed in or near the freezer compartment of the refrigerator nor directly on a frozen ice pack.
- The vaccines should not be kept in the refrigerator door, as the temperature there is more likely to fluctuate when opening and closing the refrigerator.
- The temperature of the refrigerator should be monitored by checking the thermometer regularly (at least twice daily) and by keeping a Freeze-tag® or Fridge-tag® in the refrigerator to detect if freezing temperatures have occurred. If the temperature is above 8°C or below 2°C, it needs to be adjusted as necessary to maintain the appropriate temperature.
- HPV vaccine should be administered as soon as possible after being removed from the refrigerator. Opened vials of the product should be discarded at the end of the immunization session or after 6 hours, whichever comes first.
- If transport of vaccine is required, the thermos box needs to maintain a temperature of 2–8°C.
  - Be aware that there is a considerable risk of freezing when using frozen ice packs. Therefore, frozen ice packs should be kept at room temperature for at least 5–10 minutes (until the ice inside them can be heard to move when shaken) before placing the vaccines and ice packs in the thermos. This is called "conditioning" the ice packs and it prevents the vaccine from freezing when it is placed near the ice packs. Always separate the conditioned ice packs from the vaccines with a sufficiently thick appropriate material. Remember that the risk of freezing is the most serious risk for a freeze-sensitive vaccine.
  - For brief excursions from the cold storage refrigerator, consider using water packs instead: these are ice packs kept at a temperature between 2°C and 8°C.
- HPV vaccines are sensitive to light and should be stored in the original package until ready to use.

18. **a.** Type 16
(Reference: Radhika AG, Malik R. Berek and Novak's Gynecology, South Asia Edition, 16th edition. Gurugram: Wolters Kluwer; 2022. p. 395)
Specific high-risk HPV types account for about 90% of high-grade intraepithelial lesions and cancer (HPV-16, -18, -31, -33, -35, -39, -45, -51, -52, -56, -58, -59, and -68). Type 16 is the most common HPV found in invasive cancer and in CIN 2 and CIN 3, and it is found in 47% of women with cancer in all stages. It is the most common HPV type found in women with normal cytology.

19. **b.** Type 18
(Reference: Radhika AG, Malik R. Berek and Novak's Gynecology, South Asia Edition, 16th edition. Gurugram: Wolters Kluwer; 2022. p. 396)
HPV-16 infection is not very specific; it can be found in 16% of women with low-grade lesions and in up to 14% of women with normal cytology. Human papillomavirus type-18 is found in 23% of women with invasive cancers, 5% of women with CIN 2 and CIN 3, 5% of women with HPV and CIN 1, and fewer than 2% of patients with negative findings. Therefore, HPV-18 is more specific than HPV-16 for invasive tumors.

20. **b.** Vaginal stenosis
(Reference: Radhika AG, Malik R. Berek and Novak's Gynecology, South Asia Edition, 16th edition. Gurugram: Wolters Kluwer; 2022. p. 1075)

Comparison of surgery versus radiation for stage IB/IIA cancer of the cervix:

	Surgery	Radiation
Survival	85%	85%
Serious complications	Urologic fistulas 1–2%	Intestinal and urinary strictures and fistulas 1.4–5.3%
Vagina	Initially shortened, but may lengthen with regular intercourse	Fibrosis and possible stenosis, particularly in postmenopausal patients
Ovaries	Can be conserved	Destroyed
Chronic effects	Bladder atony in 3%	Radiation fibrosis of bowel and bladder in 6–8%
Applicability	Best candidates are younger than 65 years of age, <200 lb, and in good health	All patients are potential candidates
Surgical mortality	1%	1% (from pulmonary embolism during intracavitary therapy)

21. **c.** Removal of most of the uterosacral and cardinal ligaments
(Reference: Radhika AG, Malik R. Berek and Novak's Gynecology, South Asia Edition, 16th edition. Gurugram: Wolters Kluwer; 2022. p. 1069)

22. **c.** Modified radical hysterectomy
(Reference: Radhika AG, Malik R. Berek and Novak's Gynecology, South Asia Edition, 16th edition. Gurugram: Wolters Kluwer; 2022. p. 1069)

23. **b.** Portions of distal ureter and bladder
(Reference: Radhika AG, Malik R. Berek and Novak's Gynecology, South Asia Edition, 16th edition. Gurugram: Wolters Kluwer; 2022. p. 1070)
The radical hysterectomy, performed most often in the United States, is that described by Meigs in 1944. The operation includes pelvic lymphadenectomy along with removal of most of the uterosacral and cardinal ligaments and the upper one-third of the vagina. This operation is referred to as the type III radical hysterectomy.

The hysterectomy described by Wertheim is less extensive than a radical hysterectomy and removes the medial half of the cardinal and uterosacral ligaments. This procedure is often referred to as the modified radical or type II hysterectomy. Wertheim's original operation did not include pelvic lymphadenectomy but instead included selective removal of enlarged lymph nodes.

Radical hysterectomies can be further classified as extended radical hysterectomy (type IV and type V). In the type IV operation, the periureteral tissue, superior vesicle artery, and as much as three-fourths of the vagina are removed. In the type V operation, portions of the distal ureter and bladder are resected.

24. **d.** 7,000–8,000 cGy
(Reference: Radhika AG, Malik R. Berek and Novak's Gynecology, South Asia Edition, 16th edition. Gurugram: Wolters Kluwer; 2022. p. 1075)

25. **b.** <6,000 cGy
(Reference: Radhika AG, Malik R. Berek and Novak's Gynecology, South Asia Edition, 16th edition. Gurugram: Wolters Kluwer; 2022. p. 1075)

26. **a.** 2 cm superior to the external cervical os and 2 cm lateral to the internal uterine canal
(Reference: Radhika AG, Malik R. Berek and Novak's Gynecology, South Asia Edition, 16th edition. Gurugram: Wolters Kluwer; 2022. p. 1075)

27. **b.** 3 cm lateral to point A
(Reference: Radhika AG, Malik R. Berek and Novak's Gynecology, South Asia Edition, 16th edition. Gurugram: Wolters Kluwer; 2022. p. 1075)

28. **d.** Iridium-192
(Reference: Radhika AG, Malik R. Berek and Novak's Gynecology, South Asia Edition, 16th edition. Gurugram: Wolters Kluwer; 2022. p. 1076)

Primary radiation therapy: Radiotherapy can be used to treat all stages of cervical cancer, with cure rates of about 70% for stage I, 60% for stage II, 45% for stage III, and 18% for stage IV.

Primary radiation treatment plans consist of a combination of external beam radiation therapy to treat the regional lymph nodes and to decrease the tumor volume, and brachytherapy delivered by intracavitary applicators and/or interstitial implants to provide a treatment boost to the central tumor. Intracavitary therapy alone may be used in patients with early disease when the incidence of lymph node metastasis is negligible.

The treatment sequence can depend on tumor volume. Patients usually receive 5 weeks of pelvic external beam radiation upfront, with brachytherapy introduced at week 4. In some cases, stage IB lesions smaller than 2 cm may be treated first with an intracavitary source to treat the primary lesion, followed by external therapy to treat the pelvic lymph nodes.

Larger lesions require external radiotherapy first to shrink the tumor and to reduce the anatomic distortion caused by the cancer. Tumor shrinkage >1 cm per week can be achieved with adequate external beam radiation prior to starting brachytherapy. Such a treatment strategy enables the radiation oncologists to physically implant brachytherapy applicators and achieve dosimetric radiation coverage of the tumor target volume.

In classical 2D cervix brachytherapy in cervical cancer, usual doses delivered are 7,000–8,000 cGy to point A (defined as 2 cm superior to the external cervical os and 2 cm lateral to the internal uterine canal) and 6,000 cGy to point B (defined as 3 cm lateral to point A), limiting the bladder and rectal dosage to less than 6,000 cGy.

To achieve this level, it is necessary to adequately pack the bladder and bowel away from the intracavitary source. Localization films and careful calculation of dosimetry are mandatory to optimize the dose of radiation and to reduce the incidence of bowel and bladder complications. Local control depends on delivering an adequate dose to the tumor from the intracavitary source.

29. **a.** Cisplatin
(Reference: Radhika AG, Malik R. Berek and Novak's Gynecology, South Asia Edition, 16th edition. Gurugram: Wolters Kluwer; 2022. p. 1081)

Stages IIB to IIIB invasive cancer
Therapy for patients with stage IIB or greater cervical cancer traditionally was radiation therapy. Primary pelvic radiotherapy fails to control disease progression in 30–82% of patients with advanced cervical carcinoma. Two-thirds of these failures occur in the pelvis. A variety of agents were used in an attempt to increase the effectiveness of radiation therapy in patients with large primary tumors. Because chemoradiation was superior to radiation therapy alone, chemoradiation is the preferred treatment strategy for these *patients, with cisplatin the chemotherapy agent of choice.* Nodal involvement, particularly the para-aortic lymph nodes, is the most important factor related to survival.

30. **c.** Chemoradiation, pelvic field radiation + extended field radiation + systemic chemotherapy
(Reference: Radhika AG, Malik R. Berek and Novak's Gynecology, South Asia Edition, 16th edition. Gurugram: Wolters Kluwer; 2022. p. 1068)

Management of invasive cancer of cervix by stage:

Stage	Disease	Treatment*
IA1	<3 mm – LVSI	Conization or extrafascial hysterectomy
	<3 mm + LVSI	Modified radical trachelectomy or modified radical hysterectomy + pelvic lymphadenectomy or sentinel lymph node biopsy
IA2	≥3 mm <5 mm	Modified radical trachelectomy or modified radical hysterectomy + pelvic lymphadenectomy or sentinel lymph node biopsy
IB1	≥5 mm <2 cm	Modified radical/ radical trachelectomy or modified radical/radical hysterectomy + pelvic lymphadenectomy or sentinel lymph node biopsy
IB2	≥2 cm <4 cm	Radical hysterectomy + pelvic lymphadenectomy
IB3	≥4 cm	Chemoradiation, pelvic field
IIA1	<4 cm + upper vagina	Radical hysterectomy + pelvic lymphadenectomy or chemoradiation
IIA2	≥4 cm + upper vagina	Chemoradiation, pelvic field
IIB	+ Parametria not to pelvic wall	Chemoradiation, pelvic field

Contd...

Contd...

Stage	Disease	Treatment*
IIIA	+ Lower vagina	Chemoradiation, pelvic field
IIIB	+ Pelvic wall or hydronephrosis	Chemoradiation, pelvic ± extended field
IIIC1	+ Pelvic lymph nodes	Chemoradiation, pelvic ± extended field
IIIC2	+ Para-aortic lymph nodes	Chemoradiation, pelvic + extended field + systemic chemotherapy
IVA	+ Adjacent pelvic organs	Chemoradiation, pelvic + extended field *or* pelvic exenteration
IVB	+ Distant organs	Systemic chemotherapy ± radiation, pelvic or modified held

*Treatment recommendations must be individualized based on the patient's status and specific disease variables.
(LVSI: lymphovascular space invasion; lymph: lymphadenectomy; SLN: sentinel lymph node; trachel: trachelectomy))

31. **a.** <1%

    (Reference: Radhika AG, Malik R. Berek and Novak's Gynecology, South Asia Edition, 16th edition. Gurugram: Wolters Kluwer; 2022. p. 1081)

    Stage IA1 ≤3 mm invasion: Lesions with invasion ≤3 mm have less than 1% incidence of pelvic node metastases. Within this group, it appears that the patients most at risk for nodal metastases or central pelvic recurrence are those with definitive evidence of tumor emboli in lymphovascular spaces. Therefore, patients with less than 3 mm invasion and no lymphovascular space invasion may be treated with extrafascial hysterectomy without lymphadenectomy. Therapeutic conization appears to be adequate therapy for these patients if preservation of childbearing capability is desired. Surgical margins and postconization endocervical curettage must be free of disease. If there is lymphovascular space invasion, a type I (extrafascial) or II (modified radical) hysterectomy with pelvic lymphadenectomy should be considered.

32. **b.** Cervical cancer is a clinically staged disease

    (Reference: Radhika AG, Malik R. Berek and Novak's Gynecology, South Asia Edition, 16th edition. Gurugram: Wolters Kluwer; 2022. p. 1061-2)

    The old 2008 FIGO clinical staging system of carcinoma of the cervix uteri was updated in 2018 to include imaging and pathologic findings. With the 2018 International Federation of Gynecology and Obstetrics staging system for uterine cervical cancer, imaging is formally incorporated as a source of staging information and as a supplement to clinical examination (i.e., pelvic examination, cystoscopy, and colposcopy) to obtain an accurate description of tumor spread.

    Imaging and pathology can be used, where available to supplement clinical findings with respect to tumor size and extend, in all stages.

Chapter 99

Human Papillomavirus and Vaccination

Ritu Santwani, Naisargi Patel

QUESTIONS

1. Development of recombinant human papillomavirus (HPV) vaccine based on which type of viral proteins?
   a. E6, E7
   b. E1, E2
   c. L1
   d. L2

2. All of the types of vaccine (HPV) are available in market, *except:*
   a. Hepatitis B
   b. Gardasil 4 and 9
   c. Biovac
   d. Both (a) and (c)

3. A 15-year-old girl is asking for vaccination to prevent cervical cancer. Which of these vaccines you advice?
   a. Hepatitis B
   b. Biovac
   c. Gardasil 4 or 9
   d. BCG (Bacillus Calmette-Guérin)

4. Dose schedule for Gardasil 4 vaccine in >15 years of age:
   a. 0, 1, 6 month
   b. 0, 1, 4 month
   c. 0, 2, 6 month
   d. 0, 2, 4 month

5. Gardasil 9 vaccine contains which all type of HPV strain?
   a. HPV 6, 32, 35, 40, 48, 55, 57, 62
   b. HPV 6, 11, 16, 18, 31, 33, 45, 52, 58
   c. HPV 13, 16, 18, 32, 33, 42, 55, 57, 62
   d. HPV 11, 14, 18, 33, 42, 55, 57, 62, 68

6. Human papillomavirus (HPV) vaccine is safe in pregnancy.
   a. True
   b. False

7. Which HPV genotype is most common cause of cervical cancer?
   a. HPV 11
   b. HPV 16
   c. HPV 6
   d. HPV 18

8. Which HPV genotype is most likely to harbor adenocarcinoma of cervix?
   a. HPV 11
   b. HPV 6
   c. HPV 18
   d. HPV 16

9. In which body part oncogenic HPVs are especially replicate?
   a. Cervix
   b. Brain
   c. Liver
   d. Lungs

10. All are true regarding adenocarcinoma of cervix, *except:*
    a. Microinvasive carcinomas of the cervix (MIC) site transformation zone
    b. MIC in your female
    c. MIC in oral contraceptive pill (OCP) users
    d. Associate with HPV 18

11. Women can lower their risk of getting cervical cancer.
    a. True
    b. False

12. You do not need to be screened for cervical cancer, if you have received an HPV vaccine.
    a. True
    b. False

13. Which statement among the following is false about the cervical cancer?
    a. Worldwide it is most common maiming in women.
    b. Most cases occur in developing word
    c. It is most commonly diagnosed in second decade life
    d. More common in women with high socioeconomic status

14. Which of these is a method of transmission of HPV?
    a. Sexual contact
    b. Stain to skin contact
    c. Vertical transmission
    d. All of the above

15. Which of the following is not a cervical cancer screening method?
    a. Colposcopy   b. Pap smear
    c. Primary HPV testing d. VJA/V717

16. Which of the following is used for visual inspection with acetic acid (VIA)?
    a. 1% freshly prepared acetic acid
    b. 5% freshly prepared acetic acid
    c. 10% freshly prepared acetic acid
    d. 50% freshly prepared acetic acid

17. In cervical intraepithelial neoplasia (CIN) after application of acetic acid on cervix, cervix turns in which color?
    a. Brown   b. Pink
    c. White   d. Yellow

18. Which among the following is not true regarding cervical cancer screening guidelines?
    a. Pap testing early 35 years from 21 years onward
    b. Co-testing every 5 years from 30 years onward
    c. Primary HPV testing early 5 years from 30 year
    d. Co-testing every 5 years from 21 years onward

19. Which of the following is not a risk factor for cervical cancer?
    a. Every age of intercourse b. Early menarche
    c. Smoking   d. Multiparity

20. Pap smear is useful in the diagnosis of all, *except*:
    a. Gonorrhea   b. *Trichomonas vaginalis*
    c. Human papillomavirus   d. Inflammatory changes

21. All of the following are screening methods for cervical intraepithelial neoplasia, *except*:
    a. Colposcopic-guided biopsy
    b. Pap smear
    c. Human papillomavirus DNA testing
    d. Visual inspection with acetic acid

22. A patient complaints of postcoital bleed and no growth is seen on per speculum examination; what should be the next step?
    a. Colposcopy biopsy   b. Conization
    c. Repeat Pap smear   d. Culdoscopy

23. A female attends gyne outpatient department (OPD) with history of frequent *T. vaginalis* infection. She was advised for Pap smear and she enquired for role of Pap smear in her. Give reason.
    a. It helps to screen for cervical cancer
    b. It helps to diagnose cancer in genital tract
    c. It helps to demonstrate *T. vaginalis* infection
    d. It helps to diagnose other associated genital infection in patient

24. A 37-year-old woman presented with cervical Pap smear report of High-grade squamous intraepithelial lesion (HGSIL). Colposcopy with biopsy was performed at the histopathological result revealed cervical intraepithelial neoplasia 3. What is the next step in management?
    a. Loop electrosurgical excision procedure (LEEP)
    b. Hysterectomy
    c. Cryotherapy
    d. Diathermy coagulation

25. The FIGO (International Federation of Gynecology and Obstetrics) staging of cervical cancer, which is the internationally accepted classification, is based on which of the following?
    a. Radiological examination with magnetic resonance imaging (MRI)
    b. Surgical examination
    c. Clinical examination with cystoscopy and proctoscopy
    d. None of the above

26. Approximately what proportion of women with stage IVb diseases will survive over 2 years?
    a. 50%   b. 70%
    c. 20%   d. 35%

27. On what part of the cervix do most cancers develop?
    a. Internal orifice   b. Lymph nodes
    c. External orifice   d. None of the about

28. For how long cervical cancer may stay small, not causing problem?
    a. 1–2 years   b. 2–3 years
    c. About 6 months   d. 3 or more years

29. What are the symptoms of cervical cancer in the every stage?
    a. Abdominal cramps and diarrhea
    b. Usually there are none
    c. Anemia and tiredness
    d. Nauseas

30. How many of women are likely to be survive 5 years later if cervical cancer is diagnosed and treated early?
    a. 4 out of 5   b. Almost all of them
    c. 3 out of 10   d. 10 out of 2

31. Human papillomavirus vaccines affect fertility.
    a. True   b. False

32. Human papillomavirus vaccination leads to promiscuity.
    a. True   b. False

33. Human papillomavirus vaccines cause early menopause (primary ovarian failure/premature ovarian insufficiency)?
    a. True   b. False

ANSWERS

1. **c.**
   Early gene:
   - E2:
     - Viral transcription
     - DNA replication
     - Segregation of viral genomes
   - E4:
     - HPV genome amplification
     - Virus maturation
     - Release of virions
   - E5:
     - Increase activity of E6 and E7
     - Generate aneuploidy and chromosomal instability
     - *E6:* Bind and degrade the human suppressor protein PRB

   Late genes:
   - L1:
     - Major capsid protein
     - Attachment to cell surfaces receptors
     - Highly immunogenic and induce production of type-specific antibodies against the virus
     - Minor capsid protein into capsid
     - Helps packing of viral DNA

   (References: 1-6)

2. **d.** Human papillomavirus vaccines available in market are:
   - Cervarix
   - Gardasil 4
   - Gardasil 9

   (References: 7-18)

3. **c.** (References: 7-18)

4. **c.** 0, 2, 6 month
   - Gardasil 4 and Gardasil 9 > 15 dose 0, 2, 6 month
   - Cervarix > 15 0, 1, 6 month
   - 9 to 14 years 0, 6 month

   (References: 7-18)

5. **b.**
   - Cervarix → HPV 6, 11
   - Gardasil 4 → HPV 6, 11, 16, 18
   - Gardasil 9 → HPV 6, 11, 16, 18, 31, 33, 45, 52, 58

   (References: 8-18)

6. **b.** Human papillomavirus vaccine is not recommended for use during pregnancy. People known to be pregnant should delay initiation of the vaccination series until after the pregnancy. However, pregnancy testing before vaccination is not needed. Although HPV vaccine has not been lined to causing any adverse pregnancy, if a person is found to be pregnant after starting the HPV vaccine series second and third dose should be delayed until they are no longer pregnant.

   If a person receives HPV vaccine and later learns that they are pregnant. There is no reason to be alarmed. (References: 7, 8)

7. **b.**
   - HPV 6, 11 → lower risk
   - HPV 16, 18 → High risk

   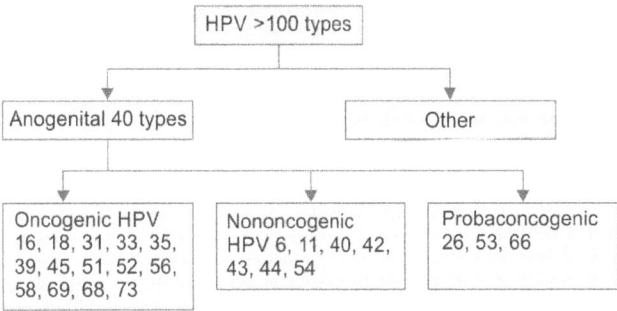

   (Reference: 19)

8. **c.**
   Squamous cell carcinoma:
   - More consistently associated with HPV infection (>95%)
   - All stages of precursor lesion show association with HPV 16

   Adenocarcinoma:
   - Less consistently associate with HPV 40%–89%
   - Endocervical glandular atypia is not associated with HPV 18
   - Minimal deviation adenocarcinoma

   (Reference: 19)

9. **a.** Human papillomavirus virus begins life cycle by infecting the basal cell of the epithelium and within these proliferating cells the viral genomes are replicated, maintained, and passed on to the daughter cells.

Viruses are transferred in seminal fluid which may result in penile cancer and laryngeal carcinoma subsequent to oral sex.
(Reference: 6)

10. **a.**
    - Squamous cell carcinoma caused by HPV 16 MIC (microinvasive carcinomas of the cervix) site is transformation zone.
    - Adenocarcinoma's most common site is endocervix.
    (Reference: 19)

11. **a.** To lower your risk, get screened as recommended, and get the human papillomavirus vaccine if you are in the age group for which it is recommended.
    (Reference: 19)

12. **b.** You should get screened for cervical cancer regularly even if you received an human papillomavirus vaccine.
    (Reference: 19)

13. **b.** Cervical cancer is second most common cancer in women in India. among the ages between 15 and 44 years. About 5% of women in general population are estimated to harbor HPV 16/18 infection at a given time and 83.2% of invasive cortical cancers are attributed to HPV 16 or 18.

- Every year 1,23,907 women are diagnosed with cervical cancer and 77,348 die from the disease in India.
(References: 20, 21)

14. **d.**
Spread of HPV infection—Genitalia to genitalia
Sexual contact—Skin to skin
                    Skin to genitalia
Nonsexual contact—Vertical transmission
                    Fomites
(a) Colposcopy is a diagnostic method.

15. **a.** Colposcopy is diagnostic method
    (Reference: 19)

16. **b.** VIA – Visual inspection with acetic acid is a naked eye examination of uterine cervix, after application of 5% acetic acid and interpreting the result after 1 minute. This is a simple and inexpensive test for the detection of cervical precancerous lesion and early invasive cancer.
    (References: 9-17)

17. **c.** The normal squamous epithelium of cervix is Pink. On application of acetic acid. Cervical intraepithelial neoplasia (CIN) lesion tells on a white color due to the increased nuclear/proteins and cytokeratins in for cervical epithelium.
    (Reference: 22)

18. **d.**

Start age	ACS-ASCCP-ASCP 2012	ACOG 2009	USPSTF 2012	USPSTF 2017
Start age	21	21	21	21
Age 2129 years	Cytology every 3 years (liquid or conventional against annual Pap)	Cytology every 2 years	Cytology every 3 years	Cytology every 3 years (liquid or conventional)
Age 30–65 years	Co-test every 5 years (preferred or every 3 years with cytology alone (acceptable against more frequent screening	Co-test every 3 years or every 3 years with cytology alone	Co-test every 5 years or every 3 years with cytology alone	Cytology every 3 years (liquid or conventional high-risk HPV testing every 5 years; or co-test every 3 years
After 65 years	Discontinue after age of 65 years if 3 negative Pap tests or 2 negative HPV tests in last 10 years with most recent test in last 5 years	Discontinue at age 65–70 years after 3 negative test in last 10 years	Discontinue after age of 65 years if adequate prior screening	Recommence screenings if prior screening is positive

(ACOG: American College of Obstetricians and Gynecologists; ACS: American Cancer Society; ASCCP: American Society for Colposcopy and Cervical Pathology; ASCP: American Society for Clinical Pathology; HPV: human papillomavirus; USPSTF: United States Preventive Services Task Force)

(References: 19, 20, 23, 24)

19. **b.** Early menarche may cause endometrial carcinoma or ovarian carcinoma.
(Reference: 19)

20. **a.** Gonorrhea can be diagnosed by clinical examination and investigation like urine analysis, gram strain smear, and culture on chocolate agar.
(Reference: 19)

21. **a.**
    - Colposcopic-guided biopsy, it is diagnostic test.
    - Screening test for cervical intraepithelial neoplasia are:
        - Pap smear
        - Liquid base cytology
        - Human papillomavirus DNA testing
        - Visual Inspection with Acetic Acid (VIA) and Visual Inspection with Lugol's Iodine (VILI)

(References: 19, 23, 25, 26)

22. **c.** *(References: 19, 23, 25, 26)*

23. **a.**
    - *Bethesda system interpretation in Pap smear:*
        - Specimen type adequately
        - General categorization
        - Automated review
        - Ancillary testing
    - *General categorization:*
        - Negative for intraepithelial lesion
        - Epithelial cell abnormality "squamous" or "glandular"

(References: 19, 23, 25, 26)

24. **a.**
    - Cervical intraepithelial neoplasia is a premalignant lesion that may exist at any one of three stages: CIN 1, CIN 2, CIN 3. If left unrelated, CIN 2 on CIN 3 can progress to cervical cancer. Instead of screening and diagnosis by the standard sequence of cytology, colposcopy, biopsy, and histological confirmation of CIN, an alternative method is to use a "screen and treat" approach in which the treatment decision is based on a screening test and treatment is provided soon.
    - Available treatments according to who guidance for CIN 2 and 3 are large loop excision of transformation zone (LLETZ) and loop electrosurgical excision procedure
    - Cold knife conization

(Reference: 19)

25. **c.** As most cases of cervical cancer occur in the developing world. Staging is based on clinical examination, although impressed imaging with magnetic resonance imaging (MRI) has added greater prediction of paramedical pelvis lymph node involvement.
(Reference: 19)

26. **c.** Roughly 20% of women with stage IVb disease will survive for 2 years.
(Reference: 19)

27. **c.** *External OS:* Most cervical cancer start in the calls of the external OS of the without treatment, this cancer can reach the small blood vessels and lymph vessels in the cervix and from there it can spread to rest of the body.
(Reference: 19)

28. **d.**
    3 or more years:
    - Most of cervical precancers and cancers develop slowly over time.
    - That is why it is important to have regular tests for cervical cancer.
    - If all women had regular pelvis examination and primary HPV tests or HPV/Pap tests, cervical precancers could be created and most invasive cervical cancer should be pretend.
    - One good way to prevent cervical cancer is to get HPV vaccination.

(Reference: 19)

29. **b.** Usually there are none.
    - Most of cases by the time symphony are noticed, the cancer has already grown and spread into nearby tissue
    - Abnormal vaginal discharge, bleeding after menopause, pelvis pain or pain during sex may be signs of cervical cancer.

(Reference: 19)

30. **a.** *(Reference: 19)*

31. **b.**
    - No; human papillomavirus vaccines do not affect fertility. They do help protect a woman's health and fertility.
    - Clinical trials before the first HPV vaccine was licensed in 2006 and safety monitoring and studies since its introduction have confirmed that the vaccine does not cause any reproductive problems in women.

- In fact, the HPV vaccine helps to protect fertility by preventing precancerous cervical growths ("lesions") and cervical cancer caused by HPV. Surgical treatment of precancerous cervical lesions can make it more difficult for a woman to become pregnant, and surgery during pregnancy can lead to premature labor and loss of a fetus. Treatment for cervical cancer (removal of the cervix and uterus, chemotherapy, and/or radiation) leaves a woman unable to bear children.

(References: 27-31)

32. b.
- No; there is no evidence that HPV vaccination has any impact on sexual activity.
- Like every vaccine, it is best to be vaccinated before exposure to the infection.
- The HPV infection is the most common sexually transmitted infection worldwide. The highest rates of HPV infection occur in sexually active men and women up to age 25 years. HPV vaccination before a person becomes sexually active reduces the risk of infection because the vaccines protect against HPV types that cause up to 90% of cervical cancer cases and 90% of genital warts.
- Several studies have found no evidence that HPV vaccination leads to increased sexual activity.

(References: 27-31)

33. b.
- No; there is no evidence of a link between early menopause (primary ovarian failure/premature ovarian insufficiency) and HPV vaccination.
- Primary ovarian failure, also known as premature ovarian insufficiency, occurs when the ovaries stop working, leading to early menopause. The cause of premature ovarian failure is often unknown, but in some cases, it may be due to cancer treatment or an autoimmune disease.
- The WHO (World Health Organization) Global Advisory Committee on Vaccine Safety (GACVS) reported in 2017 after reviewing large population level data from several countries including Denmark and the United States that it saw no evidence for a causal association between HPV vaccine and primary ovarian failure/premature ovarian insufficiency.
- About 90 million doses of HPV vaccine were administered in the United States in the period from 2009 through 2017. The United States Centers for Disease Control and Prevention (US CDC) monitoring in this period through the Vaccine Adverse Event Reporting System (VAERS) did not detect any increase in incidence of primary ovarian failure/premature ovarian insufficiency following HPV vaccination.

(References: 27-31)

REFERENCES

1. Mittal S, Banks L. Molecular mechanisms underlying human papillomavirus E6 and E7 oncoprotein-induced cell transformation. Mutat Res Rev Mutat Res. 2017;772:23-35.
2. Azuma YR, Kusumoto-Matsuo R, Takeuchi F, Uenoyama A, Kondo K, Tsunoda H, et al. Human papillomavirus genotype distribution in cervical intraepithelial neoplasia grade 2/3 and invasive cervical cancer in Japanese women. Jpn J Clin Oncol. 2014;44:910-7.
3. Choi YS, Kang WD, Kim SM, Choi YD, Nam JH, Park CS, et al. Human papillomavirus L1 capsid protein and human papillomavirus type 16 as prognostic markers in cervical intraepithelial neoplasia 1. Int J Gynecol Cancer. 2010;20:288-93.
4. Tang S, Tao M, McCoy JP, Zheng ZM. The E7 oncoprotein is translated from spliced E6*I transcripts in high-risk human papilloma virus type 16- or type 18-positive cervical cancer cell lines via translation reinitiation. J Virol. 2006;80:4249-63.
5. Biryukov J, Myers JC, McLaughlin-Drubin ME, Griffin HM, Milici J, Doorbar J, et al. Mutations in HPV18 E1^E4 impact virus capsid assembly, infectivity competence, and maturation. Viruses. 2017;9:385.
6. Oxford J, Kellam P, Collier L. Human Virology, 5th edition. Oxford: Oxford University Press; 2016. pp. 220-2.
7. Dana A, Buchanan KM, Goss MA, Seminack MM, Shields KE, Korn S, et al. Pregnancy outcomes from the pregnancy registry of a human papillomavirus type 6/11/16/18 vaccine. Obstet Gynecol. 2009;114(6):1170-8.
8. Merck & Co. Merck pregnancy registry program. Fourth annual report on exposure during pregnancy from the Merck pregnancy registry for quadrivalent human papillomavirus (types 6, 11, 16, 18) recombinant vaccine [GARDASIL/SILGARD] covering the period from first approval (June 1, 2006) through May 31, 2010. North Wales, PA: Merck & Co. In press.
9. Ali H, Donovan B, Wand H, Read TR, Regan DG, Grulich AE, et al. Genital warts in young Australians five years into national human papillomavirus vaccination programme: national surveillance data. BMJ 2013;346:f2032.
10. Markowitz LE, Dunne EF, Saraiya M, Chesson HW, Curtis CR, Gee J, et al.; Centers for Disease Control and Prevention (CDC). Human papillomavirus vaccination: recommendations of the Advisory Committee on

Immunization Practices (ACIP). MMWR Recomm Rep. 2014;63(RR-05):1-30.
11. Artemchuk H, Eriksson T, Poljak M, Surcel HM, Dillner J, Lehtinen M, et al. Long-Term Antibody Response to Human Papillomavirus Vaccines: Up to 12 Years Follow-Up in the Finnish Maternity Cohort. J Infect Dis. 2019;219(4):582-9.
12. Centers for Disease Control and Prevention. (2023). Questions about HPV Vaccine Safety. [online] Available from https://www.cdc.gov/vaccinesafety/vaccines/hpv/hpv-safety-faqs.html#A6 [Last accessed December, 2023].
13. World Health Organization. (2018). Upswing in HPV vaccination in Ireland. [online] Available from https://www.who.int/europe/news/item/18-09-2018-upswing-in-hpv-vaccination-in-ireland [Last accessed December, 2023].
14. Markowitz LE, Dunne EF, Saraiya M, et al. Human papillomavir vaccination: recommendations of the Advisory Committee on Immunization Practices (ACIP). MMWR Recomm Rep. 2014;63(No. RR-05). https:// www.cdc.gov/mmwr/preview/mmwrhtml/m6305a 1.htm 2.
15. Petrosky E, Bocchini JA Jr, Hariri S, et al. Use of 9-valent human papillomavirus (HPV) vaccine: updated HPV vaccination recommendations of the Advisory Committee on Immunization Practices. MMWR Morb Mortal Wkly Rep. 2015;64:300-4. https://www.cdc.gov/mmwr/preview/mmwrhtml/mm6411a3.htm
16. Meites E, Kempe A, Markowitz LE. Use of a 2-dose schedule for human papillomavirus vaccination-updated recommendations of the Advisory Committee on Immunization Practices. MMWR Morb Mortal Wkly Rep. 2016;65:1405-8. https://doi.org/10.15585/mmwr.mm6549a5
17. Food and Drug Administration. Prescribing information [package insert]. Gardasil 9 (human papillomavirus 9-valent vaccine, recombinant). Silver Spring, MD: US Department of Health and Human Services, Food and Drug Administration; 2018. https://www.fda.gov/media/90064/download 7. Food and Drug Administration. Prescribing information [package insert). Gardasil (human papillomavirus quadrivalent [types 6, 11, 16, and 18] vaccine, recombinant). Silver Spring, MD: US Department of Health and Human Services, Food and Drug Administration; 2015. https://www.fda.gov/media/74350/download
18. WHO: Comprehensive cervical cancer prevention and control: a healthier future for girls and women. Available: http://www.who.int/immunization/h pv/learn/comprehensive cervical cancer who 2013.pdf.
19. Berek & Novak's Gynecology. 16th edition (Chapter 16 (Page No. 912 – 945), Chapter 38)
20. Fontham, ETH, Wolf, AMD, Church, TR, et al. Cervical Cancer Screening for Individuals at Average Risk: 2020 Guideline Update from the American Cancer Society. CA Cancer J Clin. 2020. https://doi.org/10.3322/caac.21628.
21. Sundar S, Horne A, Kehoe S. Cervical Cancer. Clin Evid. 13:2285- 2292 3. Stewart BW, Kleihues P (editors) (2003) World cancer report, Lyon (France): IARC Press. 351 p
22. National Institute of Cancer Preventions & Research. 5th edition, Training Manual (Page No 5-8).
23. WHO guidelines for the use of thermal ablation for cervical pre-cancer lesions, Geneva: World Health Organization: 2019 (http://answho.int/ hitz handle/10665/329299/97892 41550558.eng.pdf).
24. Introducing and scaling up testing for human papillomavirus as part of a comprehensive programme for prevention and control of cervical cancer: a step by step guide. Geneva: World Health Organization; 2020 (www.who.int/publications/item/Bras-40075166),
25. WHO technical guidance and specifications of medical devices for screening and treatment of precancerous lesions in the prevention of cervical cancer. Geneva: World Health Organization:2020 (//.who.int//bitstream/handle/10565/331698/9789240007630-eng.pof 18, WHO handbook for guideline development, second edition. Geneva: World Health Organization
26. 2 Global strategy to accelerate the elimination of cervical cancer as a public health problem. Geneva: World Heath Organization, 2020 (tps://www.who.int/publications//tem/9789240014107)
27. Centers for Disease Control and Prevention. Questions about HPV Vaccine Safety, 2019 https://www.cdc.gov/vaccinesafety/vaccines/hpv/hpv-safety-faqs.html#A6
28. Cook EE et al. Legislation to Increase Uptake of HPV Vaccination and Adolescent Sexual Behaviors. Pediatrics September 2018;142(3):e20180458; DOI: https://doi.org/10.1542/peds.2018-0458
29. Smith LM et al. Effect of human papillomavirus (HPV) vaccination on clinical indicators of sexual behaviour among adolescent girls: the Ontario Grade 8 HPV Vaccine Cohort Study. CMAJ. 2015;187(2):E74-E81. doi: 10.1503/cmaj 140900
30. Donken R et al. Effect of human papillomavirus vaccination on sexual behaviour among young females. Can Fam Physician. 2018;64(7):509-13. https://www.ncbi.nlm.nih.gov/pmc/articles/PMC6042675/
31. Bednarczyk RA et al. Sexual activity-related outcomes after human papillomavirus vaccination of 11- to 12-year-olds. Pediatrics. 2012;130(5):798-805, doi: 10.1542/peds.2012-1516

Chapter 100: Carcinoma of Ovary

Rajshree Dayanand Katke

QUESTIONS

1. What is the most common cell origin of malignancy in carcinoma of ovary?
   a. Epithelial
   b. Mucinous
   c. Sertoli-Leydig
   d. Clear cell carcinoma

2. What is the percentage of incidence of carcinoma of ovary in India in women?
   a. 7.4%
   b. 5.3%
   c. 2%
   d. 4.2%

3. What is the role of genetic factor in the etiology of carcinoma of ovary?
   a. *BRCA1 and BRCA2* gene mutation
   b. Mismatch repair (MMR)
   c. Tumor suppressor gene *TP53*
   d. All of the above

4. Which are the most common malignancy in ovary in adolescent girls?
   a. Germ cell tumors
   b. Epithelial tumors
   c. Mucinous tumors
   d. Endometroid tumors

5. What percentage of malignant ovarian neoplasms is of germ cell origin?
   a. 5% of these tumors are malignant
   b. 3% of these tumors are malignant
   c. 8% of these tumors are malignant
   d. 6% of these tumors are malignant

6. What are the symptoms in carcinoma of ovary?
   a. Abdominal pain
   b. Abdominal distention
   c. Bowel irregularity
   d. All of the above

7. What is the most common site of primary Krukenberg's tumor?
   a. Stomach
   b. Ovary
   c. Uterus
   d. Liver

8. Individuals whose karyotypes contain a Y cell line (45,X/46,XY mosaicism or pure gonadal dysgenesis 46,XY) are predisposed to which of the following tumors?
   a. Gonadoblastomas
   b. dysgerminomas
   c. Yolk sac tumors
   d. All of the above

9. What are the histological characteristics to define borderline ovarian tumors?
   a. Complex papillary structures
   b. Multilayered epithelium
   c. Mild nuclear atypia and slightly increased mitotic activity, but do not destruct stromal invasion
   d. All of the above

10. How much is the percentage of risk of breast cancer in women with a *BRCA1* or *BRCA2* mutation?
    a. 30%–40%
    b. 5%–10%
    c. 56%–87%
    d. 40%–50%

11. What is the classical finding in serous tumor on histopathology?
    a. Psammoma bodies
    b. Howell-Jolly bodies
    c. Call-Exner bodies
    d. None of the above

12. What is percentage of invasive endometroid tumor of the ovary?
    a. 6%–8%
    b. 20%
    c. 2%
    d. 1%

13. What is rate of para-aortic lymph nodes positivity for metastasis of carcinoma of ovary stagewise?
    a. 18% in stage I, 20% in stage II, 42% in stage III, and 67% in stage IV
    b. 10% in stage I, 15% in stage II, 20% in stage III, and 30% in stage IV
    c. 30% in stage I, 45% in stage II, 60% in stage III, and 80% in stage IV
    d. 25% in stage I, 50% in stage II, 60% in stage III, and 70% in stage IV

14. **What is the first step of surgical staging in carcinoma of ovary?**
    a. Free fluid, especially in the pelvic cul-de-sac taken for cytologic evaluation
    b. If no free fluid is present, peritoneal washings should be performed with 50-100 mL normal saline
    c. Removal of tumor
    d. Both (a) and (b)

15. **What is clinical presentation of carcinoid tumors?**
    a. Flushing—80%
    b. Diarrhea and pain in abdomen
    c. Pellagra-like skin lesions—5%
    d. All of the above

16. **Regarding tumor markers, what is most common in ovarian malignancy?**
    a. Cancer antigen 125 (CA 125)
    b. CA 19.9
    c. Alpha-fetoprotein and beta-human chorionic gonadotropin
    d. All of above

17. **Alpha-fetoprotein is increased in which ovarian malignancy?**
    a. Epithelial
    b. Endometroid
    c. Germ cell tumors
    d. Breast

18. **How much is the sensitivity of serum CA 125 as a tumor marker in carcinoma of ovary?**
    a. 20%-50%
    b. 60%-70%
    c. 10%-20%
    d. 80%-90%

19. **In which conditions CA 125 is raised?**
    a. Endometriosis
    b. Carcinoma of ovary
    c. Chronic pelvic inflammatory disease and tuberculosis
    d. All of the above

20. **In mucinous ovarian malignancy which are the tumor markers used?**
    a. CA 125
    b. Carcinoembryonic antigen (CEA)
    c. CA 19.9
    d. All of the above

21. **What are the components of Risk of Ovarian Malignancy Algorithm (ROMA) index?**
    a. CA 125
    b. Human epididymis protein 4 (HE4) level
    c. Menopausal status
    d. All of the above

22. **Which of the following are components of second look laparotomy in carcinoma of ovary?**
    a. Steps are identical that of staging laparotomy
    b. Multiple cytologic specimens to be obtained
    c. Peritoneal surface biopsy to be collected
    d. All of the above

23. **Which of the following hormonal therapies are used in carcinoma of ovary?**
    a. Tamoxifen
    b. Gonadotropin agonist
    c. Aromatase inhibitors
    d. All of the above

24. **What are advantages of carboplatin as compared to cisplatin in carcinoma of ovary?**
    a. Reduced incidence of emesis
    b. Reduced incidence of sensory neuropathy
    c. Reduced incidence of ototoxicity and nephrotoxicity
    d. All of the above

25. **Which drugs used in germ cell tumor of ovary?**
    a. bleomycin, etoposide, cisplatin (BEP) regimen
    b. Tamoxifen
    c. Cyclophosphamide
    d. Methotrexate

26. **Which of the following chemotherapeutic agents used in nongestational choriocarcinoma?**
    a. Methotrexate
    b. Actinomycin D
    c. Cyclophosphamide
    d. All of the above

27. **What is role of poly(ADP-ribose) polymerase (PARP) inhibitors in carcinoma of ovary?**
    a. It targets defective DNA repair
    b. It is used in maintenance chemotherapy
    c. It is used in platinum-sensitive relapsed cases
    d. All of the above

28. **What is the surgical management of carcinoma of ovary International Federation of Gynecology and Obstetrics (FIGO) stage IA?**
    a. Total abdominal hysterectomy and bilateral salpingo-oophorectomy
    b. Supracolic total omentectomy
    c. Removal of lymph nodes
    d. All of the above

29. **Role of neoadjuvant chemotherapy is:**
    a. It decreases size of mass
    b. It decreases vascularity
    c. It is treatment option in patients who are unable to undergo primary complete resection
    d. All of the above

30. **How much is the survival rate in stage 1 of carcinoma of ovary with complete treatment?**
    a. 60%–70%
    b. 40%–50%
    c. 90%–100%
    d. 70%–80%

ANSWERS

1. **a.** Epithelial cell cancer is the most common cell origin of malignancy in carcinoma of ovary.

   About 90% of the ovarian cancers are from coelomic epithelium, these cells are from the origin of mesoderm which can undergo metaplasia.

2. **a.** Percentage of incidence of carcinoma of ovary in India in women is 7.4%.

3. **d.** Roles of genetic factor in the etiology of carcinoma of ovary are as follows:
   - *BRCA1 and BRCA2 gene mutation:* Most hereditary ovarian cancer is associated with mutations in the *BRCA1* gene, located on chromosome 17 (46). A small proportion of inherited disease has been traced to another gene, *BRCA2*, located on chromosome 13.
   - Mismatch repair (MMR)
   - Tumor suppressor gene *TP53*

4. **a.** Germ cell tumor is the most common malignancy in ovary in adolescent girls.

5. **b.** About 3% of the malignant ovarian neoplasms are of germ cell origin.

6. **d.** Symptoms in carcinoma of ovary are as follows:
   - Abdominal pain
   - Abdominal distention
   - Bowel irregularity

7. **a.** The most common site of primary Krukenberg's tumor is stomach.

8. **d.** Individuals whose karyotypes contain a Y cell line (45,X/46,XY mosaicism or pure gonadal dysgenesis 46,XY) are predisposed to gonadal ridge tumors such as gonadoblastomas, dysgerminomas, and yolk sac tumors.

9. **d.** Histological characteristics of borderline ovarian tumors are as follows:
   - Complex papillary structures
   - Multilayered epithelium
   - Mild nuclear atypia and slightly increased mitotic activity, but do not destruct stromal invasion

10. **c.** There is 56–87% percentage of risk of breast cancer in women with a *BRCA1* or *BRCA2* mutation.

11. **a.** Classical finding in serous tumor on histopathology is psammoma bodies.

12. **c.** Percentage of invasive endometroid tumor of the ovary is 2%.

13. **a.** Rate of paraaortic lymph nodes positivity for metastasis of carcinoma of ovary stagewise is 18% in stage I, 20% in stage II, 42% in stage III, and 67% in stage IV.

14. **d.** If ovarian malignancy is present and the tumor is apparently confined to the ovaries or the pelvis, surgical staging should be performed.

    Staging involves the following steps:
    - Any free fluid, especially in the pelvic cul-de-sac, should be sent for cytologic evaluation.
    - If no free fluid is present, peritoneal washings should be with 50–100 mL of saline.
    - A systematic exploration of intra-abdominal surfaces and viscera is performed.
    - Suspicious areas or adhesions present on the peritoneal surfaces should be sampled for biopsy.
    - The diaphragm should be sampled for cytologic assessment.
    - The omentum should be resected from the transverse colon (infracolic omentectomy).
    - The retroperitoneal spaces should be explored to assess the pelvic and paraaortic lymph nodes.

15. **d.** Clinical presentation of carcinoid tumors includes following:
    - Flushing—80%
    - Diarrhea and pain in abdomen
    - Pellagra-like skin lesions—5%

16. **d.** Tumor markers in ovarian malignancy are as follows:
    - Cancer antigen 125 (CA 125)
    - CA 19.9
    - Alpha fetoprotein
    - Beta-human chorionic gonadotropin

17. **c.** Alpha fetoprotein level is increased in germ cell tumors.
18. **a.** Sensitivity of serum CA 125 as a tumor marker in carcinoma of ovary is 20%–50%.
19. **d.** Conditions in which CA 125 is raised are as follows:
    - Endometriosis
    - Carcinoma of ovary
    - Chronic pelvic inflammatory disease
    - Tuberculosis
20. **d.** Tumor markers used in mucinous ovarian malignancy are:
    - CA 125
    - Carcinoembryonic antigen (CEA)
    - CA 19.9
21. **d.** Components of Risk of Ovarian Malignancy Algorithm (ROMA) index includes:
    - CA 125
    - Human epididymis protein 4 (HE4) level
    - Menopausal status
22. **d.** The second-look laparotomy technique is identical to that for the staging laparotomy.

    Operation is performed through a vertical abdominal incision. The incision is taken below the level of the umbilicus, so that if pelvic disease is detected in the absence of any palpable upper abdominal disease, a smaller incision might suffice. The incision is extended cranially as per need:
    - Multiple cytologic specimens to be obtained
    - Peritoneal surface biopsy to be collected, particularly in any areas of previously documented tumor
23. **d.** Hormonal therapies used in carcinoma of ovary are as follows:
    - Tamoxifen
    - Gonadotropin agonist
    - Aromatase inhibitors
24. **d.** Advantages of carboplatin as compared to cisplatin in carcinoma of ovary are as follows:
    - Reduced incidence of emesis
    - Reduced incidence of sensory neuropathy
    - Reduced incidence of ototoxicity and nephrotoxicity
25. **a.** Chemotherapeutic agents used in germ cell tumor of ovary includes bleomycin, etoposide, cisplatin (BEP) regimen.
26. **d.** Chemotherapeutic agents used in nongestational choriocarcinoma are as follows:
    - Methotrexate
    - Actinomycin D
    - Cyclophosphamide
27. **d.** Roles of poly (ADP-ribose) polymerase (PARP) inhibitors in carcinoma of ovary are as follows:
    - It targets defective DNA repair.
    - It is used in maintenance chemotherapy.
    - It is used in platinum-sensitive relapsed cases
28. **d.** Surgical management of carcinoma of ovary (FIGO) stage IA includes:
    - Total abdominal hysterectomy and bilateral salpingo-oophorectomy
    - Supracolic total omentectomy
    - Removal of lymph nodes
29. **d.** Neoadjuvant chemotherapy is a treatment option in patients who are unable to undergo primary complete resection.

    Neoadjuvant chemotherapy decreases the size of mass and vascularity.
30. **c.** Survival rate in stage 1 of carcinoma of ovary with complete treatment is about 90%–100%.

REFERENCES

1. Berek JS. Novaks Gyanecology.Lippincott Williams & Wilkins, 2000.
2. Kumar S, Padubidri VG , Daftary SN. Shaws Textbook of Gyanecology 18th Edition.

Chapter 101

Germ Cell Tumors

Vandana Solanki, Vertika Singh

QUESTIONS

1. An 8-year-old girl, not achieved menarche, presented with abdominal distension and a lump 10×5 cm, globular, irregular margins with restricted up and down mobility.
   CT scan showed a mass of 15.52 × 11.52 × 10.73. Serum LDH was raised.
   Laparotomy was done on a smooth bosselated mass with cut section solid fleshy and tan was removed. 11 months later, she came with a CT scan showing an 8 × 5 cm hypoechoic preaortic mass with mildly dilated pelvicalyceal system what is next step of management?
   a. FNAC from mass
   b. Second look laparotomy
   c. Chemotherapy
   d. Follow-up after 1 week

2. A 4-year-old female from Haryana presented with abdominal lump for 1 months and bleeding per vagina on and off for 7 days. On abdominal examination, a hard 20 × 20 cm mass is felt with indistinct margins and restricted mobility. Tumor markers are within normal limits. MRI was suggestive of a solid and cystic (mixed) lobulated mass 19 × 19 × 16 cm in abdominopelvic region suggestive of teratoma. Which of the following statements is *incorrect*?
   a. Tumor markers are positive in mixed variants
   b. Elevated AFP levels are associated with presence of embryonic hepatic and intestinal components
   c. Contralateral involvement is common and routine wedge resection is advised in all patients
   d. In premenopausal females, fertility preserving operations are recommended

3. A 7-year-old girl presented to the gynecology OPD with abdominal pain for 2 months and vaginal bleeding as spotting for 15 days. On examination, patient had a mass of 16 × 16 cm with indistinct margins and restricted side-to-side mobility in the pelvic region. Patient had tanner stage 2 breast and pubic hair development. Tumor markers AFP and beta-HCG were raised. CT scan showed a 16 × 16 × 18 cm solid mass with areas of hemorrhage and necrosis displacing bowel. On the basis of the above clinical picture, which is correct?
   a. The patient has embryonal carcinoma which is secreting estrogen
   b. Shows Shiller dual bodies in HPE
   c. The above tumor may rarely secrete alpha-1 antitrypsin
   d. Triphasic teratoma

4. Which of the following is incorrect regarding GCT?
   a. Most of the germ cell variants are unilateral tumors
   b. They account for about 70 percentage of all ovarian neoplasms in first 20 decades of life
   c. They are slow growing in nature
   d. Better prognosis

5. A 12-year-old female presented in gynecology OPD with a mass of 10×14 cm solid mass with an intact capsule in right ovary on the CT scan.
   Patient had abnormal facial hair, acne, and deep voice.
   Tumors markers were positive for LDH.
   What is the plan of management in such a patient?
   a. Total abdominal hysterectomy and B/l salpingo-oophorectomy
   b. Unilateral salpingo-oophorectomy
   c. Unilateral oophorectomy and inspection of contralateral side
   d. Bilateral oophorectomy

6. Which of the following is incorrect regarding dysgerminoma?
   a. Dysgerminomas comprise 30–40 percentage of all GCT
   b. They are commonly associated with precocious puberty and virilization is seen
   c. They are seen to arise from gonadoblastomas in gonadal dysgenesis
   d. Seen only in males

7. A 21-year-old female with history of primary amenorrhea currently on estrogen and progesterone supplements for menstruation and menstruating with a 46 XY karyotype presented with pain in lower abdomen. Patient is 164 cm tall with tanner stage 4 breast development and adult distribution of pubic hair. CT scan showed a 5 × 5 × 4 cm solid mass involving the right ovary. Laparotomy was done and HPE was suggestive of dysgerminomas. Which of the following statements is correct?
   a. 15% of dysgerminomas are seen in phenotypic females with abnormal gonads
   b. Malignancy can be associated with patients who have pure gonadal dysgenesis but not in those with mixed gonadal dysgenesis and androgen insensitive syndrome
   c. In most cases, dysgerminomas arise from gonadoblastomas
   d. Malignancy in gonadoblastomas is rarely seen if left in situ

8. A 22-year-old G1P0+0 34 week single live intrauterine pregnancy came with dull on and off pain in abdomen for 1 month and an MRI suggestive of a solid mass 10 × 12 cm mass with a vascular pedicle arising from left ovary. On examination, a 12 × 12 cm is palpable separate from uterus. Patient is admitted and tumors markers are done which are suggestive of raised Serum LDH.
   What would the line of further management?
   a. Immediate termination of pregnancy
   b. Elective LSCS along with laparotomy
   c. Chemotherapy should be started
   d. Chemotherapy after delivery

9. What is the most common mode of spread of dysgerminomas?
   a. Blood   b. Transcoelomic
   c. Lymphatic   d. Direct invasion

10. What is the treatment of metastatic disease in case of dysgerminomas?
    a. Bilateral salpingo-oophorectomy
    b. BEP regimen for four cycles
    c. Unilateral l salpingo-oophorectomy only
    d. Unilateral salpingo-oophorectomy with resection of suspicious lesion followed by BEP for four cycles

11. Which of the following is a correct statement?
    a. Dysgerminomas during pregnancy need termination of pregnancy
    b. Chemotherapy is contraindicated in pregnant females with dysgerminomas
    c. Surgery for dysgerminomas to be done after delivery
    d. Chemotherapy is given in same doses in pregnancy with dysgerminomas as in nonpregnant

12. A 13-year-old girl came in gynecology OPD with complaints of a hard mass in right flank for about 2 months. On examination, it was 12 × 8 cm with irregular margins. Laparotomy was done and the mass was sent for HPE which was later suggestive of dysgerminoma components and Schiller–Duval bodies. Which of the following is correct?
    a. The least common component is endodermal sinus tumor
    b. The most frequent combination is dysgerminomas and embryonal carcinoma
    c. Elevated levels of serum levels of AFP and HCG are a characteristic of these tumors
    d. Most important prognostic factor is size of the primary tumor and its most malignant component

13. Which of the following are incorrect statement regarding recurrence in dysgerminomas?
    a. Lesions larger than 10–15 cm are more likely to recur
    b. Lesions appear before 20 years recur more
    c. Microscopic patterns suggesting numerous mitosis, anaplasia, and a medullary pattern recur more
    d. None of the above

14. A 20-year-old married female, married life—2 years, came to the emergency room 1month ago with abdominal distension and intermittent pain for past 20 days. Urine pregnancy test was done which was negative. Examination showed a 15 × 18 cm solid mass with irregular margins, felt separate from uterus in left adnexa. CT scan showed a mass of 12 × 15 cm with solid and cystic

components with abnormal vessels in left adnexa and mild ascites. The levels of AFP were elevated. Which of the following statements is true for the above clinical scenario?
- Statement A—in rare cases, these tumors also secrete alpha-1 antitrypsin
- Statement B—biopsy of suspicious lesions of contralateral ovaries are advised
- Statement C—the median age group of presentation is 16-18 years
- Statement D—hysterectomy and contralateral salpingo-oophorectomy has been seen to improve outcome
   a. B and D
   b. A and C
   c. A and D
   d. C and D

15. Most common malignancy to develop in pure benign teratomas:
   a. Adenocarcinoma
   b. SCC
   c. Sarcoma
   d. Mixed mesodermal tumor

16. Which of the following is incorrect statement about immature teratomas?
   a. The most frequent site of metastasis is peritoneum
   b. They are highly chemosensitive tumors
   c. Contralateral involvement is common needing routine wedge biopsy of opposite ovary
   d. Tumor markers AFP and HCG are negative

17. Most important prognostic factor of immature teratoma is:
   a. Stage
   b. Site
   c. Size
   d. Grade

18. 5 year survival rates with all stages of pure immature teratoma are:
   a. 80-90%
   b. 60-70%
   c. 50-60%
   d. 70-80%

19. Which of the following is an incorrect statement regarding endodermal sinus tumor?
   a. Contralateral salpingo-oophorectomy has no significant effect on outcome
   b. Chromosomal analysis in premenarcheal patients is of no significance
   c. They secrete alpha-1 antitrypsin
   d. AFP levels correlate to extent of disease

20. A 26-year-old G3P1+1(L1) 10week pregnancy came to the emergency room with abdominal pain and dizziness. On examination, there was tenderness in left iliac fossa. On per vaginum examination, a mass of 6×6 was felt in left fornix with tenderness, uterus was approximately 10 weeks in size. USG showed a viable 10 week 3 day fetus and a 7 ×5 cm ovary with large heterogeneous area and normal Doppler study raising suspicion of ovarian torsion. Detorsion was done and a bosselated tumor was removed. HPE showed dysgerminoma with stage 1A. What is the next line of management?
   a. Follow-up
   b. MRI followed by laparotomy at 14-16 weeks
   c. Adjuvant chemotherapy
   d. Immediate termination of pregnancy

21. Best treatment modality for endodermal sinus tumor of the ovary:
   a. Unilateral salpingo-oophorectomy
   b. Bilateral salpingo-oophorectomy and hysterectomy in postmenopausal females
   c. Unilateral salpingo-oophorectomy with 1 cycle of BEP every 15 days
   d. Unilateral salpingo-oophorectomy with frozen section followed by four cycles of BEP given every 21 days

22. What percentage of leukemia is associated with etoposide treatment in cases of germ cell tumors receiving BEP regime?
   a. 0.4-0.5%
   b. 4-5%
   c. 2-3%
   d. 0.3-0.4%

23. Which of the following statements is incorrect about polyembryoma?
   a. They comprise embryoid bodies
   b. They are common in premenarcheal girls
   c. They are associated with elevated HCG and AFP
   d. Pseudopuberty is a feature not seen with these tumors

24. What chemotherapy regimen is commonly used in choriocarcinoma of ovary?
   a. BEP
   b. MAC
   c. VAC
   d. ACE

25. The most frequently seen mixed germ cell tumor combination is:
   a. Dysgerminomas and endodermal sinus tumor
   b. Embryonal carcinoma and dysgerminomas
   c. Dysgerminomas and polyembryoma
   d. Dysgerminomas and pure immature teratoma

26. **Most important prognostic factor of mixed germ cell tumors is:**
    a. Size of entire tumor only
    b. Size of most malignant component
    c. a and b both
    d. Grade

27. **Embryonal carcinoma is histologically different from choriocarcinoma of ovary:**
    a. Syncytiotrophoblast present in embryonal carcinoma and cytotrophoblast absent
    b. Syncytiotrophoblast absent in embryonal carcinoma and cytotrophoblast present
    c. Both types of cells are present in embryonal carcinoma
    d. Both types of cells are absent in embryonal carcinoma

28. **Which of the following statements is incorrect regarding embryonal carcinoma of ovary?**
    a. They secrete AFP, HCG, and estrogen
    b. They are most commonly seen in the group age 4-28 years
    c. Treatment of choice is bilateral oophorectomy followed by BEP for 4-6 cycles
    d. Precocious puberty is seen

29. **Which of the following is correct about radiotherapy in dysgerminomas?**
    a. Dysgerminomas are not very radiosensitive
    b. Radiotherapy for dysgerminomas is associated with loss of fertility
    c. Radiotherapy is given routinely in doses 2,500-3,000 Gy
    d. It is the first-line management in dysgerminomas for metastatic disease

30. **What is the recurrence rate in the 1st year after treatment for dysgerminomas?**
    a. 88%   b. 90%
    c. 66%   d. 75%

ANSWERS

1. **c.** Chemotherapy
   Dysgerminomas are confined to single ovary hence unilateral salpingo-oophorectomy is advised. Follow-up is done by physical examination every 2 months for first 12 months and CT scan at 6 and 12 months. For occult metastatic disease, chemotherapy by BEP regimen for 4-6 cycles is recommended.
   (Reference: Bereck's and Novack's, 16th edition)

2. **c.** Contralateral involvement is rare and routine wedge resection or biopsy is not recommended in cases of pure immature teratoma.
   The pure mature teratoma is seen in age <20 years, comprises 10-20% of all ovarian malignancy. Precocious puberty is seen.
   "In postmenopausal females, total abdominal hysterectomy and bilateral salpingo-oophorectomy may be performed with complete staging."
   "In premenopausal females as immature teratomas are confined to one ovary, unilateral oophorectomy and fertility sparing surgery is performed."
   (Reference: Berecks and Novacks, 16th edition)

3. **a.** The above features, i.e., elevated AFP and beta-HCG, precocious puberty, and irregular bleeding due to elevated estrogen are seen in embryonal carcinoma
   Embryonal carcinoma is extremely rare tumors commonly seen in age group 4-28 with median 14 years. Treatment involves unilateral oophorectomy followed by combination chemotherapy with BEP.
   (Reference: Berecks and Novacks, 16th edition)

4. **c.** Germ cell tumors are *rapidly growing* tumors leading to better prognosis due to early detection. They are derived from primordial germ cells of the ovary. In the first 2 decades, almost 70% tumors are germ cell tumors.
   (Reference: Berecks and Novacks, 16th edition)

5. **c.** The age of the patient and elevated serum LDH point toward the diagnosis of dysgerminomas...the treatment modality for dysgerminomas is unilateral oophorectomy (fertility preserving) and contralateral inspection at 10-15% cases can show bilateral tumor.
   (Reference: Berecks and Novacks, 16th edition)

6. **d.** Dysgerminomas are seen in both sexes and can arise from extragonadal sites
   (Reference: Berecks and Novacks, 16th edition)

7. **c.** The above clinical scenario is suggestive of Swyer syndrome with pure gonadal dysgenesis.
   5% dysgerminomas are seen abnormal gonads of phenotypic females.
   More than 50% of gonadoblastomas develop malignant chances if in situ.
   Malignancy can be associated with patients who have pure gonadal dysgenesis, mixed gonadal dysgenesis, and androgen insensitive syndrome.
   (Reference: Berecks and Novacks, 16th edition)

8. b. Elective LSCS with laparotomy
Presence of dysgerminomas is not an indication of termination of pregnancy
   With stage 1 a patient can continue pregnancy after tumor removal.
   Chemotherapy can be safely given in nonpregnant doses in second and third trimester.
(Reference: Berecks and Novacks, 16th edition)

9. c.

10. d. Unilateral salpingo-oophorectomy with resection of suspicious lesion followed by BEP for 4-6 cycles.
(Reference: Figure 39-20 page 1136, Berecks and Novacks, 16th edition)

11. d. Presence of dysgerminomas is not an indication of termination of pregnancy.
   With stage 1 a patient can continue pregnancy after tumor removal.
   Chemotherapy can be safely given in nonpregnant doses in second and third trimester.
(Reference: Berecks and Novacks, 16th edition)

12. d. Most important prognostic factor is *size of the primary tumor* and its most malignant component
   The most frequent combination is *dysgerminomas and endodermal sinus tumor.*
   These tumors may secrete AFP, HCG, or both or neither depending upon its components.
   The most common component of mixed malignancy was dysgerminomas which occurred in 80%, followed by EST in 70%, immature teratoma in 53%, choriocarcinoma in 20%, and embryonal carcinoma in 16%.
(Reference: Berecks and Novacks, 16th edition)

13. d. Lesion >10-15 cm, lesions appearing before 20 years, microscopic patterns suggesting numerous mitosis, anaplasia, and a medullary pattern recur more
(Reference: Berecks and Novacks, 16th edition)

14. b. The above clinical scenario is suggestive of endodermal sinus tumor.
   Median age of presentation is 16-18 years.
   "Abdominal or pelvic pain is seen in 75% of cases. 10% cases present as asymptomatic pelvic mass". "*EST is 100% unilateral hence biopsy of opposite side is contraindicated*". Microscopic characteristics are Schiller dual bodies described as "a cystic space lined with a layer of flattened or irregular endothelium into which projects a glomerulus like tuft with central vascular core. *Most ESTs secrete AFP and rarely alpha-1 antitrypsin.*"
   "*The addition of hysterectomy and contralateral salpingo-oophorectomy does not alter the outcome and is not indicated.*"
(Reference: Berecks and Novacks, 16th edition)

15. b. SCC

16. c. These are rarely contralateral and routine wedge biopsy of opposite ovary is not recommended
(Reference: Berecks and Novacks, 16th edition)

17. d. The most important prognostic factor of immature teratoma is grade.
(Reference: Berecks and Novacks, 16th edition)

18. d. 5-year survival rate with all stages of pure immature teratoma is 70-80% and 90-95% with surgically staged stage 1 disease.
(Reference: Berecks and Novacks, 16th edition)

19. b. "*The association of EST with gonadal dysgenesis must be appreciated and chromosomal analysis should be performed preoperatively in premenarcheal patients.*"
(Reference: Berecks and Novacks, 16th edition)

20. b. "When a stage 1A cancer is found, tumor can be removed intact and pregnancy can be continued. For patients with more advanced disease, continuation of pregnancy depends upon the gestational age of fetus. Chemotherapy can be given safely in second and third trimester in the same doses as given in non-pregnant patient without apparent detriment to fetus."
(Reference: Berecks and Novacks, 16th edition)

21. d. The treatment involves surgical exploration, unilateral salpingo-oophorectomy, and frozen section for diagnosis. *The addition of hysterectomy and contralateral salphingo-oophorectomy does not alter the outcome and is not indicated.*
   "Any gross metastasis should be resected but thorough surgical staging may be omitted because all patients need chemotherapy. Bilaterality does not occur."
   3-4 cycles of BEP should be given every 3 weeks as primary chemotherapy for EST.

22. a. "*The incidence of leukemia is approximately 0.4-0.5% representing a 30-fold increase in likelihood in patients receiving a cumulative etoposide.*"
(Reference: Berecks and Novacks, 16th edition)

23. **d.** Pseudopuberty is seen with these tumors. Polyembryoma are extremely rare tumors of ovary, composed of embryoid bodies.

They tend to occur in very young premenarcheal girls with signs of pseudopuberty and elevated levels of AFP and HCG.
(Reference: Berecks and Novacks, 16th edition)

24. **b.** Choriocarcinoma of ovary most commonly occurs in younger than 20 years. Histologically, it is similar to gestational choriocarcinoma. There is presence of isosexual precocity in 50% patients. They have elevated levels of beta-HCG. They show complete response to methotrexate, actinomycin, and cyclophosphamide (MAC) chemotherapy. BEP regimen can be used alternatively. The prognosis is poor as most patients have metastasis to distant organs at the time of diagnosis.
(Reference: Berecks and Novacks, 16th edition)

25. **a.** The most common component of mixed malignancy was dysgerminomas which occurred in 80%, followed by EST in 70%, immature teratoma in 53%, choriocarcinoma in 20% and embryonal carcinoma in 16%.

The most frequent combination is dysgerminomas and endodermal sinus tumor.
(Reference: Berecks and Novacks, 16th edition)

26. **c.** Most important prognostic factor is size of the primary tumor and its most malignant component.
(Reference: Berecks and Novacks, 16th edition)

27. **d.** *Embryonal carcinoma is extremely rare* tumor that is distinguished from choriocarcinoma of ovary by the absence of cytotrophoblastic and syncytiotrophoblastic cells.
(Reference: Berecks and Novacks, 16th edition)

28. **c.** The treatment of choice is unilateral oophorectomy followed by combination chemotherapy with BEP.
Reference: Berecks and Novacks, 16th edition

29. **b.** Dysgerminomas are very radiosensitive and doses of 2,500–3,500 cGy may be curative even for gross metastasis. Loss of fertility is a problem with radiation and is rarely used as first line.
(Reference: Berecks and Novacks, 16th edition)

30. **d.** *"About 75% recurrences occur within first year after initial treatment*, most common sites being peritoneal cavity and retroperitoneal lymph nodes. These patients should be treated with chemotherapy. If prior chemotherapy with BEP was given, second-line options like paclitaxel, ifosfamide, cisplatin or vinblastine, ifosfamide, and cisplatin."
(Reference: Berecks and Novacks, 16th edition)

Chapter 102: Menopause General: Part 1

Rao Preethi Venkatachala, Ruchika Garg

QUESTIONS

1. **The following hormones play an important role in hot flashes:**
   a. Kisseptin, Neurokinin B, Dynorphin receptors
   b. Follicle stimulating hormone (FSH), luteinizing hormone (LH), thyroid stimulating hormone (TSH)
   c. Kisseptin, Neurokinin B, LH
   d. LH, CRH, Dynorphin receptors

2. **The most effective treatment for vasomotor symptoms of menopause is:**
   a. Systemic estrogen therapy
   b. Paroxetine
   c. Gabapentin
   d. Isoflavones

3. **Hormonal changes during menopause include all, *except*:**
   a. Increase in FSH
   b. Decrease in estrogen
   c. Increase in inhibin
   d. Decrease in AMH

4. **A tissue selective estrogen complex approved for treatment of vasomotor symptoms in menopausal women with uterus includes:**
   a. Combination of conjugated estrogen and paroxetine
   b. Combination of conjugated estrogen and bazedoxifene
   c. Combination of conjugated estrogen and gabapentin
   d. Combination of conjugated estrogen and clonidine

5. **Dyspareunia and vulvovaginal atrophy of menopause is best treated with:**
   a. Ormeloxifene
   b. Ospemifene
   c. Raloxifene
   d. Clomiphene

6. **Genitourinary syndrome of menopause is treated by all, *except*:**
   a. Low-dose vaginal estrogen therapy
   b. Vaginal use of DHEA
   c. Ospemifene
   d. Vaginal use of progesterones

7. **Risk factors for osteoporosis include all, *except*:**
   a. Systemic corticosteroid use
   b. Hypothyroidism
   c. Hyperparathyroidism
   d. Smoking

8. **Osteoporosis is defined when bone mineral density of the woman shows a T score of:**
   a. ≥ -1
   b. between -1 and -2.5
   c. ≤ -2.5
   d. ≥ -2.5

9. **Management of osteoporosis includes:**
   a. Alendronate
   b. Sildenafil citrate
   c. Bupropion
   d. Thyroxine

10. **Findings of Women's Health Initiative EPT trial include all, *except*:**
    a. 34% reduction in hip fractures with hormone therapy
    b. Hazard ratio was increased for coronary heart disease, pulmonary embolism, and stroke
    c. Increased risk of breast cancer
    d. Increased risk of colorectal cancer

11. **The criteria for diagnosing menopause in healthy women aged over 45 years include all, *except*:**
    a. No periods for 12 months and not using hormonal contraceptives
    b. Is based on symptoms in women without a uterus
    c. Increased FSH in women using combined estrogen and progestogen contraception or high-dose progestogen
    d. AMH is not used for diagnosis

12. **Features of menopausal transition as per STRAW include all, *except*:**
    a. Fertility problems
    b. Menstrual irregularity
    c. Vasomotor symptoms
    d. Declining bone density

13. **Feature of late menopause as per STRAW classification is:**
    a. Worsening risk of cardiovascular disease
    b. Menstrual irregularity
    c. Vasomotor symptoms
    d. Decline in antral follicle count

14. **FSH cannot be used to titrate estrogen dosage in menopausal women on hormone therapy because of loss of:**
    a. Inhibin
    b. AMH
    c. LH
    d. Progesterone

15. **Absolute contraindication for hormone therapy in postmenopausal woman is:**
    a. Venous thromboembolism
    b. Fibrocystic disease of breast
    c. Rheumatoid arthritis
    d. Uterine leiomyoma

16. **The circulating estradiol levels after menopause is:**
    a. 40-400 pg/mL
    b. 30-200 pg/mL
    c. 20-80 ng/dL
    d. 10-20 pg/mL

17. **The mood changes during menopause are due to:**
    a. Decline in estrogen at menopause affects neurotransmitters that regulate mood
    b. Vasomotor symptoms
    c. Vicissitudes of life
    d. All of above

18. **A diagnosis of metabolic syndrome requires the presence of all, *except*:**
    a. Increased waist circumference
    b. Increased blood pressure >130/85 mm Hg
    c. Increased HDL
    d. Increase in fasting blood sugar level >100 mg/dL

19. **In women who have undergone hysterectomy with bilateral salpingo-oophorectomy, the combined estrogen progestogen therapy is indicated in all, *except*:**
    a. Endometriosis
    b. Endometrioid tumor of ovary
    c. Early stage of endometrial carcinoma
    d. Breast carcinoma

20. **In women in whom hysterectomy with bilateral salpingo-oophorectomy has been performed for endometriosis, the following hormone therapy regimen is recommended:**
    a. Estrogen therapy
    b. Progestogen therapy
    c. Combination of estrogen progestogen therapy
    d. Androgen therapy

21. **Osteoporosis is least likely to occur in which of the following women?**
    a. Asian
    b. Those who lead a sedentary lifestyle
    c. Smokers
    d. Obese women

22. **Hormone therapy is not useful in:**
    a. Vaginal atrophy
    b. Hot flashes
    c. Prevention of osteoporosis
    d. Prevention of coronary heart disease

23. **Estrogen therapy for postmenopausal symptoms causes an increase in:**
    a. LDL
    b. VLDL
    c. Total cholesterol
    d. Triglycerides

24. **Estrogen administration in a menopausal woman increases the:**
    a. Gonadotropin secretion
    b. LDL cholesterol
    c. Bone mass
    d. Colorectal cancer

25. **A 48-year-old lady suffering from AUB-A underwent hysterectomy. She wishes to take hormone therapy. Physical examination and breast examination are normal. But DEXA of hip and spine shows a T score of <−2.5. The treatment of choice is:**
    a. Progesterone
    b. Testosterone
    c. Estrogen + progesterone combination
    d. Bioidentical hormones

26. **Denosumab is a monoclonal antibody approved for the treatment of:**
    a. Postmenopausal osteoporosis
    b. Vasomotor symptoms
    c. Psychological symptoms
    d. Genitourinary symptoms

27. **The risk for starting tissue selective estrogen complex (conjugated estrogen/bazedoxifene) includes all, *except*:**
    a. Breast cancer
    b. Endometrial cancer
    c. Colorectal cancer
    d. Stroke

28. **As per the WHI trial, no increase in risk of coronary heart disease is seen:**
    a. Within 10 years of menopause
    b. If aged >60 years
    c. Regardless of age
    d. Regardless of years postmenopause

29. **The "Timing Hypothesis" of WHI trial proposes that:**
    a. Early initiation of hormone therapy is associated with less atherosclerosis in blood vessels
    b. Late initiation of hormone therapy is associated with less atherosclerosis in blood vessels
    c. Does not support the early versus late intervention trial with estradiol (ELITE) trial
    d. Hormone therapy for 5 years is associated with faster progression of subclinical atherosclerosis when initiated within 6 years of menopause

30. **Hormone therapy has no effect on carotid artery intimal thickness when initiated in women more than _____ years after menopause.**
    a. 6
    b. 10
    c. 4
    d. 2

ANSWERS

1. **a.** *(Reference: Page 444, Novaks)*
2. **a.** *(Reference: Page 444, Novaks)*
3. **c.** *(Reference: Page 443, Novaks)*
4. **b.** *(Reference: Page 444, Novaks)*
5. **b.** *(Reference: Page 447, Novaks)*
6. **d.** *(Reference: Page 447, Novaks)*
7. **b.** *(Reference: Page 448, Novaks)*
8. **c.** *(Reference: Page 448, Novaks)*
9. **a.** *(Reference: Page 449, Novaks)*
10. **d.** *(Reference: Page 450, Novaks)*
11. **c.** *(Reference: NICE Guidelines)*
12. **d.** *(Reference: Page 1436, Speroff, 9th edition)*
13. **a.** *(Reference: Page 1436, Speroff, 9th edition)*
14. **a.** *(Reference: Page 1442, Speroff, 9th edition)*
15. **a.** *(Reference: Page 453, Novaks)*
16. **d.** *(Reference: Page 1455, Speroff, 9th edition)*
17. **d.** *(Reference: Page 1477, Speroff, 9th edition)*
18. **c.** *(Reference: Page 1489, Speroff, 9th edition)*
19. **d.** *(Reference: Page 1526, Speroff, 9th edition)*
20. **c.** *(Reference: Page 1526, Speroff 9th edition)*
21. **d.** *(Reference: Page 448, Novaks)*
22. **d.** *(Reference: Page 450, Novaks)*
23. **d.** *(Reference: Page 1511, Speroff, 9th edition)*
24. **c.** *(Reference: Page 1727, Speroff, 9th edition)*
25. **c.** (Reference: Page 1729, Speroff, 9th edition)
26. **a.** *(Reference: Page 450, Novaks)*
27. **c.** *(Reference: Page 449, Novaks)*
28. **a.** *(Reference: Page 450, Novaks)*
29. **a.** *(Reference: Page 451, Novaks)*
30. **b.** *(Reference: Page 451, Novaks)*

REFERENCES

1. Malik R, Radhika AG. Berek & Novak's Gynecology South Asian edition, Second impression. Gurugram: Wolters Kluwer (India) Pvt. Ltd.; 2022.
2. Taylor Hugh S et al. Speroff's Clinical Gynecologic Endocrinology and Infertility. Ninth edition. Wolters Kluwer, 2020.
3. National Institute for Health and Care Excellence. (2019). Menopause: diagnosis and management, 2023. [online] Available from: https://www.nice.org.uk/guidance/ng23. [Last accessed December, 2023].

Chapter 103: Menopause General: Part 2

Ashwini Bhalerao-Gandhi

QUESTIONS

1. **Premature menopause is defined as menopause that occurs before the age of:**
   a. 40 years
   b. 35 years
   c. 43 years
   d. 45 years

2. **Menopause is referred to as "Late Menopause" if it occurs after the age of:**
   a. 50 years
   b. 51 years
   c. 52 years
   d. 55 years

3. **Cause of premature ovarian failure is:**
   a. Chromosomal defect
   b. Autoimmune disorders
   c. Toxins like chemotherapy/radiotherapy
   d. All of the above

4. **Late onset of menopause is associated with following factors:**
   a. Increased BMI and multiparity
   b. Type I diabetes mellitus and stress
   c. Increased BMI and high altitude living
   d. Smoking

5. **The time period during which a woman's body makes the natural transition to menopause making the end of the reproductive years is known as:**
   a. Climacteric
   b. Menopause
   c. Premature menopause
   d. Perimenopausal transition

6. **Description of hot flushes is as follows:**
   a. A sudden feeling of warmth in the upper body, which is usually most intense over the face, neck, and chest. The duration is between seconds to 2–3 minutes
   b. Sudden feeling of heat to arms and legs. The duration being seconds to 2–3 minutes
   c. Feeling of heat all over the body accompanied by headaches and anxiety
   d. Feeling of heat all over the body. The duration being minutes to 2 hours

7. **Women who are postmenopausal are prone for all, *except*:**
   a. Osteopenia
   b. Dyslipidemia
   c. Weight loss
   d. Fat redistribution

8. **Neuroendocrinal charges occurring in menopausal women are responsible for:**
   a. Brain fog
   b. Mood disturbances
   c. Hot flushes and night sweats
   d. All of the above

9. **Sarcopenia occurs due to following risk factors, *except*:**
   a. Sleep disorders
   b. Low protein intake
   c. Low physical activity
   d. Menopausal state

10. **In the WHI randomized trial, a lower rate of following disease was detected:**
    a. Colon cancer
    b. CHD
    c. Breast cancer
    d. Stroke

11. **Vitamin D deficiency is associated with all, *except*:**
    a. Type I diabetes mellitus
    b. Cardiovascular disease
    c. Cancer
    d. Renal stones

12. **Vitamin D deficiency leads to following skeletal changes:**
    a. Osteomalacia
    b. Osteopenia
    c. Osteoporosis
    d. All of the above

13. **Postmenopausal women should undertake following exercise program:**
    a. Balance exercise
    b. Endurance exercise (aerobic)
    c. Strength exercise
    d. All of the above

14. Which are absolute contraindications for HMT?
    a. Cancer breast, Cancer endometrium
    b. Pregnancy
    c. Thromboembolism
    d. All of the above

15. The musculoskeletal health is adversely affected in postmenopausal women because:
    a. Estrogen deficiency accelerates age-related deterioration
    b. Bones have estrogen receptors
    c. Skeletal muscles have estrogen receptors
    d. All of the above

16. The risk of falls is reduced by which of the following factors?
    a. Hip joint support
    b. Eyesight check-ups
    c. Walking stick
    d. Vitamin D supplementation
    e. All of the above

17. Following are the risk factors for osteoporosis, *except:*
    a. Alcohol use   b. Smoking
    c. Low calcium intake   d. Obesity
    e. Turner's syndrome

18. The drug which is FDA approved for treatment of moderate-to-severe dyspareunia is:
    a. Tibolone   b. Ospemifene
    c. DHEA   d. Genistein

19. Following groups are at higher risk of having low vitamin D level, *except:*
    a. People who have lighter skin
    b. Infants and young children <4 years
    c. Older people aged 65 years and above
    d. Pregnant and breastfeeding women

20. What are the indications for DEXA?
    a. Postmenopausal women <5 years of menopause with risk factors for fractures
    b. Radiological evidence of osteopenia and presence of vertebral compression fracture
    c. Women with fragility fractures
    d. All of the above

21. AMH level indicating very low fertility is ___ ng/mL.
    a. <0.3   b. 0.3–2
    c. >6.5   d. 2–4

22. In which conditions, transdermal administration of estrogen is preferred?
    a. Increased risk for choletlithiasis
    b. Hypertriglyceridemia
    c. Hypertension
    d. All of the above

23. Following progesterone is not associated with high breast cancer risk:
    a. Medroxyprogesterone
    b. Dydrogesterone
    c. Micronized progesterone
    d. Both b and c

24. Tibolone therapy should be administered in following women:
    a. Women who are at least 1 year postmenopausal
    b. Recently menopausal women
    c. Women who are at least 10 years postmenopausal
    d. Perimenopausal women

25. Use of raloxifene is approved for:
    a. Treatment of CA breast
    b. Treatment of osteoporosis
    c. Prevention and treatment of osteoporosis
    d. None of the above

26. Following conditions are risk factors for carcinoma breast, *except:*
    a. Exposure to intense radiation
    b. Diet high in vegetables and fruits
    c. Long-term use of estrogen plus progestogen
    d. History of breast cancer in mother or sister

27. Risk factors for ovarian carcinoma are all, *except:*
    a. Use of oral contraceptive pills
    b. Infertility treatment with clomiphene citrate
    c. Family history of ovarian carcinoma
    d. Women who are BRCA-1 positive

28. The most common malignancy in women is:
    a. Carcinoma esophagus
    b. Carcinoma breast
    c. Carcinoma cervix
    d. Carcinoma endometrium

29. Following are risk factors for Ca endometrium, *except:*
    a. Multiparity   b. Chronic anovulation
    c. Tamoxifen   d. Late menopause

30. Ovaries beyond menopause:
    a. Have no role to play
    b. Retain some reproductive function
    c. Continue to be an endocrine organ
    d. None of the above

ANSWERS

1. **a.** Premature menopause is defined as menopause that occurs at age >2 standard deviation below the mean estimated for the reference population. The age of 40 years is used frequently as an arbitrary limit below which the menopause is said to be premature.

2. **d.** Some women experience late menopause in their late 50's or 60's. The timing is greatly influenced by genetics, lifestyle, menstrual cycle patterns, and medications.

3. **d.** Premature ovarian failure is a syndrome of amenorrhea of >4 months, low sex steroid levels, elevated gonadotropin levels among women younger than 40 years of age.

4. **a.** Overweight and obese women have a 50% higher risk of late menopause than other women. Fat tissue produces and stores estrogen, which delays its depletion. The timing and number of pregnancies a woman had may delay onset of menopause.

5. **d.** Perimenopause is the transitional period before menopause. During this period, levels of estrogen start to decrease. This period can last for over a decade and causes symptoms in a majority of women.

6. **a.** Hot flushes, also known as vasomotor symptoms, cause intense heat and sweat in the face, neck, and chest. The skin may turn red as if blushing. Occurrence is lowest prior to entering the menopausal transition, increasing in the early transition and higher still in the late transition near the final menstrual period.

7. **c.** Menopause onset is associated with increased total fat and abdominal (visceral) fat and decreased energy expenditure and fat oxidation.

8. **d.** Menopause is the last phase in the cascade of events occurring both in the central nervous system (CNS) and in the ovaries. Several neuroendocrine changes and hypoestrogenism play a key role in causing vasomotor symptoms, mood disturbances, brain fog, etc.

9. **a.** Sarcopenia is age-related progressive loss of muscle mass and strength. Being physically inactive and eating an unhealthy diet can contribute to the disease.

10. **a.** The women's health initiative (WHI) randomized, placebo controlled trial evaluating estrogen plus progestin identified more risks than benefits for the use of combined hormone therapy. However, during the intervention phase of the trial, there was a statistically significant 44% lower rate of colorectal cancer diagnoses in the estrogen plus progestin group.

11. **d.** Research suggests that vitamin D could play a role in the prevention and treatment of a number of different conditions including diabetes, hypertension, glucose intolerance, and multiple sclerosis.

12. **d.** The consequences of vitamin D deficiency are secondary hyperparathyroidism and bone loss, leading to osteoporosis and fractures. Mineralization defects may lead to osteomalacia in the long term, and muscle weakness, causing falls and fractures.

13. **d.** Weight bearing exercises, such as walking and running, as well as moderate weight training help to increase bone mass. In postmenopausal women, moderate exercise helps to preserve bone mass. In postmenopausal women, moderate exercise helps to preserve bone mass in the spine and prevents fractures. Exercise also helps to improve mood. Hormones called endorphins are released in the brain.

14. **d.** Contraindications to MHT include a history of breast cancer, CHD, a previous venous thromboembolic event or stroke, active liver disease, unexplained vaginal bleeding, endometrial cancer, or transient ischemic attack.

15. **d.** Menopause has an adverse impact on overall musculoskeletal health. It is associated with osteoporosis, osteoarthritis, and sarcopenia.

    Poor musculoskeletal health has multifactorial etiology, but hormones play a major role.

16. **e.** Loss of balance and increased body sway are important risk factors for falls in the postmenopausal women. The age-associated increase in the incidence of osteoporotic fractures results from a combination of increased fall risk and reduced bone strength.

17. **d.** Osteoporosis is caused by a reduction in bone mass. White and Asian women, especially older women who are postmenopausal are at highest risk. Age, race, lifestyle choices, medical conditions, and treatments are predisposing factors for osteoporosis.

18. **b.** Ospemifene is used to treat women with moderate-to-severe dyspareunia and vaginal dryness caused by

menopause. Low estrogen levels may cause changes in the vulvar and vaginal areas that lead to atrophy and dryness. It is a selective estrogen receptor modulator (SERM) with agonist actions on vaginal tissue, endometrium, and bone.

19. **a.** People with dark skin, postmenopausal women, pregnant, and lactating women are prone for vitamin D deficiency. Risk factors for vitamin D deficiency are sun exposure due to latitude, season, time of day, clothing, sunscreen use, skin pigmentation, obesity, some chronic illnesses, etc.

20. **d.** DEXA scan is recommended to diagnose osteoporosis. All women 65 years and older and men 70 years and older should be screened for asymptomatic osteoporosis. Individuals at any age with osteopenia or fragility fractures on imaging studies, individuals 50 years and older with fracture with minimal or no trauma should undergo DEXA scan.

21. **a.** Anti-Müllerian hormone (AMH) is now recognized as the most reliable marker of ovarian reserve status. Decreased serum AMH levels are a reflection of decreased ovarian reserve and very low or undetectable AMH levels in women with amenorrhea strongly suggest ovarian failure.

22. **d.** Orally administered hormones are first metabolized by the liver before entering the systemic circulation and metabolites are excreted in the bile and urine. Transdermally administered estrogen avoids this first-pass metabolism and can therefore be given in lower doses for equivalent physiologic effects. Transdermal estradiol does not increase the risk of venous thromboembolism, and does not increase the risk of stroke.

23. **d.** The increased risk of developing breast cancer is linked to combined MHT. The type of progestogen also makes a difference. Risk increases when preparations containing some types of progestogen (norethisterone/medroxyprogesterone) were taken for more than a year. The lowest risk is with dydrogesterone/micronized progesterone.

24. **a.** Tibolone can be used by postmenopausal women who have not experienced a natural period for at least 1 year. If taken sooner, irregular bleeding may be experienced. Women can also transition from cyclical or combined continuous MHT onto tibolone.

25. **c.** Raloxifene is an FDA-approved second-generation selective estrogen receptor modulator, a drug with an estrogen-agonistic effect on bone, increasing bone mineral density and mass by decreasing bone resorption. It is indicated in the treatment and prevention of postmenopausal osteoporosis.

26. **b.** A woman's risk for breast cancer is higher if she has a mother, sister, or daughter or multiple family members who have had breast or ovarian cancer. Women who had radiation therapy to the chest or breasts have a higher risk. MHT taken for >5 years can raise risk for breast cancer. Certain OCS taken for a long time also has been found to raise the risk. Older women with obesity also have a higher risk.

27. **a.** Genetics, parity, environment, hormonal factors, and inflammation play an important role in the development of ovarian cancer. Women who had breast, uterine, or colorectal cancer have a higher risk. Half of all ovarian cancers are found in women 63 years of age or older. Women who use oral contraceptive pills for 5 or more years have about a 50% lower risk of developing ovarian cancer than women who have never used oral contraceptives.

28. **b.** Some of the cancers that most often affect women are breast, colorectal, lung, cervical, endometrial, ovarian, and skin. About 1 in 8 women will get invasive breast cancer in their lifetime. In India, cancer cervix is most common in especially rural area, but in metro cities—cancer breast is the most common.

29. **a.** Most of the risk factors linked to endometrial cancer come from too much exposure to estrogen hormone. Multiparous women are known to have a lower risk of developing either ovarian or endometrial cancer than nulliparous women. This is due to the lack of ovulation leading to decreased estrogen levels and increased progesterone levels during pregnancy.

30. **c.** The ovaries continue to have an endocrine function after menopause. Estrogen production is reduced but higher amounts of androgens are secreted. The primary estrogen produced changes from estradiol (E_2) to estrone (E_1) after menopause.

Chapter 104: Vaginal Discharge

Dhara Singh, Ruchika Garg

QUESTIONS

1. False statement regarding color, consistency, and pH of vaginal discharge:
   a. During puberty—white and thick mucus, pH—3.5-4.7
   b. During menstruation—white, clear, copious, and elastic, pH—3.5-4.7
   c. During pregnancy—white/slightly gray and musty smell, pH—3.5-4.7
   d. Menopause—copious and thick, pH—4.5-5.8

2. Noninfective cause of vaginal discharge:
   a. Foreign body (IUCD, Tampoon)
   b. Endometritis
   c. Erosive lichen planus
   d. All of the above

3. Infective causes of vaginal discharge are all, *except*:
   a. Bacterial vaginosis (BV)
   b. *Chlamydia trachomatis*
   c. Fusobacterium
   d. *Neisseria gonorrhea*

4. A 17-year-old girl is being treated at the OPD for vaginal discharge. Bacterial vaginosis is assumed to be the cause. Which of the following findings matches BV?
   a. pH < 4.5
   b. Frothy vaginal discharge
   c. Predominance of anaerobes
   d. Flagellated organisms

5. An unpleasant odor and vaginal discharge are reported by a 27-year-old lady. An erythematous vagina and punctures of the cervix are discovered during the speculum examination. What is the most probable diagnosis among the following?
   a. Candidal vaginitis
   b. Trichomonal vaginitis
   c. Bacterial vaginosis
   d. Human papillomavirus

6. Six hours after the inoculation, which of the following organisms may be separated from a wet surface?
   a. *Candida albicans*
   b. *Trichomonas vaginalis*
   c. *Gardnerella* species
   d. Peptostreptococci

7. An oral antibiotic regimen for cystitis in a 26-year-old woman was finished 1 week ago. Itching, burning, and a yellowish vaginal discharge have been bothering her for the past day, she claims. The best therapy is which one of the following?
   a. Metronidazole
   b. Erythromycin
   c. Fluconazole
   d. Hydrocortisone

8. A 19-year-old female comes to OPD with excessive vaginal discharge.

   Microscopic examination of discharge shows increase in WBC, clumps of bacteria, and loss of normal lactobacillus. Slide is shown below. Correct statement is:

   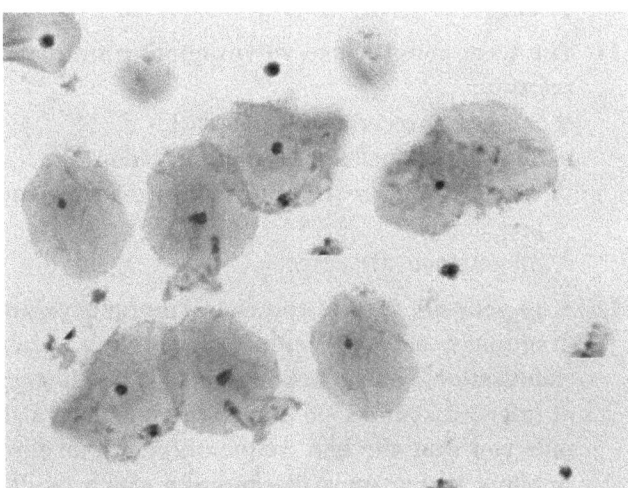

a. This type of discharge has pH < 4.5
b. This slide resembles ground-glass appearance
c. Can occur in female who are not sexually active
d. This type of discharge shows decrease in WBCs

9. A 35-year-old diabetic woman comes to gynecology OPD with history of pruritus and vaginal soreness. She also tells you that she is on oral contraceptive pills. You examine the patient and per speculum the picture you see is given below. Which type of organism you expect?

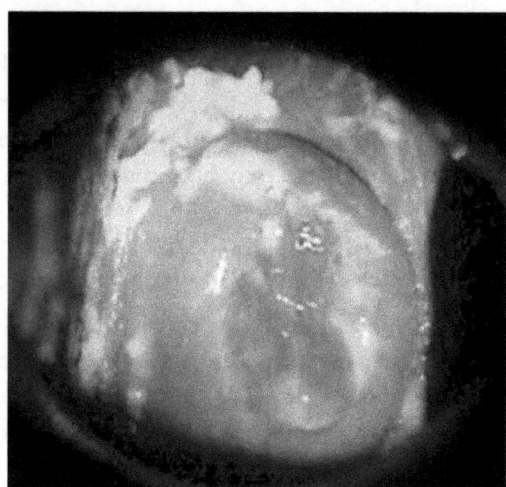

a. *Candida albicans*   b. *Mycoplasma hominis*
c. *Gardnerella vaginalis*   d. *N. Gonorrhea*

10. Which findings justify vulvovaginal candidiasis?
    a. Pruritus, dyspareunia and abnormal vaginal discharge is specific symptom
    b. Discharge is often fowl smelling
    c. Discharge is thin and nonadherent
    d. Diagnosis is done by 10% KOH microscopy

11. The term complicated vulvovaginal candidiasis refers to:
    a. Episodes is recurrent (>4 per year)
    b. Suspected nonalbicans candida infection
    c. Women with predisposing factor (diabetes and pregnancy)
    d. All statement are correct

12. A 30-year-old female comes to emergency with diagnosed case of ectopic pregnancy. After stabilization, you got to know that she had history of infertility conceived after treatment. She also tells you that she had frequent episode of fowl smelling frothy vaginal discharge for which she did not took any treatment. Which type of infection she might me suffering since last year?
    a. Bacteria vaginosis
    b. Vulvovaginal candidiasis
    c. Trichomonas vaginitis
    d. Atrophic vaginitis

13. Which statement regarding *Neisseria gonorrhoeae* is false?
    a. Organism known to survive in swimming pools and hot tubs
    b. Usually associated with PID, urethritis, and dysuria
    c. Culture in New York agar medium is common diagnostic test
    d. Co-existing Chlamydia is present in 50% patients

14. A slide examination of vaginal discharge is done (image shown below) of a female who come to OPD with vaginal discharge. The microscopic examination revealed the organism as *Chlamydia trachomatis*. Which type of discharge is associated with this type of infection?

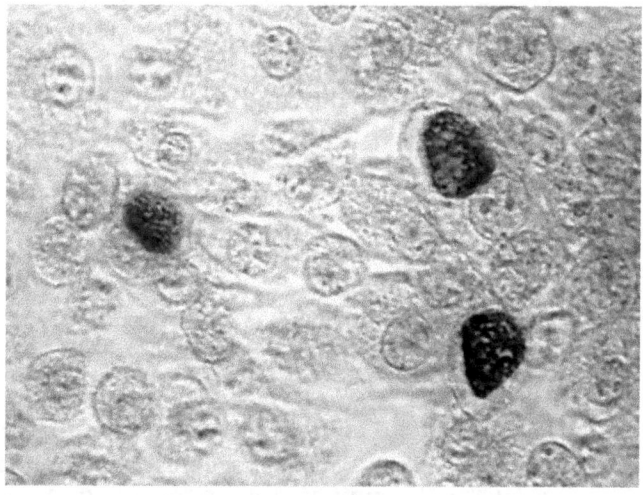

a. Fowl smelling purulent discharge
b. A thick adherent discharge
c. Frothy vaginal discharge
d. Odorless mucoid vaginal discharge

15. Which statement justifies atrophic vaginitis?
    a. Atrophy of vaginal mucosa due to increased estrogen level.
    b. pH is usually <4.7
    c. Patient usually has urinary symptoms
    d. Discharge is thick and copious

16. A 45-year-old patient comes to day care OPD with purulent discharge and vulvovaginal burning and microscopic examination reveals overgrowth of gram-positive cocci, usually streptococci. The correct diagnosis is:
    a. Chronic cervicitis
    b. Atrophic vaginitis
    c. Desquamative inflammatory vaginitis
    d. Trichomonas vaginitis

17. Match the following type of vaginitis with the risk factor:
    a. Bacterial vaginosis
    b. Trichomoniasis
    c. Vulvovaginal candidiasis
    d. Atrophic vaginitis

    I. Menopause
    II. Uncontrolled diabetes
    III. New/multiple sexual partners
    IV. Lifetime frequency of sexual activities

    Options:
    a. a-I, b-III, c-IV, d-II
    b. a-III, b-IV, c-II, d-I
    c. a-II, b-IV, c-III, d-I
    d. a-II, b-IV, c-III, d-I

18. Amine odor on whiff test is present in which of the following types of vaginal infection?
    a. Bacterial vaginosis
    b. Chlamydia trachomatis
    c. Vulvovaginal candidiasis
    d. a and b

19. Which vaginal infection correctly matches the microscopic appearance of its vaginal discharge?
    a. Gonorrhea—Spherical intracellular bacteria
    b. Trichomoniasis—Flagellated parasites
    c. Chlamydia trachomatis—Gram-negative diplococci
    d. Bacterial vaginosis—Presence of B Blastospheres

20. Amsel's criteria of bacterial vaginosis does not include:
    a. Homogenous gray white discharge
    b. pH of vaginal discharge <4.5
    c. Fishy odor
    d. Clue cells present on wet mount microscopy

21. True about Nugent score is all, *except*:
    a. Gold standard test for bacterial vaginosis
    b. Score >6 is bacterial vaginosis
    c. Score <4 is normal
    d. Total score is between 2 and 8

22. Match the correct option regarding Hay–Ison criteria for bacterial vaginosis:
    1. Grade 0   2. Grade 2
    3. Grade 3   4. Grade 4

    I. Bacterial vaginosis
    II. Intermediate flora
    III. Not related to BV, indicated recent use of antibiotics.
    IV. Not related to BV, Gram positive cocci only
    a. 1-I, 2-II, 3-III, 4-IV
    b. 1-III, 2-II, 3-I, 4-IV
    c. 1-I, 2-IV, 3-III, 4-II
    d. 1-IV, 2-II, 3-III, 4-III

ANSWERS

1. **d.** Menopause—copious and thick, pH—4.5–5.8
2. **d.** All of the above
3. **c.** Fusobacterium
4. **c.** Predominance of anaerobes
5. **b.** Trichomonal vaginitis
6. **b.** *Trichomonas vaginalis*
7. **c.** Fluconazole
8. **b.** This slide resemble ground glass appearance
9. **a.** *Candida albicans*
10. **d.** Diagnosis is done by 10% KOH microscopy
11. **d.** All statement are correct
12. **c.** Trichomonas vaginitis
13. **a.** Organism known to survive in swimming pools and hot tubs
14. **d.** Odorless mucoid vaginal discharge
15. **c.** Patient usually has urinary symptoms
16. **c.** Desquamative inflammatory vaginitis
17. **b.** a-III, b-IV, c-II, d-I
18. **d.** a and b
19. **b.** Trichomoniasis—Flagellated parasites
20. **b.** pH of vaginal discharge <4.5
21. **d.** Total score is between 2 and 8
22. **b.** 1-III, 2-II, 3-I, 4-IV

REFERENCES

1. Akinbiyi AA, Watson R, Feyi-Waboso P. Prevalence of *Candida albicans* and bacterial vaginosis in asymptomatic pregnant women in South Yorkshire, United Kingdom. Outcome of a prospective study. Arch Gynecol Obstet. 2008;278(5):463-6.
2. Zhou Y, Wang W, Sun Y, Qian W, Liu Z, Wang R, et al. Corrigendum to "The prevalence and risk factors of psychological disturbances of frontline medical staff in China under the COVID-19 epidemic: workload should be concerned". [Journal of Affective Disorders 2020;277:510-514.]. J Affect Disord. 2022;299:721.
3. Miller KE. Diagnosis and treatment of *Chlamydia trachomatis* infection. Am Fam Physician. 2006;73(8): 1411-6.
4. Machado D, Castro J, Palmeira-de-Oliveira A, Martinez-de-Oliveira J, Cerca N. Bacterial Vaginosis Biofilms: Challenges to Current Therapies and Emerging Solutions. Front Microbiol. 2016;6:1528.
5. Sherrard J, Wilson J, Donders G, Mendling W, Jensen JS. 2018 European (IUSTI/WHO) International Union against sexually transmitted infections (IUSTI) World Health Organisation (WHO) guideline on the management of vaginal discharge. Int J STD AIDS. 2018;29(13):1258-72.

EU GSPR Authorised Reprsentative
Logos Europe, 9 rue Nicolas Poussin
1700, La Rochelle, France
Phone: +33 (0) 6 67 93 73 78
E-mail: contact@logoseurope.eu

www.ingramcontent.com/pod-product-compliance
Ingram Content Group UK Ltd.
Pitfield, Milton Keynes, MK11 3LW, UK
UKHW052155041025
463590UK00011B/172